ANATOMY AND PHYSIOLOGY FOR NURSES

Jane Ryman 1980

ANATOMY AND PHYSIOLOGY FOR NURSES

By

T. W. A. GLENISTER

C.B.E., T.D., M.B., B.S., D.Sc., Ph.D.(Lond.)

*Professor of Anatomy in the University of London
at Charing Cross Hospital Medical School*

and

JEAN R. W. ROSS

B.Sc., M.B., Ch.B.(Edin.)

*Senior Lecturer in Anatomy, Charing Cross Hospital
Medical School, London*

THIRD EDITION

WILLIAM HEINEMANN MEDICAL BOOKS LTD
LONDON

First published 1965
Second Edition 1974
Third Edition 1980

© by T. W. A. Glenister and Jean R. W. Ross, 1980

ISBN 0 433 12102 5

Printed in Great Britain by
Butler & Tanner Ltd, Frome and London

CONTENTS

LIST OF COLOURED ILLUSTRATIONS

PREFACE TO THE THIRD EDITION

THE policy set out in the prefaces to the two previous editions has been adhered to. This has meant continuing throughout the text the process of clarification and correction, particularly in the light of the comments received from students using the previous editions. Believing, as we do, that Anatomy and Physiology should be presented as the integrated study of the living human body, we have included among the twenty-two new illustrations fifteen radiographs, a most useful means of displaying living anatomy. With the increasing availability of ultrasound scanning facilities, and with the advent of Computerized Axial Tomography, we thought it appropriate to supplement the revised section on radiological anatomy with descriptions and illustrations referring to these newest methods of body-imaging. We also thought it necessary to introduce new material, such as surfactant, the prevention of Rh disease in infants and the Limbic System, all subjects not included in previous editions, but of increasing importance for the understanding of disorders and of their correction.

With the dropping of eponyms from embryological and histological nomenclature, as well as from anatomical terminology, new terms are coming increasingly into common use. Throughout the text, the accepted Paris Nomenclature has been used. It has also been necessary to adopt the S.I. unit system throughout with explanations, where appropriate, and with the units previously in use quoted in brackets.

For the new illustrations we are most indebted to the Department of Medical Illustration of Charing Cross Hospital Medical School and to Dr. J. McIver who supplied the scans. We wish to thank most warmly Miss Ninetta Martyn of William Heinemann Medical Books Ltd., who has been so very helpful in all aspects of the preparation of this third edition.

T. W. A. G.
J. R. W. R.

London, January 1980

PREFACE TO FIRST EDITION

THERE is no point in giving nurses a course of instruction in the basic subjects of Anatomy and Physiology that may be academically satisfying, but which is far in excess, as regards content and complexity, of the needs of a nursing career. However, experience in teaching members of the Nursing Profession has shown us repeatedly and clearly that, more often than not, students and indeed qualified nurses, studying for the Tutor's Diploma, are overwhelmed by the mass of information presented to them. This is because to master it is too often for them merely a feat of memory, without understanding. While floundering in attempts to comprehend complexities, they frequently miss the significance of broad outline and general principle.

The aim of this book is therefore to provide a well-illustrated, concise text, which tries to explain as well as to inform, at the same time covering the subject matter necessary for passing examinations.

It is hoped that in studying the human body as a dynamic, developing, functioning and eventually ageing entity in which structure and function are closely related, nurses will acquire a sound knowledge of the basic subjects of Anatomy and Physiology. This will enable them to take an intelligent interest in the exercise of their profession and will provide sound roots on which to graft knowledge culled in other disciplines. With this end in view, the applications of Anatomy and Physiology to the clinical subjects are pointed out, but care is taken to leave the amplifications and the use of further examples to the Tutor, who can adapt them to the needs of the particular stage of training of the student. Though it may seem illogical to deal with growth changes at the end of the book, we thought that the significance of growth changes could be appreciated only after the disposition of adult structures had been studied.

A proportion of the material presented in this book may seem to some teachers superfluous to the needs of nurses. Nevertheless, we feel justified in including something of the more 'academic' aspects of the subjects because we are convinced that, quite often, even an outline of bodily structure and function fails to make sense unless the underlying principles of, say development, are understood. In addition, we think that a text of this nature should provide information for the more interested student who 'wants to know'. Now that it is becoming accepted that the teaching of Anatomy and Physiology should not be confined to the preliminary part of the course, but should extend throughout the training period, there will be an increasing number of student nurses who want to satisfy themselves about the anatomy and physiology of the diseases and their treatments which they encounter in the course of their nursing duties.

In an attempt to meet these widely varied requirements we have presented the more academic topics in smaller print. The labelling of some diagrams, too, is more elaborate than the text they illustrate.

The nomenclature used, namely the Nomina Anatomica 1961, is that which has been accepted internationally. When a term differs from that still in current use in this country, the latter has been included in brackets. Throughout the text, terms are printed in bold type and definitions are in italics.

We feel that much of the value of this book lies in the large number of illustrations which have been designed and executed with great originality and skill by Mr. Frank Price, to whom we are greatly indebted for his friendly cooperation. We also wish to express our sincere thanks to Mr. Owen R. Evans and to the late Dr. J. Johnston Abraham, both of Messrs. William Heinemann Medical Books Ltd. Their encouragement and understanding have made the writing of this book not only possible but enjoyable.

T. W. A. G.
J. R. W. R.

London, June 1965

PREFACE TO THE SECOND EDITION

IN preparing this second edition we acknowledge the helpful comments and appreciative reviews of the first edition from our colleagues in the nursing profession. They have enabled us to clarify and correct many passages. The approach and the format of the book have been welcomed by nurses and it seemed advisable to retain the layout and style of presentation.

We have included new background information and given more extensive coverage to subjects which are expanding rapidly, such as cytology, immunology and genetics with something of the biochemical basis.

Many of the existing illustrations have been modified and improved and 28 new illustrations are included.

We wish once again to express our thanks to Mr. Frank Price for his help and skill with the illustrations and to Mr. Owen Evans for his continued interest and encouragement. We also wish to thank Miss Martyn of William Heinemann Medical Books Ltd., for all her help in the preparation of this edition.

T. W. A. G.
J. R. W. R.

London, January 1974

SECTION I

CHAPTER I

THE IMPORTANCE AND RELEVANCE
OF ANATOMY AND PHYSIOLOGY

THE plain facts of anatomy and the somewhat esoteric speculations of physiologists may strike the student nurse as far removed from the devoted service which this very same student wishes to give to sick people. Yet, if something of the reasons for different nursing procedures and for what goes on at the bedside, or in the clinic, are to be understood, Medicine and Surgery must form an integral and obvious part of the course of instruction. These applied sciences make sense only if they are seen in the light of the basic subjects which form the subject of this book. From the very outset the student of nursing must appreciate that Medicine, Surgery, Pathology and Therapeutics are concerned with the recognition and correction of deranged structure and function. This is impossible without a clear knowledge of normal structure and function, and of how structure is closely related to function, and indeed is often an expression of function.

The Scope of Anatomy

Anatomy is the study and knowledge of the structure of the body. Considered as an exercise in memorizing the form, position and relations of an organ or origin, course and distribution of a nerve, the subject can be as dead as the cadaver the anatomist dissects. On the other hand, if looked upon as the study of how and why a structure has its particular shape or position in the living body, and how these features can be related to normal function, and indeed to disease and its symptoms, then anatomy becomes the study of a living, dynamic, beautifully organized whole.

We find therefore that anatomy embraces the study of embryology, that is the formation and development of the individual before birth, the study of growth changes during childhood and adolescence, of the mature body and of the degenerative changes associated with ageing.

Comparative anatomy, which compares the structure of the human body

1

with the structure of animals, tells us something of the place of Man in nature and may throw some light on his possible biological ancestry. The anatomist, in his quest for more knowledge about the human body, is not restricted to the use of a scalpel to cut up a cadaver. Ever more powerful microscopes have enabled him to develop the sciences of cytology and histology, which teach us about the structure of cells and tissues, and to extend enormously the range of knowledge we have concerning the structure of the body. By the use of special methods (see below) the living human body can be studied, and this plays a great part in teaching us how the structure of the body reflects its function.

Scope of Physiology and Biochemistry

Physiology and Biochemistry are in no danger of being looked upon as 'dead' subjects, for they deal with the study of the function and the chemistry of the living body. There are limits, both moral and practical, to the information obtainable by the direct study of the human body in health and disease. Physiologists and Biochemists are therefore often constrained to study in animals the phenomena which interest them. If their findings seem to apply consistently throughout the animal kingdom, or at any rate to a substantial number of mammals (the large subdivision of the animal kingdom in which the mothers suckle their young—Man is a mammal), then it is often justifiable to assume that the same kind of process takes place in the human body.

The subdivision of basic medical science into the compartments of anatomy, physiology and biochemistry is quite artificial, because nowadays it is true to say that the subjects overlap one another so much, that many topics of great interest fall within the scope of all three, and no worker in any of the three disciplines can afford to ignore the other two. In other words, structure and function cannot be considered in isolation from each other.

SOME CHARACTERISTICS OF HUMAN LIFE

The study of the basic physical and chemical feature of the human body reveals a wealth of logical relationships of form and function. In order to understand and appreciate human life, it is also necessary to be aware of the intricacy of the systems by which life is controlled. Just to study the components of the body in physical terms leaves one with a picture only of the structure of the body and of its parts. It will be obvious that the structure is organized, but the characteristic features of life will be missed unless one looks for the activity that goes on within the structure.

A living thing behaves the way it does because it is organized to prevent its dissolution into its surroundings. Thus, the activity which is characteristic of a living being is directed towards the preservation of an efficient individual and, through him or her, of the species. Life is characterized by a capacity for maintaining stability and continuity.

The study of the anatomy and physiology of Man is therefore properly concerned with the examination of all the mechanisms by which human life is maintained. This involves more than considering everyday activities like breathing and eating, but also includes those concerned with the defence of life and repair of the body as well as the problem of ageing. The continuity of life in a species depends on reproduction, which results in the formation and growth of new individuals. This involves the replication and addition of new material to the organism and this again is a characteristic of life.

The body is made up of chemical elements and these are organized into molecules (such as carbohydrates, proteins and fats, see p. 37). These are not merely mixed together in the body, but are arranged into units of organization known as cells. The cells are organized into tissue and organs, which in turn make up the body. All these add up to little more than a corpse, unless one takes into account that in a living human being matter continually enters and leaves the body. While many materials in the body have a rapid turn-over, others enter and leave the body at a slow rate and others to a negligible extent. The essence of a living body is that it consists of atoms of ordinary chemical elements caught up and made part of that body for a while. The living activity takes up these atoms and organizes them in a characteristic way. The life of an individual consists essentially of the activity he imposes on the materials he is made of. It is reasonable to make the concept of activity the focal point of the idea of life. In this way, the ageing of an individual is seen as a change in the activity of the individual and of his constituent parts, and not as a gradual change in the substance of his body.

Homeostasis

As has been said already, the activity of a living organism tends towards the preservation of the organization of the whole system, i.e. living activities are directed towards the end of self-maintenance. Although the individual molecules comprising the living organism change continuously, the manner of proceeding, which is living, is preserved intact.

The maintenance of the remarkable constancy of the general pattern of organization within the individual (though with certain gradual changes) is called homeostasis. The term is sometimes used more specifically to describe the maintenance of the 'internal environment' of the individual, especially the composition of his blood and of the fluid bathing his tissues, but the concept can be applied more widely to living matter in general and the maintenance of its pattern of activities, which ensure its continuity.

The activities that go on in the body are thus directed to provide the materials necessary for maintaining its particular shape and organization. The fact that the whole organism does not fade away into its surroundings is achieved by continuous expenditure of energy to keep the various materials in place and to renew them. As the materials of the body are not kept in closed containers the body can maintain its composition only by constantly replacing the materials that are lost with others of the same kind.

The means by which living organisms prevent themselves from dissolution are very varied. For example, Man is an organism containing much water and salt, but he lives in an environment containing relatively little water and most of that lacking in salt. He must therefore have within his organization various mechanisms that prevent undue loss of water and, since he cannot avoid losing water altogether, there must be mechanisms that ensure that the lost water is replaced. On the other hand, if too much water is taken in, the excess needs to be eliminated. Energy is required to carry out these activities and, to provide this energy, further activities are necessary to collect food for fuel and oxygen to burn it, thus making the energy available.

Perhaps the next question one might ask is, 'Where does the information come from, that is necessary for the organization associated with life?' This leads straight to the problem of the origin of life.

One of the features of living things is that they have a tendency to become increasingly complex. Also in the course of evolution, the survival and successful reproduction of those living organisms endowed with characteristics, which enabled them to thrive in various environments, has resulted in the appearance of a diversity of species equipped with increasing information about ways and means of keeping alive. This information is transmitted to succeeding generations, in other words, inherited, by means of genes.

Prior to the advent of Man, evolution operated only by heredity, but human evolution has resulted in the ability to use tools and in a faculty to use language as a means of communication. The latter, combined with the invention of symbols to express language, has enabled Man to store and transmit information supplementary to that available through genetic inheritance.

SI Units

In all scientific work measurement plays an important part. Recently, the system of units based on the **metre** (m), **kilogram** (Kg) and **second** (s), has been adopted internationally and is known as the Système International d'Unités, the SI unit system.

The Calorie is not included in the SI system. Heat, being a form of energy, is measured, like work done, in **joules** (J)

$$1000 \text{ joules} = 1 \textbf{ kilojoule (kJ)}$$
$$1 \text{ Calorie} \quad = 4\cdot2 \text{ kilojoules}$$

Temperature is measured in **degrees Celsius** (°C). The values correspond with the former degrees centigrade.

The term micron is omitted from the SI unit system. **Micrometre** (μm) which is the same size, is used instead.

$$1 \text{ μm} = \frac{1}{1000} \text{ mm}$$

Nanometre (nm) is the unit used for measurements in electron microscopy.

$$1 \text{ nm} = \frac{1}{1000} \text{ μm}.$$

Millilitre (ml) is used instead of cubic centimetre.

The unit for pressure is the **pascal** (Pa)

$$1000 \text{ pascals} = 1 \textbf{ kilopascal (kPa)}$$

The pressures of gases and the blood pressure have been measured conventionally in millimetres of mercury (mmHg)

$$1\text{mm Hg} = 133 \text{ Pa}$$

The use of the millimetre of mercury is still authorized for measurements of blood pressure, but this is under revue.

Throughout the text SI units have been used, with values in other, more familiar, units in brackets.

METHODS OF STUDYING THE BODY AND ITS FUNCTIONS

MACROSCOPIC EXAMINATION: By this is meant the examination of the body with the naked eye, that is without magnifying optical aids; it consists mainly of dissecting the embalmed bodies of deceased persons (cadavers).

MICROSCOPIC EXAMINATION: This is the study of the cells and tissues of the body with the aid of microscopes. This method has revealed, and is revealing, details of the minute structure of the body. This knowledge has helped us to understand many aspects of the functions of the various parts of the body.

EMBRYOLOGY: This is the study of the development of the individual before birth. It explains much about the arrangement of the structures of the body and helps to show how congenital malformations (defects with which babies may be born) develop.

COMPARATIVE ANATOMY AND PHYSIOLOGY: For ethical reasons, there is a limit to the study and experimentation to which the human body can be subjected. Much work is therefore carried out on animals. In this way, general biological principles are established, many of which are applicable to Man.

LIVING HUMAN ANATOMY, PHYSIOLOGY AND BIOCHEMISTRY: The living human body can be studied in many ways and some of the main ones will be mentioned.

Inspection consists of looking at the body and of considering such features as its form, proportions, degree of development, posture and movements.

Palpation consists of examining the body with the hands. This enables the examiner to determine the texture, position, form and mobility of many structures and organs.

Percussion, which is a special way of tapping on the surface of the body, enables one to determine whether the underlying part is hollow or solid. The size of some organs can be made out in this way.

Auscultation consists of listening, usually with a **stethoscope,** to the sounds produced by the flow of air, blood and other fluids in some organs of the body, or produced by movements of whole organs, or by parts of them.

BASIC OBSERVATIONS: The temperature, pulse rate, rate of respiration and the blood pressure can be measured.

EXAMINATION OF BODY FLUIDS: It is relatively easy to collect samples of urine, blood, cerebrospinal fluid, stomach contents, etc. The chemical constituents of these fluids can be analysed and this provides information about the normal and abnormal functioning of the organs producing the fluids.

ENDOSCOPY: Special instruments can be inserted into various orifices (openings) in the body, enabling the observer to determine the appearances of the interior of such organs as the external ear, the pharynx and larynx, the bronchi, the œsophagus, the stomach, the rectum, the vagina and the bladder. Because the cornea and lens of the eye are transparent, the interior of the eye can be examined by looking into it with an **ophthalmoscope.**

RADIOLOGY: **X-rays** can be used to produce pictures (**radiographs**) of bones and of most of the internal organs. X-rays alter a photographic plate in the same way that light rays do when an ordinary photograph is taken. They have an advantage over light rays in that they are able to penetrate solid objects to some extent. They pass easily through the soft tissues of the body, but not so easily through bone, expecially where it is thick. Bones show up well on radiographs because they are opaque to X-rays (they are **radio-opaque**) and cast heavy shadows on the photographic plate (Figs. 54 and 57). Some of the internal organs cannot be seen on radiographs until they have been filled with a substance known as a **contrast medium.** Such a substance may transmit the X-rays either better than do the body tissues, for example a gas like air or oxygen, or less well, for example compounds of barium and of iodine (Figs. 184 and 199). The contrast medium makes the outline of the cavity of the organ stand out clearly on the radiograph.

Air and oxygen are used for radiographs of joints and of the ventricles of the brain. Barium sulphate, given by mouth, is used for the alimentary tract because it is insoluble and cannot therefore be absorbed. Compounds of iodine, which are excreted by the liver in the bile, are given to the patient by mouth or by intravenous injection for pictures of the gall bladder and bile duct. Other compounds of iodine, which are excreted by the kidneys, are given by intravenous injection for pictures of the urinary tract (Fig. 199). Oily fluids containing compounds of iodine are introduced through special instruments for pictures of the bronchial tree, and of the uterus and uterine tubes.

X-rays are not perceived by the human eye as light is. However, when they fall on certain substances they cause them to shine or fluoresce. A screen coated with such a substance fluoresces when X-rays fall on it. If a patient stands in front of the **fluorescent screen,** an X-ray shadow picture of the patient is seen on it. The movements of organs like the heart, lungs and intestines can be watched, as can the filling and emptying of organs like the stomach.

By the use of these techniques a great deal has been learned about normal living anatomy. The pictures are of living organs in their normal relationships.

Computerized tomography (CT, or computerized axial tomography, CAT) is a recent technique and this gives clearer and more detailed pictures than the traditional radiographs, which show images of the different structures superimposed on one another.

Computerized tomography uses, instead of photographic film, highly sensitive detectors to take many thousands of measurements of the strength of X-ray beams after they have passed through the body. During a single scan, measurements are recorded from only a thin horizontal plane passing through the body. The readings are fed into a computer, which in a few seconds converts the stream of electronic information into a television-like picture of a cross section of the body. Fig. 196 is an example of such a scan.

ULTRASOUND SCANNING: This method of creating a scan picture of internal organs uses high-frequency sound waves. They are transmitted into the body and are then reflected at the interfaces between internal structures. The echoes so produced are mapped to make a picture. An ultrasound scan is illustrated in Fig. 197.

The ultrasound technique is valuable because it differentiates between soft tissues. It also has the great advantage that ultrasound waves are nonionizing (unlike X-rays) and, as far as is known, are no biological hazard. For these reasons ultrasound scans are particularly useful for examining the pregnant uterus.

ELECTRICAL INVESTIGATION: As various parts of the body function, electrical changes take place, and these can be measured with complicated electrical equipment; this has taught us much about the functioning, in health and disease, of the brain (**electro-encephalography**); the heart (**electro-cardiography**) and muscles (**electromyography**).

RADIOACTIVE ISOTOPES: The way in which certain chemical compounds circulate and are used in the body may be studied by injecting radioactive forms of the compounds and then tracing them round the body with instruments which detect or measure radioactivity.

THE EXPERIMENTAL APPROACH: This consists of observing how the body and its constituent parts react to changes in the surrounding conditions. The various diseases to which the body is subject have produced what might be termed 'Nature's experiments' and the study of the body's reactions to disease has, as a result, taught us much about the way in which the body functions.

Changed circumstances can, of course, be brought about artificially; that is, experiments can be performed. There is a limit to what may be done to a human being in this way, and so, much of this kind of work is carried out on animals. Some of the knowledge gained in this way is directly applicable to Man.

It is now possible to grow organs, or portions of them, or individual cells in the laboratory. These *in vitro* (literally in glass) experiments have been used increasingly to study how organs, tissues and cells react to particular influences. Their surroundings can be regulated accurately and the results of deliberate changes in them can be observed directly. In the body so many different factors act on the object of study, that it is often impossible to know what causes a given reaction.

'THE NORMAL'

The basic medical sciences of Anatomy, Physiology and Biochemistry are concerned with the study of the **normal** structure and function of the body.

What is 'Normal'?

The normal cannot be defined with precision. Consider a single attribute such as height. A person may be short or tall or, like most people, of medium height, and yet in all three cases may be considered normal; the normal height therefore covers a **range of variation.** In the same way, the normal functioning of the body varies from one person to another, and in the same person at different times. Take the heart rate as an example (p. 363). Most adults have a heart rate of about 70 beats per minute; in children it is considerably faster, in elderly people and athletes considerably slower. In each of these cases the rate is faster during exercise than during rest. Thus the normal heart rate has a range of variation. *The abnormal is what lies outside the accepted range of normal variation.* For example, an excessively short person is a dwarf and an excessively tall person exhibits gigantism. If the heart rate is outside the range of normal variation for given circumstances, it is a sign that function is deranged, that is, that the person is ill.

In many instances the normal can be clearly distinguished from the abnormal. In other cases the limits of normality merge with the beginnings of abnormality and there is no clear line of demarcation.

INDIVIDUAL VARIATION

The range of normal variation is responsible for the differences, often striking, by which we distinguish at a glance one normal person from another.

There is normal individual variation in every detail of structure and function of the body. Some variable characteristics are inherited by an individual from previous generations, for example height, hair and eye colour, and blood groups. On the other hand, the environment influences the development of other variations, for example, regular use of certain muscles causes them to respond by enlarging, so producing individual variations which reflect different ways of life.

The normal variation in the general configuration of the body is worth noting: some people are short and broad, others are tall and thin, and others again are intermediate (Fig. 1). Variations in normal functioning, and even in mental outlook, are associated with these different body types.

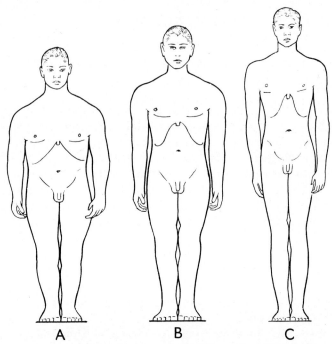

Fig. 1. Schemes to show variations in the general configuration of the body: A, short, broad individual with wide subcostal angle; B, intermediate type of body-build; C, tall, thin individual with narrow subcostal angle.

Asymmetry

A slight asymmetry of the proportions and movements of the two sides of the body is so common as to be regarded as normal. This can be confirmed by critical examination of almost every face. Some of the asymmetry of the body is associated with individual right- or left-handedness.

SEX DIFFERENCES

There are differences of structure and function between men and women. Most of these differences are related to the different reproductive functions of the two sexes, and find expression in the **primary sexual characteristics** which affect the configuration of the reproductive organs (see Chapter XVII), and **secondary sexual characteristics** which involve several other organ systems.

Not only is the **texture of the skin** different, but the **distribution pattern of hair** is characteristic in the two sexes. Thus a man grows hair on the face and chest, and in the pubic region the hair is distributed over a triangular area the apex of which reaches the vicinity of the navel or umbilicus. Also men tend to become bald as they grow older. On the other hand, not only do women not go bald and not grow hair on face or chest, but the triangle of hair over the pubic region is inverted when compared with that of the male.

On the whole, women lay down more **subcutaneous fat** (possibly as a store for pregnancy and lactation) so that they withstand cold better than do men.

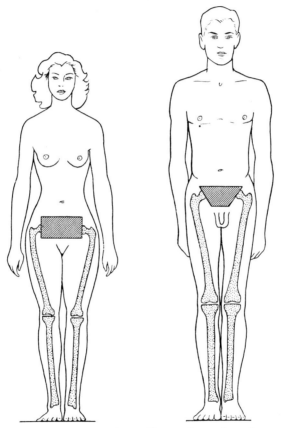

Fig. 2. Scheme to show differences in the bodily configuration of a woman compared to that of a man. The cylindrical shape of the woman's pelvic cavity and the more funnel-shaped male equivalent, as well as the relative positions of the lower limb bones are represented diagrammatically.

Also, whereas in men the fat is distributed evenly over the body surface, in women it tends to be localized in the region of the limb girdles. This, in conjunction with breast development, gives the **female figure** its characteristic hour-glass shape (Fig. 2).

The **pattern of growth** is different in the two sexes and this is described in detail in Chapter XIX. Not only are **stature** and **muscular development** usually greater in the male, with the result that the **bones** of men are heavier and have more prominent markings and ridges on them, but men also tend to have larger **brains** and consequently larger **skulls.** The **clavicles** lie more horizontally in women than in men. As the **pelvis** of a woman is designed to allow the passage of a baby's head during the birth process, it is necessary for the outlet below to be approximately the same size as the inlet above. Thus the cavity of a woman's pelvis is more or less cylindrical (Fig. 2). In a man, however, no such consideration need be taken into account, and the whole construction of the pelvis is devoted to ensuring stability with the result that the male pelvic cavity is funnel shaped (Fig. 2). This in turn affects the shape of the **hips,** so that in a woman the hips are further apart. The result of this is that the neck of the thigh bone (**femur**) is bent more on the shaft than in a man. The angle between the bones of the forearm and the line of the humerus (**the carrying angle**) is consequently also increased. In addition women have a more marked **lumbar curvature.**

Because of the special construction of the female hip region (p. 151), a woman is unable to extend her thigh (i.e. carry it backwards) to the same extent as a man. This means that, in order to take a stride of the same length as that taken by a man of comparable stature, a woman must rotate her pelvis to compensate for her restricted extension at the hip (Fig. 3). This is why the gait of man and that of woman differ characteristically.

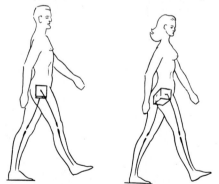

Fig. 3. Scheme to show the rotation of a woman's pelvis, when she takes a stride of the same length as that taken by a man of comparable stature.

As will be seen in a subsequent section, the **mechanism of respiration** can be broken down into a thoracic and a diaphragmatic component. Women use the former mainly, and men the latter. This is possibly associated with reproductive function, for a pregnant woman has to accommodate a baby and its accessory structures, such as the placenta, in her womb. This restricts considerably the space available in the abdominal cavity and makes movements of the diaphragm more difficult.

The difference between the reproductive functions of men and women is reflected in the different way their respective reproductive glands affect, or are affected by, the other endocrine glands of the body. The cyclial nature of the female reproductive processes causes **cyclical variations** in many physiological processes in a woman. Another important sex difference is that women are more subject to anæmia (insufficient red corpuscles or hæmoglobin in the blood—see pp. 393 to 397) perhaps because of their periodic loss of blood. The **red blood count** of a woman is almost invariably lower than in a man.

It is noteworthy that, in general, women have a greater **resistance to environmental changes** than do men. They are less susceptible to exposure to cold, to X-rays and to certain diseases, though more susceptible to others. Their **expectation of life** is better, their **expenditure of energy** is more efficient and it need hardly be pointed out that the **psychological outlook** of a woman is different from that of a man.

AGE DIFFERENCES

Physiology and Anatomy are customarily described in terms of the mature adult. The physiology and anatomy of babies, children, adolescents and of the elderly differ in important ways, and these differences are discussed in Chapters XIX and XX.

RACIAL VARIATION

The human species is divided into sub-groups called races. It may be presumed that each characteristic of every population represented, at some time, an adaptation to a particular environmental factor, though its present significance may be very difficult to identify. Diversity is important as various types of people are needed to make up a human community that is rich in adaptability potential. A population that is homogeneous from a genetic point of view is at risk because it may be overcome by any number of factors, be it an infection or any other change in the environment to which it fails to adapt.

It seems then that there are many hereditary characters that are useful under certain conditions, and human populations differ considerably in superficial features, which they themselves recognize and to which they attach importance. These include skin colour, type of hair, facial characters and general body build.

Although races do not constitute clearly identifiable discrete groups, some major differences between peoples have come to be recognized. At the **caucasoid** extreme are fair skin, thin nose, thin lips and a considerable amount of wavy hair. **Negroid** peoples, on the other hand, have dark skin, broad noses, thick everted lips and short, black, tightly curled hair. The third, **mongoloid** group has yellow or reddish skin, slanted eyes, a rather flattened nose and straight black hair which is sparse on the body. A fourth, smaller **australoid** group, is characterized by a dark skin, but the other features of body form and hair resemble the caucasoid features.

THE SYSTEMS OF THE BODY

A system consists of the different parts of the body which work together to carry out some specific function or functions which are similar or complementary.

The following systems are described in subsequent chapters:

The **skeletal system** consists of bones, joints and ligaments. Its function is to support the body and yet allow movement.

The **system of skeletal muscles** comprises those muscles which are attached to the bony skeleton and are under voluntary control. These muscles move the parts of the body in relation to each other and move the body in relation to its surroundings.

The **nervous system,** consisting of the brain, spinal cord and the peripheral nerves, controls the body and enables all parts to act together in harmony. It perceives the nature of the surroundings and enables the body to react in a suitable way.

The **organs of special sense** assist the nervous system by receiving information through the nose (smell), mouth (taste), eyes (sight) and ears (hearing).

The **integumentary system** consists of the skin and its various appendages such as nails, hair and sweat glands. It both protects the body from the outside world and is a means of contact with this environment.

The **respiratory system** consists of the lungs and the air passages which connect them with the exterior. Air passes to and from the lungs where oxygen is absorbed into the blood-stream and the waste gas, carbon dioxide, is eliminated. A secondary function of this system is voice production and speech.

The **cardiovascular** or **circulatory system** comprises the heart and blood vessels of the body. It maintains the blood supply to every part of the body and so ensures a constant supply of oxygen and food materials to the cells and, equally important, the regular removal of waste products from them.

The **blood and lymphatic systems** comprise the tissues responsible for producing the formed elements of the blood, the cells that provide the defence mechanisms of the body, and the filtering tissues in the body.

The **alimentary system** comprises a series of tubular organs concerned with the ingestion, transport, digestion and absorption of food and the elimination of its residues, together with the associated glands which secrete digestive juices.

The **urinary system** consists of the organs which produce, store and void urine. It is the principal means of excretion of waste products from the body.

The **endocrine system** comprises a number of glands which, having no ducts, secrete substances called hormones into the blood-stream and so influence organs which may be situated at a considerable distance from the gland which produced the hormone.

The **reproductive system** consists of the organs concerned with procreation.

THE SUBDIVISIONS OF THE BODY

The human body is divided into the following parts: the **head**; the **neck**; the **trunk,** which is divided into the chest or **thorax** and the belly or **abdomen**; a pair of **upper limbs** and a pair of **lower limbs.**

TOPOGRAPHICAL NOMENCLATURE

If the body is to be described adequately, it is necessary to establish certain readily understood conventions about the position, relations and movements of the various parts of the body.

The arbitrary position of the body chosen for all descriptions is known as the **anatomical position** (see Fig. 51). The body is viewed from in front; it is standing upright; the head held up, the arms held straight by the sides of the body with the palms of the hands facing forwards and the thumbs on the outside; the feet are on the ground with the toes pointing forwards and the legs are straight. The aspect of the body which faces the viewer is known as the **ventral** or **anterior surface,** and the surface at the back, i.e. hidden from the viewer, is known as the **dorsal** or **posterior surface.** The upper end of the body is called **superior,** and the lower **inferior.** These adjectives can be used to describe the relation of one part of a body to another, so that 'in front of' is known as 'anterior to'; 'behind' as 'posterior to'; 'above' as 'superior to'; and 'below' as 'inferior to'. Thus the head is superior to the neck; the hand inferior to the arm; the navel anterior to the backbone; the navel inferior to the chest, but superior to the leg, etc.

Superficial and deep are used to indicate the relative depth of structures from the surface of the body or of a limb. Structures in a limb are either nearer to the root of the limb or further away from it, so that we talk of the foot as being at the **distal** end of the lower limb, and the thigh at its **proximal** end. An imaginary line running through the centre of the whole length of the body, or of a limb, is known as the **axis** of the body or limb. In considering the side to side relation of the various parts of the body to its axis, those nearer to the axis are said to be **medial**, and those further away **lateral**. A structure situated actually on the axis is said to be **median**. A line along, or parallel to, the axis is **longitudinal**, and one across it at a right angle is **transverse**. In considering movements, *bending the body, or a limb, so that the ventral surfaces come together,*

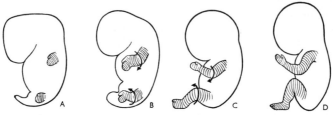

Fig. 4. A scheme to show the development and rotation of the limbs: A, limb buds growing out laterally from the trunk of an embryo. The dorsal surfaces of the limb buds face the observer. B, limbs of the embryo becoming flexed in the region of the developing elbow and knee. C, upper limb rotating laterally and lower limb rotating medially. D, the root of the upper limb has moved closer to the back of the fetus and the whole limb has rotated laterally, so that its ventral surface faces forwards with the thumb on the lateral side of the hand. The lower limb has rotated medially, so that the original ventral surface faces backwards and the big toe comes to lie on the medial side of the foot.

is known as **flexion.** *Bending them so that the dorsal surfaces come nearer to each other, is known as* **extension.**

Applying these terms to the lower limb presents an initial difficulty. Bending the knee is flexion; that is, the approximation of seemingly posterior or dorsal surfaces of the limb. These surfaces are, however, really ventral surfaces which altered their position during development, when the lower limb rotated (Fig. 4).

Bringing a structure in towards the axis of the body, or of a limb, is known as **adduction,** and carrying it away from the axis is known as **abduction.** Flexion, extension, adduction and abduction can be combined in sequence to produce a circular movement known as **circumduction.** Twisting about an axis is known as **rotation.**

Theoretically the body can be cut through in many different ways; this gives rise to the concept of different **planes of section** (Fig. 5). If the body is sectioned along its axis, i.e. longitudinally, two main possibilities come to mind: either the body is cut down its midline into right and left halves, i.e. in the **sagittal plane** (named from the sagittal suture in the skull (p. 123),

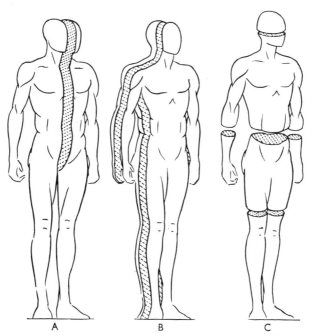

Fig. 5. Scheme to illustrate planes of section of the body: A, sagittal plane; B, coronal plane; C, transverse or horizontal planes.

which runs from front to back) (Fig. 40), or it is cut in a plane at right angles to the first, resulting in a front and a back half of the body, i.e. it has been sectioned in the **coronal plane** (named from the coronal suture in the skull (p. 123), which runs from side to side (Fig. 41)). If cut across horizontally, the body has been sectioned in the **transverse plane.**

CHAPTER II

THE CHARACTERISTICS OF THE HUMAN BODY COMPARED WITH OTHER SPECIES

MAN has been known for centuries as a rational animal and, though his anatomy and physiology resemble those of other mammals (animals that suckle their young) in many respects, certain features that distinguish Man are worth considering.

Man's ability to use tools and language is linked to the possession of a brain capable of processing quantities of information greatly in excess of the capacity of the brain of any other creature. The extraordinary development of the human brain is also associated with consciousness and the power of thought. From the point of view of Human Biology, and indeed of Medicine, it is brain activity that characterizes human life. This is not to say the 'Brain' and 'Mind' are synonymous, but consciousness together with the deepest expressions and insights of the spiritual person are only possible through the activity of the human brain.

Man is thus primarily distinguished by consciousness and capacity for rational thought and reflection. He constitutes a person in relation with other persons and with the environment in which he finds himself. He searches for meaning and assumes responsibility for fashioning the world to his own advantage and for human relations.

Like other creatures, the human individual is the result of the interplay of evolution, genetics and the environment, but to some extent other animals are more adaptable to environmental changes. When an animal finds itself in an altered environment, if it survives at all, it usually adjusts itself quickly to the new conditions. Man, however, is less flexible in his physiology. He adapts much more by inventiveness and cultural development. Whereas other animals adapt by biological compensations, Man adjusts on the whole as a toolmaker— by artificial means, by inventions.

Basic Structure of Vertebrates

First let us consider the fundamental pattern of bodily structure in vertebrates (animals with a backbone). Looked at from an evolutionary and developmental point of view, the body is seen to be elaborated and modified from a

18

simple basic pattern. This consists of a head and trunk made up of **segments** which are essentially similar, and which are, so to speak, arranged along a flexible **axial rod** (**notochord**) which becomes a backbone.

Each segment is made up of the following parts (Plate 7): a section of the **central nervous system** which is in the form of a tube lying dorsal to the axial rod; part of the body wall containing **skeletal muscle** arranged in two main masses—one dorsal to the axial rod, for bending the axial rod backwards or dorsally, that is an **extensor muscle mass**; the other ventral to the axial rod, for bending the axial rod forwards, or ventrally, that is a **flexor muscle mass**; and a **segmental nerve** which connects the muscle masses of each segment to the section of the neural tube of that segment. Each segmental nerve divides into an **anterior** and a **posterior primary branch** or **ramus**. The anterior primary ramus supplies the ventrally placed flexor muscle mass, the posterior primary ramus supplies the dorsally placed extensor muscle mass. Near the cranial (head) end of the trunk, and near the caudal (tail) end of the trunk a number of segments are modified to form the **limbs** and the connecting and supporting **limb girdles.**

The **upper limb,** or **forelimb,** develops from the lower cervical (neck) segments and its girdle is known as the **pectoral girdle**; the **lower** or **hindlimb** develops from lumbosacral segments and its girdle is known as the **pelvic girdle.** It is important to realize that the limbs grow out laterally, or sideways, from the **ventral** half of the trunk and consequently the nerves to the limbs are derived from the nerves supplying that ventral part of the trunk, namely the anterior primary divisions of the segmental nerves. Bones develop along the axis of each limb dividing the muscle tissue in it into a dorsal muscle mass and a ventral muscle mass (Fig. 120). Following the same principles as were applied to the trunk muscles and nerves, it is found that in the limbs the muscles lying **dorsal** to the bones are **extensor** in function and are supplied by **posterior** divisions of the anterior primary rami of segmental nerves. In the same way the muscles lying **ventral** to the bones are **flexors** and are supplied by **anterior** divisions of the anterior primary rami. If the limbs remain as lateral outgrowths from the trunk, it will be readily understood that the leading, or **preaxial,** digit (thumb and big toe) has the same relative position in all limbs, and the only method of progression possible to the animal is one in which bending of the trunk sideways is associated with the bringing forward of the forelimb of one side and the hindlimb of the other (Fig. 6, A). Such animals force air into their lungs by means of a swallowing movement.

In a **mammal,** which runs well and efficiently on four legs, the arrangement is very different. The trunk muscles are used for balance and support, and also for breathing by a suction mechanism. The **hindlimb** is **rotated** or twisted inwards so that it becomes an efficient **pushing** limb which no longer needs to be dragged forwards by bending the trunk sideways. This results in the **preaxial** or leading digit (the big toe) lying on the **medial** or inner side of the foot and the originally ventrally placed flexor musculature comes to lie at the back of the limb (Figs. 4, D and 6, B). In **Man**, with the adoption of the **upright posture,** the equivalent of the forelimb is an upper limb which is not required for supporting the trunk and so is free to become a **prehensile,** or grasping limb. It is rotated or twisted a little so that the leading or preaxial digit (the thumb)

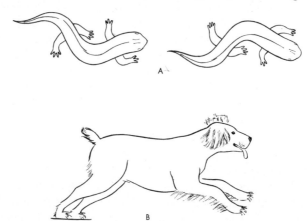

Fig. 6. Scheme illustrating the method of propulsion, A in a primitive animal such as a salamander, and B, in a mammal such as a dog.

In A, the trunk is twisted first one way, then the other, to carry the limbs forwards. In B, the trunk is propelled forwards by the hindlimbs, the forelimbs being used to support the weight of the body while the hindlimbs are carried forwards.

comes to lie on the outer or lateral side of the limb. The extensors and flexors are placed on the posterior and anterior aspects of the limb respectively (Fig. 4, C and D).

Some Essentially Human Characteristics

Prolonged Gestation, Childhood and Maturation

The period of gestation, that is, the length of time the unborn child is carried in the mother's womb, is very long when the size of the human body is taken into consideration. (Huge mammals, such as elephants and whales, have longer gestation periods.) Again, it is remarkable that from a quarter to a third of the average lifespan of Man is spent growing and maturing to adulthood. This means that children are dependent on their parents much longer, and the reproductive phase of human life starts much later after birth, than is the case with other mammals.

Brain, Head Size and Face

In relation to the size of the human body, the brain is far larger than in any animal. Correspondingly, the bones protecting this brain form a skull of relatively enormous capacity. The skull consists of two main parts: the brain case and the facial skeleton with the jaws. The brain case has been developed in Man to such an extent that it overshadows the jaw skeleton. As a result, Man has a forehead produced by the bulging of the brain case over the eyes, and a forward-looking relatively 'flat' face which replaces the protruding snout of animals; the jaw bones supporting the teeth are relatively small, but the lower jaw is more prominent and gives Man a chin. The large size of the human head produces several biological problems of which two may be mentioned: firstly the great weight of the head requires special mechanical arrangements for its support, e.g. the foramen magnum, through which the brain is continuous with the spinal cord, is on the lower surface of the skull which, in turn, is situated on top of the cervical vertebræ and is thus directly supported by them; secondly the relatively large size of the human baby and, especially, of its head, means that a woman's pelvis must have a special configuration to allow it to pass through during labour.

Upright Posture

Although some animals, such as apes and bears, can adopt an upright posture, they are all much more dependent on their forelimbs both for support and for progression than Man, who relies entirely on the lower limbs for progression, i.e. walking and running. The upper limbs are then completely free for prehension (grasping objects). This completely alters the mechanics of weight transmission from that of a four-legged animal.

Extra strain is placed upon the vertebral column, especially its lumbar region, and upon the bones and joints of the lower limb. The strain of weight bearing in the upright posture is the reason for the common derangements of these regions in Man. Especially in those who are overweight, it accounts for the prevalence of backache, of arthritis in the hip and knee joints, and of painful feet.

EFFECTS ON NECK, TRUNK, PELVIS AND PERINEUM: The number of vertebræ in Man's vertebral column is reduced. There are only twelve thoracic vertebræ compared with the thirteen found in the basic mammalian pattern, and only five instead of seven lumbar vertebræ. In addition Man's vertebral column has special curves (p. 133) to give it extra strength and resilience in the upright posture. The musculature of the back, which in Man is important for the control of the vertebral curvatures, is characteristically well developed.

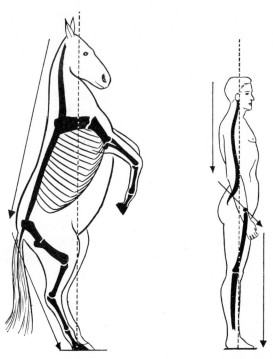

Fig. 7. Scheme illustrating the lines along which weight is transmitted when a horse rears up on its hindlimbs and when a man stands erect; the line of gravity is indicated by an interrupted line. In Man, the line of the vertebral column and that of the lower limb bones lies close to the line of gravity, so that relatively little muscular effort is required to maintain the erect posture. In the horse, the line of gravity falls well in front of the line of the vertebral column and of that of the hindlimbs, hence a strong effort by the extensor musculature is required to maintain the erect position.

Whereas the chest of most mammals is flattened from side to side, that of Man is flattened from front to back (Fig. 7). This has the effect of bringing the centre of gravity of the body backwards, nearer to the line of the vertebræ that have to sustain the weight. The human pelvis is modified by a great expansion of its upper part (the iliac wings) so that this can contribute to the support of the viscera and also afford an extensive attachment for the very large gluteal (buttock) muscles required to maintain an upright posture.

The fact that Man and higher apes have no tail may be related to the fact that the upright posture creates problems of support in the lower part of the pelvis, that is in the perineum. The musculature there, which in lower animals is used to control the tail, is used in these higher forms to provide a muscular support, or floor, to the pelvic cavity. The capaciousness of the human pelvis has already been mentioned. Its configuration differs from that found in animals in that the front, or pubis, comes to lie more or less opposite the sacrum. (In the upright posture the tip of the coccyx is on the same horizontal plane as the upper part of the pubic symphysis.)

EFFECTS ON THE UPPER LIMB: As already mentioned, the adoption of the upright posture leaves the upper limb free to become **prehensile.** Associated with this, the limb undergoes **lateral torsion,** or twisting, and is brought alongside the trunk. The scapula or shoulder blade is now situated at the back of the trunk rather than at the side. The human forearm is relatively long and capable of a remarkable degree of the twisting movements known as **pronation** and **supination** (p. 166). Relatively short fingers are combined with a large thumb which can perform a high degree of **opposition,** the movement which brings the thumb into contact with each of the other fingers in turn. Opposition is essential for nearly all the useful movements of the human hand.

EFFECTS ON THE LOWER LIMB: The great length and strength of the lower limb are associated with its straightening out by extension at the hip and knee joints. The buttock muscles, which keep the hip extended and the quadriceps femoris, which extends the knee, are very well developed in Man. The big toe, which plays an important rôle in the human mode of walking, is characteristically very large. In addition, the bones of the foot are comparatively fixed (when compared with those of the hand), and arranged to form arches which give a special resilience to the human gait.

CHAPTER III

AN INTRODUCTION TO BIOCHEMISTRY*

Biochemistry is the study of the chemical processes which occur in living tissues.

Chemistry is a science which deals with matter, which in turn may be defined as anything that possesses weight. Chemistry studies the nature and composition of matter; the breaking down, or analysis, of complex matter into simpler forms; the building up, or synthesis, of complex matter from simple constituents; and the laws that govern the interaction between the different kinds of matter.

Chemistry covers such a wide field that many different branches are recognized. Among them are inorganic chemistry, organic chemistry and biochemistry.

Inorganic chemistry developed as the study of matter surrounding us. It has been shown that all matter consists of about a hundred distinct simple substances, the **elements.** *An element is a substance from which no simpler substance can be obtained by any chemical reaction.* Some elements occur in nature uncombined with other elements, for example, metallic gold, but most substances are **compounds.**

A **compound** *is the chemical combination of two or more elements.* A compound is not a mere mixture of elements, but consists of elements joined together in a particular way and in definite proportions which are always the same for a given compound.

Usually a compound bears no resemblance to the elements of which it is composed. For example, common salt or sodium chloride is a white crystalline solid; it is a chemical compound of sodium and chlorine. Sodium is a soft shiny metal and chlorine is a green pungent gas. Both are very harmful to living things. Sodium chloride, however, is harmless and indeed essential to the body (p. 570).

An **atom** *is the smallest portion of a chemical element that can exist in a chemical compound or take part in a chemical reaction.* Individual atoms rarely exist alone. In an element they are combined with similar atoms and in a compound with atoms of other elements.

A **molecule** *is the smallest portion of matter that is capable of separate existence.* A molecule of a compound, therefore, is composed of dissimilar atoms, and in the molecule of an element all the atoms are the same.

---

* Only some of the simplest concepts and definitions are included. For fuller expositions the student is referred to textbooks of chemistry and biochemistry.

Organic chemistry is a branch of chemistry which began by the study of compounds elaborated only by living organisms, plant or animal. Chemists have since learned to synthetize many of these compounds in the laboratory, so that the original definition no longer holds. The substances all contain the element carbon, so that organic chemistry is now defined as the chemistry of the carbon compounds. Most of these organic compounds are formed from five of the elements—carbon, hydrogen, oxygen, nitrogen and sulphur. A few contain a small number of other elements.

Chemical Formulæ

To make reference to the elements quick and easy, each is known by a symbol, and this symbol represents one atom of the element. The elements found in the human body are listed below with their symbols:

Carbon	C	Potassium	K
Oxygen	O	Sodium	Na
Hydrogen	H	Magnesium	Mg
Nitrogen	N	Iron	Fe
Calcium	Ca	Copper	Cu
Phosphorus	P	Manganese	Mn
Chlorine	Cl	Zinc	Zn
Sulphur	S	Iodine	I

These symbols are used in **formulæ** to show which elements and how many atoms of each unite to form a given compound. Thus two atoms of hydrogen and one of oxygen are needed to make one molecule of water which is, therefore, written H_2O. Sodium chloride is $NaCl$.

Most inorganic compounds can be specified by such simple molecular formulæ. Many thousands of different organic compounds, however, are built up from only five main elements. Many very different compounds may, therefore, have the same molecular formula, e.g. five have the formula C_6H_{14}. In the organic compounds the three dimensional pattern in which the atoms of the different elements are joined is all-important. For a formula to convey the identity of an organic compound it must show something of the grouping and pattern of the elements. Such a formula is a **structural formula.** For example, acetic acid whose molecular formula is $C_2H_4O_2$, has the structural formula $CH_3 \cdot COOH$. In fact, all organic acids have the special group —COOH in the molecule, so that an acid can be recognized at once, no matter how complicated the rest of the formula. A special group of this kind is known as a **radical**. Certain other radicals and ways of joining radicals together are easily written down in this way. Each radical has distinctive properties which it confers on the compound containing it.

Amines are organic compounds which are built on a certain pattern and contain nitrogen. If part of that pattern is replaced by —COOH the substance becomes an **amino acid.** Thus $CH_2(NH_2)COOH$ is a simple amino acid. Amino acids join together in long chains to form proteins.

Name of group	Formula	Characteristic of
Carboxyl	—COOH	Organic acids
Hydroxyl	—OH	Alcohols
Amino	—NH$_2$	Amino acids
Peptide linkage	—CO·NH—	Proteins

CHEMICAL CHANGE

When a substance undergoes a chemical reaction its constituent elements are not destroyed, but the appearance of the resulting substance may be entirely changed.

Chemical reactions are of different kinds. Two or more substances may combine together to form a new substance, e.g. clean, bright, hard iron combines with the oxygen and water vapour in damp air to form a reddish brown powder called rust or hydrated iron oxide. A single substance may decompose into two or more substances, e.g. sugar when heated strongly changes into carbon, which is black, and water vapour. Two substances may react together to give two different substances.

All chemical reactions take place more quickly if the temperature is raised, and, conversely, more slowly if the temperature is lowered. This is true, within limits, of the biochemical reactions in the body.

Oxidation and Reduction

When oxygen is added to a substance, or when hydrogen is taken away from it, it is said to be **oxidized.** Conversely, when a substance loses oxygen, or when hydrogen is added to it, it is **reduced.** Every oxidation involves a corresponding reduction of some other substance. Oxidation and reduction reactions are of great importance in the biochemistry of the body. The oxidation of food provides most of the energy required for the functioning of the body. Direct addition of oxygen is not common; oxidation of organic substances in the body usually involves the removal of hydrogen. This is often accomplished by oxygen itself, which in the process is reduced to water, H_2O. In the body, oxidation is carried out in the presence of enzymes (see below) called oxidases and dehydrogenases. The oxidation of food materials to carbon dioxide and water is accomplished in many complicated stages, each stage having its own specific enzymes.

Hydrolysis

Hydrolysis *is a chemical reaction in which a complex compound is broken down into simpler ones by combining with water.* Proteins are hydrolysed to give amino acids (p. 42); fats are hydrolysed to give an alcohol and a fatty acid (p. 40); and polysaccharides are hydrolysed to give sugars. Such reactions occur in the body in the presence of the appropriate enzymes (see below) which are called **hydrolases.** Examples are pepsin and trypsin which act on proteins, lipase and phosphatase which act on fats and amylase which acts on polysaccharides.

ENZYMES

Some chemical reactions can be made to take place quickly, even at a low temperature, by the addition of a small amount of a substance, called a **catalyst,** *which, though it speeds up the reaction, is not changed or used up in so doing.* In biochemistry it has been found that organic catalysts, made by the living cells, are essential for promoting the multitude of biochemical reactions associated with 'living'. These *organic catalysts are called* **enzymes.** Each different biochemical reaction has its own specific enzyme. An enzyme may work inside the cell in which it was produced, for example those concerned with the oxidation of carbohydrate in muscle cells (p. 181) or it may be secreted from the cell to work elsewhere, for example the enzymes in the digestive juices (p. 460).

EFFECT OF TEMPERATURE ON ENZYMES

Enzymes work best at body temperature, 37°C (98·4°F). If the body temperature is lowered, the actions which they catalyse progress more slowly. This is the basis of the cooling technique used in surgical operations on the heart. When the temperature is low, cell metabolism proceeds very slowly, very little oxygen is needed, and the blood supply to the tissues can be cut off for short periods without harm to the cells, not even to the very sensitive nerve cells in the central nervous system (p. 116).

At temperatures above 37°C enzymes are increasingly inactivated and so the biochemical reactions become slower. In burns some of the cells exposed to the heat are killed even though they are not charred, because their enzymes are destroyed.

EFFECT OF pH ON ENZYMES

Enzymes are very sensitive to the pH (p. 31) of their environment. Even a small alteration in the pH may stop their action.

ENERGY

Every chemical reaction is associated with the taking in or giving out of **energy.** Energy has many different forms, e.g. heat, light, electricity and motion. The energy liberated from chemical reactions in the body is used to maintain the body temperature, for mechanical work and for other purposes. The energy comes from the breaking down of the complex organic substances in our food, i.e. the energy has been 'stored' as potential energy in the foodstuffs. It should be noted that this energy comes from the sun in the form of light and heat which enables plants to synthetize the complex organic compounds from the water and carbon dioxide present in the air. Even if the food is meat or fish, the potential energy it contains is there because of the activity of the plants eaten by the animal or fish whose flesh it is. Only plants are able to use directly the energy from the sun. It follows, therefore, that the animal kingdom, man included, is entirely dependent on plants for making available from the sun the energy which is necessary for life.

MEASUREMENT OF ENERGY

One form of energy can be changed directly or indirectly into any other form. Heat and work are two of these forms and both are measured in units called **joules** (J). One thousand joules make a kilojoule (kJ). Previously the unit of measurement for heat was the Calorie (C).

$$1 \text{ Calorie} = 4 \cdot 2 \text{ kilojoules (approx.)}$$

The potential energy of any foodstuff can be determined by measuring the heat produced when a given amount is completely burnt in oxygen. For example 1 gram of mixed carbohydrate yields 17 kilojoules (4 Calories) (see also fats, p. 40; proteins, p. 43). In the body, of course, this energy might be used as heat to keep the body warm but equally it could be used to do work in causing a muscle to contract (see also p. 180).

THE RELEASE OF ENERGY

When coal or wood is burnt in an open fire, we see that heat and light are given off and ashes are left. What happens is that once the fuel, i.e. the coal or wood, has been raised to a high enough temperature it begins to react with the oxygen in the air—a chemical reaction has started. The complex organic materials combine with oxygen from the air and break down to form the simple substances, carbon dioxide and water, which escape up the chimney in gaseous form. The ashes are the inorganic substances which were present in the fuel and which did not react in the same way with the air. The energy given out during this chemical reaction appears as heat and light. (Note: this energy came originally from the sun. In the case of coal, it was stored up by the giant plants of prehistoric times; in the case of wood, more recently.)

We 'burn' fuel in our bodies in an essentially similar way. The fuel is the organic material in our food, mainly the carbohydrate and the fat. This reacts with oxygen to form carbon dioxide and water with the release of energy which appears as heat or work. A difference is that the chemical reaction is carried out at body temperature—a temperature very much lower than that which is necessary for ordinary 'burning'. The reaction takes place in the cytoplasm of living cells and is made possible by the presence of enzymes (p. 27).

IONIZATION

Many substances when they are dissolved in water split up or **dissociate** *into electrically charged particles called* **ions.** Such substances which dissociate into ions are called **electrolytes.**

Sodium chloride, dissolved in water, dissociates into sodium ions, Na^+, and chloride ions, Cl^-. These ions, present only when the salt is dissolved, and each possessing its own characteristic electric charge are altogether different from sodium and chlorine atoms. Copper sulphate, $CuSO_4$, dissolved in water dissociates into the copper ion, Cu^{++}, and the sulphate ion, SO_4^{--}. The ion of copper carries two positive charges and the sulphate ion carries two negative charges. A compound ion like SO_4^{--} is an example of a **radical** (p. 25). Ions carrying positive charges (e.g. Na^+, Cu^{++}) are called **cations** and those carrying negative charges are called **anions.**

Substances vary very much in the extent to which they dissociate when they are dissolved in water.

ACIDS

Acids are substances which, when dissolved in water, dissociate into one or more hydrogen ions, H^+, and an anion whose nature varies with the acid.

Hydrochloric acid HCl gives H^+ and Cl^-
Sulphuric acid H_2SO_4 gives $2H^+$ and SO_4^{--}
Nitric acid HNO_3 gives H^+ and NO_3^-
Acetic acid CH_3COOH gives H^+ and CH_3COO^-

A property common to all the substances we call acids is the ability to form hydrogen ions when they are dissolved in water.

Different acids vary in the extent to which they dissociate. Hydrochloric acid becomes almost completely ionized; that is to say, it forms a great many hydrogen ions (and chloride ions too, of course). Acids which ionize like this are called **strong acids.** Acetic acid dissociates very little and forms few hydrogen ions, most of its molecules remaining intact. Acids which do not form ions readily are called **weak acids.**

ALKALIS

Alkalis are substances which when dissolved in water dissociate into one or more hydroxyl ions, OH^-, and a cation whose nature varies with the alkali.

Sodium hydroxide (caustic soda), NaOH, gives OH^- and Na^+.

A property common to all the substances we call alkalis is the ability to form hydroxyl ions when they are dissolved in water.

Like acids, different alkalis dissociate to different extents. Sodium hydroxide ionizes freely, forming many hydroxyl ions (and sodium ions) and is called a **strong alkali,** whereas ammonium hydroxide (household ammonia) ionizes very little, forms few hydroxyl ions (and ammonium ions), and is called a **weak alkali.**

SALTS

If a solution of any acid and a solution of any alkali are mixed together we find that water is formed and also a substance called a **salt,** of which common salt is a good example.

$$HCl + NaOH = NaCl + H_2O$$
$$\text{acid} + \text{alkali} = \text{salt} + \text{water}$$

HYDROGEN ION CONCENTRATION; pH

Water itself dissociates to a very small extent into ions, each molecule giving one hydrogen and one hydroxyl ion. In pure water the concentration of hydrogen ions and hydroxyl ions is exactly the same.

$$H_2O = H^+ + OH^-$$

We have seen that a substance is an acid if it produces hydrogen ions when dissolved, and an alkali if it produces hydroxyl ions. In pure water the acidity due to the hydrogen ion and the alkalinity due to the hydroxyl ion cancel each other out. Pure water is therefore neutral.

A solution is acid if it contains more hydrogen ions than hydroxyl ions; it is alkaline if it contains more hydroxyl ions than hydrogen ions.

To indicate the acidity or alkalinity of solutions a scale is used; the figures range from 1 to 14, preceded by the symbol pH.

A solution is neutral when the pH is 7.

A solution is acid when the pH is less than 7.

A solution is alkaline when the pH is more than 7.

The pH of a solution is a measure of the hydrogen ion concentration. It is important to note that the greater the hydrogen ion concentration, that is, the more acid the solution, the smaller is the figure for pH. The more alkaline the solution the higher is the figure for pH.

INDICATORS

Certain dyes have the property of being one colour at a given pH and a different colour at another pH, changing colour as the pH is altered. Litmus, for example, is mauve in neutral solutions (pH 7), pink in acid solutions (pH less than 7) and blue in alkaline solutions (pH more than 7). By using a range of indicators the pH of any solution can be found.

BUFFER SOLUTIONS

The pH of living tissues varies within very narrow limits. The pH of the blood is about 7·4, and in health is never less than 7·3 nor more than 7·5. In 'acidosis' it falls below 7·3 and at 7·0 may be fatal. In 'alkalosis' it rises above 7·5 and at 7·6 may be fatal. The pH must be maintained almost constant in spite of the fact that there are constantly being added lactic acid from the oxidation of fat and carbohydrate (p. 181); and amino acids, fatty acids, etc., from the digestion of food.

Blood is able to take in acid or alkali without alteration in the pH because it contains substances which act as **buffers.** These buffer substances 'mop up' at once any hydrogen ions or hydroxyl ions which are added to the solution by combining with them to form undissociated molecules.

A buffer solution is a solution which tends to maintain its pH constant in spite of the addition of moderate amounts of acid or alkali. Buffers act as 'shock absorbers' preventing sudden changes of pH.

Blood plasma, red blood corpuscles, tissue fluid and indeed all the cells of the body contain such buffering substances. Although these buffers function well for a time, the pH is altered to an increasing extent as all the available buffers are used up. The kidney plays an important part in reconstituting them (see also p. 494).

Different substances are found acting as buffers in different places. For example in the blood plasma important buffers are carbonic acid with sodium bicarbonate, sodium salts of phosphoric acid and proteins with their sodium salts. In the red blood corpuscles hæmoglobin with its potassium salt and potassium salts of phosphoric acid act as buffers.

COLLOIDS

There are two kinds of solution, namely true (or crystalloidal) and colloidal. The essential difference is in the size of the particles of the dissolved substance.

Common salt and sugar form true solutions in water: their molecules and ions are roughly the same size as the water molecules, so small as to be completely invisible. Substances forming true solutions may or may not dissociate.

Particles too small to be seen with the naked eye, but large enough to be seen under a light microscope, can be shaken up in water to form a suspension. Soon they settle to the bottom, showing that the mixture was not a proper solution.

Particles intermediate in size between the molecules of a true solution and the fine dust in a suspension, do not settle out of a solution although they are very large in comparison with the water molecules all round them. This is because, constantly bombarded from all directions by water molecules, they are small enough to be kept in a state of constant random movement, known as **Brownian Movement.** They can be seen with an electron microscope but not with a light microscope. *These particles of intermediate size form a* **colloidal solution,** *and are known as* **colloids.**

DIFFUSION

If a lump of sugar is placed in a glass of water it gradually disappears. Even if the water is kept perfectly still, the dissolved sugar molecules mix with the water until they are spread evenly through it. This spreading to form a homogeneous solution is called **diffusion.**

In such an experiment the water, which does the dissolving, is called the **solvent** and the sugar, which dissolves in it, is called the **solute.**

Diffusion occurs because the molecules of both the solvent and solute are in a state of constant motion, colliding endlessly with each other and with the walls of the vessel. After each collision the molecules set off in a different direction. Given enough time, therefore, the random movement of the molecules results in their becoming uniformly mixed.

OSMOSIS

Osmosis is the diffusion of a liquid through a membrane.

If we take a cylinder (Fig. 8) and tie a membrane, for example a piece of parchment, over one end, partly fill the cylinder with water, and place it in a beaker of water, so that the two water surfaces are at the same level (Fig. 8, A),

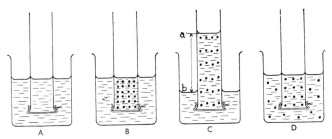

Fig. 8. To illustrate osmosis: A, pure water in a beaker separated by a semipermeable membrane from pure water in the cylinder; B, sugar (indicated by dots) solution in the cylinder, with water in the beaker; C, the osmotic pressure, a b, developed by the sugar solution; D, the result after a time, if the membrane is not truly semipermeable.

nothing appears to happen even if the apparatus is left indefinitely. In fact, water molecules are colliding with both surfaces of the parchment and some are passing from the cylinder into the beaker and equal numbers are passing from the beaker into the cylinder.

If now we put into the cylinder instead of pure water, a solution of sugar (Fig 8, B), we find that after a time the surface level in the cylinder rises. This is because the sugar molecules are not able easily to pass through the membrane, while water molecules pass freely from the beaker into the cylinder as before. Water molecules in the cylinder are hindered from colliding with and passing through the membrane because sugar molecules are in the way. More water therefore passes into the cylinder than out of it, and the fluid level rises (Fig. 8, c). This osmosis produces a pressure which is called the osmotic water attraction of the sugar solution or **osmotic pressure.** In this experiment it would be represented by the difference between the fluid levels *a* and *b* (Fig. 8, c).

This rise results in the development of a hydrostatic pressure in the cylinder, i.e. pressure due to the weight of the extra water in it. The hydrostatic pressure forces water molecules from the cylinder into the beaker more and more strongly as it becomes higher. Eventually the hydrostatic pressure equals the osmotic water attraction (osmotic pressure) of the sugar solution and no more extra water enters the cylinder.

A membrane such as we have postulated above, which allows passage to solvent molecules but not to solute molecules, is a **semipermeable membrane.**

The osmotic pressure of a solution may be defined as equivalent to the hydrostatic pressure set up when the solution and pure solvent are separated by a semipermeable membrane.

If a membrane is not a true semipermeable membrane, but allows molecules of solute to pass slowly, an osmotic pressure is still set up, but it is transient. Water molecules diffuse much more quickly than solute molecules so that the hydrostatic pressure rises as before. As time passes, however, the solute molecules diffuse into the pure solvent until a balance is set up when the concentration of sugar molecules in the beaker equals that in the cylinder (Fig. 8, D). In such a case the transient osmotic pressure is due to the difference between the rate of osmosis of the solvent compared with that of the solute.

The osmotic pressure of a solution depends on the **number** of particles (molecules or ions) of the solute or solutes in a given volume—the higher the number the greater the osmotic pressure irrespective of their size. That is to say, the more concentrated the solution, the greater its osmotic pressure, no matter whether the particles are large or small. If several different solutes are present, the total osmotic pressure is the sum of their separate pressures. Electrolytes have a higher osmotic pressure than non-electrolytes because the osmotic pressure depends on the number of solute particles, and each of the ions of a dissociated electrolyte counts as one such particle.

If two solutions of different osmotic pressure are separated by a semi-

permeable membrane, water will pass from the solution of low osmotic pressure
to that of high osmotic pressure until the osmotic pressures on the two sides of
the membrane are the same.

INORGANIC SUBSTANCES OF GREAT IMPORTANCE IN HUMAN PHYSIOLOGY

Water

Electrolytes

Trace elements

WATER

Many substances are indispensable to the living body, but water performs
a greater number of essential functions in living tissues than any other substance. Two-thirds of the adult body consists of water. It is an essential part of
the protoplasm of every cell, and it is the main constituent of all the body fluids
—tissue fluid, blood plasma, lymph and cerebrospinal fluid. Biochemical reactions take place in the body only in the presence of water; that is, the cease-
less chemical changes which are inseparable from 'living', depend on water. The
body can absorb its food materials only after they are dissolved in water, and the
poisonous waste products of metabolism can be eliminated only if they are dissolved in water. The gaseous exchanges in the lungs can take place only if the
gases are first dissolved in water. Water is very important in the regulation of
body temperature.

The body loses water continuously in the breath, as sweat, in urine and in
fæces. A total of about 3 litres is lost each day in average conditions (p. 571).
Water is not stored in the body, and therefore it must be taken in at frequent
intervals, to compensate for this loss. Men have survived two months without
food, when water was available. Deprivation of water as well as of food may be
fatal in two days.

The biologically important properties of water are:

Solvent. Water has remarkable power to dissolve substances. It forms true solutions and colloidal solutions. In addition certain substances which by themselves are
insoluble in water, like fats, can be brought into solution in the presence of special
compounds called 'hydrotropic substances', of which cholic acid found in bile is one
example.

Thus water is the universal solvent for the compounds of the body.

Heat buffer. More heat is needed to raise the temperature of water than of almost any other substance. This means that heat liberated from chemical reactions in the body raises the body temperature by a minimum amount.

Latent heat of vaporization. In changing from liquid water to gaseous water vapour, water takes in a large quantity of heat. The evaporation of water from the surface of the skin is therefore an efficient way of losing heat from the body.

Ionizing medium. Water allows many compounds to form ions easily. This increases the range of possible chemical reactions.

Catalyst. Water accelerates very many chemical reactions. In the body all chemical reactions occur in the presence of water.

Lubricating action. In joints, in the serous cavities and at other sites where friction might occur, watery solutions form good lubricants.

ELECTROLYTES

The body fluids, notably the plasma, and the cytoplasm of the cells of the body, have dissolved in them a number of simple inorganic substances of the kind which dissociate in solution, namely electrolytes. They are very important, because upon their proper concentrations depends the normal functioning of the body cells according to the laws of osmosis. Because of their buffering properties they help to keep the pH within its very narrow normal range.

The most important electrolytes are **sodium bicarbonate, potassium bicarbonate, sodium chloride, potassium chloride** and **calcium phosphate.** They form the following ions:

Bicarbonate ion	HCO_3^-
Sodium ion	Na^+
Chloride ion	Cl^-
Potassium ion	K^+
Phosphate ion	PO_4^{---}
Calcium ion	Ca^{++}

TRACE ELEMENTS

Small amounts of certain other elements are essential to the body.

Iron (Fe), forms an essential part of hæmoglobin.

Iodine (I), is indispensable to the body for the formation of thyroxine, the hormone of the thyroid gland.

Fluorine (Fl) in very small quantities is believed to help to maintain tooth structure and prevent caries.

Magnesium (Mg), Copper (Cu), Manganese (Mn) and Zinc (Zn) are also found in very small amounts and are known to be necessary for health.

Analysis of the human body shows that 65% is water. Of the remaining solid 35%, most is organic matter. The elements found in these solids of the human body are listed below, and the amount given is the percentage of the total body weight:

Carbon	18·5	Chlorine	0·16
Oxygen	6·5	Sulphur	0·14
Hydrogen	2·7	Potassium	0·10
Nitrogen	2·6	Sodium	0·10
Calcium	2·5	Magnesium	0·07
Phosphorus	1·1	Iron	0·01
		Copper	Trace
		Manganese	Trace
		Zinc	Trace
		Iodine	Trace

ORGANIC SUBSTANCES OF GREAT IMPORTANCE IN HUMAN PHYSIOLOGY

Three main groups of organic compounds are to be considered, namely carbohydrates, fats and proteins.

CARBOHYDRATES

Carbohydrates form the main bulk of our food. They are cheap, easily digested and quickly metabolized. They provide one of the main sources of energy for the body in a form which can be used quickly.

The carbohydrates contain only carbon, hydrogen and oxygen. In most cases, for every carbon atom in the molecule (and there may be very many) there are two hydrogen atoms and one oxygen atom, i.e. hydrogen and oxygen in the proportions which form water; hence the name carbohydrate.

There are three main classes of carbohydrates, namely monosaccharides, disaccharides and polysaccharides.

1. Monosaccharides

These are the simple sugars, each one a single sugar unit. They are colourless crystalline solids and have a sweet taste. Examples are glucose, galactose and fructose.

Glucose is also called dextrose or grape sugar. From it most of the carbohydrates of importance in human biochemistry are built, and it is in the form of glucose that the carbohydrates are carried in the blood. It is found in fruit and in honey and can be obtained by breaking down starch and glycogen. Pure glucose dissolves very easily in water. It is not as sweet as ordinary household sugar (cane sugar).

Galactose is one of the monosaccharides in the disaccharide lactose (milk sugar). It combines with lipids to form cerebrosides which are important constituents of the myelin in the myelin sheaths of nerves (p. 224). Most of the galactose ingested is converted to glucose by the liver.

Fructose is also called lævulose or fruit sugar. It is found in sweet fruits and honey and is one of the monosaccharides in sucrose (cane-sugar). It is found in the seminal fluid (p. 530) and in amniotic fluid (p. 71). Most of the fructose eaten is converted to glucose by the liver.

2. Disaccharides

These are two simple sugar units joined together. They can be broken down readily into their constituent units. Examples are:

Maltose formed from glucose and glucose.

Lactose (milk sugar) formed from glucose and galactose.

Sucrose (cane sugar, household sugar) formed from glucose and fructose.

3. Polysaccharides

These are compounds consisting of a large number of sugar units joined together. Examples are starch, glycogen and cellulose, all of which are built from glucose units. Their molecules are very large, so they form colloidal solutions in water, except for cellulose which is insoluble.

Starch is found in many vegetable cells, e.g. potato, wheat and rice, and forms a large part of our food. In the process of digestion it is broken down by stages into the glucose units of which it is built.

Glycogen, also called animal starch, is the form in which carbohydrate is stored in the animal body. Starch gives a blue colour when mixed with iodine, and glycogen a red-brown colour.

Cellulose forms the walls of vegetable cells. The glucose units are joined differently from those in starch and glycogen. Cellulose is insoluble in water and cannot be broken down by the process of digestion in Man. Considerable quantities are ingested in vegetable food and this adds bulk to the intestinal contents, thus stimulating peristalsis.

CHEMICAL REACTIONS OF CARBOHYDRATES IN THE BODY: During digestion, carbohydrates are broken down by hydrolysis to simple sugar units, for only these can be used by the body. Many enzymes assist in this process. Ptyalin in the saliva and amylase in the pancreatic juice act on starch breaking it down to maltose. Maltase then changes maltose to glucose. Similarly lactase and sucrase act on lactose and sucrose respectively.

In the body cells, the oxidation of glucose is one of the principal sources of energy.

Glucose + oxygen = carbon dioxide + water + ENERGY

One gram of carbohydrate in the food yields 17 kilojoules (4 Calories).

Certain sugars, because of the structure of their molecules, can reduce alkaline solutions of cupric salts, which are blue, to cuprous oxide which is an insoluble reddish brown powder. This is the **basis of Benedict's test for sugar in the urine** (p. 496). The 'Clinitest' for glucose is a proprietary adaptation of Benedict's test.

These **reducing sugars** (i.e. those which give a positive Benedict reaction) include glucose, galactose, fructose, maltose and lactose.

Starch and sucrose do not reset in this way.

Many other substances besides the reducing sugars can act as reducing agents in these tests, e.g. aspirin excreted in the urine.

FATS AND RELATED COMPOUNDS (LIPIDS)

This is a large class of compounds all of which are insoluble in water, but soluble in 'fat solvents' like ether, acetone and benzene.

Fats in our food are an important source of energy in compact form. To derive the same amount of energy from carbohydrates more than twice as much must be eaten. The body stores energy by storing fat. In addition, fat stored in a layer under the skin acts as an insulator to prevent loss of heat from the body.

Fats are built up mainly from carbon, hydrogen and oxygen, but a few contain phosphorus or nitrogen or both. The following kinds of fats and their derivatives deserve mention:

1. True fats (neutral fats or simple lipids)
2. Phospholipids (compound lipids)
3. Sterols.

True Fats

True fats are the esters of glycerol with fatty acids.

Glycerol is one of a group of organic compounds, known as alcohols, whose characteristic is the presence of the hydroxyl group (OH). Glycerol has in fact three hydroxyl groups and is a sticky colourless liquid with a sweet taste.

A **fatty acid** is a relatively simple organic compound which contains one of the carboxyl (COOH) groups characteristic of organic acids. The commonest fatty acids found in natural fats like butter, lard and olive oil are palmitic acid, stearic acid and oleic acid. Butyric acid is found in butter.

If all the carbon atoms in a fatty acid are joined to as many other atoms as they can be, and in particular if all the places for hydrogen atoms in the molecule are filled, that fatty acid is **'saturated'**. If some of the places for hydrogen are vacant the fatty acid is **'unsaturated'**. For example, palmitic, stearic and butyric acids are saturated; oleic acid is unsaturated.

When a fatty acid and an alcohol react together, an **ester** *and water are formed.* Many such esters are pleasant smelling and are used as artificial fruit essences and perfumes. Others, in which the alcohol involved is glycerol, are the true fats.

The true fats, then, found in ordinary food materials and in the body are the esters of glycerol with such fatty acids as palmitic acid, stearic acid, oleic acid and butyric acid, namely palmitin, stearin, olein and butyrin.

Fats from natural sources are always a mixture of these different esters. The properties of a given natural fat depend on the particular esters present. Vegetable fats contain a high proportion of esters of unsaturated fatty acids, and these tend to be more liquid at atmospheric temperature than the esters of saturated fatty acids, which are found in greater proportion in animal fats. Olein, from the unsaturated oleic acid is liquid; the greater the proportion of olein the softer and more fluid the natural fat. Olive oil contains 75% olein; beef suet, which is hard, contains 25% olein.

PROPERTIES OF TRUE FATS: True fats are insoluble in water, are lighter than water and, therefore, float on its surface. If the surface tension is lowered, for example by bile salts, the fats can form emulsions (p. 479). They are soluble in the 'fat solvents', e.g. ether, chloroform, benzene and carbon tetrachloride and also in each other.

A fat is solid or liquid at room temperature according to the proportions of the different esters present. The more unsaturated fat it contains, the softer and more fluid it is.

If fatty acids like stearic acid, palmitic acid and oleic acid are made to react, not with an alcohol, but with an alkali like caustic soda, salts are formed, in this case sodium stearate, sodium palmitate and sodium oleate, which are soaps.

CHEMICAL REACTIONS OF FATS IN THE BODY: Fats are hydrolysed to give glycerol and fatty acids, for example in the intestine during digestion. These substances may combine again to form fat with the elimination of water.

Fats are oxidized to form carbon dioxide and water with the release of energy. One of the first stages in the oxidation of fats is **desaturation,** which takes place in the cells of the liver. The saturated fatty acids are changed, by removal of hydrogen atoms, into unsaturated fatty acids. One gram of fat oxidized to carbon dioxide and water gives 38 kilojoules (9 Calories).

In the body, oxidation to carbon dioxide and water can be completed only in the presence of carbohydrate. In starvation and in diabetes mellitus the carbohydrate stores are exhausted and fats are oxidized only to acetone (and similar substances) instead of to carbon dioxide and water. Acetone is poisonous and is excreted in the urine where it can be discovered by testing, and in the breath where it may be recognized by its characteristic sweetish smell. This condition is known as **ketosis.**

Phospholipids

Phospholipids are compounds of glycerol and fatty acids, but in addition their molecules contain phosphorus and nitrogen.

These complex fatty compounds are found in every animal and plant cell, and especially in the brain. Cell membranes are mainly composed of phospholipids which play an important part in the transfer of substances into and out of the cell.

Sterols

Sterols, like alcohols have a hydroxyl group and are found free or as esters of fatty acids. All have molecules built up from the same basic pattern—the steroid nucleus. There is a carbon atom at each angle of the structural formula given below.

HO

The following are all examples of this group:

Cholesterol is found in many tissues and is a main constituent of gall stones.

Ergosterol is present in the skin where it is converted into Vitamin D by ultra-violet light.

Bile acids help to emulsify fat in the intestine.

Sex hormones. Œstrogens, progesterone and testosterone are all sterols.

Corticosterone, the hormone of the adrenal cortex, is closely related to the sex hormones.

PROTEINS

Proteins are complex organic compounds with very large molecules, and all contain nitrogen. Proteins are essential constituents of every cell of the body. In addition they help to form supporting and protective structures like bones, cartilage, skin, nails and hair. (In plants the carbohydrate cellulose supports and protects.)

Proteins are essential in the diet for the growth and repair of the body and for pregnancy and lactation. They supply nitrogen in the only form in which it can be used. They also supply sulphur in an available form and also certain amino acids (see below) which the body cannot synthetize.

Proteins consist of carbon, hydrogen, oxygen and nitrogen, and many contain, in addition, sulphur or phosphorus. Protein molecules are very large and form colloidal solutions. Proteins are built up by joining simpler units called amino acids (see below) into long chains. An amino acid contains at least one carboxyl group, COOH, and at least one amino group, NH_2. When two amino acids join, the carboxyl group of one reacts with the amino group of the other with the formation of water

$$-COOH + -NH_2 = -CO\cdot NH- + H_2O$$

The link joining the two amino acids $-CO\cdot NH-$ is the **peptide linkage.**

The compound formed from two amino acids is a **dipeptide;** from three, a **tripeptide,** and from many amino acids a **polypeptide.** A protein molecule is formed by joining several hundred amino acid molecules of about twenty different kinds in this way.

Protein molecules can be broken down by hydrolysis into their constituent parts. In digestion this occurs with the help of enzymes, the proteolytic enzymes, such as pepsin, trypsin and erepsin. Proteins are broken down by stages—first to proteoses, then to peptones, to polypeptides and finally to their constituent amino acids.

The different proteins found in food vary greatly in their usefulness to the body according to the different amino acids they contain. Proteins of animal origin, from meat, fresh eggs and milk contain all the essential amino acids (see below) and are said to have a high **biological value.** Food providing these proteins is expensive and, in the third world, in short supply. Proteins of vegetable origin are said to have a low biological value because, though they may contain the essential amino acids, one or more of these may be in such small proportion that adequate growth and repair cannot be achieved. Some mixtures of vegetable proteins, especially if they include proteins from pulses (peas, beans, lentils etc.) can provide enough of all the essential amino acids.

Amino Acids

Every amino acid molecule contains at least one carboxyl group and at least one amino group NH_2; the rest of their molecules vary considerably. Twenty different amino acids are found in the proteins of the body (see table). Some of them can be built up by the cells from ingested substances. *Others cannot be synthesized by the body* and so they must be provided in the food. These are the **essential amino acids** which are found in proteins of animal origin and in less satisfactory proportions in vegetable protein.

Amino acids found in proteins:

Essential	*Not essential*
Leucine	Alanine
iso-Leucine	Arginine
Lysine	Aspartic acid
Methionine	Cystine
Phenylalanine	Glutamic acid
Threonine	Glycine
Tryptophan	Histidine
Valine	Hydroxyproline
	Proline
	Serine
	Tyrosine
	Ornithine

Histidine is an essential amino acid for infants. Methionine and cystine are the sulphur-containing amino acids.

The amino acids taken in by the body from the proteins in the food are used by the body cells to build up the proteins the body needs for its cells and its supporting structures. Hence proteins are often called 'body building' foods. Any amino acids in excess of these needs are deaminated, i.e. the nitrogen is removed from them (p. 478), in the liver, and the remaining parts of the amino acid molecules are converted to glucose. Proteins, therefore, besides being used for body building, are a useful source of energy. One gram of protein in the food, used only to produce energy, yields 17 kilojoules (4 Calories).

Some Proteins Found in the Body

Albumins and **globulins** are usually found together, as they are, for example, in plasma, muscle, milk and egg white. They form colloidal solutions which coagulate when they are heated. The white of an uncooked egg is transparent and fluid. When the egg is boiled, the white, composed of albumins and globulins, becomes white and solid. This property is the basis of the testing of urine for albumin by heating it. (To prevent other substances in the urine from giving a white cloud, the urine must first be made acid.)

Scleroproteins form most of the supporting structures in animals. Examples of scleroprotein follow:

Collagen forms the fibres in white fibrous connective tissue and in fibro-cartilage.

Elastin forms the elastic fibres of connective tissue.

Ossein is found in bones and teeth.

Keratin is found in hair and nails, and in wool, horn, real silk and feathers.

Conjugated Proteins

Conjugated proteins are built up from amino acids, but have in their molecules some other component in addition. Some examples are given:

Caseinogen found in milk is a protein containing phosphoric acid.

Mucin, which lubricates the alimentary and respiratory tracts, is a protein combined with a polysaccharide.

Nucleoproteins are compounds of proteins with nucleic acid (see below). They are found in all cell nuclei and in the cytoplasm of cells.

Hæmoglobin is a compound of the protein globin with hæm which is an organic compound containing iron. Hæm gives hæmoglobin its characteristic red colour and the property of being able to carry oxygen.

Nucleic Acid

Nucleic acids are found in all cell nuclei and in the cytoplasm of cells. The nucleic acid in the nucleus is the main constituent of the chromosomes (p. 51) which carry, in this chemical code form, all the information necessary for the activity of the cell. This includes the nature and extent of any specialization of the cell, and in this way the chromosomes determine the characteristics of the whole organism. Those nucleic acids, found in the nucleolus and nuclear sap and in the cytoplasm of the cell, are the means by which the chemical codes on the chromosomes control the synthesis of proteins, especially of enzymes, in the cytoplasm. These proteins, in turn, determine the activities of the cell.

The remarkable properties of the nucleic acids depend on their structure. There are two nucleic acids, namely deoxyribonucleic acid, D.N.A., found only in the chromosomes, and ribonucleic acid, R.N.A., found both in the nucleus and in the cytoplasm.

The chemical structure characteristic of nucleic acids is a double helix, a double spiral formed by two sugar phosphate chains linked together by paired bases called purines and pyrimidines (Fig. 9). Each nucleic acid has four different bases, namely two purines and two pyrimidines. A purine always pairs with a pyrimidine in the opposite chain.

D.N.A. and R.N.A. have a similar structure but the constituents differ. In D.N.A. the sugar is deoxyribose and the pyrimidines are thymine and cytosine. In R.N.A. the sugar is ribose and the pyrimidines are uracil and cytosine. Both D.N.A. and R.N.A. contain the purines adenine and guanine. In the double helix of D.N.A. adenine always pairs with thymine and guanine with cytosine. In R.N.A. adenine always pairs with uracil and guanine with cytosine.

D.N.A. and R.N.A. double helices are able to reproduce themselves with great accuracy. The double helix can be thought of as a zip-fastener which

during replication gradually 'unzips' from one end to the other. The free un-
zipped bases attract their complementary bases from the surroundings and then
these bases are joined up by another sugar phosphate chain, so that two helices
result, both identical with the original one.

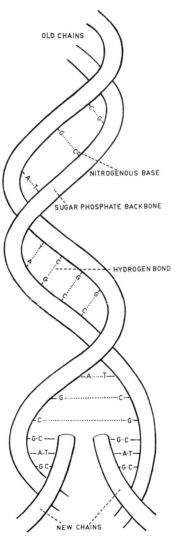

Fig. 9. Scheme of part of a D.N.A. spiral. Replication is taking place in the lower part.

Within a cell, the genetic code in the D.N.A. is given expression in protein synthesis. The process is summarized in Fig. 10 and is carried out by R.N.A. First, messenger R.N.A. is formed in the nucleus. In very much the same way as replication occurs, a chain of R.N.A. is synthetized which is exactly complementary to a section of D.N.A. This messenger R.N.A. passes out into the

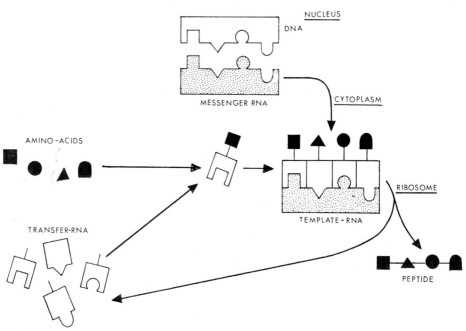

Fig. 10. Scheme showing how the D.N.A. of the nucleus orders the synthesis of a peptide in the cytoplasm from amino acids with the help of messenger-R.N.A, transfer-R.N.A. and template-R.N.A. (Modified from Emery's Textbook of Medical Genetics.)

cytoplasm where it becomes part of a ribosome (p. 93), in which protein synthesis takes place. Here it may be called template R.N.A.

The cytoplasm contains transfer R.N.A. It is thought that there are several varieties, each of which attaches itself to a particular amino acid from the cytoplasm. Each transfer R.N.A. then attaches itself to a point in the template R.N.A. into which it alone fits. In this way specific amino acids are brought close together in a particular order and join up to form polypeptides (p. 42) and then proteins.

The Genetic Code

Proteins are formed of only twenty **different** amino acids. Genetic information is stored within the D.N.A. molecule in the form of a triplet code. Each amino acid is represented by three of the possible four nitrogenous bases p. 44 arranged in a particular order. The three bases so arranged form the **codon** for that particular amino acid. Within the D.N.A. molecule the codons are arranged to represent the pattern of amino acids in polypeptides and proteins. It is thought that a gene (p. 52) may be the sequence of codons for a particular polypeptide.

The chemical basis of inheritance and development

The genetic make up of an individual depends on the chromosomes inherited from both parents. It is determined at the time of fertilization when the chromosomes from the sperm join the chromosomes of the ovum to form the nucleus of the first cell of the new individual.

These chromosomes contain D.N.A. The D.N.A. contains codons arranged in specific patterns and each particular pattern is a gene. This first cell contains all the genes, that is, the whole of the chemical code, needed to enable it to grow and develop into an adult with all the characteristics of the species and with individual inherited characteristics too. The D.N.A. in the nucleus causes the formation of messenger R.N.A., which, as we have seen, enables the ribosomes in the cytoplasm to synthetize matching amino acids and then particular proteins. The special enzymes (which are proteins) for given necessary reactions in the cell are made in this way and so the activity of the cell is determined, determined that is, by the D.N.A. in the nucleus. All the activities of this first cell, and of all the cells which result from its growth and repeated multiplication are regulated in this way. The chemical code in the form of D.N.A., thus controls the development of the whole individual, by controlling the synthesis of the proteins of which he is built. These proteins are species specific, and are organized to form a member of one species only, because the chemical code of one species is different from that of all other species.

The accurate replication of D.N.A. (p. 45) in the chromosomes during the prophase of mitosis (p. 53) is essential, so that all the cells of an individual will carry exactly the same code.

CHAPTER IV

AN OUTLINE OF EARLY HUMAN DEVELOPMENT

GENERAL CONSIDERATIONS

ALTHOUGH the activities associated with life are directed towards maintaining the integrity of the individual member of the species, these activities are not permanently successful and the individual, be he animal or man, ages and in the end, dies.

However, the pattern of activity which is the essential characteristic of life, although it fails for the individual with his limited lifespan, nevertheless continues indefinitely in the group, race or species of which the individual forms a part. So, what is maintained by the processes of life is a species made up of interbreeding individuals.

The process by which this continuity within the species is attained is known as reproduction.

The significance of reproduction

Reproduction produces a population that is able to change very slowly by gradually producing new types, who can adapt themselves and survive in changing circumstances.

Although an individual can adapt himself to some extent to his environment, it is essential to produce repeatedly new individuals, each slightly different from the other, if the species is to contain individuals suited to the conditions prevailing at any period in a changing environment. It follows that the continuous production of new individuals necessitates the death of some, who already exist, if overcrowding is to be avoided. Also the diversity of the types produced by reproduction would be restricted if the same individuals went on reproducing indefinitely.

The essence of reproduction is the passing on of instructions for organization of the life of the species, race or group, to a new unit belonging to it.

By means of reproduction, the activity that characterizes the life of the species is started again. At first, the new life is relatively simple, incomplete and not able to look after itself wholly. As it develops, the new being gradually reaches an adult state in which can be made the necessary adjustments to maintain his individual life for a relatively long time. In order to ensure survival of the race, the new individual must be like his predecessors, but not exactly like. There is no biological advantage in replacing individuals by others that are identical. The aim of reproduction is the production of a range of types. This is achieved by variations in the hereditary instructions transmitted from one generation to the next and also ensured by sexual reproduction by which each new individual inherits his bodily features and organization from two parents, one male and the other female. In Man, as in some other animals, there are special biological mechanisms to ensure that the process actually mixes different hereditary strains (see pp. 54 and 56). Thus, the sociological provisions against incest have a sound biological basis.

In reproduction, there is passed on a chemical 'blue-print' of the instructions for organization, in coded form, simple enough for it to be combined with that derived from another individual. The power of the male reproductive cell, the **sperm,** and of the female reproductive cell, the **ovum,** to make copies in this way lies primarily in their nuclei. The chemical composition of the nucleus (see p. 44 and p. 90) controls the activity that goes on in a cell throughout its life. The essential feature of sexual reproduction is that nuclear material from a male and from a female make a single new nucleus. The differences between adult males and females are largely directed towards achieving the fusion of two nuclei, one derived from each sex.

The task of parents is not limited, of course, to providing reproductive cells or **gametes.** It includes nourishing and bringing up the offspring .The mother at first nourishes the offspring with her body, then with her milk and later by giving it food. The father contributes by providing for the whole family.

The consideration of sexual reproduction, resulting in an offspring inheriting bodily features from both its parents, inevitably leads us to a consideration of the **biological laws of inheritance** or **genetics.**

Before the individual is ready to undergo the not inconsiderable rigours and indeed dangers attending upon the process of birth, several critical phases of development take place. First the egg, provided by the mother, has to be encountered and **fertilized** by a sperm, provided by the father, before **conception,** that is the initiation of a new individual, can even take place. The resulting **conceptus** (product of conception) or **zygote** has then to be conveyed to the mother's womb, where it must attach itself and embed itself within the lining of the womb by a process known as **implantation.** It is a noteworthy thought that perhaps one third of all conceptions fail to effect this critical process satisfactorily and are lost, often without the mother even realizing it.

Having become satisfactorily implanted, the **embryo** must establish channels of supply and disposal with its mother, and this is done by developing a **placenta** which, though made by the embryo, is not an integral part of its body. It links the embryo to the mother as long as the embryo remains in the womb, but at birth the placenta is cast off by both baby and mother. The development of the placenta is associated with the formation of a **primitive vascular system** which distributes the supplies, obtained from the mother, throughout the embryo.

At about the same time another critical process, which is known as **organization,** takes place. This is concerned with the sorting out and rearranging of the various cells, so that an embryo comes to have a head and a tail end, a front, a back, a right and a left side. In other words the **axis of the body** is laid down. A splitting of the axis may occur, thus giving rise to one kind of identical twins. If the separation is incomplete, conjoined or siamese twins result.

The rest of the first three months of pregnancy is concerned with further specialization and sorting out of cells into tissues, organs, systems and limbs by a process known as **differentiation.** This leads to the formation of a small individual which has the appearances of a human baby (see Fig. 28) and can be recognized as such. It is now known as a **fetus.** During this phase of differentiation the developing embryo is particularly susceptible to disturbances of development. If the mother becomes infected by certain organisms, such as the German measles virus, the embryo may be harmed. The parts of the embryo which are affected most are just those which are differentiating most actively at the particular time when the mother is suffering from the disease. Thus, if the disease affects the mother 6 to 8 weeks after conception, the baby's eyes may be damaged, but if the disease occurs a couple of weeks later, the baby may be born deaf. During the first three months of pregnancy the **hormones,** or internal secretions, produced by the mother's pituitary gland and by her ovaries play a very important role in maintaining the lining of the womb, and so in helping the embryo to become established within the womb so that it can differentiate satisfactorily.

At the end of the first three months, the placenta largely takes over the production of the endocrine secretions necessary for maintaining the pregnancy and bringing it to a successful conclusion. It is not surprising to find that this take-over period is a somewhat unstable one and, if the hormonal balance is upset too much, the embryo, which has now reached the stage of being a fetus, may be expelled from the womb, that is, **aborted.** Indeed a high proportion of the spontaneous abortions in clinical practice occur at this time, namely 10 to 12 weeks after conception.

The last six months of the pregnancy, i.e. about two-thirds of it, is concerned mainly with **growth** and **maturation** of the fetus which will enable it to survive when it is eventually detached from its mother.

It has already been explained that the placenta is made by the fetus and it should be realized that the placenta provides a membrane barrier between the blood of the fetus, which circulates into and through the ramifications of the placenta, and the blood of the mother that bathes the exterior of the placenta (Plate 2 and Figs. 22 and 23). It is therefore common practice to refer to **the placental barrier** and this exists from implantation till term. **Term** is the end of pregnancy and is followed by **parturition,** the process of **birth.**

It normally takes an average of **266 days** for a human being to develop from a single-celled fertilized egg to a baby of over two-hundred million cells.

PRODUCTION OF GAMETES

The name gametes is used to denote the cells which both male and female produce to enable them to reproduce the species. These **gametes** or **sex cells** are known as **sperms** or **spermatozoa** when produced by a male and, the corresponding cell produced by the female is known as an **egg** or **ovum** (Fig. 12).

The coming together and fusion of a sperm with an ovum is known as **fertilization** or **conception,** and this is the coming into existence of a new individual of the species. This individual consists at first of one cell.

Details of cell structure are given in the chapter on histology. It suffices to state here that a cell is the basic functional unit of which the body is made up. Its envelope or wall is known as the cell membrane and inside this is contained a semi-liquid substance called cytoplasm. In the middle of the cytoplasm there is a more or less spherical structure known as the nucleus. The nucleus can be looked upon as the headquarters of the cell and it contains all the necessary equipment for instructing the cell about the performance of its functions.

Genes and Chromosomes

In the nucleus of the newly conceived one-celled individual are located threadlike structures known as **chromosomes.** These are arranged in pairs, one member of each pair having been derived from the father and the other from the mother.

The chief importance of the chromosomes lies in that they make it possible for potential characteristics to be transmitted to the offspring, for it is in the chromosomes that are located the minute physico-chemical packages, that are the basic hereditary materials, and which are called **genes.** These hereditary particles contain the instructions for the design of all the parts of the new baby.

The physico-chemical instructions are in the form of giant **nucleic acid molecules** (see p. 44), whose components behave rather like the letters of an alphabet—just as varying sequences of letters spell different words, in this instance, varying sequences of the molecular components spell different instructions.

The nucleus of each human cell contains **46 chromosomes.**

Mitosis

In many tissues the cells divide, not only during the period of growth and development, but continue to do so throughout life. A skin cell for instance divides once every three or four days. This means that during a lifetime such a cell divides something like 10,000 times. This is not true of the cells of all tissues and, on the whole, the more specialized the tissue, the less frequently the cells making it up divide. Thus, nerve cells in the brain probably do not divide again after the baby is born.

Normally, when cells divide in the body, the two daughter cells resulting from the division each contain 46 chromosomes, and the process of dividing the nucleus in this multiplicative fashion, i.e. one cell with 46 chromosomes giving rise to two cells with 46 chromosomes each, is known as **Mitosis.**

The fact that the cells of some tissues divide so often during the lifetime of the individual means that there is much room for error, yet in fact the process of cell division is extremely well regulated and the occurrence of mistakes during cell division is very rare.

The process of mitosis consists of a continuous series of events which, for the sake of convenience when describing them, are separated somewhat artificially into stages and these are as follows (see Plate 1):

Interphase is the period during which the cell is said to be 'resting' between two divisions. The word 'resting' is misleading because a lot of activity is going on in the cell during this stage and a considerable part of this activity is concerned with the next division of the cell. During interphase the cell nucleus contains the normal number of chromosomes which is characteristic for the species. The number is described as **diploid,** or **2N,** because it is made up of two sets of matched chromosomes, one set having been derived from each parent. Another feature of this phase is that during it the chromosomes are long and difficult to see. While the cell is said to be 'resting' it is in fact growing to

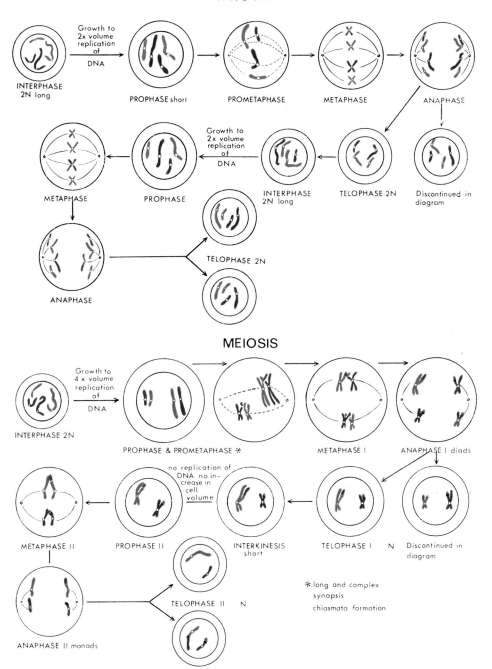

Plate 1. Mitosis and meiosis.

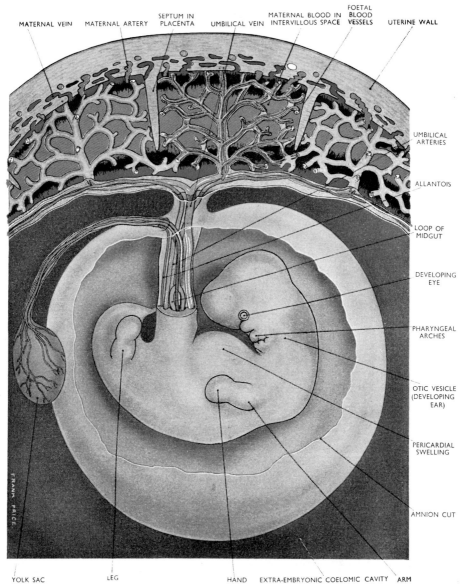

MATERNAL VEIN   MATERNAL ARTERY   SEPTUM IN PLACENTA   UMBILICAL VEIN   MATERNAL BLOOD IN INTERVILLOUS SPACE   FOETAL BLOOD VESSELS   UTERINE WALL

UMBILICAL ARTERIES

ALLANTOIS

LOOP OF MIDGUT

DEVELOPING EYE

PHARYNGEAL ARCHES

OTIC VESICLE (DEVELOPING EAR)

PERICARDIAL SWELLING

AMNION CUT

YOLK SAC   LEG   HAND   EXTRA-EMBRYONIC COELOMIC CAVITY   ARM

FRANK PRICE

Plate 2. A schematic representation of the structure of the placenta and of its relations to the embryo. (Modified freely from Hamilton, Boyd and Mossman's *Human Embryology*.)

[*facing page 53*

twice the size it was just after the previous division and the D.N.A. of the chromosomes is being replicated (see p. 45).

Prophase is a period during which the chromosomes become clearly visible in the nucleus because they have become short, much thicker and take up stains much more readily.

Prometaphase is the phase during which the nuclear membrane disappears and the 'mitotic spindle', which is responsible for the movement of chromosomes during mitosis, is established from the centrosome of the cell. The centrioles of the centrosome (see p. 94), which have reproduced themselves, come to lie at the opposite poles of the spindle.

Metaphase, which is the stage at which the chromosomes are best seen. At first each resembles the letter 'X' in shape, because each chromosome has divided longitudinally into two daughter chromosomes, or **chromatids,** though these remain attached to one another at the **centromere.** Late in metaphase the centromere divides and the two daughter centromeres, with their associated chromatid, begin to move apart towards the opposite poles of the spindle.

Anaphase is the period during which the newly formed daughter chromosomes move to the opposite poles of the spindle.

Telophase is the phase during which the two groups of daughter chromosomes each become surrounded by a newly constituted nuclear membrane and the cell cytoplasm is divided into more or less equal parts to surround each of the daughter nuclei, which enter the interphase stage once more.

Meiosis

It will be appreciated that, if the coming together and fusion of a sperm and an ovum at fertilization is to result in a cell with a nucleus containing 46 chromosomes, then the sperm and the ovum should contribute only 23 chromosomes each to the new cell produced by conception (conceptus or zygote). It follows from this that, when the gametes (sperms or ova) are produced, somehow the number of chromosomes in them must be reduced from the usual 46 to 23 (the **haploid,** or **1N,** number). The special division which leads to the production of 2 daughter cells containing only 23 chromosomes is known as **meiosis** (Plate 1).

This kind of cell division takes place only in the sexual glands (**gonads**) responsible for the production of gametes, namely in the **testis** or testicle of the male and in the **ovary** in the female.

Further details of the production of sperms and ova are considered in the chapter describing the reproductive system.

Meiosis takes place in two steps, each of which has a prophase, metaphase, anaphase and telophase (Plate 1). In the first step, called the **meiosis I** or the **reduction division,** the prophase is very long and complex. The chromosomes are divided longitudinally into two chromatids during this phase although the centromeres do not divide. During prophase the homologous chromosomes (see below) become arranged in pairs (**synapsis**) and an exchange of parts between the chromatids of homologous chromosomes may occur (Plate). This process is referred to as **crossing over** and provides for most of the great variety of recombinations of hereditary characters seen in the offspring of biparental reproduction. The points of breakage and reunion on the chromosomes are known as **chiasmata.**

At metaphase the members of each pair of homologous chromosomes then separate and at anaphase migrate to opposite ends of the spindle, so that each daughter nucleus receives at telophase only one member of each pair. Each one of these chromosomes consists of two chromatids joined by a centromere and is known as a **diad.**

The second step, called **meiosis II** or the **maturation division** follows the same stages. At metaphase the centromeres divide and the chromatids separate to migrate into separate nuclei. The resulting chromosomes made up of one chromatid only are known as **monads.**

The period between meiosis I and meiosis II is referred to as **interkinesis.**

ELEMENTS OF GENETICS

As has already been described (p. 51), the 46 chromosomes in the nucleus of the human cell are arranged in 23 pairs, each consisting of a chromosome of paternal origin and one of maternal origin. On these complementary or **homologous chromosomes** are situated the corresponding genes, one derived from the father and the other from the mother. These pairs of genes control contrasting characters in an individual and are known as **alleles.** One pair of alleles will determine, for instance, whether the individual will be tall or short, and another pair whether dark or fair. Any one normal individual can have two, and only two alleles. There may however be many different alleles scattered in a population.

When a pair of genes is considered, it is often found that one of them always exerts its influence, irrespective of what the other member of the pair is. Such a gene is **dominant.** Other genes exert their effects only if the other member of the pair allows it so to act. These are **recessive.** An example would be that a gene producing tallness (T) might be the dominant and the gene responsible for shortness (*t*) might be the recessive (see Fig. 11 and p. 56). When these two genes come together the offspring will then always be tall and will be short only if both his genes are for shortness. It follows that three possibilities exist: either an individual contains two genes each of which is for tallness, i.e. *TT* (this individual is said to be **homozygous** for the dominant), or each of which are for shortness *tt* (this individual is said to be homozygous for the recessive) and the third possibility is that the individual inherited the dominant from one parent and the recessive from the other, in fact his genetic constitution is mixed, i.e. *Tt*

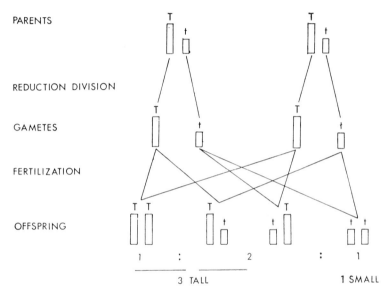

Fig. 11. Scheme showing the pattern of transmission of contrasting characters (tallness *T*, shortness *t*) from heterozygous parents.

(this individual is said to be **heterozygous**). This heterozygous individual will appear outwardly to be exactly like the one homozygous for the dominant gene, that is their **phenotypes** (bodily characteristics) are the same, although their **genotypes** (genetic constitution in this case *Tt* and *TT*) are different.

In view of what has been said above, it will be understood that a homozygous *TT* can produce only gametes bearing the dominant *T*, a homozygous *tt* can produce only gametes bearing the recessive *t*, but the heterozygous individual produces gametes half of which carry the dominant *T* and half of which carry the recessive *t*. As well as controlling body characteristics and functions, genes may be **responsible for defects, malformation, malfunction or disease.**

GENETIC VARIATION

All the biological characteristics of an individual are produced by the nucleic acid in his genes as this controls the enzymes that produce and direct his organization (see p. 44). Most characters are influenced by many enzymes and hence by many genes. Although the inheritance of tallness has been used as an example of the simple transmission of characters which is easy to follow, the height of a man is in fact affected by many factors: by the amount of growth in length of the bones, by the actions of the pituitary gland, by the effectiveness of digestion, to quote but a few.

A few inherited characters are the result of the operation of only one, or of only a few enzymes, and hence as the result of the operation of only one gene, but usually the character is the product of a particular combination of genetically determined factors. Such inheritance is described as **multifactorial.**

To complicate the matter further, most genes seem to have more than one effect—they are **pleiotrophic.** Important examples in Man are that the gene producing the blood group A increases the liability of the individual to cancer of the stomach, whereas people of Group O seems to be more liable to duodenal ulceration.

The variation in transmission of characters, which is so biologically advantageous, is achieved by such processes as **genetic recombination** and **mutation.** Genetic recombination consists of the exchange of genes between homologous chromosomes in the course of every meiosis. Mutation, on the other hand, is a rare sporadic change in an individual gene so that its effects are different. It must be stressed however, that mutations observed to occur in Man are almost invariably deleterious and result in a disability or disordered function rather than in any improvement.

A heterozygous individual possessing a recessive defective gene does not suffer from the condition caused by this gene, because the effect is counteracted by the corresponding dominant normal gene on the homologous chromosome. Such a heterozygous possessor of a defective gene is known as a 'Carrier'. However, the carrier may transmit the defective gene to an offspring not possessing a compensating normal gene and so it will be afflicted by the abnormality (see Fig. 13).

SEX DETERMINATION AND SEX LINKAGE

Of the 23 pairs of chromosomes, 1 pair is concerned with determining the sex of the individual. These two chromosomes are called the **sex chromosomes.**

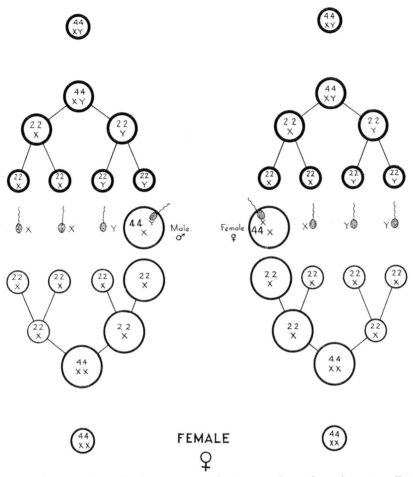

Fig. 12. A scheme to show the development of sperms and ova from the germ cells of the male and female respectively, and to show the determination of the sex of the offspring at fertilization. In the male, the germ cells contain 44 chromosomes + an X and a Y chromosome (total 46) and they divide to give rise to sperms containing 22 chromosomes + either an X or a Y chromosome (total 23). In the female, the germ cells contain 44 chromosomes + $2X$ chromosomes (total 46) and they divide to give rise to ova all containing 22 chromosomes + an X chromosome (total 23). Note that the production of the ovum is associated with the formation of three small polar bodies. At fertilization, if a Y-bearing sperm fuses with the ovum, the offspring contains a total of 46 chromosomes, i.e. 44 chromosomes (22 from each parent) + an X (from the mother) and a Y chromosome (from the father) and it is male. If fertilization is effected by an X-bearing sperm, the offspring also contains a total of 46 chromosomes including, in this case, $2X$ chromosomes (one from each parent) and it is female.

The two chromosomes are similar in the female who has $2X$ chromosomes, but a male has an X chromosome and a small Y chromosome; thus the female state is represented as XX and the male as XY (see Fig. 12). The nucleus of a cell that is not dividing does not show its chromosomes, but such nuclei do show a small particle of darkly staining chromosomal material—**sex-chromatin**—when they contain two X chromosomes (see Fig. 30). It is thus possible to tell the sex of an individual, from soon after fertilization and throughout life, by looking at the nuclei of the individual's cells with a miscroscope.

When the gonads are producing gametes, the pair of sex chromosomes is split and distributed to the gametes which, in the female, all bear X chromosomes, but in the male, half the gametes bear an X chromosome and the other half a Y chromosome (Fig. 12).

If an X-bearing sperm joins an ovum (also X bearing) in fertilization, the resulting conceptus or zygote will be XX, i.e. a female. If a Y-bearing sperm

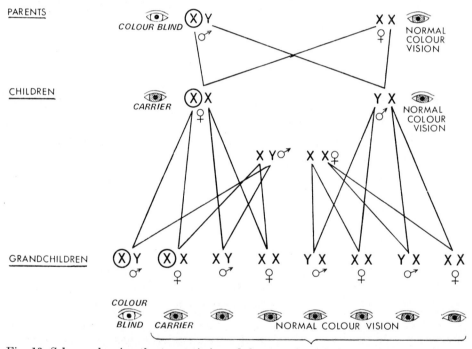

Fig. 13. Scheme showing the transmission of the gene for colour blindness through two generations. The iris of colour blind individuals is shown white; the iris of those with normal colour vision is cross-hatched. The X chromosome bearing the abnormal gene is encircled.

effects fertilization the offspring will be XY or male, i.e. sex is determined at the moment of conception. It must be noted that the sex chromosomes also bear genes other than those concerned with the determination of the sex of the individual; these characters are said to be sex-linked and are responsible for the phenomenon of **sex-linked inheritance** (Fig. 13).

As is well known, the condition of colour blindness is for practical purposes confined to men, the reason being that the gene responsible for the condition is located on the X chromosome. The gene is a recessive so that the other X chromosome of a woman can counteract the colour blind effect. A man, however, has a Y and an X chromosome, so, if his X chromosome bears the gene for the defect, there is no other X chromosome present to counteract the colour blind effect. It will also be noted that, as the gene for this condition is on an X chromosome, colour blindness is inherited from the mother of the affected male. Other conditions such as baldness are called **sex-limited** because although, not determined by the sex-chromosomes, the gene responsible for the condition only expresses itself in an individual who produces male sex hormones.

HUMAN GENETICS AND MEDICINE

From all that has been said earlier in this chapter and in the chapter introducing the subject of Biochemistry it will be understood very readily that the subject of human genetics is, and is likely to be of increasing relevance to clinical medicine.

It is important to assess the relative importance and interplay of genetic and environmental factors in normal development, and their rôle in the causation of congenital malformations and other diseases transmitted from parent to offspring by defective genes. Parents also wish to obtain adequate information on the risk of an abnormality occurring if there is a history of such a condition in the family. This helps them to put the risk into perspective, both in relation to the chance of the offspring being severely handicapped and in relation to the outlook for the child, should he prove to be affected.

In the case of most hereditary disease, the presence or absence of the defective gene in either parent and the probability of its transmission to the children can only be assessed as the result of careful examination of the history of the health of the parents and near relatives together with a precise diagnosis in affected individuals. Occasionally, it will be clear that the condition is transmitted by a single dominant gene (p. 54), in which case half the germ cells of the affected parent will possess the defective gene and the risk of the children being affected can be expressed as a 1 : 2 risk. In the case of a recessive gene, particularly if the condition is determined by multifactorial inheritance (p. 56), then the prediction is much more difficult and has to be made on the basis of more elaborate estimates which are beyond the scope of this account. It should, however, be appreciated that risks expressed as 1 : 10, 1 : 20, 1 : 30 etc. should be seen in the context that any pregnancy has a 1 in 50 random chance of resulting in the birth of a severely deformed or handicapped child.

Identification of genetic and chromosomal abnormalities

At present, the genes of an individual cannot be examined and only their manifestations, or **expression,** can be observed. This expression may take the form of a recognizable abnormality, either structural or biochemical (**inborn errors of metabolism**). A number of these genetic abnormalities can be identified by the biochemical analysis of the body fluids or of the cells of affected individuals. Sometimes carriers of the defective gene can be recognized in the same way, though the abnormality may be minimal.

Some abnormalities, however, are the result of the affected person possessing chromosomes that are so abnormal that the examination of the chromosomes under a microscope reveals the basic defect. This may take the form of an extra chromosome, an absent chromosome, chromosomes with bits missing, chromosomes with extra bits stuck on and deformed chromosomes. It seems that any alteration in the total amount of chromosomal material in the nucleus, or in the individual chromosome, results in relatively gross abnormality of the individual possessing these chromosomes.

Karyotypes and Chromosomal Analysis

When a cell enters mitosis (p. 52) the chromosomal material in its nucleus becomes more obvious and each chromosome becomes visible along its whole length. In metaphase, each chromosome resembles the letter 'X' in shape, each half consisting of **a chromatid** joined to its partner by a centromere.

By means of special techniques illustrated in Fig. 14 the cells from the blood, or indeed from other parts of the body, can be induced by culture techniques to undergo mitosis. They are then fixed in metaphase, and the chromosomes are spread out on a slide, examined and photographed (Fig. 15). The outline of each chromosome is then cut out from the photograph and these are arranged in pairs and in sequence as shown in Figs. 14, 16 and 17. It will be seen that the chromosomes are arranged in order of size and according to whether the centromere is near the middle of the chromatids or nearer to one end of them. Each chromosomal pair is numbered 1 to 22 and they are arranged into groups A, B, C, D, E, F, and G according to their size and shape. In addition there are

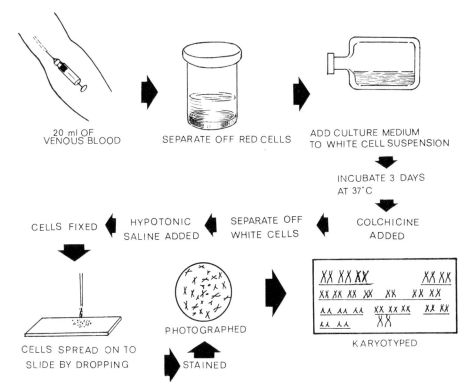

Fig. 14. Diagram showing the steps in the preparation of a karyotype. (After Emery's Elements of Medical Genetics.)

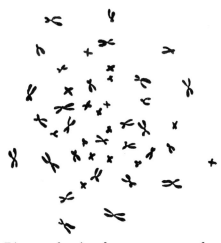

Fig. 15. Diagram showing chromosomes spread on a slide.

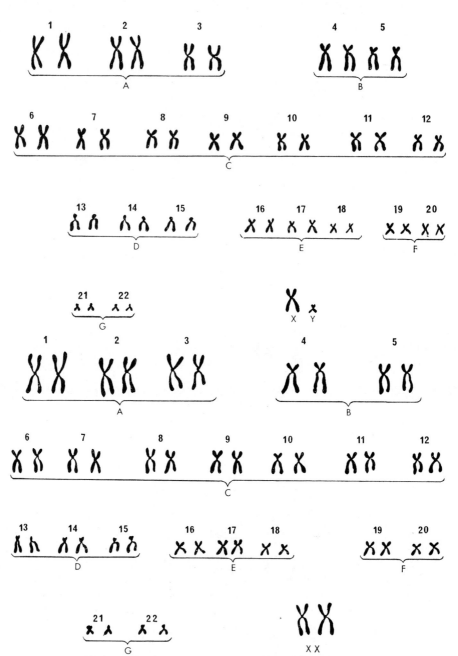

Fig. 16. Chromosomes arranged in karyotypes: male above; female below.

2X chromosomes in females and an X and a Y chromosome in males. These are the **sex-chromosomes** and the other twenty-two pairs make up the **autosomes.** Setting out of the chromosomes in the arrangement just described is known as a **karyotype** and reveals whether the individual's chromosomes are free from gross defect.

In certain abnormalities, the number (Fig. 17) or shape of the chromosomes may be altered and this may be caused by a number of processes:

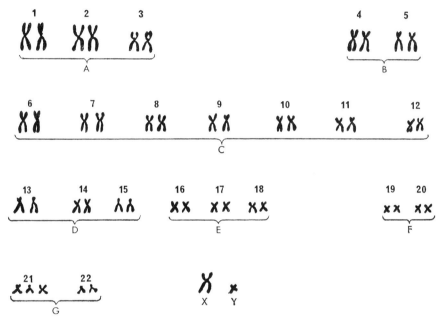

Fig. 17. The karyotype of a case of Down's syndrome due to trisomy of 21.

Non-disjunction during meiosis may result in a chromosomal pair not separating properly and both members of the pair arriving in one of the daughter germ cells, whereas the other daughter cell will lack that particular chromosome altogether. In this way, the cell with the extra chromosome will, if it is fertilized, possess three chromosomes of a type instead of the normal two, and this condition is known as **trisomy.**

Deletion refers to the loss of a chromosome or of part of a chromosome, and this may occur either in the course of meiosis, when the germ cells are being produced, or it may happen when the chromosomes of developing germ cells are subjected to noxious environmental influences, such as ionizing radiation.

Sometimes a piece from one chromosome breaks off and then sticks to another chromosome, either in its own or in another group. This is known as a **translocation.**

As well as looking at the karyotype of an individual in post-natal life, it is now possible to look at the karyotype of cells shed by the fetus into the amniotic fluid. Amniotic fluid is obtained by **amniocentesis** i.e. drawing off the fluid through the suprapublic portion of mother's abdominal wall and through the uterine wall between the 14th and 16th weeks of pregnancy. Examination of the cells obtained from this amniotic fluid may enable one to diagnose a chromosomal abnormality prior to the birth of the infant.

FERTILIZATION

The female genital or reproductive tract undergoes cyclical changes and, on an average, four weeks are required to complete the cycle. The most obvious manifestation of the cycle is that every 4 weeks there is a loss of blood from the genital tract which is known as 'a period' or **menstruation.** Under normal circumstances the ovary releases one ovum (**ovulation**) 14 days before menstruation, which takes place only if the ovum is not fertilized and the lining of the womb, which has been prepared for the reception of a fertilized ovum or zygote, is shed—hence the bleeding.

The fact that ovulation has taken place is indicated by a rise in the **basal body temperature** of the woman (temperature taken in the mouth or rectum before rising in the morning). A chart illustrating this rise is illustrated in Fig. 222. If ovulation is followed by fertilization, this rise of temperature is maintained throughout pregnancy. If fertilization does not occur, the temperature remains slightly elevated till a couple of days before menstruation, when it falls to the lower pre-ovulation level.

If sperms are introduced into the woman's genital tract within 48 hours of the ovulation (i.e. the ovum being shed) one of the sperms may penetrate the ovum and fertilize it. There will then be no menstruation 2 weeks later and this will probably be the first indication to the woman that she is pregnant. No more menstruation will occur until after the birth of the offspring.

The characteristic of the **ovum** or egg is that it is a relatively large cell containing a lot of cytoplasm round the nucleus. It cannot move itself (i.e. it is non-motile) and has to rely on the structures of the female genital tract to transport it.

Sperms, on the other hand, consist of a head, a middle piece and a tail which is very active and can propel the sperm. The head, which accounts for most of the bulk of the sperm, consists mainly of the nucleus of the male gamete. A sperm carries very little cytoplasm.

Whereas it is usual for a woman to produce one ovum each month of her reproductive life, except during pregnancies, a man continuously produces millions of sperms. It is usual for **sexual intercourse (copulation)** to result in the depositing of as many as 300 million sperms in the genital tract of the woman. These sperms then swim up the genital tract of the woman. For fertilization to take place, only one of them need penetrate the ovum in the upper part of the uterine tube. Fertilization is thought to take place and to be possible only **within 24 hours of ovulation** and within 48 hours of copulation. This is because an ovum remains fertilizable for less than 24 hours and because sperms retain their fertilizing capacity in the female genital tract for 48 hours only. At **fertilization** one sperm penetrates the ovum, the head of the sperm becomes detached from the tail and the sperm nucleus travels to the centre of the ovum where it meets the nucleus of the ovum. The two nuclei fuse, thus re-establishing the number of chromosomes at 46. The fused ovum and sperm, or **fertilized ovum,** is called a **zygote.**

The zygote, containing its full complement of chromosomes and genes, already possesses all the instructions which determine the features of the species, the future configuration of the body and face which will give it the 'family likeness', the future colour of the eyes, skin and hair, as well as the sex of the new individual. There are instructions determining whether this individual will be short or tall, fat or lean. Also determined at this stage are the proneness to certain diseases and whether the baby will be born with certain malformations. Some aspects of temperament and intelligence are determined at the very beginnning of life. Each new human being is thus a distinct entity, never being entirely like the parents or ancestors, but being a blend of the genetic heirlooms bequeathed to it by its parents.

DEVELOPMENT AFTER CONCEPTION

Cleavage

Within a matter of hours the zygote starts to divide by mitosis, a process known as **cleavage,** as a result of which a progressively larger number of progressively smaller cells called **blastomeres** are produced. When there are about 16 blastomeres the zygote is known as a **morula** (Fig. 18).

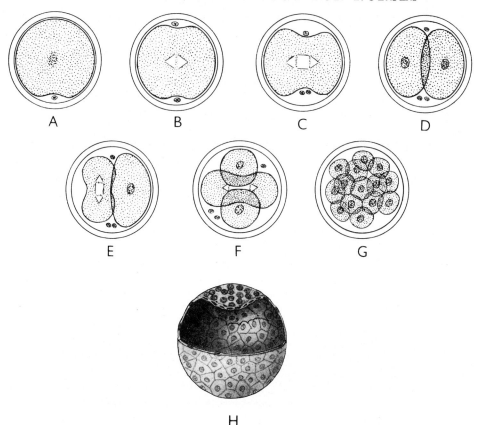

Fig. 18. A scheme illustrating cleavage of the zygote (A) to form a blastocyst (H). A, B and C show stages of the first cleavage division of the zygote, with spindle formation and migration of an equal number of chromosomes to each of the two blastomeres (D); E shows the second cleavage division occurring in a plane at right angles to the first; F shows formation of the four cell stage; G morula; H blastocyst, with upper half opened to show the inner cell mass and blastocystic cavity; polar bodies are shown in A, B, C, D, E and F.

TWINNING

It has been stated above that a woman usually produces one ovum a month and human pregnancies usually result in the birth of one baby. Occasionally a woman sheds more than one ovum at about the same time and, if both of these are fertilized, twinning will occur. As these twins are the product of the fertilization of different eggs by different sperms, they will be no more like one another than any other brother or sister, and are known as **fraternal twins.**

If, however, the cleavage of a single zygote results in the formation of two or more individuals, the result will be **identical twins** as they have the same genetic make-up. They will necessarily be of the same sex.

About 1 in 80 human pregnancies leads to the birth of twins. Some families however, appear to have a genetic predisposition to twinning.

PASSAGE OF THE ZYGOTE TO THE UTERUS

As has already been described, fertilization, which occurs in the outer portion of the uterine tube (Fig. 19) leads to **cleavage** and formation of a

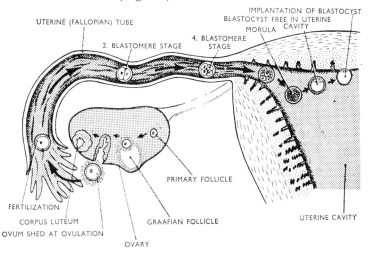

Fig. 19. A schematic representation of the development, maturation and rupture of an ovarian follicle. Successive stages in the passage of the ovum into the uterine tube, fertilization and subsequent development of the zygote, up to the stage of implantation, are shown.

ball of cells called a **morula.** This morula acquires a cavity filled with fluid and becomes a **blastocyst.** While these changes are taking place in the developing egg, it is wafted along the **uterine tube** towards the cavity of the **uterus** or **womb.** It has become a blastocyst by the time it reaches this cavity, the journey having taken about 4 or 5 days.

IMPLANTATION

After a further 2 or 3 days have elapsed, the blastocyst becomes attached to the lining epithelium of the uterus. It then sinks into the uterine lining, the

endometrium, to become embedded in it. This is called **implantation,** and is usually reckoned to take place 7 to 8 days after fertilization.

At the time of implantation, the blastocyst is a hollow ball of cells, the cavity being filled with fluid. At one pole of the blastocyst there is a clump of cells known as the **inner cell mass,** which will give rise to the embryo proper, and the remainder of the cells forming the shell of the cyst constitute what may now be called **trophoblast** (Fig. 20). These are the cells that carry out the

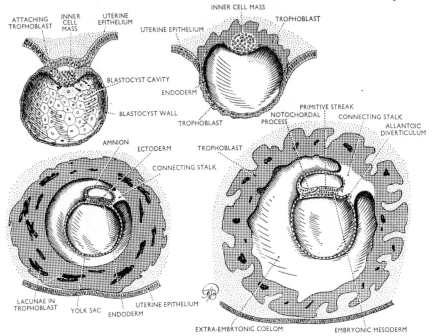

Fig. 20. Diagrams of successive stages in the development and implantation of a blastocyst, leading to the formation of a chorionic vesicle.

burrowing of the blastocyst into the endometrium which has been prepared to receive it. As the implantation process takes place, the surface of the blastocyst becomes roughened by the trophoblast cells growing irregularly to give rise to short cellular sprouts. At the same time spaces, called **lacunæ,** appear between the cells of the expanding trophoblastic shell. To start with, trophoblastic sprouts are present over the whole surface of the blastocyst, and they grow out into the maternal tissues which at this stage are very vascular. These small sprouts actually break through the lining of the maternal capillaries and so come to be bathed directly by the mother's blood, which now also percolates through the trophoblastic lacunæ. From this stage on, till the end of pregnancy interchanges of oxygen, food, excretory products and carbon dioxide can take place between the zygote and the mother.

Before this stage, the zygote was using up its built-in reserves of food, and absorbing nutriment from the fluid produced by the lining of the uterine tube and by the glands of the endometrium. As it was burrowing into the maternal tissues it was using the breakdown products of the maternal tissues it had destroyed.

It will be appreciated that, while the zygote is living as a free individual within the maternal genital tract, it is very small and chemical substances can diffuse to all its constituent parts. After implantation, the blastocyst starts to grow at a remarkable rate and becomes too big for simple diffusion to be adequate for the needs of all its constituent parts. The need for a heart and vascular system to pump and distribute the supplies round the developing organism becomes evident. As implantation proceeds, the structure of the blastocyst becomes much more complicated and it is converted into a **chorionic vesicle** containing an **embryo** (Fig. 20).

Decidua

After the blastocyst is implanted the endometrium is known as **decidua,** because this lining of the womb is shed at the birth of the fetus. The actual decidua to which the blastocyst is attached is the **decidua basilis.** As the blastocyst sinks into it, the superficial portions of the decidua close in over the superficial pole of the blastocyst and form the **decidua capsularis.** The rest of the uterine lining is the **decidua parietalis** (see Fig. 22, B).

EMBRYONIC PHASE OF DEVELOPMENT

FORMATION OF PRIMARY TISSUES

At the beginning of the implantation phase the **blastocyst** has been seen to consist of a hollow ball of cells which was thickened in one place by the presence there of an **inner cell mass** (Fig. 20). The cells in the inner aspect of this mass become flattened and are known as **endodermal cells** (Fig. 20). These cells spread right round the inside of the trophoblastic shell so that the blastocyst has become a two-layered structure—trophoblast on the outside, endoderm on the inside. The enclosed cavity is now known as the **primary yolk sac** (Figs. 20 and 21). A split appears next within the inner cell mass and the resulting cavity is known as the **amniotic cavity.** This separates the trophoblast from the embryo itself which now consists of two layers (Fig. 21), an upper layer of

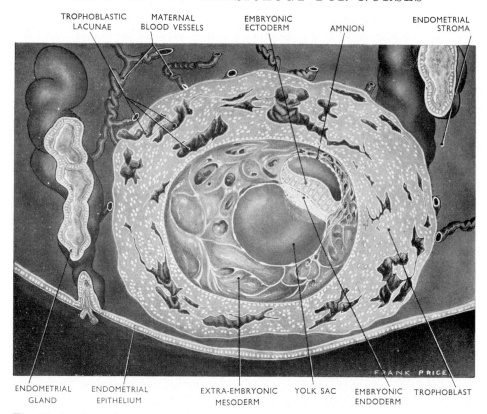

TROPHOBLASTIC LACUNAE · MATERNAL BLOOD VESSELS · EMBRYONIC ECTODERM · AMNION · ENDOMETRIAL STROMA

ENDOMETRIAL GLAND · ENDOMETRIAL EPITHELIUM · EXTRA-EMBRYONIC MESODERM · YOLK SAC · EMBRYONIC ENDODERM · TROPHOBLAST

FRANK PRICE

Fig. 21. A schematic representation of an early human embryo in its chorionic vesicle, implanted in endometrium. (Modified from Hamilton, Boyd and Mossman's *Human Embryology*.)

ectodermal cells continuous with the cells lining the amniotic cavity and a lower or inner layer of **endodermal cells** already described above. It will be seen from the diagrams (Figs. 20 and 21) that the embryo is in the form of a disc composed of the two layers just described. A third layer of cells now appears between the trophoblast and the endoderm of the yolk sac, extending also round the amnion. This is the **primary extra-embryonic mesoderm.**

FORMATION OF CONNECTING STALK AND CHORION

The **primary extra-embryonic mesoderm** proliferates to form quite a thick layer of loosely arranged primitive connective tissue cells called **mesenchyme.** A split appears in this mesenchyme which results in the formation of the **extra-embryonic cœlom** (Figs. 20 and 21). This split extends almost the whole way round the yolk sac and amniotic cavity, so that one layer of the mesenchyme is in contact with the trophoblast and the other surrounds the yolk sac and amniotic cavity. The split does not, however, extend round completely in the region of the future caudal or tail end of the embryo—this region where the primary mesoderm is not split is known as the **connecting stalk** (Fig. 20). From now on, the trophoblast and the layers of mesenchymatous mesoderm related to it constitute what is known as the **chorion** (Fig. 22).

Soon after the establishment of the body stalk, an outgrowth or diverticulum from the yolk sac endoderm grows into it (Fig. 20); this diverticulum is the **allantois.**

THE FETAL MEMBRANES

The **fetal membranes** *are developed from the original blastocyst, but do not form part of the embryo or fetus proper.* They consist principally of membranes that cover the embryo or fetus and separate it from its mother. The main ones are the **amnion,** the **chorion** and the **placenta** with its **umbilical cord.** The mode of formation of the **amnion** has already been described. It later expands to occupy the whole of the extra-embryonic cœlomic cavity (Fig. 22) and so comes to provide a complete covering for the embryo, yolk sac and body stalk. The **amniotic cavity** is filled with **amniotic fluid,** and the embryo or fetus comes to be completely surrounded by it (Fig. 22) so as to be protected and supported. The **chorion,** consisting of trophoblast and the outer layer of mesoderm, forms a membrane that completely surrounds the embryo, or fetus, and its accessory structures, and effectively separates them from the maternal tissues. The chorion forms a spherical **chorionic vesicle** and at birth, both chorion and the amnion are ruptured to liberate the fetus.

The chorion undergoes further development and fetal blood vessels grow into it. These blood vessels are continuous with those inside the embryo through the connecting stalk which develops into the **umbilical cord** (see Plate 2 and Fig. 22).

The Placenta

The lacunæ between the trophoblastic cells, forming the wall of the chorionic vesicle, extend and coalesce to form a **chorionic labyrinth.** The trophoblastic **trabeculæ** which surround the spaces of this labyrinth are initially arranged irregularly, but they soon tend to be disposed radially within the chorion. The trophoblastic trabeculæ become recognizable as columns that branch as they

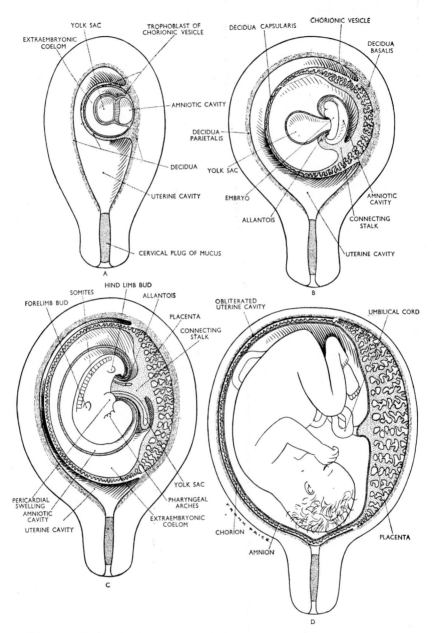

Fig. 22. Diagrams illustrating the relations of the embryo and fetus to the chorionic vesicle, fetal membranes, decidua and uterine cavity at different stages of intra-uterine life. A and B represent the relations during the presomite and somite phases of embryonic development; C the relations when the placenta is established; D the definitive arrangements during the fetal phase.

reach out to the periphery of the trophoblastic shell (see Fig. 23). These columns are now called **villi** and the chorionic labyrinth between them, which is filled with maternal blood, is also called the **intervillous space.** The maternal blood is supplied to the intervillous space by branches of the uterine artery in the endometrium and drained away by uterine veins (Plate 2 and Fig 23).

While a villus consists of a column of trophoblast it is called a **primary villus.** Subsequently, the extræmbryonic mesoderm of the chorion invades the column to give it a core of embryonic connective tissue around which the trophoblast becomes organized into an inner layer of cellular **cytotrophoblast (Langhans Layer)** and an outer layer where the cells boundaries fuse and disappear to form a syncytium, **syncytiotrophoblast.** Such a villus is known as a **secondary villus.** When a set of embryonic vessels has become established in the mesodermal core of the villus, it is known as a **tertiary villus.**

The cellular trophoblast at the periphery of the chorionic vesicle maintains the attachment of the vesicle to the maternal tissues and is known as the **cytotrophoblastic shell,** whereas the endometrium adjoining this shell is known as the **boundary zone.** This boundary zone is traversed by the maternal blood on its way to and from the intervillous space.

It will be seen from what has been described above, and from the arrangements of blood vessels depicted in Plate 2 and Fig. 23, that the fetal blood circulating in the vessels within the villi is separated from the maternal blood in the intervillous space by tissue composed of several layers. These layers are the wall of the fetal blood vessels, the connective tissue of the villus and the trophoblast covering it. All the substances exchanged between the maternal blood and the fetal blood must pass through this barrier, which in the developed placenta is called the **placental barrier. Fetal blood and maternal blood do not mix.**

The interstitial growth of the cytotrophoblastic shell provides a mechanism for circumferential extension of the chorionic vesicle. Expansion of the shell increases the volume of the intervillous space by encroachment upon the surrounding decidua. The area of trophoblast exposed to maternal blood in the intervillous space is also increased by the sprouting of branch villi from the primary stems. These then also pass through the successive stages of being primary, secondary and eventually vascularized tertiary villi.

The villi which are directed towards the decidua basalis enlarge and branch elaborately, while those that are directed towards the decidua capsularis degenerate about two months after implantation has been effected (see Fig. 22). In this way the chorion which protrudes along with the decidua capsularis into the uterine lumen becomes smooth and almost avascular, the **chorion læve,** whereas the chorion in contact with the decidua basalis, where the villi persist

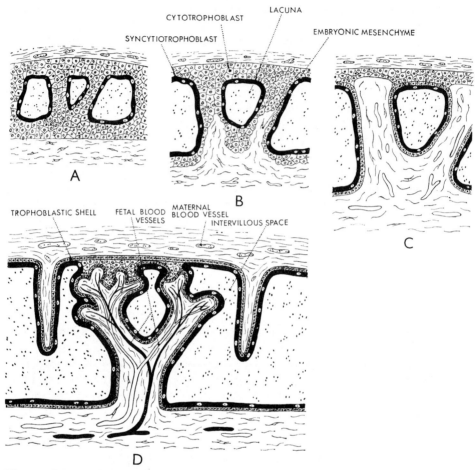

Fig. 23. Scheme showing the stages in the development of the placenta and its villi. A, primary villi; B, secondary villi; C, early tertiary villi; D, definitive arrangement.

and continue to develop, becomes the **chorion frondosum.** This chorion frondosum progressively assumes the discoidal shape of the definitive **placenta.**

Growth in thickness as well as in circumference continues in the placenta until the end of the fourth month, after which only circumferential growth continues until almost the end of pregnancy. It should also be noted that after the third month of pregnancy, the thickness of the placental barrier tends to diminish as the result, first of the disappearance of the cytotrophoblastic,

Langhans layer covering the villi, and subsequently by the progressive thinning of the syncytiotrophoblastic and mesenchynal components of the barrier.

The mature placenta has the form of a flattened circular cake about 20 cm across and about 3 cm thick. At full maturity, the ratio of infant weight to placental weight is about 6 : 1, so that the placenta usually weighs about 500 grams at term.

The placenta is essentially a structure which provides a large area of apposition between the maternal and fetal circulations for the exchange of materials. These transfers are controlled by the placental membrane, or barrier, which separates these two circulations.

However, it should not be overlooked that, as the amnion covered by chorion læve and decidua capsularis expands, the lumen of the uterine cavity is obliterated by fusion of the decidua capsularis with the decidua parietalis (Fig. 22). As a result the **chorio-amnion** becomes closely related to the decidua parietalis. This provides a large area of apposition between maternal and fetal tissues, and some exchanges between mother and fetus can also take place here.

FUNCTIONS OF THE PLACENTA

1. **Endocrine function.** The placenta is the site of synthesis of chorionic gonadotrophic hormones, and of œstrogenic and progestational hormones (see chapter on female genital system).

These hormones at first reinforce, and then gradually take over the function of similar hormones secreted by the mother to ensure that the pregnancy is maintained. From the end of the third month of pregnancy, the placenta has completely taken over the production of these pregnancy maintaining hormones. If the placenta does not take over this function effectively, the deficiency may lead to a miscarriage. As is well known, this is most common during the first three months of pregnancy.

2. **Placental transfer**. The placenta affords a barrier through which water and other substances pass to and from the fetus. Oxygen passes to the fetus, and carbon dioxide and other waste products are eliminated from it. Amino acids and sugars can pass through it fairly readily. Protein such as γ-globulins, which confer some passive immunity to the fetus against certain diseases, are also conveyed across the barrier. Electrolytes such as sodium, potassium and iron can pass across to the fetus as can water-soluble vitamins; fat-soluble vitamins are poorly transferred. Steroid hormones, which includes sex hormones, pass across readily. Babies are often born showing signs of having been stimulated by the mother's hormones, e.g. the baby's breasts may be engorged

and actually produce a secretion 'witch's milk' because they have responded to the hormones that were preparing the mother's breasts for lactation.

3. **Protection.** The placenta prevents some noxious substances from reaching the fetus; most bacteria do not cross the barrier. However, many viruses,

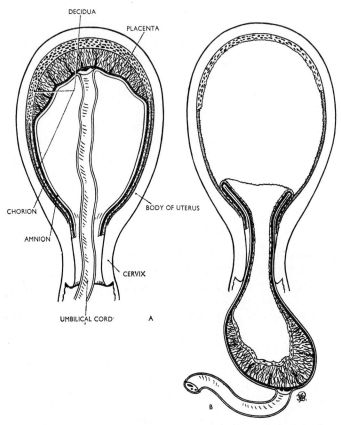

Fig. 24. Diagrams showing A, the relations of the fetal membranes to the uterus after the fetus has left it and B, the separation of decidua with these fetal membranes during the third stage of labour.

such as those of German measles, and the spirochætes that cause syphilis can cross the barrier to affect the developing embryo or fetus. It should also be realized that some drugs, e.g. morphine and anaesthetics, cross the barrier easily and affect the fetus.

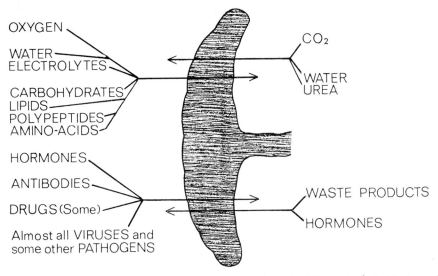

OXYGEN

WATER
ELECTROLYTES

CARBOHYDRATES
LIPIDS
POLYPEPTIDES
AMINO-ACIDS

HORMONES

ANTIBODIES

DRUGS (Some)

Almost all VIRUSES and
some other PATHOGENS

CO₂

WATER
UREA

WASTE PRODUCTS

HORMONES

Fig. 25. Diagram showing the exchanges across the placenta. The maternal side is on the left and the fetal side on the right of the illustration.

The Umbilical Cord

The umbilical cord connects the fetus to the placenta. It stretches from the umbilicus, in the anterior abdominal wall of the fetus, to near the middle of the placenta. Sometimes it is attached to the placenta at or near the edge, or even to the chorion beyond the edge of the placenta.

The umbilical cord, whose surface is covered by amnion, is twisted and irregular, and contains **two arteries** and **one vein** embedded in jelly-like connective tissue, called **Wharton's jelly.** Blood belonging to the fetus circulates in these arteries and vein (Plate 2).

At term, the umbilical cord is usually approximately the same length as the baby, about 54 cm (slightly over 20 inches), but it may be much longer or shorter.

After birth, the muscle in the walls of the umbilical vessels contracts so as to occlude them. Nevertheless, as a precaution against the baby losing blood, the umbilical cord is tied before it is cut. The stump of the cut umbilical cord separates from the baby's abdominal wall within a few days of birth, the site of its former attachment being indicated by a scar, the **navel** or **umbilicus.**

DETERMINATION OF AXIS AND DEVELOPMENT OF GERM LAYERS OF EMBRYO

The development of the embryo has so far been described up to the stage when the embryo consisted of a two-layered disc (Fig. 21) with the amniotic cavity above it and the yolk sac below it. The upper layer is known as **ectoderm** and the lower layer as **endoderm.** This disc gives no indication of which part is the head and which the tail end of the embryo.

The next phase of development is concerned with the **organization** of the embryo into an individual with a head end, with a tail end, with a right and a left side, with a front and with a back. The embryo is then at the **primitive streak stage.**

PRIMITIVE STREAK STAGE

A groove, the **primitive streak,** appears in the ectoderm of the future caudal (tail) half of the embryo. It lies along the cranio-caudal axis and from this stage on the individual has bilateral symmetry, i.e. the right and left halves are mirror images of each other. Associated with this laying down of the **embryonic axis,** a cellular rod arises from the cranial end of the primitive streak and grows forward between the ectoderm and endoderm towards the future head end of the embryo. This rod is the **notochord** (Fig. 26). From the margins of the primitive streak, cells bud off and are insinuated between the ectoderm and endoderm so forming a third, middle layer called the **secondary mesoderm.** This mesoderm is pushed out not only sideways, but forwards on either side of the notochord, and backwards towards the tail. Two small areas are, however, avoided by the mesoderm and at these sites the ectoderm and endoderm remain in contact with one another. The cranial of these two areas is just in front of the notochord and is known as the **bucco-pharyngeal membrane** (its thickened endodermal component is known as the **prechordal plate**). The area caudal to the primitive streak is known as the **cloacal membrane.**

Head and Tail Folds

The growth forwards of the notochord induces the overlying ectoderm to thicken and form a **neural plate** which becomes a **neural groove,** when its midline portion sinks below the level of the dorsal surface of the embryo (Plate 7). The margins of the neutral plate become raised to form the **neural crest.** The neural groove closes to form a **neural tube,** which gives rise to the brain and spinal cord (Figs. 26 and 27).

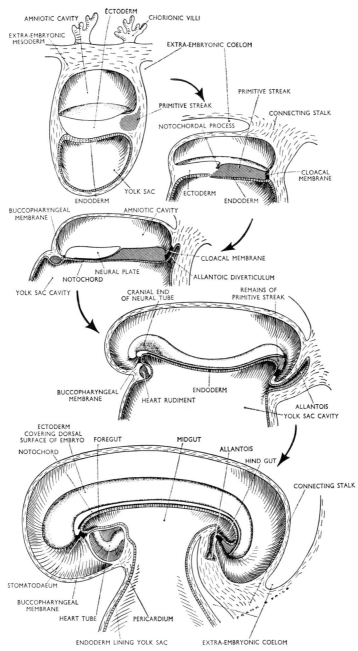

Fig. 26. Schemes to show the development of the embryonic disc into an embryo with a definite cranio-caudal axis.

Rapid growth of the head and tail regions of the embryo causes these to bulge up and curl over to form **head-** and **tail-folds** (Figs. 26 and 27). This has the effect of pulling up the buccopharyngeal and cloacal membranes from their previous horizontal to a vertical position. Further growth forward of the head-fold region, and backwards of the tail-fold region, draws out the related portions of the **endoderm**. The cranial extension is a tube known as the **foregut** which extends forward as far as the buccopharyngeal membrane; the caudal extension reaches the cloacal membrane and is known as the **hindgut** and the middle portion of embryonic endoderm forms the roof of the yolk sac and constitutes the **midgut** (Fig. 26). It will be remembered that the **allantois** (p. 71) is a caudal outgrowth from the yolk sac endoderm into the **connecting stalk**. Its origin from the yolk sac is thus related to the hind gut and the site where they join is known as the **cloaca**. The mesoderm in the floor of the foregut gives rise at this stage to the **developing heart** (Fig. 26) and the shelf behind this structure, in the angle between the foregut and the bulging midgut is called the **septum transversum**.

SOMITE EMBRYO

When the embryo is now examined (Fig. 27), it is seen that there are regularly arranged blocks of mesoderm on each side of the midline. These blocks are known as **somites,** and they are a manifestation of the fact that the embryo is made up of a series of similar segments (Fig. 27 and Plate 7).

Each segment has the same basic structure and consists of:

IN THE MIDLINE a portion of the **neural** tube dorsally
a portion of **notochord** immediately ventral to it
a portion of the **gut** ventrally.

LATERALLY a **somite** on each side of the neural tube
a **segmental nerve** joining the neural tube to the somite
the **intermediate cell mass** lateral and ventral to the somite
the **lateral plate mesoderm** lateral and ventral to the intermediate cell mass.

The somites, the intermediate cell mass and the lateral plate mesoderm are all developed from the primitive streak and constitute the secondary mesoderm.

This basic pattern is modified differently at various levels of the neck and trunk to give rise to the adult pattern, but evidence of this original segmentation is still found in the segmental arrangements of the spinal nerves, the arrangement of the vertebræ and ribs and in the body wall musculature. It should be noted that the segmental nerve establishes its connection with the somite at this early stage and, whatever position the somite assumes, the nerve supply from the original level is maintained. This explains how the diaphragm which is derived from cervical somites receives its nerve supply from the neck region (Phrenic nerve, p. 271).

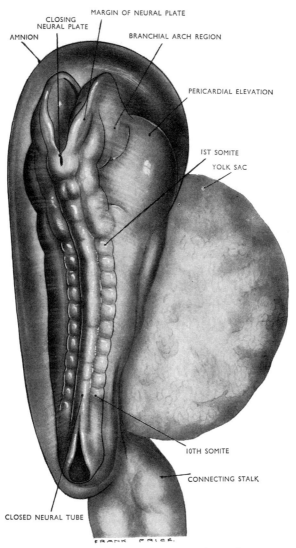

Fig. 27. Dorsal view of a 10-somite embryo.

Fate of the Germ Layers

In the presomite and somite stages of development, the **three basic germ layers—ectoderm, mesoderm** and **endoderm**—are relatively distinct and fairly easily recognized. For practical purposes, it is true to say that all the tissues of the body are derived from one or other of these three layers.

ECTODERM GIVES RISE TO THE EPITHELIAL CONSTITUENTS ONLY OF THE FOLLOWING:

1. The epithelium of the skin, that is the epidermis, and its appendages, i.e. nails, hair follicles, sebaceous glands, sweat glands and mammary glands.
2. The epithelium of the mucous membrane lining the lips, cheeks, gums, part of the floor of the mouth surrounding the root of the tongue, the hard palate, the nasal cavities with the sinuses extending from them, and also the enamel of the teeth.
3. The epithelium of the lower part of the anal canal and of the terminal parts of the urogenital tract.
4. The anterior lobe of the pituitary gland, which develops as an outgrowth from the roof of the primitive mouth.
5. The epithelium of the cornea and the lens of the eye.
6. The epithelium of the outer ear and of the outer layer of the ear drum.
7. The central nervous system (but not its blood vessels), the retina of the eye and the optic nerves, the epithelium at the back of the iris and the muscle tissue in the iris.
8. The sensory epithelia of the olfactory and auditory organs.
9. The neural crest and its derivatives.

The **neural crest** is the raised margin of the neural plate where the latter is continuous with the ectoderm covering the back of the embryo (Plate 9). As the neural plate folds up to form the neural tube, the neural crest cells leave it and migrate to different parts of the embryo to form:

(a) Sympathetic ganglion cells and the cells of the suprarenal medulla.
(b) The sensory ganglion cells of cranial and spinal nerves.
(c) Neurilemma (Schwann cells) around peripheral nerve fibres.
(d) The cells of the pia and arachnoid layers of the meninges.
(e) Some connective tissue elements in the head region.
(f) Melanoblasts—the cells responsible for pigmentation in the body.

ENDODERM GIVES RISE TO THE EPITHELIAL CONSTITUENTS ONLY
OF THE FOLLOWING:

1. The epithelium of the alimentary tract, except for the beginning and end,
   and the epithelium of the ducts and secretory cells of the glands derived
   from it (including liver, pancreas, thyroid, parathyroid and thymus).
2. The epithelium of the mucous membrane lining the pharyngo-tympanic
   (Eustachian) tube, middle ear, inner layer of ear drum and mastoid
   cavity.
3. The epithelium of the mucous membrane lining the larynx, trachea,
   bronchi and bronchioles, and the epithelium lining the alveoli of the lung.
4. The epithelium of the mucous membrane lining the bladder (except the
   trigone), most of the female and male urethra and glands derived from it
   (e.g. the prostate gland and the bulbourethral glands in the male and the
   greater vestibular glands in the female); the lower part of the vagina.

MESODERM GIVES RISE TO THE REMAINING TISSUES OF THE BODY:
As described on p. 78 the mesoderm in the embryo (**intra-embryonic
mesoderm**) is developed from the **primitive streak** and is known as **secondary mesoderm** in contradistinction to primary mesoderm, which develops in
the extra-embryonic part of the blastocyst wall (p. 70) before the primitive
streak has appeared in the embryonic disc.

As described on p. 80 the secondary mesoderm comprises the **somites, the
intermediate cell mass** and the **lateral plate mesoderm.**

The **somites** give rise to three components: **the sclerotome; the dermatome; the myotome.**

The **sclerotome** part of the somite migrates medially and surrounds the
notochord where part of the sclerotome forms the **axial skeleton.** The rest
forms **mesenchyme,** the precursor of all connective tissues.

The **dermatome** gives rise to the connective tissue elements of the skin
(the **dermis**) and so confers a segmental pattern on the innervation of the skin.

The **myotome** gives rise to the **skeletal muscles** and accounts for the
segmental innervation of muscles. It divides into a dorso-medial part, which
becomes to the dorsal extensor musculature, and an anterolateral part, which
becomes the body wall muscles, the trunk flexors and the muscles of the
limbs (Plate 7 and Fig. 120).

The **intermediate cell mass** gives rise to urogenital organs.

The **lateral plate mesoderm** splits into two layers:

The outer layer—**somatopleure**—lines the ectoderm of the body wall.

The inner layer—**splanchnopleure** or **visceropleure**—covers the gut.

DEVELOPMENT OF BODY CAVITIES: The cavity between the layers of the lateral plate mesoderm is known as the **intra-embryonic cœlom.**

The cranial portion of this cœlom is related to the developing heart where it forms the **pericardial cavity**: behind this the cavity is related to the developing lungs and forms the **pleural cavity**: the part of the cœlom caudal to the septum transversum is related to the developing gut and gives rise to the **peritoneal cavity.**

It will be readily understood that the **somatopleure** gives rise to the **parietal layer** and the **splanchnopleure** to the **visceral layer** of these **serous membranes.** Their cells lining the cœlomic cavity become flattened to form simple squamous epithelium (p. 102) called **mesothelium.**

It follows that the **parietal layer** is supplied by **nerves supplying the body wall,** i.e. the anterior primary rami of spinal nerves. (The body wall muscles having been insinuated between the skin and the somatopleure); the **visceral layer** is supplied by the **nerves supplying the viscera,** i.e. autonomic nerves (Plate 7 and Fig. 120).

FURTHER STRUCTURES DERIVED FROM LATERAL PLATE MESODERM: Part of the peritoneal mesothelium is specialized to form **germinal epithelium** for the gonads, it forms the **cortex of the suprarenal** and also the **paramesonephric (Müllerian) duct.**

In addition it gives rise to **mesenchyme.** In the **somatopleure** this mesenchyme gives rise to **connective tissue** which separates the developing skin from the mesothelium of the parietal layer of the serous membrane. At a later stage skeletal muscles derived from somites migrate into this mesenchymatous layer to complete the body wall. In the **splanchnopleure,** the mesenchyme not only gives rise to **connective tissue** separating the endoderm of the primitive gut from the mesothelium of the visceral layer of the serous membrane, but it gives rise also to the **smooth muscle wall of the viscera.**

Mesenchyme

This embryonic tissue consists of cells which have many cytoplasmic processes, and which produce a jelly-like intercellular substance and fibrils to form embryonic connective tissue. In the head region part of the mesenchyme is derived from the **neural crest,** but elsewhere it is developed from mesoderm. As has been described on p. 70 mesenchyme is developed from **primary mesoderm** in the extra-embryonic parts of the blastocyst wall, but in the embryo, it is the **secondary mesoderm** from the primitive streak which gives rise to mesenchyme. The cells of mesenchyme are remarkable in that they can develop into many different tissues in the body. As well as giving rise to **connective tissues,** they develop into **cardiac** and **visceral muscle** and give rise to the **cardiovascular system.**

DERIVATIVES OF MESENCHYME IN GENERAL (Plate 3):

1. Connective tissue proper, cartilage, bone (including dentine).
2. Myocardium and visceral musculature.
3. Endocardium and endothelium of blood vessels.
4. Lymph nodes, vessels and spleen.
5. Bone marrow, blood cells.
6. Fascia, tendons, synovial membranes.

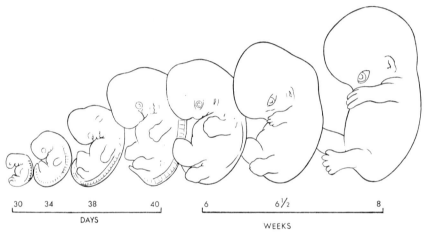

| 30 | 34 | 38 | 40 | 6 | 6½ | 8 |
DAYS

WEEKS

Fig. 28. The development of the external form from the somite embryo to the fetal stage.

CONGENITAL MALFORMATIONS

A pregnant woman has about a **1 in 50** chance of producing a malformed baby at term. A number of congenital malformations are incompatible with life and babies so affected die. Of the remaining malformations, a considerable number are amenable to surgical treatment and correction.

From what has been said in preceding sections, it will be realized that congenital malformations may be due to a number of different factors and causes. Some congenital abnormalities are due to defective genes and are therefore **hereditary**: others are due to **environmental factors.**

To understand how the latter operate, it is necessary to appreciate that the first three months, and particularly the first two months of pregnancy are devoted to the formation and specialization of the various parts of the embryo. This progressive specialization is known as **differentiation.** Now it is just when tissues and organs are actively differentiating, that they are particularly vulnerable to noxious substances such as infective organisms, certain drugs, X-rays, etc. It is thus during the first two months of pregnancy that malformations are particularly liable to be induced. This is why it is so important not to expose mothers to these hazards in early pregnancy.

Further aspects of growth and of the development of function during prenatal life are considered in Chapter XIX.

CHAPTER V

THE TISSUES OF THE BODY

What is Histology?

TISSUES may be defined as assemblages of cells and fibrous elements, in which one particular type of cell or fibre usually predominates, organized to form the material basis of the organs or functional systems of the body. By strict definition **histology** is the science of tissues, but by common usage it has come to refer as well to the study of the structure and function of cells (**cytology**), and of the disposition of tissues within organs (**microscopic anatomy**). Instruments that magnify—**microscopes** of various kinds—are used to examine the different parts of the body to obtain information about their detailed structure. The tissues are often treated with stains to make the various constituents easier to see, and this aspect of histology has led to the study of the chemical reactions of cells and tissues (**histochemistry**). Histology plays an important part in the correlation and integration of the basic medical sciences. The details revealed by microscopes form a natural extension of structure as studied with the naked eye in **anatomy.** The relation of structure to function provides an obvious bridge which leads to **physiology,** and the chemical reactions of histochemistry give an insight into the chemical reactions taking place in the body, the study of which is known as **biochemistry.** Histology also forges an important link with **pathology,** which deals with the structure and function of the body in disease, and it is stating the obvious to say that the normal must be known before the abnormal can be understood.

HOW MAY TISSUES BE STUDIED?

The simplest way is to dissect the body and observe what the tissues look like and their relation to one another. This naked-eye study forms part of **macroscopic anatomy.**

If a tissue is to be looked at with the aid of a microscope, the observer may want to study the appearances and reactions of living tissue or cells. Various instruments and ingeniously designed apparatus exist, which enable the observer to study such things as the blood flow through the capillaries in the tissues of an anæsthetised animal. Alternatively, portions of tissue may be removed from the body and looked at with a microscope, but, when light is shone through living tissues, not much detail can be seen unless use is made of the different phases of light waves with special equipment such as the **phase-contrast microscope.** Much information is being obtained about the nature and behaviour of cells by observing them with the aid of this kind of microscope, when they are kept alive and growing outside the body in **tissue cultures.** Such cells, grown outside the body, are no longer part of the integrated organism and they often behave in an abnormal way. Nevertheless, tissue culture is a convenient way of studying the reactions of cells and tissues to different surroundings.

The more usual routine methods of studying the structure of tissues entail fixing small pieces of tissue after they have been removed from the body. This **fixation** has the effect of killing the cells in the fragment of tissue, at the same time preserving it in the hope of preventing decomposition and maintaining the relationships of the tissue constituents to one another. Most **fixatives,** for example formalin and alcohol, act by precipitating the proteins in the tissue—a process comparable to boiling an egg. (In a hard-boiled egg the yellow and white constituents are 'fixed' in their normal relation to one another). In order that the fixed tissue may be cut thinly enough to be transparent for viewing through a microscope, the fragment is usually **embedded** in wax before thin slices or **sections** are cut. These are then mounted, that is stuck on glass slides. The wax which supports the tissue is dissolved out and the section is stained with dyes which make the different parts of cells and tissues clearly visible. The wavelength of light limits the **magnification** of a light microscope to between 1000 and 2000 times. Ultra-violet light has been used to obtain greater magnification and the greatest magnification—well over 100,000 times—is obtained when a beam of electrons is shone through the tissue, a technique known as **electron microscopy,** which magnifies structures so much that it is possible to see large molecules.

Microdissection has enabled parts of cells to be dissected out and examined, and **micropipettes** can be used to obtain minute specimens of fluid from tissues so that they may be analysed chemically. **Micro-electrodes** can be inserted into individual cells so that electrical recordings can be made while the cell performs its functions.

These methods, and many others, are being used extensively to try to determine how the body and its organs and tissues function and how these functions are related to structure.

THE MICROSCOPIC STRUCTURE OF THE BODY

The body is composed of three main components—namely, cells, intercellular substances and fluids.

Cells *are the smallest units of living matter which can lead an independent existence and reproduce themselves.* All cells are made of protoplasm which has a jelly-like consistency. Most of the cells in the body measure from about 10 to 25 micrometres (microns μ) in diameter (1 micrometre, $\mu m = \frac{1}{1000}$ mm). The constituent parts of cells are usually described in terms of a smaller scale of

measurement used in electron microscopy. On this scale the unit is the nanometre (nm) and 1 nm = $\frac{1}{1000}$ μm.

Intercellular substances (p. 94) *are non-living materials made by cells
and lying between them.* Though some intercellular substances are soft, others
are firm or hard and they give the body its shape.

Fluids. Several kinds of fluid are found in the body. **Tissue fluid** (p. 95)
bathes every cell and fills all the spaces between cells and intercellular substances. **Blood** (p. 392) and **lymph** (p. 406) are confined in vessels in which they
circulate. The body fluids provide the cells with the substances they need for
living, and remove the waste products of their metabolism.

Protoplasm is a colloid and its most abundant component by far is water.
Most people know that, in addition to water, our diet must contain three basic
foodstuffs—protein, fat and carbohydrate—certain salts and minerals, and
small amounts of other compounds such as vitamins. This is because protoplasm
itself consists of these substances. Apart from water, proteins are the most
abundant and important constituents of protoplasm. Our diet does not require
as great a proportion of protein as this might suggest, because fats and carbohydrates are used as fuel to provide energy, and dietary proteins are required
only for synthesis of such protoplasm as is necessary for the maintenance of cells
and to allow growth.

Protoplasm has seven **basic properties**:

1. **Irritability**: This is the faculty of being able to respond to a stimulus.
2. **Conductivity**: This is the ability of protoplasm to transmit a wave of
   excitation from the point where a stimulus is received to another part of
   the cell.
3. **Contractility**: This is the ability of the protoplasm of a cell to rearrange
   itself so that the cell, or part of a cell, is shortened in one direction.
4. **Absorption** and **assimilation**: Absorption is the ability of protoplasm
   to take in substances from the surroundings. Fluids and dissolved substances may diffuse directly through the cell wall. Fluids may also be
   taken in as droplets (i.e. by **pinocytosis**) and solids can be ingested as
   tiny particles (i.e. by **phagocytosis**). Assimilation is the incorporation
   of absorbed material into the protoplasm. This is usually brought about
   by the activity of the protoplasm in breaking down the ingested material
   and using it up.
5. **Excretion** and **secretion**: Protoplasm has the ability to discharge
   material from a cell. If the material is a waste product, then the process
   is **excretion**; if the material is useful to the body, then the process is
   known as **secretion**.

6. **Respiration:** This is the ability of protoplasm to effect the interaction of food substances and oxygen to form carbon dioxide and water with the liberation of energy.

7. **Growth** and **reproduction:** Growth is the ability of protoplasm to increase in amount. When the protoplasm in a cell increases, the cell grows larger. As it grows larger and larger, the point is reached when the outer surface is only just big enough in area to allow the exchange of enough of the materials necessary for the large amount of protoplasm inside the cell. Further growth is impossible unless the cell divides into two smaller cells, when the same amount of protoplasm is surrounded by a much larger surface area. These smaller cells in turn grow until they too must divide, that is, reproduce themselves. When growth occurs by means of enlargement of the cells the process is called **hypertrophy.** When growth is by multiplication of cells it is called **hyperplasia.**

It will be appreciated that these seven characteristic properties of protoplasm are not always developed to the same extent in every cell. For instance irritability and conductivity are best developed in nerve cells; contractility in muscle cells; absorption in certain cells of the intestine; phagocytosis in macrophages; excretion in kidney cells; secretion in the cells of glands; growth and reproduction in the germ cells (p. 522) and in the cells of tissues that have to be constantly replaced such as epithelia and blood-forming tissues.

THE CELL AND ITS CONSTITUENTS

Protein by itself is unable to carry out the business of life. Living requires the cooperation of many parts of a cell and it is necessary to consider how the instructions contained in the D.N.A. of the nucleus regulates the ordered interaction of the parts of the cell (see p. 44).

Cells themselves associate with other cells to form tissues and organs which together constitute an individual, who is a functional living separate member of the species. The cell is thus a unit of living matter, made of protoplasm integrated within itself, capable of homeostatic reactions, provided with mechanisms for defence and for repair of parts, able to replicate itself and destined to age and eventually to die as an entity.

The cells that make up the body show considerable variation in size, shape and function, but there are a number of basic structural features which are common to the majority of cells when they are observed through microscopes (see Fig. 29).

The tiny mass of protoplasm, which is the individual cell, is surrounded by a cell membrane, or **plasmalemma,** which has a thickness of about 8 nm. Electron-microscopy suggests that the plasma membrane is a three-layered structure and this, combined with biochemical analysis, has indicated that the outermost and innermost layers are composed mainly of protein, whilst the middle layer contains lipid molecules. It appears that the outer layer of the plasmalemma is more complex in composition than the inner one, and its surface possesses glycoproteins, polysaccharides and carbohydrates which are associated with the immunological and other properties of the cell surface. The external surface also regulates the movement of molecules into and out of the cell protoplasm. The cell surface plays a vital rôle in maintaining the homeostatic equilibrium of the cell.

It is misleading to think of the cell membrane as a simple envelope surrounding the cell contents. It is in fact continuous with a complex system of protoplasmic membranes inside the cell. In addition the cell may show a number of surface specializations: in the regions where certain types of cells are in contact with each other, the plasmalemma is highly modified to form **junctional complexes** or **desmosomes** which function as intercellular bridges. In addition, on the free surface of a cell, the cell membrane is frequently thrown up into numerous minute projections called **microvilli.**

The protoplasm inside the cell membrane is called the **cytoplasm.** Within the cytoplasm, and distinct from it, is a more or less spherical mass of protoplasm, the **nucleus.** The nucleus of the cell is a kind of headquarters which, to a considerable extent controls the characteristics and functioning of the cell. The nucleus is surrounded by a **nuclear envelope,** or **nuclear membrane,** which is bilaminar, the inner and outer layers being continuous with each other at the margins of holes in the membrane, called **nuclear pores.** It is likely that the pores provide a transfer mechanism from the nucleus to the cytoplasm.

Within the nucleus there is **nuclear sap,** or **nucleoplasm,** in which are found granules of a substance called **chromatin** because it readily takes up certain dyes, so that the nucleus has colour (chroma) in stained preparations. A nucleus also usually contains one or more tiny spheres which have a similar affinity for these dyes. Such a sphere is called a **nucleolus** and is concerned with the regulation of the cellular metabolism. The essential function of the nucleus is to allow the genetic information to be preserved and to pass it on in its original form from one generation of cells to another. In addition, it has to direct R.N.A. synthesis for the production of a large number of proteins in the cell.

The morphological appearances of the nucleus will depend on the various phases of the cell cycle and the description given here refers to the non-dividing cell.

The chromatin, which is seen in nuclei, is in fact located in thread-like structures called **chromosomes,** which become visible as threads when a cell is dividing (see Plate 1 and p. 52).

In the chapter dealing with development, it was explained that the cells of a female body contain two X sex chromosomes, whereas the cells of a male

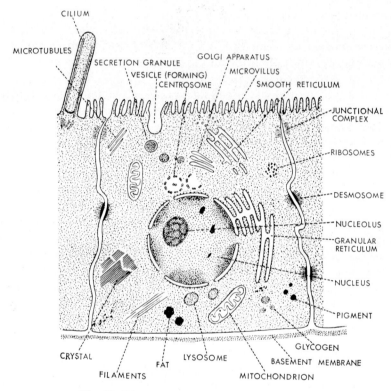

Fig. 29. Diagram of a cell and of its contents.

body contain one X and one Y chromosome. The bulk of an X chromosome is greater than that of a Y chromosome, therefore female cells contain more chromatin than male cells, and this is manifested by the presence, within the nucleus of every female cell, of a small particle of chromatin known as **'sex-chromatin'** (Fig. 30). Thus, by looking at cells with the aid of a microscope, it is possible to determine whether they originated in a male or in a female body, since only the cells of the latter contain sex-chromatin.

Both chromatin and nucleoli take up basic dyes because they are made up of **nucleoproteins** which contain **nucleic acid.** There are two types of this acid, **ribonucleic acid or R.N.A.,** which is found in nucleoli, and **deoxyribonucleic acid or D.N.A.,** which is found in chromosomes. The D.N.A. molecule forms the basis of the chemical composition of **genes** (see p. 52) and provides the means of storing genetic information within the cell, i.e. the means of making a cell look and behave like the particular cell it is. D.N.A., therefore, plays an important part in cell division and in ensuring that a given cell produces two similar daughter cells.

It has already been mentioned that there is R.N.A. in the nucleoli of nuclei, but this same substance is also present in varying quantities in the cytoplasm of the cell. In general, more of it is present when a cell is active, for example, when it is secreting or when it is growing.

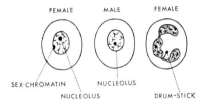

Fig. 30. Diagram to show the presence of sex-chromatin in the form of a particle in a typical cell from a human female, and in the form of a 'drum-stick' in a woman's granular leucocyte. Cells from males do not contain these structures.

The cytoplasm of the cell is highly heterogeneous and reflects the complexity of cell organization. It contains many structures, called **organelles,** which form part of the living constituents of the cell. Small particles, **ribosomes** and **microsomes,** are concerned with protein synthesis. **Mitochondria** carry respiratory enzymes and are looked upon as the throttle mechanism or power-packs of the cell. The mitochondrion possesses a striking structure consisting of an outer and an inner membrane system. There is generally a large number of infoldings of the inner membrane which form **cristæ.** Mitochondria show a considerable variation in their size and shape, and are concerned with fatty acid metabolism as well as with cell respiration processes.

The cytoplasm also contains a whole system of membranes—the **endoplasmic reticulum**—which act as sites of biochemical synthesis and are capable of forming a sophisticated cytoplasmic vacuolar system. The granular endoplasmic reticulum carries ribosomes, associated with R.N.A., and possibly passes their products to the smooth membranes of the **Golgi network** (see below), which itself may be concerned with the secretory activity of the cell. The endoplasmic reticulum is also associated with the nuclear envelope.

There is evidence to support the possibility that the endoplasmic reticulum is continuous with the plasmalemma which extends into the cell cytoplasm. The endoplasmic reticulum also forms the nuclear envelope during stages of cell division. It should be noted that there is a striking increase in the amount of endoplasmic reticulum in relation to protein synthesis occurring in active cells.

The **Golgi apparatus or network** appears as a complex of crescent-shaped and smooth surfaced membranes forming flattened sacs or **cisternæ.** Numerous small and large vesicles are also associated with this region and they may be derived from the cisternæ. The Golgi complex may sometimes be seen to be an extension of the smooth endoplasmic reticulum system. The sac-like structures forming the Golgi region often become filled with secretion products of the cell and these are possibly conveyed to the plasmalemma by the vesicles formed in the region.

The cytoplasm also contains the **centrosome** in which are located the **centrioles** concerned with cell division. The **basal granules** of the motile **cilia** are to be found in the cytoplasm when these are present.

Microtubules and **lysosomes** may also be observed. The latter contain a high concentration of digestive enzymes which are separated from the cell cytoplasm by a membrane sac. Their function is to digest various substances and they are particularly prominent in cells engaged in digestive processes.

Particular types of cell may have characteristic features in their cytoplasm. Thus muscle fibres contain contractile **myofibrils.**

Particular types of cell may have characteristic cell **inclusions.** These are particles, such as iron pigment, which have been taken into the cell for storing, or they may be reserve materials in the form of droplets or granules of fat or carbohydrate.

INTERCELLULAR SUBSTANCES

Many kinds of cells produce substances which they extrude and maintain in the spaces between the cells. These substances are known as **intercellular substances** of which there are two types—one is formless or **amorphous,** examples being **ground** and **cement substances;** the other is **formed** and consists of fibres which may be very fine (**reticulin**), coarse and inelastic (**collagen**), or elastic (**elastin**).

In general, the older a tissue the more formed intercellular substance it contains, and the smaller the proportion of elastic fibres present. In other words, with age tissues become tough and lose their elasticity.

It should be noted that amorphous intercellular substances are made up of large complex molecules of carbohydrate nature known as **mucopolysaccharides.** In general, the more complex they are the more solid the intercellular substance is. They can be reduced to simpler compounds by a process known as **depolymerization.** This renders them more liquid and facilitates the **diffusion** and **spreading** of substances within the tissue. This is important, because some bacteria produce **spreading factors,** which are enzymes that depolymerize intercellular substances, and so facilitate the spread of the infection within a tissue.

TISSUE FLUID

In the spaces between cells, as well as intercellular substances, there is a considerable amount of fluid which is known as **tissue fluid.** Basically, it is a solution of substances being transported to the cells from the blood-stream and from the cells back to the blood. Thus it enables food substances and oxygen to diffuse to the cell, and waste products to diffuse back to the blood. If a tissue contains too little tissue fluid, it shrinks and is said to be **dehydrated;** if it contains too much, the tisssue swells and is said to be **œdematous** (œdema or dropsy—water-logging).

Homeostasis. Every cell is bathed by tissue fluid on which it depends for all its requirements. The tissue fluid is the **internal environment** in which the cell lives. No matter how the external environment of the organism alters, the characteristics of this internal environment must be kept within narrow limits or the cells stop functioning and die. *Homeostasis is the constancy of the internal environment* (see also p. 3).

The cells are constantly removing substances like oxygen and food materials from the tissue fluid, and adding others like waste products to it. It is obvious that there must be some means of replenishing the food materials and removing the waste products, if the composition of the tissue fluid is to remain the same. This is accomplished by the blood, which flows past close to every cell, in capillaries which are also bathed by the tissue fluid. Substances pass from the blood plasma into the tissue fluid and from the tissue fluid into the plasma by osmosis (p. 33). Indeed, water, the main constituent of tissue fluid, reaches the tissue spaces in this way, and we speak of the production and removal of tissue fluid according to whether the volume of the tissue fluid is being increased or decreased.

Tissue Fluid Production and Removal

Tissue fluid is being produced and removed constantly, and in health production exactly equals removal, a constant optimum volume remaining in the tissue spaces.

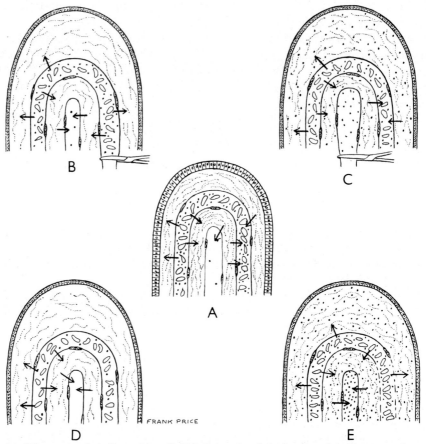

Fig. 31. Schemes to show how tissue fluid is formed and drained, and to illustrate the mode of action of the factors concerned in its production. In each diagram there is a centrally placed lymphatic vessel and a capillary loop containing blood. The arterial end of the loop is to the left and the venous end to the right. This loop is surrounded by connective tissue cells and intercellular substance bathed in tissue fluid. The colloids are represented by coarse-dots. The arrows indicate the direction in which fluid and crystalloids are passing. A, the normal process; B, the effects of blocking the venous end of the capillary; C, the effects of blocking the lymphatic outflow; D, the effects of diminishing the colloid content of the blood; E, the effects of accumulating colloids in the tissue spaces. (Modified from Ham's *Histology*.)

A **capillary** (p. 354) is a very thin-walled vessel (only one flat cell thick) one end of which is continuous with an arteriole and the other with a venule (Plate 23). The hydrostatic pressure within a capillary at its arterial end is sufficient to force out water and dissolved crystalloids (small molecules) into the surrounding tissue spaces. However, as the capillary wall acts more or less like a semipermeable membrane (p. 34), the blood colloids (large molecules, mostly proteins), are retained within the capillary. At the venous end of the capillary, the hydrostatic pressure within it has fallen considerably, and at the same time the concentration of the colloids in the capillary has increased because of the loss of water. This has the effect of increasing the osmotic pressure (p. 34) sufficiently to suck water back into the capillary. In addition there are lymphatic vessels in the tissue spaces (Fig. 31) and a proportion of the tissue fluid is reabsorbed into them. These lymphatics have the advantage of having in their walls minute holes, which allow the passage into them of any colloids which may have escaped into the tissue spaces. Were it not for lymphatics, colloids would gradually accumulate in the tissues.

Water-logging of the tissues, **œdema,** can be caused in many ways.

1. **By blockage of a vein** (Fig. 31, B): this increases the amount of tissue fluid produced by increasing the hydrostatic pressure within the capillary, most notably at its venous end. This prevents reabsorption of tissue fluid because the osmotic pressure of the colloids (sucking in water) is not sufficiently great to overcome the raised hydrostatic pressure (pushing out water). Also, as the vein is blocked, the outflow of blood from the capillary is obstructed.
2. **By blockage of lymphatics** (Fig. 31, C): this eliminates one of the channels through which fluid is usually removed and also prevents the colloids, which have escaped into the tissue spaces, from being removed. This tends to equalize the osmotic pressure inside the capillary with that outside, and removes one of the main factors concerned with sucking fluid back into the capillary.
3. In some instances, e.g. in the glomeruli of the kidney (p. 492), filtration may be increased by **raising the hydrostatic pressure** at the arterial end of a capillary, but this is a mainly theoretical rather than an actual consideration.
4. **Colloids may be deficient,** as in kidney disease, when the colloids are lost in the urine (Fig. 31, D). This again means that the osmotic pressure gradient at the venous end of the capillary is insufficient to draw water back into it.

5. Colloids may escape in quantity into the tissue spaces because the **capillary wall has been damaged,** e.g. in burns and in infections (Fig. 31, E). This causes fluid to be retained in the tissues because the osmotic gradient at the venous end of the capillary has been eliminated as in (2).

Maintenance of Homeostasis

Clearly homeostasis depends on circulating blood. However, the blood is only the vehicle which carries to the cells the substances they need, from sites where they are taken in by the body or are manufactured by the body. On the other hand, the blood also carries away from the cells the waste substances to sites where they can be eliminated from the body.

Homeostasis therefore depends on:—

1. Adequate circulation of the blood.
2. Adequate supplies of oxygen (i.e. proper functioning of the lungs), water, food materials (glucose, amino acids, lipids, inorganic salts), heat, regulators (vitamins and hormones) and protective substances (antibodies).
3. Adequate elimination of waste products, namely of carbon dioxide by the lungs and of urea, uric acid and creatinine by the kidneys.
4. Maintenance of the pH of the plasma at 7·4 by means of buffering substances (p. 32) in the first instance, and by the lungs (p. 343) and especially by the kidneys (p. 494) in the long run.

THE FOUR PRIMARY TISSUES OF THE BODY

The whole body is made up of four basic types of tissue (Table 1):

1. **Epithelial tissue** or **epithelium** which is designed to provide coverings and linings for the surfaces of the body. All the glands of the body develop from epithelial surfaces, so that they too are epithelial.
2. **Connective tissue,** is concerned with connecting and supporting the various parts of the body.
3. **Muscular tissue** which provides the motor power in the body.
4. **Nervous tissue** which conducts impulses from one part of the body to the other.

EPITHELIAL TISSUE

A CLASSIFICATION OF THE TISSUES

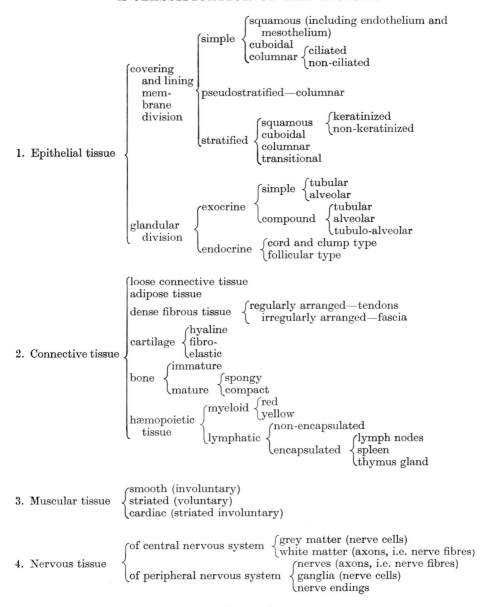

1. Epithelial tissue
   - covering and lining membrane division
     - simple
       - squamous (including endothelium and mesothelium)
       - cuboidal
       - columnar
         - ciliated
         - non-ciliated
     - pseudostratified—columnar
     - stratified
       - squamous
         - keratinized
         - non-keratinized
       - cuboidal
       - columnar
       - transitional
   - glandular division
     - exocrine
       - simple
         - tubular
         - alveolar
       - compound
         - tubular
         - alveolar
         - tubulo-alveolar
     - endocrine
       - cord and clump type
       - follicular type

2. Connective tissue
   - loose connective tissue
   - adipose tissue
   - dense fibrous tissue
     - regularly arranged—tendons
     - irregularly arranged—fascia
   - cartilage
     - hyaline
     - fibro-
     - elastic
   - bone
     - immature
     - mature
       - spongy
       - compact
   - hæmopoietic tissue
     - myeloid
       - red
       - yellow
     - lymphatic
       - non-encapsulated
       - encapsulated
         - lymph nodes
         - spleen
         - thymus gland

3. Muscular tissue
   - smooth (involuntary)
   - striated (voluntary)
   - cardiac (striated involuntary)

4. Nervous tissue
   - of central nervous system
     - grey matter (nerve cells)
     - white matter (axons, i.e. nerve fibres)
   - of peripheral nervous system
     - nerves (axons, i.e. nerve fibres)
     - ganglia (nerve cells)
     - nerve endings

TABLE 1

Functions

The main functions of epithelial tissue are protection, absorption and secretion.

Protection. Epithelium forms the **covering** and **lining membranes** of the body and so protects the other body cells. The epithelium of the skin protects from some of the hazards of the external environment, such as drying, ultra-violet light, abrasion and bacteria. The epithelium of the alimentary canal protects from the contents of the canal which include powerful digestive juice and, in places, bacteria. The epithelium of the urinary tract protects from the hypertonic urine. The structure of these covering and lining membranes is very closely related to the nature of the protection they must provide (p. 102).

Absorption. Food must be taken into the body from the outside world, and, since epithelium covers the body surfaces, it is obvious that some parts of it, notably the epithelium lining the alimentary canal, must have the property of absorption. An absorbing epithelium is only one cell thick and often has a **'brush border'** (p. 102).

Secretion. Some of the cells of epithelia have developed the ability to secrete products which enable the functions of protection and absorption to be carried out more efficiently. The mucus secreted on to some epithelial surfaces protects the surface cells from drying air currents or from digestive juices. The digestive juices secreted by other cells break down food materials until they are easily absorbed.

Glands (p. 103) are made of epithelial cells which have become specialized for secretion.

There are, therefore, two main kinds of epithelial tissue, namely—covering and lining membranes (p. 102) and glands (p. 103).

Some General Characteristics of Epithelia

Power of regeneration. Epithelia, because they form covering and lining membranes, are subject to wear and tear, and therefore are in continuous need of repair and replacement. This tissue tends, therefore, to contain a relatively high proportion of dividing cells. It is during cell division that changes in the genetic make-up of any cell may occur (**mutation**) (see p. 56). The changes are mostly unfavourable. One of the possible changes is that the new cell no longer differentiates normally, but divides giving rise to a new line of undifferentiated, rapidly dividing cells, namely **cancer cells.** Epithelial cells because they divide often are more likely to undergo this change and produce a cancer.

Avascularity. Epithelia contain no blood vessels; the nearest blood vessels are in the related connective tissue (Fig. 32). If the epithelium is thick, the superficial cells are at a considerable distance from the nearest blood vessel, and it may be difficult for oxygen and food substances to reach them by diffusion.

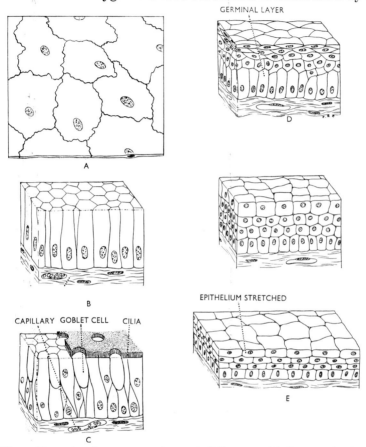

Fig. 32. Three-dimensional representations of different epithelia. A, simple squamous epithelium, shown in plan view because of extreme thinness; B, columnar epithelium; C, pseudostratified, ciliated, columnar epithelium; D, non-keratinized, stratified squamous epithelium; E, transitional epithelium.

If the surface of the epithelium is **dry,** the superficial cells die and are converted to a horny, scaly material called **keratin.** If the surface is **moist,** the oxygen dissolved in the wet film may be sufficient to enable the superficial cells to survive and not be keratinized. For example, the epidermis of the skin is keratinized but the epithelium lining the inside of the mouth is not.

Cohesion. The cells constituting an epithelium must be held together if an intact surface is to be preserved. This is effected by small cytoplasmic processes (**tonofibrils**) binding the cells together or by other 'locking devices' near the surface of cells called **terminal bars** or by **desmosomes.** In addition the cells are 'set' in cement substance which contains reticular fibres and forms a **basement membrane** (Fig. 29).

1. Covering and Lining Membranes

Simple epithelium is only **one cell thick** and is found on surfaces where the wear and tear is not great.

(a) **Simple squamous epithelium** is found where wear and tear is minimal. It is composed of a single layer of flat or squamous cells (Fig. 32, A). The peritoneum and the endothelial lining of blood vessels are examples.

(b) **Simple columnar epithelium** is found where wear and tear is a little greater, for example lining the gut. Tall columnar cells stand packed together on a basement membrane (Fig. 32, B).

The structure of these columnar cells varies according to the other functions they perform, so that several varieties of columnar cells are recognized:

Ciliated columnar epithelium. Short hair-like processes called **cilia** project from the surface of each cell. The cilia beat in harmony and move mucus and foreign particles along the surface.

Goblet cells are columnar cells which are specialized to secrete mucus. The mucus accumulates in the cytoplasm until the cell walls bulge, making the cell look like a goblet.

'Brush border'. A striated border or brush border is found on the surface of cells engaged in absorption. The electron microscope has shown that the striations are really minute finger-like projections, **microvilli,** some 3000 on every cell, which increase the area of the cell membrane through which diffusion can therefore take place more easily.

(c) **Simple cuboidal epithelium** is found in a few sites, for example, covering the ovary. It is like columnar epithelium but the cells are not as tall.

Stratified epithelium *is composed of more than one layer of cells* and is found on surfaces which are subjected to considerable wear and tear, for example in the mouth and on the skin. While it is admirable for protection, it is unsuited to absorption and secretion.

Stratified squamous epithelium (Fig. 32, D) is made up of many layers of cells, and derives its name from the fact that the surface cells are flat squames. The deepest cells called the **germinal layer,** lie on the basement membrane and are columnar. They divide frequently and each new set of daughter cells pushes the cells above them nearer to the surface. As the cells approach the surface they become progressively flatter. The cells on the surface are rubbed off by general wear and tear and are continuously replaced by cells from below.

Keratinized stratified squamous epithelium. It was explained on p. 101 that if the surface of the epithelium is dry, as on the skin, the surface cells, far from the blood capillaries, die and are converted to the horny scaly material, **keratin.** Keratin forms a waterproof protective layer (Fig. 133).

Non-keratinized stratified squamous epithelium. If the surface is kept moist, as in the mouth, the superficial cells survive until they are rubbed off, and so do not form keratin.

Transitional epithelium is not unlike stratified squamous epithelium but differs in some important respects (Fig. 32, E). It lines hollow viscera which must expand and whose lining needs to be watertight. It is found lining parts of the urinary tract. The most superficial cells, instead of being flattened, are large and rounded, and can spread out when the organ they line expands, so greatly increasing their surface area without breaching the continuity of the lining.

Pseudostratified epithelium is really a simple columnar epithelium, but it looks at first as if it were stratified, because, although all the cells stand on the basement membrane, they are of unequal height, and the nuclei lie at different levels (Fig. 32, C). This type of epithelium is found characteristically as **pseudostratified ciliated columnar epithelium** lining the respiratory tract.

2. Glands

Glands, be they ductless (**endocrine**) or equipped with ducts (**exocrine**), develop as a rule from epithelial surfaces (Fig. 33).

When they grow from epithelium, they push the connective tissue underlying the epithelium before them. As the epithelial buds grow, connective tissue and blood vessels are left behind between the advancing columns and form the basis of fibrous partitions (**septa**) between the lobes of the gland. These septa convey blood vessels to the interior of the gland.

The parts of the cellular columns nearest the surface become the ducts and the cells of the tips of the columns eventually specialize to form secretory units. The ducts remain less specialized, and if damaged, they can regenerate and even give rise to new secretory units.

The endocrine glands form the subject of a subsequent chapter (p. 507).

GLANDS WITH DUCTS: These are either **simple,** when each duct leads from a single secretory unit, or **compound** if a number of small ducts from many secretory units unite to form a larger duct.

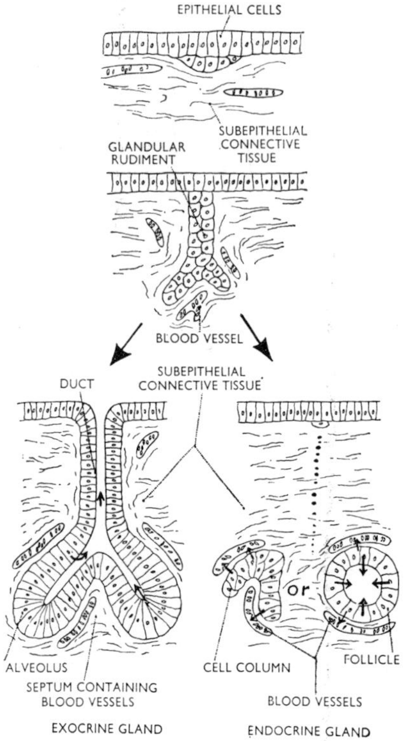

Secretory units may be (a) **tubular,** or (b) **globular** in which case they are called **acini** or **alveoli.**

MECHANISM OF SECRETION: Cells secrete in three ways, and three corresponding kinds of glands are described:

1. **Epicrine glands.** The cells secrete their products on to their surfaces. Examples are the salivary glands and the tear glands.
2. **Apocrine glands.** The cells lose part of their cytoplasm in the process of secretion. Examples are the sweat glands and the mammary glands.
3. **Holocrine glands.** During secretion the cell disintegrates and the whole of its cytoplasm is included in the secretion. The sebaceous glands of the skin are an example. Of course the cells are replaced by division of the remaining cells.

Salivary glands, which are epicrine, are made up of two types of secretory units: the one type—**serous**—produces a watery secretion, the other—**mucous**—produces a sticky secretion.

Fig. 33. Diagrams illustrating the development of exocrine and endocrine glands.

The parotid gland contains only serous acini but the submandibular and sublingual glands are mixed, containing both serous and mucous acini.

CONNECTIVE TISSUE

There are many varieties of connective tissue (see Plate 3). They are characterized by the large amount of intercellular substance which is produced by the cells. All connective tissue cells develop from the primitive connective tissue of the embryo, the **mesenchyme.**

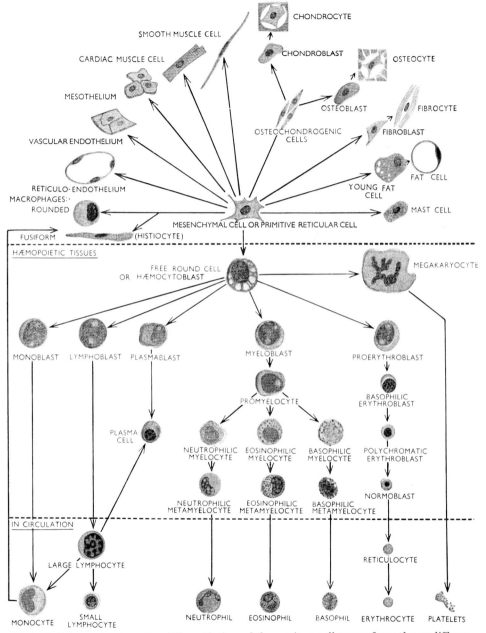

Plate 3. Scheme to show the differentiation of the various cell types from the undifferentiated mesenchymal cell. Cells of the blood and their precursors are shown below the upper interrupted line. Cells found normally in the circulating blood are shown below the lower interrupted line. (Modified from Ham's *Histology*.)

[*facing page 104*

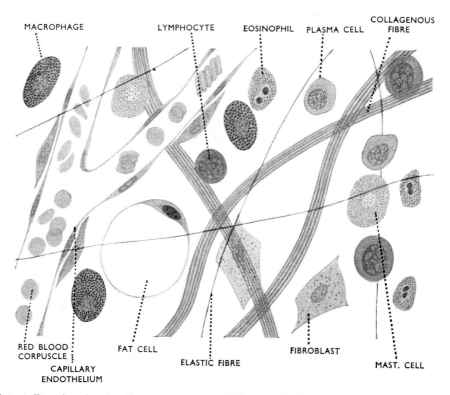

MACROPHAGE LYMPHOCYTE EOSINOPHIL PLASMA CELL COLLAGENOUS FIBRE

RED BLOOD CORPUSCLE FAT CELL FIBROBLAST MAST. CELL

CAPILLARY ENDOTHELIUM ELASTIC FIBRE

Plate 4. Drawing showing the arrangements of fibres and cells in a stained preparation of loose connective tissue. (Modified from Hamilton's *Text-book of Human Anatomy*.)

[*facing page 105*

Loose connective tissue or **areolar tissue** (Plate 4). The cells, called **fibroblasts** lie in semi-fluid amorphous intercellular substance which is traversed by collagenous and elastic fibres. It also contains **macrophages,** cells which ingest foreign particles and play an important part in body defence, and **mast cells** which contain heparin and histamine. Areolar tissue is the packing material which fills in the intervals between the more specialized cells in a tissue, between the tissues in an organ and between the organs of the body.

Dense connective tissue or **fibrous tissue.** This tissue is made up chiefly of bundles of collagenous fibres between which the fibroblasts lie (Fig. 34). There is little amorphous intercellular substance. The collagen makes it tough and strong. **Regular** fibrous tissue is made of parallel bundles of collagen fibres. Tendons are an example. **Irregular** fibrous tissue has bundles of collagen fibres running in different directions as for example in sheets of deep fascia.

Adipose tissue. Many of the connective tissue cells in the body specialize to store fat. Droplets of fat appear in the cytoplasm and coalesce to form a single large globule of fat which pushes the cytoplasm and nucleus to the periphery of the cell (Plates 3 and 4). An aggregation of such fat-storing cells is known as adipose tissue.

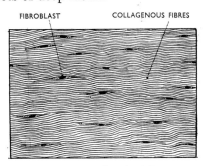

FIBROBLAST   COLLAGENOUS FIBRES

Fig. 34. Drawing showing the arrangement of fibres and cells in dense regular connective tissue.

Cartilage

Cartilage or gristle consists of cells, **chondrocytes,** which are separated by a considerable amount of amorphous intercellular substance in which formed fibres are embedded. The chondrocytes lie in spaces called **lacunæ** and, at the boundary of cartilage with another tissue, the cartilage is enveloped by a connective tissue membrane called **perichondrium.**

The perichondrium consists of two layers, an outer fibrous layer containing blood vessels and an inner layer which consists of cells—**chondroblasts.**

A characteristic feature of cartilage is that, generally speaking, it is avascular in the sense that it contains no capillaries, so that the chondrocytes depend on diffusion through the intercellular substance for nutrition and for disposal of products of metabolism.

The type of cartilage described has a somewhat glassy, translucent appearance and is known as **hyaline cartilage** (Fig. 35, B). Hyaline cartilage, covers the articular surfaces of bones and forms parts of the skeleton, for example the costal cartilages. The number of collagen fibres in hyaline cartilage may be increased to make it stronger and it is then known as **fibrous cartilage** (Fig. 35, A). This is found in intra-articular discs and at the attachment of tendons to bone. At some sites in the body, cartilage needs to be **elastic** and this is achieved by the incorporation of numerous elastic fibres (Fig. 35, C). Such sites are the epiglottis and the pinna of the ear.

Cartilage, being strong and resilient, acts as a support for the softer tissues.

DEVELOPMENT OF CARTILAGE: Mesenchymal cells condense together and then start secreting intercellular substance to form young cartilage, while the most peripheral cells of the condensation form perichondrium. While the cartilage is young and plastic, the cells in the centre of the cartilaginous substance can divide and produce more cells that secrete intercellular substance. This process is known as **interstitial growth.** The chondroblasts of the perichondrium can also lay down young cartilage around the periphery of the cartilage and this process is known as **appositional growth.**

Calcification of cartilage. Calcification occurs in some hyaline cartilage, notably in the cartilage models of bones before they undergo ossification (p. 108).

As cartilage matures the older cells begin to secrete an enzyme (p. 27) called **phosphatase.** This enzyme liberates an excess of phosphate ions in the tissue fluid trapped in the intercellular substance. The excess of phosphate ions causes the formation of solid calcium phosphate salts in the intercellular substance, that is the cartilage becomes calcified.

This process has an unfortunate result, however, for the chondrocytes. Although the cartilage is made stronger, the calcified intercellular substance no longer allows diffusion to and from the chondrocytes to take place efficiently so that the chondrocytes die. Calcified cartilage is not a living tissue and is therefore not satisfactory for permanent support.

Bone

Bone is similar to cartilage in that cells, **osteocytes,** lie in **lacunæ** surrounded by much intercellular substance which contains calcium salts. But **bone differs from cartilage** in being richly supplied with blood vessels. No osteocyte is more than 0·5 mm from a capillary, and although the osteocytes lie in lacunæ, the lacunæ are connected by numerous tiny tunnels, **canaliculi,** in the intercellular substance. Tissue fluid seeps through them to the osteocytes so that the vital supplies are maintained.

The intercellular substance of bone is mainly collagen impregnated with solid calcium salts. The collagen gives bone resilience and the calcium salts make

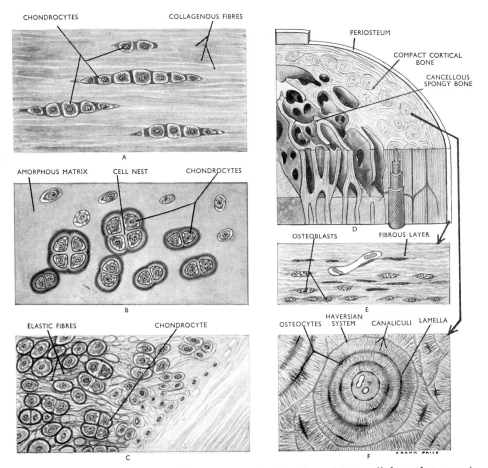

Fig. 35. Drawings illustrating the arrangements of cells and intercellular substances in different types of cartilage and bone. A, fibrous cartilage; B, hyaline cartilage; C, elastic cartilage; D, a section of the shaft of a long bone; E, periosteum; F, compact bone. Haversian systems are now called osteons.

it hard and strong. Bone is, therefore, an even better support for the soft tissues than is cartilage. The calcium in bone makes it radio-opaque and so it shows up well on radiographs (p. 7).

Bone, being rigid, can undergo only appositional growth.

Periosteum. Just as cartilage is surrounded by perichondrium, bone is surrounded by periosteum which consists of an outer **fibrous layer** and an inner layer, the **osteogenic layer,** composed of cells called **osteoblasts** (Fig. 35, E).

TYPES OF BONE: There are two types of bone, **compact bone** (cortical bone) which is strong and solid, and consists of **osteons** (Haversian systems) (Figs. 35, D and F), and **spongy bone** (cancellous bone) which consists of openly arranged small slender beams called **trabeculæ.** They are arranged like the structure of a sponge, but spongy bone is, of course, hard, like all bone, and not soft as the name might suggest. The trabeculæ develop along the lines of stress in the bone (Figs. 61 and 63).

Bone Development and Growth

Bone develops in two ways:

1. **Intramembranous ossification,** in which bone is laid down in a membranous precursor or model.
2. **Endochondral ossification,** in which ossification takes place in a model made of hyaline cartilage.

In both processes, some of the mesenchymal cells become specialized to form a special intercellular substance, namely collagen impregnated with calcium salts, which is characteristic of bone. These cells are **osteoblasts.** The region in which they first start to form bone in the membranous or cartilaginous model is called the **centre of ossification.** Like all mesenchymal cells, osteoblasts have processes which link adjoining cells. Once they have surrounded themselves and their processes with intercellular substance, the osteoblasts withdraw their processes and become rounded **osteocytes** lying inside bony lacunæ. The tiny tunnels left where their processes originally were, remain as the **canaliculi.**

1. INTRAMEMBRANOUS OSSIFICATION: This occurs in most of the flat bones of the skull. Mesenchymal cells come together to form a dense membrane. Some of the cells in the centre become osteoblasts and start to lay down bone, forming the centre of ossification. The ossification extends outwards in an irregular pattern, its margin consisting of radiating spicules. As further layers of bone are formed on the surface of the spicules by appositional growth, the trabeculae of spongy bone are formed.

The cells on the surface of the membrane become the osteogenic cells of the periosteum. They lay down layers of compact bone on the surface of the developing bone.

2. ENDOCHONDRAL OSSIFICATION: First a cartilaginous model of the future bone is formed. This is surrounded by perichondrium. In the cartilaginous model, the most centrally placed cells are the oldest. In a long bone the oldest

cells are in the middle of the shaft. As was explained above, mature cartilage cells cause calcification of the intercellular substance between them and this leads to their death.

The perichondrium now assumes osteogenic properties and is then known as periosteum. It forms a cuff of bone round the middle of the shaft, and capillaries and osteoblasts grow in from the periosteum to lay down bone on the scaffolding of calcified acellular cartilage. In this way, the shaft of the bone begins to ossify from the **primary centre of ossification.** The process extends towards the two ends of the young bone which still consist of cartilage. This cartilage continuously grows, leaving a trail of maturing cartilage cells which cause calcification. This in turn is followed by the extending ossification.

The arrangement of the cells in the intercellular substance, and their relation to the blood vessels, is striking in compact bone formed in this way. Long narrow tunnels contain blood vessels. Round the tunnels layers of intercellular substance alternate with rings of lacunæ containing osteocytes. Such a system is an **osteon** (Haversian system) (Fig. 35, F). The osteons in compact bone, and the bony trabeculæ in spongy bone develop always in the lines of the stresses and strains to which the bone is subjected (Fig. 61).

Eventually, the cartilage cells in the centre of the cartilaginous ends of the developing bone mature also and cause calcification. Blood vessels and osteoblasts invade the calcified cartilage from the periphery and from the shaft to set up a **secondary centre of ossification,** or **epiphysis,** in the centre of the cartilaginous end. The cartilage persists on the surfaces of the ends of the bone to form the **articular cartilage.**

The cartilage left between the epiphysis and the shaft is in the form of a disc of **epiphyseal cartilage.** By its continued growth it allows the bone to grow. Eventually the epiphyseal cartilage too is replaced by bone, when the epiphysis is said to fuse with the shaft. When this happens the bone stops growing.

Growth in the girth of the bone is by appositional growth from the periosteum, and as the bone grows blood vessels are incorporated into the bony substance to ensure its blood supply.

The part of the bone ossified from the primary centre of ossification is known as the **diaphysis;** those parts ossified from secondary centres are known as **epiphyses** and the region of the bone adjoining an epiphysis, where growth is taking place, is known as the **metaphysis.**

Students should not visualize the epiphyseal cartilage as a smooth disc. Its surface is in fact made up of a series of pegs which extend into the shaft and so help to anchor the epiphysis to the shaft.

Although a long bone has an epiphysis at each end, one appears earlier than the other. The first one to appear is usually the last to fuse, so that the bone grows more at this end which is known as the **growing end of the bone.** It is important to know which end is the growing end, because injury or interference with its blood supply is more likely to cause serious deformity by stopping growth. Also, tumours of bone usually occur at the growing ends of bones. **Epiphyses** develop where bones are subject to the stresses and strains of **pressure** or of **traction.** The epiphyses at the ends of long bones are pressure epiphyses. The epiphyses for the trochanters of the femur and for the tuberosities of the humerus are traction epiphyses (Fig. 233).

RESORPTION OF BONE—REMODELLING: As a bone grows it has to be remodelled. The expanded ends of the younger bone have to be reshaped to form part of the cylindrical shaft of the older bone and to establish the marrow cavity. Obviously, in addition to the laying down of new bone, some of the old bone must be removed. In the same way, during growth of the vault of the skull, bone is being formed continuously on the outside but is being removed on the inside. This removing of bone is called resorption. It is effected by large multinucleated cells called **osteoclasts.** The process of altering the disposition of bone during growth is known as remodelling.

BONE AS A LIVING TISSUE: It is essential to realize that bone is a living tissue. The activity of the osteoclasts is not confined to growing bones. In all bones, at all times, resorption of the intercellular substance continues, and is exactly equalled by the activity of osteoblasts laying down new bone.

SOME FACTORS AFFECTING BONE GROWTH: Bone growth and development is affected by intrinsic **genetic factors** which determine the general shape and texture of the bone. The **pull of muscles** plays a rôle in determining the markings of muscle attachment. **Posture** may affect the shape of bones by altering the stresses and strains. **Hormones** are important. The **parathyroid hormone** controls the mineral content of bones. The **growth hormone** of the anterior pituitary, the **sex hormones** (p. 578) and the **thyroid hormone** all affect bone growth. **Dietary factors** include **Vitamin D** which is important in preventing rickets, a condition in which the bones are too pliable so that they bend under the body weight. **Vitamin C** is also important for the laying down of collagen in bone.

HÆMOPOIETIC TISSUE

Hæmopoietic tissue is concerned with the formation of the **blood corpuscles.** Blood itself may be regarded as a connective tissue in which the cells are represented by the red and white blood corpuscles, and the intercellular substance by the **plasma.**

There are two types of **hæmopoietic tissue**—myeloid tissue and lymphatic tissue:

Myeloid tissue is found in red bone marrow.

Lymphatic tissue is found in lymph nodules, in lymph nodes and in organs such as the spleen and thymus gland.

The two types of tissue are similar, both being derived from **mesenchyme** and both containing two main kinds of cells, namely **hæmocytoblasts,** which produce the cells of the blood, and **reticulo-endothelial** cells which provide a filter for body fluids.

Reticulo-endothelial tissue

This tissue is designed for filtering body fluids and consists of **reticulo-endothelial cells,** some of which lay down intercellular substance in the form of a very fine network or **reticulum.** Other reticulo-endothelial cells are flat and form the endothelial walls of wide irregular capillaries called **sinusoids** which traverse the reticulum. The name reticulo-endothelial is therefore derived from the microscopic structure of the tissue. The sinusoids contain blood or lymph (pp. 112 and 113).

The reticulo-endothelial cells are able to ingest particles, that is, they are **phagocytic** and they do not always remain part of the sinusoid wall, but may become **free** phagocytes.

SITUATION: Reticulo-endothelial tissue is found scattered in many sites in the body. It is found in the myeloid tissue of red marrow and in lymphatic tissue such as the lymph nodes and the spleen. (In myeloid tissue, and in the spleen and hæmal lymph nodes, the sinusoids contain blood. In other lymphatic tissue the sinusoids contain lymph.)

Reticulo-endothelial cells are found in the walls of the sinusoids of the liver where they are known as **stellate cells** (Kupffer cells).

The free phagocytic reticulo-endothelial cells are very similar to the wandering **macrophages** (**histiocytes**) found scattered through areolar tissue, and to the **monocytes** of the blood.

FUNCTIONS: Reticulo-endothelial cells, especially those in the spleen, ingest and destroy the worn-out cells of the blood.

Reticulo-endothelial cells ingest foreign particles, for example bacteria and dust from the air reaching the lungs, and so provide an important defence mechanism.

Reticulo-endothelial cells probably also aid in defence by producing antibodies.

Myeloid Tissue or Red Bone Marrow

The **hæmocytoblasts** of red bone marrow produce red blood corpuscles (**erythropoiesis**); they produce granular leucocytes (**leucopoiesis**); they also produce platelets and possibly some monocytes. The **reticulo-endothelial tissue** filters the bood.

SITUATION: In the adult, red marrow is found in only some of the bones, namely in flat bones like the sternum, ribs and skull bones, in vertebræ and in the ends of the long bones.

In children up to four years old, all the bone marrow is red, but, as the child grows older, the red marrow in the shafts of the long bones is gradually replaced by yellow marrow until the adult pattern is reached. Yellow marrow is really resting marrow. It looks yellow because it contains fat instead of developing blood corpuscles. In the fetus, blood cells, including lymphocytes, are formed in the liver and spleen before the red marrow is fully developed. Even in adult life, if the need for extra blood cells should become great, these former sites of blood formation become active again.

STRUCTURE: In red bone marrow, between the trabeculæ of the spongy bone, are found all the different kinds of cells associated with the development of red blood corpuscles, granular leucocytes and platelets. They are supported by a fine network of reticular fibres produced by reticulo-endothelial cells. Throughout the tissue is a network of wide sinusoidal capillaries whose walls are formed by reticulo-endothelial cells. As blood passes through, new cells enter it through the walls and some of the old cells are removed by the reticulo-endothelial cells.

STERNAL PUNCTURE: It is often necessary to examine samples of red bone marrow to see whether the formation of the blood cells is taking place normally. The red marrow is obtained by puncturing the cortical bone of the sternum and drawing out some of the red marrow cells into a syringe.

FUNCTION: In the red bone marrow there are cells derived from mesenchyme, called **haemocytoblasts**, which develop there in three different ways to form either red blood corpuscles (p. 394), granular leucocytes (p. 394), or platelets (p. 396) (see Plate 3).

Lymphatic Tissue

The **hæmocytoblasts** of lymphatic tissue produce non-granular white blood corpuscles, i.e. **lymphocytes** and **monocytes**. The reticulo-endothelial tissue filters mainly lymph, although in the spleen and in hæmal lymph nodes it filters blood.

LYMPHATIC NODULES: The unit of lymphatic tissue is the **lymphatic nodule** (Figs. 161 and 162). The centre of the nodule, the **germinal centre,** contains hæmocytoblasts which in turn give rise to **lymphoblasts** and **monoblasts.** These in turn develop into lymphocytes and monocytes respectively (Plate 3). These lymphocytes and monocytes form a closely packed layer of cells round the more loosely arranged germinal centre. Those at the periphery enter adjacent sinusoids and are carried away by the lymph.

Types of Lymphatic Tissue

1. LYMPHATIC TISSUE DESIGNED TO FILTER TISSUE FLUID: This is essentially diffuse and is usually situated beneath epithelium covered surfaces through which organisms could gain access to the body's tissues. Examples of this type are found in the mucous membrane of the alimentary tract and of the respiratory tract (Fig. 161).

2. LYMPHATIC TISSUE DESIGNED TO FILTER LYMPH: Lymph is contained in lymph vessels, in which a one way circulation is ensured by means of **valves.** Set on the course of lymph vessels are encapsulated masses of lymphatic tissue called **lymph nodes** (Fig. 162, p. 408). As the lymph percolates through the meshes of the node, foreign particles and bacteria are filtered off by the reticulo-endothelial cells, and lymphocytes and monocytes are added to it.

3. LYMPHATIC TISSUE DESIGNED TO FILTER BLOOD: The main blood filtering organ is the **spleen** (p. 410). Blood is also filtered in a few **hæmal lymph nodes** situated mainly behind the peritoneum. They filter blood instead of, or in addition to, lymph.

MUSCULAR TISSUE

Muscle cells are specialized for contraction. All muscle cells are long and narrow, so that the shortening of the cell, which occurs during a contraction, may be as effective as possible. Because of their shape, **muscle cells** are often called **muscle fibres.** (In nervous tissue a nerve fibre is only a process, i.e. the axon, of a nerve cell. In connective tissue a fibre is not part of a cell at all, but is composed of intercellular substance.)

There are three types of muscle:

1. Smooth Muscle

Smooth muscle consists of small spindle-shaped cells with centrally placed elongated nuclei (Fig. 36, c). The cytoplasm contains poorly marked longitudinally disposed fibrils—**myofibrils** that consist of long chains of protein molecules which are responsible for the contraction of the cell.

This kind of muscle is designed for comparatively slow contraction, over relatively long periods of time, with little expenditure of energy so that it does not tire easily. Its contraction is not under voluntary control, hence it is also known as **involuntary muscle.** Among the muscle fibres are fibroblasts and reticular and collagenous fibres which act as a harness for it.

2. Striped Muscle

Striped muscle (Fig. 36, A and B) consists of large, cylindrical cells often several centimetres in length, each containing several nuclei which are placed at the periphery of the cell. The cell exhibits marked **cross striations** (hence its name). Striped muscle cells, like smooth muscle cells, have **myofibrils** running the length of the cell. Every myofibril in striped muscle, however, is made up of many short segments called **sarcomeres,** each of which has light and dark

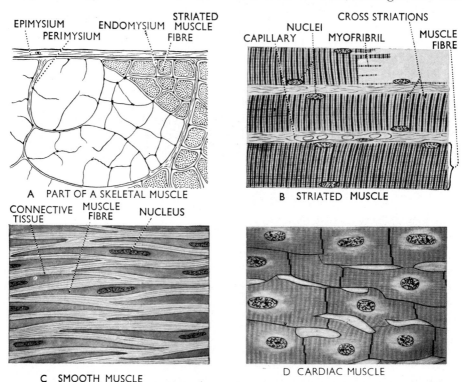

A   PART OF A SKELETAL MUSCLE

B   STRIATED MUSCLE

C   SMOOTH MUSCLE

D   CARDIAC MUSCLE

Fig. 36. Schemes illustrating the different types of muscular tissue and some of the relations of it to connective tissue.

bands across it (Fig. 36, B). The myofibrils are placed so that the light and dark bands are exactly in line with the light and dark bands of adjacent myofibrils, so that the cytoplasm of the whole cell appears to have cross striation.

Striped or striated muscle is designed for strong contraction, over relatively short periods of time, and its contractions involve a considerable expenditure of energy. It needs, therefore, a rich blood supply to bring food materials and oxygen to it, and to dissipate the heat generated, as well as to dispose of metabolites. The richness of the blood supply is witnessed by the fact that capillaries run between individual muscle fibres. In spite of this, striped muscle tires quickly. Contraction of this type of muscle is usually under voluntary control, hence it is also called **voluntary muscle.**

Each striped muscle cell is surrounded by a fine sheath of reticular fibres, the **endomysium.** Muscle cells are bound into bundles by connective tissue called

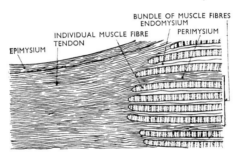

Fig. 37. Drawing of a portion of the junction between a muscle and its tendon.

the **perimysium.** The bundles in turn are held together within a fibrous sheath, the **epimysium,** which encloses a whole muscle. These layers of connective tissue provide a harness for the muscle fibres. At the ends of the muscle they are continuous with the fibrous tissue in the **tendon** (Fig. 37) or blend with the periosteum of a bone, at the same time sending some fibres through into the intercellular substance of the bone itself to give a really firm attachment. Where tendons are attached to bone, the fibrous tissue is often reinforced by cartilage to form fibro-cartilage (see p. 106).

3. Cardiac Muscle

Cardiac muscle differs from the previous two types, not only in structure, but in function. The heart starts beating 3 or 4 weeks after conception and goes on beating until death. Thus it can never 'rest' and, in addition, it must be able to conduct impulses in such a way that the various parts of the heart contract in the correct sequence to produce an ordered and effective heart-beat.

Cardiac muscle fibres are cylindrical with centrally placed nuclei (Fig. 36, D). They have cross striations like striped muscle. The fibres branch and anastomose with adjacent fibres, and this allows an impulse to spread from one fibre to another as well as along the length of a fibre.

CONDUCTING SYSTEM OF THE HEART: In order to convey the cardiac impulse from the atria to the ventricles in the necessary way (p. 361), some cardiac muscle fibres are modified to conduct rather than to contract. They are the large, hypertrophied, unstriped **Purkinje fibres,** and they constitute the **atrio-ventricular bundle** (of His).

NERVOUS TISSUE

The nervous system is made up of nerve cells, or **neurones,** and special connective tissue cells, called **neuroglia,** which provide a supporting network of fibres for the neurones in the central nervous system. Neuroglia is important because the majority of tumours within the central nervous system arise from this tissue. Such a tumour is called a **glioma.**

The **neurone** or **nerve cell** *is the functional unit of the nervous system;* it is described in more detail on p. 223. It consists of a large cell body, from which extend several short processes called **dendrites.** These convey nervous impulses towards the cell body. From the cell there usually extends also one long process, **the axon,** which conveys impulses away from the cell body. Axons may branch, and, within the central nervous system (p. 227), axons and their branches are collected together in bundles called **tracts,** whereas outside the central nervous system, they are grouped together to form **peripheral nerves** (see p. 228).

Coverings of peripheral nerves. In the same way that muscle fibres are covered by layers of connective tissue (p. 115), **axons** within peripheral nerves are covered, not only by a **myelin sheath** and a **neurilemmal sheath** (described on p. 224), but each axon is separated from its neighbouring fibres by a layer of fibrous tissue called **endoneurium.** A number of axons are bound together within a nerve by a layer of connective tissue, called **perineurium,** to form **fascicles.** The fascicles are bound together to form a **peripheral nerve** by a layer of connective tissue termed the **epineurium.**

Although the other details of the structure of nervous tissue are described in the chapter dealing with the Nervous System, attention is drawn here to the fact that nervous tissue is particularly sensitive to, and easily damaged permanently by oxygen-lack. **Many structural arrangements in the body and several physiological phenomena** make sense when it is realized that they are **designed to ensure an adequate supply of blood to the brain.**

SECTION II

CHAPTER VI

THE SKELETAL SYSTEM

BONES

THE STRUCTURE OF BONES

Bone, whether developed in membrane or in cartilage (p. 108) is of two kinds—**compact** (or cortical) and **spongy** (or cancellous) (see also p. 108).

Compact bone is dense and uniform. Spongy bone, on the other hand, is of an open texture, made of thin interlocking plates of bone with spaces between. These spaces contain bone-marrow (p. 112), (Fig. 38).

The skeleton consists of many separate bones connected at joints. The bones differ greatly in size and shape, but the four main types are **long, short, flat and irregular.**

A **long bone** has a cylindrical shaft, each end of which is expanded for articulation with adjacent bones and for the attachment of muscles. The humerus and femur are good examples (Fig. 39). If such a bone is cut lengthwise (Fig. 38) it is seen that the shaft is hollow and that a thick layer of compact bone forms its walls. In life, the cavity is filled with **yellow marrow** (p. 112) (cf. the 'marrow bone' from the butcher). The expanded ends of a long bone have a thin outer covering of compact bone and the interior is filled with spongy bone containing **red marrow** (p. 112). Certain bones of the hand and foot have the shape and structure of long bones but, because they are very small, they are known as miniature long bones.

A **short bone** is small, and roughly cubical in shape. The bones of the carpus and tarsus are examples. They have an outer layer of compact bone surrounding the spongy interior and its contained red marrow.

A **flat bone** is thin, rather than flat, and is composed of two plates of compact bone with a layer of spongy bone, containing red marrow, between. The bones of the vault of the skull, the scapula and the ribs are examples.

Irregular bones cannot be classified in the other groups and are of various shapes. They include the vertebræ and many of the bones of the

117

skull. An outer layer of compact bone covers the spongy, marrow-containing interior.

The external surfaces of bones are fairly smooth but smoothest of all are those areas, the joint surfaces, by which one bone articulates by means of a

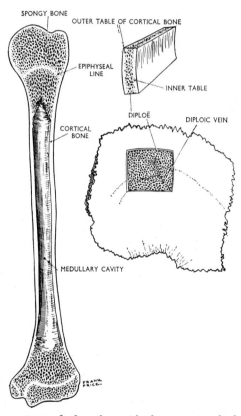

Fig. 38. The internal structure of a long bone (the humerus) and of a flat bone (the parietal bone of the skull).

synovial joint with an adjacent bone. Rough areas, ridges and prominences are found especially where the strong fibrous tissue of tendons and ligaments is attached to the bone, for example, the trochanters of the femur. The external surfaces of bones are moulded too by adjacent soft tissues. For example, arteries and veins often form grooves in bone, and even the sulci and gyri of the brain mould the inside of the vault of the skull.

Radiology of Bones

Because bones contain calcium they show up clearly on radiographs. The thick layer of compact bone in the cylindrical hollow shafts of long bones and the spongy or cancellous bone of their expanded ends can be clearly seen (Figs. 54 and 61). The trabeculæ in the cancellous bone are laid down in the lines of stress.

THE FUNCTIONS OF BONES

Support

Because they combine strength and elasticity, bones support well the soft tissues of the body. The vertebral column is a good example in that it supports the trunk, but all the bones of the body act in this way to some extent. Where bones have to withstand great stresses, they are bigger and stronger than elsewhere. The femur and tibia are thick and strong to carry the body weight.

Attachment of Muscles

To work effectively, muscles must have firm attachments. Bones provide that. The shape of many bones is modified to provide an extensive area for the attachment for muscles. For example, the scapula (Fig. 52) and the ilium (Fig. 59) are flattened to give a large surface area for muscle attachment, and such projections as the spines of the vertebræ and the spine of the scapula also provide extra anchorage sites.

Levers

Bones form a series of mechanical levers which are used when the muscles move one part of the body in relation to another and when the body is moved in relation to its environment.

Protection

Bones play an obvious part in protecting delicate and important organs. The skull protects the brain; the vertebral canal of the spine protects the spinal cord; the rib cage protects the thoracic and upper abdominal viscera.

Calcium Storage

Bones act as a reservoir for calcium which can be withdrawn when it is needed.

Blood Formation

The red marrow, which is found throughout the bones of children up to 4 years old, and in the ends of the long bones, in the flat bones and in some short and irregular bones of the adult, produces the red blood corpuscles, the platelets and the granular leucocytes of the blood.

Bones and Surface Anatomy

Some bones lie deep in the body, covered by muscles and fat. Other bones are nearer the surface and, in many places, parts of them can be felt easily in the living subject so that their shapes can be traced out. Such bones form good landmarks on the surface of the body and can be used as reference points on the skin of a living person in tracing the outline of hidden organs. That is to say, these bony landmarks are of great importance in surface anatomy (Figs. 51 and 58).

Patients confined to bed may be liable to develop pressure sores over bony points subjected to continuous pressure which interferes with the blood flow. Vulnerable regions are the sacrum, the ischial tuberosities, the heels and the elbows.

THE SKELETON

The skeleton consists of the bones of the head and trunk and the bones of the limbs.

THE SKELETON OF THE HEAD AND TRUNK

This comprises the skull, the mandible, the thirty-three vertebræ of the vertebral column, twelve pairs of ribs and the sternum (Figs. 39 and 40).

The skeleton of each limb consists of the limb girdle, a single long bone in the proximal segment, two parallel long bones in the next segment and then the small bones of the hand or foot. In the upper limb the girdle is formed of the clavicle and scapula. The humerus articulates with the scapula, the radius and ulna articulate with the humerus, and the hand with the radius. The lower limb girdle consists of the hip bone or innominate bone, which articulates with the hip bone of the opposite side and with the sacrum. The femur articulates with the hip bone, and the tibia with the femur. The fibula lies alongside the tibia. The foot, composed of small bones, articulates with the tibia and fibula.

The Skull

The skull consists of a number of bones joined by immovable joints called

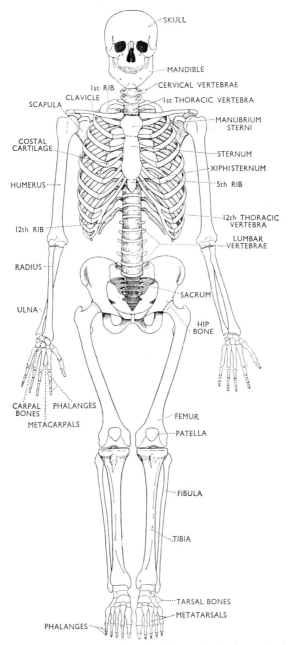

Fig. 39. The skeleton, seen from the front. The left arm is in the anatomical position. The right arm is pronated.

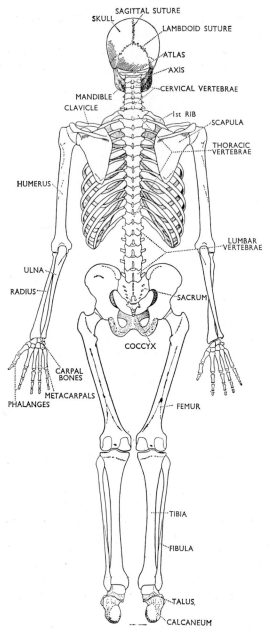

Fig. 40. The skeleton, seen from behind.

sutures (p. 158). The names and positions of these bones are illustrated in
Figs. 41, 42, 43 and 44.

The skull has two regions, the bony box (the **calvaria**) which protects the
brain, and the skeleton of the face, which is fixed to the lower anterior part of
the brain box.

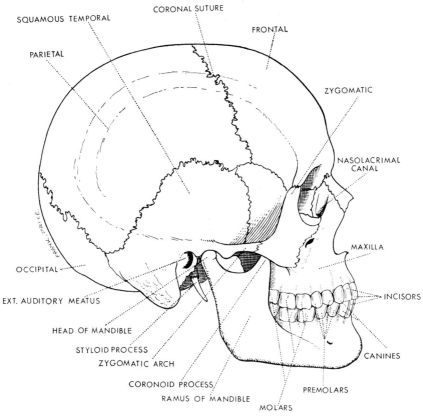

Fig. 41. The skull and mandible, seen from the right side.

THE CALVARIA: From the outside it can be seen that the roof and sides of
the brain box are formed by a number of curved flat bones (Fig. 41)—anteriorly the **frontal bone,** behind that the **parietal bones** and posteriorly the
occipital bone. The frontal bone is jointed to the two parietal bones by the
coronal suture. The **sagittal suture** unites the two parietal bones and the
lambdoid suture is between the parietal bones and the occipital bone (Fig. 40).

On the side of the brain box the **squamous part** of the **temporal bone** can be seen. It is connected to **the petrous part,** the very hard bone, pyramidal

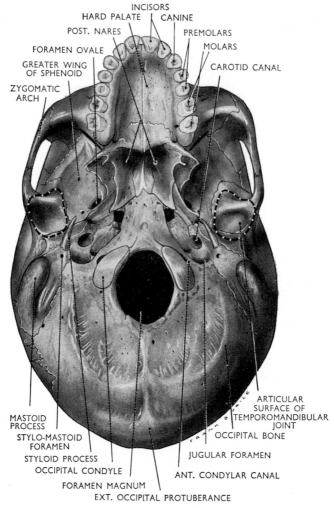

Fig. 42. The skull seen from below. The third molars (wisdom teeth), have not erupted.

in shape which helps to form the base of the skull and which contains the middle ear and the internal ear (p. 304). Below the squamous temporal, a large oval hole, the **external auditory meatus** can be seen. To its edges the cartilaginous external ear is attached. In front of the external auditory meatus, part of the temporal bone, a bar called the **zygoma**, stretches forwards. On the under

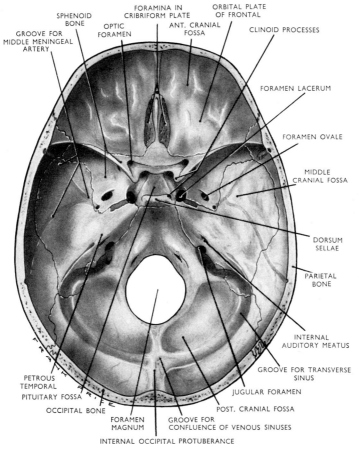

Fig. 43. The base of the skull, seen from above.

surface of its attachment the smooth area for articulation with the mandible can be seen (Fig. 42). This area is nearly circular in outline, but is deeply hollowed out in its posterior part, just in front of the meatus, and convex anteriorly. Behind and below the meatus is the prominent rounded **mastoid process** of the temporal bone which can be palpated in the living subject.

The floor of the brain box is called the **base of the skull** (Fig. 42) and is formed from behind forwards, by part of the occipital bone, by the petrous

(p. 124) part of the temporal bone, by the **sphenoid bone** and by backward projections from the frontal bone which, at the same time, form the roof of the two orbits. The base of the skull contains many holes through which blood

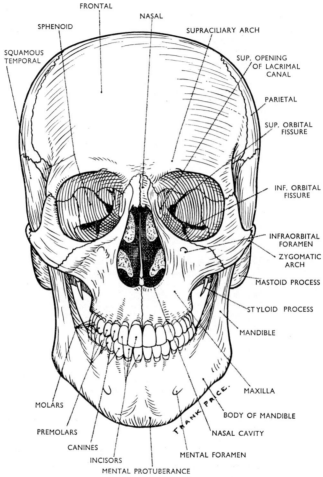

Fig. 44. The skull and mandible, seen from the front.

vessels and nerves enter and leave the skull. The largest, the **foramen magnum** (Fig. 42) in the occipital bone, transmits the spinal cord. The two **occipital condyles** project downwards one on each side of the foramen magnum. The smooth articular surfaces articulate with the atlas (p. 132). On the occipital bone, in the midline, where the back of the brain box turns under to become the base is an irregular prominence, the **external occipital protuberance.** This landmark is easily felt in the living subject.

The floor of the interior of the brain box is divided into three fossæ (Fig. 43). The **anterior cranial fossa,** bounded mainly by the frontal bone, contains the frontal lobes of the cerebral hemispheres. Near the midline, only the **cribriform** (sieve like) **plate** of the **ethmoid bone** separates this part of the cranial

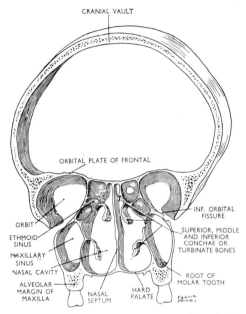

CRANIAL VAULT

ORBITAL PLATE OF FRONTAL

INF. ORBITAL FISSURE

ORBIT

ETHMOID SINUS

SUPERIOR, MIDDLE AND INFERIOR CONCHAE OR TURBINATE BONES

MAXILLARY SINUS

NASAL CAVITY

ROOT OF MOLAR TOOTH

ALVEOLAR MARGIN OF MAXILLA

NASAL SEPTUM

HARD PALATE

Fig. 45. A coronal section through the skull, to show the relationships of the cranial cavity, the nasal cavity, the orbits, the mouth and some of the paranasal sinuses.

cavity from the uppermost part of the nasal cavity. The **middle cranial fossa,** whose floor is formed by the sphenoid bone and the petrous temporal bone, holds the temporal lobes of the cerebral hemispheres. Several parts of the complex **sphenoid bone** can be identified. The central part is the **body** of the sphenoid. It is continuous posteriorly with the occipital bone and carries, on its upper surface, projections which form a hollow, the **hypophyseal fossa** in which the pituitary gland lies. From the body, the paired **greater wings** of the sphenoid extend laterally to form the anterior limit of the lateral part of the middle cranial fossa, and above it the narrow **lesser wings** stretch laterally to form the sharp posterior boundary of the anterior cranial fossa. The **posterior**

cranial fossa, bounded by the petrous temporal bones and the occipital bone contains the pons, medulla oblongata and cerebellum. Wide grooves for the transverse and sigmoid sinuses (p. 376, and **Fig.** 43) can be seen as well as that for the superior sagittal sinus which extends upwards to the roof.

THE SKELETON OF THE FACE (Fig. 44): Below the anterior part of the brain box are two cavities, each shaped like a cone lying on its side. These are the **orbits** which contain the eyeball and its associated structures. The margin

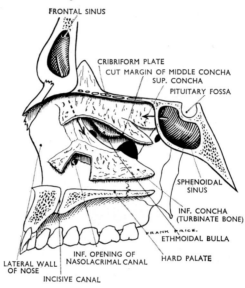

FRONTAL SINUS

CRIBRIFORM PLATE

CUT MARGIN OF MIDDLE CONCHA

SUP. CONCHA

PITUITARY FOSSA

SPHENOIDAL SINUS

INF. CONCHA (TURBINATE BONE)

ETHMOIDAL BULLA

HARD PALATE

INF. OPENING OF NASOLACRIMAL CANAL

LATERAL WALL OF NOSE

INCISIVE CANAL

Fig. 46. The lateral wall of the nasal cavity, seen from inside. Part of the middle concha has been removed to show the sinuses opening into the middle meatus. Part of the inferior concha has been removed to show the nasolacrimal canal opening into the inferior meatus.

of the orbit is easily felt in the living subject. The roof of the orbit is formed mainly by part of the frontal bone which separates it from the anterior cranial fossa above. The floor of the orbit is formed mainly by the maxilla (p. 128). Between the orbits and forming their medial walls, is the **ethmoid bone** (Fig. 45) which surrounds the upper part of the nasal cavity (p. 129). The **maxilla,** the most massive bone of the face lies below orbit and to the lateral side of the nasal cavity. Its lowest part carries the upper teeth (p. 432) and forms the **hard palate** (Fig. 45), which is a horizontal shelf of bone, separating the mouth from the nasal cavity. The lower surface of the hard palate and the part of maxilla carrying the upper teeth can be examined in the living mouth.

The **zygomatic bone** forms the most prominent part of the cheek. It extends upwards to form the lateral margin of the orbit and backwards to meet the zygomatic process of the temporal bone, thus completing the **zygomatic arch** (Fig. 41).

The **nasal cavity** is much more extensive than the appearance of the external nose (i.e. the part visible on the face) suggests. It extends from the **external nares,** which open to the exterior in front, to the **posterior nares** which communicate with the pharynx behind. The floor is the palate which separates the nose from the mouth. The roof is formed by the **cribriform plate**

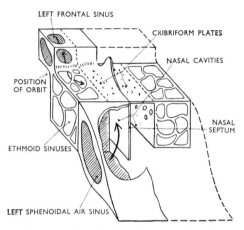

LEFT FRONTAL SINUS

CRIBRIFORM PLATES

NASAL CAVITIES

POSITION
OF ORBIT

NASAL
SEPTUM

ETHMOID SINUSES

LEFT SPHENOIDAL AIR SINUS

Fig. 47. A scheme of the frontal, ethmoidal and sphenoidal sinuses and their relation to the nasal cavity.

of the ethmoid. It also slopes downwards posteriorly, where it is formed by the body of the sphenoid, and in front, where it is formed by the two small **nasal bones** (Fig. 44) which are part of the external nose and can be palpated in the living face. The rest of the external nose has a less rigid cartilaginous skeleton.

The nasal cavity is narrow from side to side, compared with its other dimensions, especially in the upper region which is bounded by parts of the **ethmoid bone** (Fig. 45). The nasal cavity is divided vertically by a thin midline partition, the **nasal septum** (Fig. 45), which is bony behind and cartilaginous in front. From each lateral wall three horizontal bony shelves, each curled like a scroll (Fig. 45) project into the cavity. They are arranged one above the other and are called the inferior, middle and superior **conchæ** (turbinates).

Certain of the bones adjacent to the nose are hollow. The cavities are the **paranasal sinuses** and all of them communicate with the nasal cavity. They serve to lighten the bones and act as resonating chambers for the voice. The **maxillary sinus** in the maxilla (Fig. 45) is lateral to the lower part of the nose and below the orbit. Its opening is high up on its medial wall. The **frontal sinus** (Fig. 46) is in the frontal bone, adjacent to the midline and extending upwards. The **ethmoidal sinuses** (Figs. 45 and 47) are multiple small cavities in the

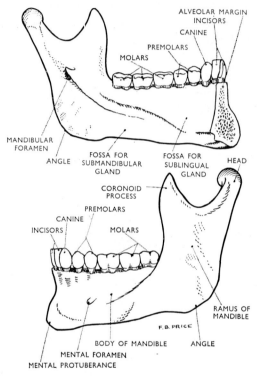

Fig. 48. The mandible, seen from the inside (upper diagram), and from the outside (lower diagram).

ethmoid bone, and the **sphenoidal sinus** occupies the body of the sphenoid (Figs. 46 and 47).

In the anterior part of the infero-medial angle of the orbit a shallow groove, the **lacrimal fossa**, leads down to the upper end of a canal, the **naso-lacrimal canal**, which conveys tears from the eye (p. 289) into the lowest part of the nasal cavity (Figs. 41 and 46).

Mandible. The mandible (Fig. 48) consists of a curved horizontal part, the **body**, which carries the lower teeth and at each end of the body, a vertical part, the **ramus** which, by means of its ovoid **head**, articulates with the skull. The lower border of the body meets the ramus at the **angle of the jaw**. This angle can be felt easily in the living subject in front of and below the lobe of the ear.

Hyoid bone. The hyoid bone is slender and is shaped like the letter U (Fig. 136, D and E). It lies in front of the neck at the root of the tongue, below the mandible and above the larynx. The **body** of the hyoid bone is in front, with a **greater horn** projecting backwards from each end, and a **lesser horn** pointing upwards from the junction of the greater horn with the body.

The hyoid does not articulate with any other bone, but gives attachment to ligaments and muscles, notably to some of the muscles of the tongue, to the middle constrictor of the pharynx and to the infrahyoid muscles (Fig. 89).

The hyoid bone can be palpated in the neck above the larynx. It can be felt to move upwards with the larynx during swallowing.

The Vertebral Column

The vertebral column supports the trunk and protects the spinal cord. It is built of small separate bones, the **vertebræ**, thirty-three in all, connected firmly by joints and ligaments to give a strong but flexible column. The vertebral column has five regions, namely the **cervical region** with seven vertebræ, the **thoracic region** with twelve, the **lumbar region** with five, the **sacral region** with five and the **coccygeal region** with four. In the adult the five sacral vertebræ are fused to form one bone, the **sacrum**, and the four coccygeal vertebræ are rudimentary and partially fused to form the **coccyx** (Fig. 50).

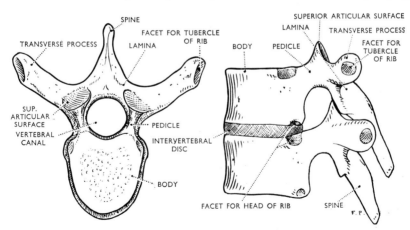

Fig. 49. A typical vertebra (from the thoracic region) seen from above; two typical vertebrae articulated and seen from the side.

Each **vertebra** (Fig. 49) consists of the **body** in front and the **neural arch** behind. The body is a short cylinder of bone with flat upper and lower surfaces. It is connected to the adjacent verebral bodies by cartilaginous joints (p. 159) and forms with them the weight-bearing part of the column. Each half of the neural arch is made up of a cylindrical **pedicle** which is attached to the upper part of the back of the body, and a flatter **lamina.** The two laminæ join in the midline posteriorly to complete the arch. The **spine** projects backwards from this point. On each side where the pedicle joins the lamina, a **transverse process** projects laterally. The spine and the transverse processes are for attachment of muscles. In the thoracic region the transverse processes also articulate with the ribs and help to support them. Near the roots of the transverse processes a pair of **superior articular processes** projects upwards and a similar pair, the **inferior articular processes,** projects downwards. The superior articular processes of one vertebra are connected by small synovial joints with the inferior articular processes of the vertebra above.

When the vertebræ are articulated, the series of neural arches forms the **vertebral canal** which protects the spinal cord and the roots of the spinal nerves. In the articulated column a foramen is present between adjacent pedicles. These foramina are the **intervertebral foramina** through which the spinal nerves emerge.

REGIONAL CHARACTERISTICS:

Cervical vertebræ. Every transverse process of the cervical vertebræ has a foramen through which pass the vertebral vessels. The first cervical vertebra is the **atlas** and the second the **axis.** These two are considerably modified to support the skull and to enable it to move on the vertebral column (Fig. 68).

The atlas has no body but is ring shaped, with a bony arch in front and another behind, these being connected by a lateral mass on each side. Each lateral mass articulates by a facet on its upper surface with the occipital condyle of the skull and by a facet on its under surface with the axis.

The axis, the second cervical vertebra, has projecting from the upper surface of its body, a peg-like process, the dens, which articulates with the back of the anterior arch of the atlas.

Thoracic vertebræ have facets on the bodies and on the transverse processes for articulation with the ribs.

Lumbar vertebræ have massive bodies for bearing the weight of the trunk.

Sacrum. Though the sacral vertebræ are fused to form a single bone, some of their individual parts, e.g. the bodies and the spines, can be identified. The anterior and posterior sacral foramina seen respectively on the front and on the back of the sacrum, transmit the branches of the sacral nerves (p. 278). The upper part of the body of the first sacral vertebra projects forwards (Fig. 50) and is called the **sacral promontory**. On each side of the sacrum is an area, ear-shaped in outline, for articulation with the hip-bone at the sacro-iliac joint.

Coccyx. Vestiges of the individual vertebræ can be seen.

THE VERTEBRAL COLUMN AS A WHOLE: The articulated vertebral column presents four well-marked curves in the sagittal plane (Fig. 50). The **thoracic curve** and the **sacral curve** are concave forwards, and are present in the early embryo. The **cervical** and **lumbar curves** are convex forwards and develop after birth, the cervical when the child begins to lift its head and the lumbar when the child begins to stand up.

The curves give added elasticity to the column and help to make weight bearing easier.

Exaggeration of the thoracic curve is **kyphosis** and exaggeration of the lumbar curve is **lordosis**. Abnormal lateral curves are **scoliosis**. So that balance may be maintained, any curvature of the vertebral column is accompanied by a corresponding curve in the opposite direction above or below or both.

The Skeleton of the Thorax

This comprises the twelve thoracic vertebræ, twelve pairs of ribs and the sternum.

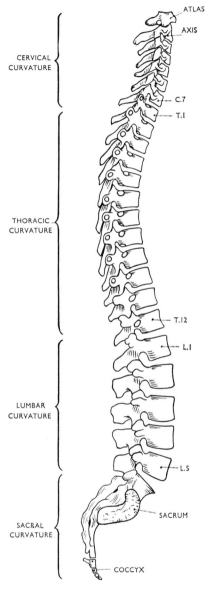

Fig. 50. The vertebræ, arranged to show the curves of the vertebral column, seen from the right side.

vertebræ, twelve pairs of ribs and the sternum.

Ribs. Each rib is a very elongated flat bone. A typical rib has a long narrow curved **shaft** with an internal and an external surface. At the posterior end is a small rounded knob, the **head,** which bears two articular facets, one for articulation with the vertebra of its own number and one for the vertebra above. The head is joined to the shaft by a narrow **neck.** On the shaft close to the neck is a prominence, the **tubercle** which articulates with the transverse process of the vertebra of its own number. To the anterior end of each rib is attached a bar of hyaline cartilage, the **costal cartilage,** which may articulate with the sternum or with the costal cartilage above.

The first seven pairs of ribs are **true ribs;** their cartilages articulate in front with the sides of the sternum. The eighth, ninth and tenth pairs are **false ribs;** their cartilages articulate each with the cartilage above. The eleventh and twelfth pairs are **floating ribs;** their cartilages have no articulation but are embedded in the muscles of the abdominal wall.

Sternum. (Fig. 39). The sternum is an elongated flat bone situated in the midline of the upper part of the front of the thorax. It has a **body,** with which the **manubrium,** its upper part, articulates by means of a permanent cartilaginous joint. The sternum is angulated at this joint which is easily felt under the skin and is called the **sternal angle** (angle of Louis). The **xiphoid process** is a flat irregular triangle of cartilage or bone which juts down from the lower end of the body into the anterior wall of the abdomen. It is joined to the body by the **xiphisternal joint.**

The medial ends of the clavicles articulate with the upper lateral angles of the manubrium. The costal cartilages of the first seven pairs of ribs articulate with the sides of the sternum, the first pair just below the clavicle, the second at the level of the sternal angle, the others with the body. Like other flat bones, the sternum contains red marrow even in the adult. Samples of bone marrow are often obtained by puncturing the sternum and withdrawing some of the marrow into a syringe, so that the blood forming cells can be examined.

The articulated bones of the thorax form a cage (Figs. 39 and 40), which protects the heart, lungs and upper abdominal viscera. The cage is barrel-shaped, but narrower above than below, longer behind than in front and compressed from front to back, so that it is wider from side to side. The bodies of the vertebræ project forwards into the cavity (see p. 588).

The upper end of the thorax communicates with the neck at the **inlet.** This is bounded by the first thoracic vertebra, the first pair of ribs and the upper border of the manubrium. The inlet slopes from above downwards and forwards. The lower end of the thorax, the **outlet,** is bounded by the xiphisternal joint, the lower six pairs of costal cartilages, which form the '**costal**

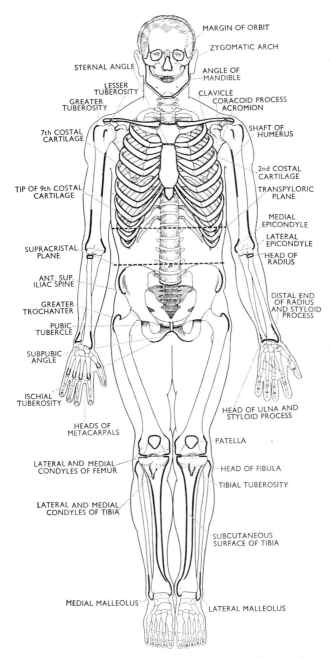

MARGIN OF ORBIT

ZYGOMATIC ARCH

STERNAL ANGLE

ANGLE OF MANDIBLE

LESSER TUBEROSITY

GREATER TUBEROSITY

CLAVICLE
CORACOID PROCESS
ACROMION

7th COSTAL CARTILAGE

SHAFT OF HUMERUS

2nd COSTAL CARTILAGE

TIP OF 9th COSTAL CARTILAGE

TRANSPYLORIC PLANE

MEDIAL EPICONDYLE

LATERAL EPICONDYLE

SUPRACRISTAL PLANE

HEAD OF RADIUS

ANT. SUP. ILIAC SPINE

GREATER TROCHANTER

DISTAL END OF RADIUS AND STYLOID PROCESS

PUBIC TUBERCLE

SUBPUBIC ANGLE

ISCHIAL TUBEROSITY

HEADS OF METACARPALS

HEAD OF ULNA AND STYLOID PROCESS

PATELLA

LATERAL AND MEDIAL CONDYLES OF FEMUR

HEAD OF FIBULA

TIBIAL TUBEROSITY

LATERAL AND MEDIAL CONDYLES OF TIBIA

SUBCUTANEOUS SURFACE OF TIBIA

MEDIAL MALLEOLUS

LATERAL MALLEOLUS

Fig. 51. The skeleton superimposed on an outline of the body seen from the front. The parts of the bones which can be felt easily are marked heavily.

margin', the shafts of the twelfth ribs and the twelfth thoracic vertebra. The outlet is closed by the diaphragm (p. 198).

Surface anatomy. Much of the thoracic cage can be identified by palpation in the living subject, although it is largely covered by muscles of the upper limbs and abdominal walls to which it gives origin. The **suprasternal notch** between the medial ends of the clavicles is easily identified. A finger drawn downwards from it over the front of the sternum encounters a horizontal ridge which represents the **sternal angle**. The **second costal cartilage** articulates with the sternum at this angle and can be identified. The other costal cartilages, ribs and intercostal spaces can then be numbered. The **costal margin** can be palpated and the tips of the eighth, ninth and tenth costal cartilages are identified as irregularities. The **tip of the ninth costal cartilage** lies in the transpyloric plane at the level of the first lumbar vertebra (p. 205). In the lower part of the back of the neck one vertebral spine is more prominent than any other. It is the **seventh cervical**. The thoracic spines can then be numbered from it. Note that the middle thoracic spines slope downwards so much that the tip of a given spine is at the level of the lower part of the body of the vertebra below.

THE SKELETON OF THE LIMBS

The Skeleton of the Upper Limb

Shoulder girdle. The shoulder girdle connects the free upper limb with the trunk. It consists of two bones, the clavicle and the scapula.

Scapula (Fig. 52). The scapula or shoulder blade is a flat bone, triangular in outline. One of its flat surfaces faces one side of the upper part of the back of the thorax. The **spine** of the scapula projects from the posterior surface (Fig. 53) and ends laterally in a prominence, the **acromion** which overhangs the shoulder joint. The **acromion** articulates with the clavicle. The upper lateral angle of the scapula carries the **glenoid fossa** which is a very shallow hollow, oval in outline, for articulation with the head of the humerus. Medial to the glenoid fossa the **coracoid process** (Fig. 52) projects forwards from the upper border of the scapula.

The flat surfaces and prominent spine of the scapula present extensive areas for attachment of the muscles which connect the shoulder girdle with the trunk and with the free upper limb.

The spine, the acromion, the coracoid process, the medial border and the inferior angle can be felt in the living subject. To feel the coracoid process

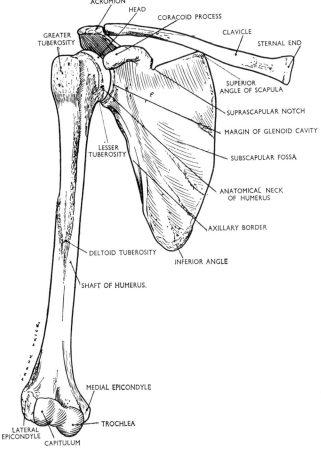

Fig. 52. The right clavicle, scapula and humerus, seen from the front.

palpate deeply in the hollow below the lateral third of the clavicle and move the shoulder girdle so that the coracoid process moves under the examining fingers.

Clavicle. The clavicle (Fig. 52) is a slender long bone which articulates at its lateral end with the acromion of the scapula and at its medial end with the manubrium of the sternum. It helps to brace the shoulder away from the trunk, in this way facilitating free movement of the upper limb.

The clavicle can be palpated throughout its length.

Humerus. The humerus is the bone of the upper arm. It is a typical long bone (p. 117). The upper end consists of the head and the greater and lesser

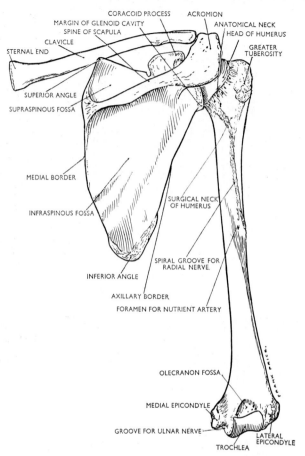

Fig. 53. The right clavicle, scapula and humerus, seen from behind.

tuberosities. The **head** is rounded and smooth for articulation with the glenoid fossa of the scapula at the shoulder joint. The **greater tuberosity** and the **lesser tuberosity** are prominences close to the lateral aspect of the head. They are for the attachment of muscles. Between them is a groove, the **intertubercular** (bicipital) **groove,** in which the tendon of the long head of the biceps muscle lies. The head is separated from the tuberosities laterally and from the shaft by an ill-defined groove, the **anatomical neck.** The narrower region which connects the head and tuberosities with the shaft is called the **surgical neck** (Fig. 52).

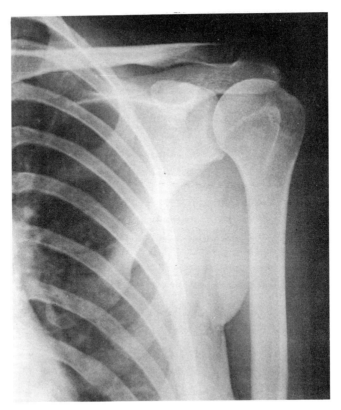

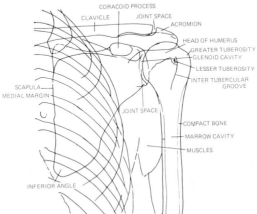

CORACOID PROCESS

CLAVICLE   JOINT SPACE

ACROMION

HEAD OF HUMERUS

GREATER TUBEROSITY

GLENOID CAVITY

LESSER TUBEROSITY

INTER TUBERCULAR
GROOVE

SCAPULA

MEDIAL MARGIN

JOINT SPACE

COMPACT BONE

MARROW CAVITY

MUSCLES

INFERIOR ANGLE

Fig. 54. A radiograph of the shoulder region, posterior view, showing the clavicle, scapula, humerus, acromioclavicular joint and shoulder joint.

The **shaft** is cylindrical. Half way down on the lateral aspect is a rough area, the **deltoid tuberosity,** for insertion of the deltoid muscle. On the back of the shaft, extending obliquely downwards from the medial to the lateral side, is a shallow groove, the spiral groove, in which the radial nerve lies.

The lower end of the humerus is flattened in front and behind. It carries the **capitulum,** the **trochlea** and the **medial** and **lateral epicondyles** (Figs. 52 and 71). The capitulum, towards the lateral side, is smooth and rounded for articulation with the head of the radius. The trochlea, more medial, is pulley-shaped and articulates with the trochlear notch of the ulna. The medial and lateral epicondyles, are for attachment of muscles. Above the trochlea on the back of the bone is a deep hollow, the **olecranon fossa,** into which the olecranon of the ulna fits when the arm is extended at the elbow joint. On the front of the bone the **coronoid fossa** above the trochlea, and the **radial fossa** above the capitulum accommodate the coronoid process of the ulna and the head of the radius respectively in flexion at the elbow joint.

The greater tuberosity and the medial and lateral epicondyles can be felt easily in the living subject.

Radius and **ulna.** The radius and the ulna are the bones of the forearm. Both are typical long bones. In the anatomical position, i.e. with the forearm in the supine position, they are parallel, with the radius on the lateral side (often, therefore, called the radial side) and the ulna on the medial (or ulnar) side.

Radius. The proximal end of the radius is the **head** which is a short cylinder connected with the shaft by the narrow **neck** (Fig. 55). The sides of the head are smooth to articulate with the radial notch of the ulna at the superior radio-ulnar joint. The proximal surface of the head is smooth and a little concave to articulate with the capitulum of the humerus at the elbow joint.

The cylindrical shaft has a sharp edge along its medial aspect, to which the interosseous membrane is attached. Just below the neck, on the medial side of the shaft, is the very prominent **tuberosity of the radius** into which the biceps is inserted.

The lower end of the radius is relatively thick and broad and articulates by its distal surface with the proximal row of carpal bones. The medial surface of the distal end of the radius carries the **ulnar notch,** to articulate with the head of the ulna. The base of the triangular cartilage of the wrist joint is attached to the ridge which separates these two articular surfaces (Fig. 73). The **styloid process** points downwards from the lateral side of the lower end of the radius.

Ulna. The proximal end of the ulna bears the **olecranon process** in line with the shaft, the **coronoid process** on the front of the upper end of the shaft and the **trochlear notch** between these two processes (Fig. 55). The trochlear notch articulates with the trochlea of the humerus. The processes give attachment to muscles.

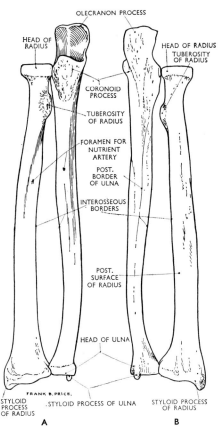

Fig. 55. The right radius and the right ulna seen A, from the front and B, from behind.

The lateral aspect of the coronoid process carries a smooth notch, the **radial notch** for articulation with the head of the radius.

The shaft is cylindrical, and along the sharp border on its lateral aspect is attached the interosseous membrane which connects it with the shaft of the radius.

The lower end is smooth and rounded and is called the **head.** (*Note that the* term 'head' as applied to bones refers to the shape of the part, not to a position at the proximal end of a bone.) It articulates with the ulnar notch on the distal end of the radius and with the upper surface of the triangular cartilage of the wrist joint. From the medial part of the lower end of the ulna the **styloid process**

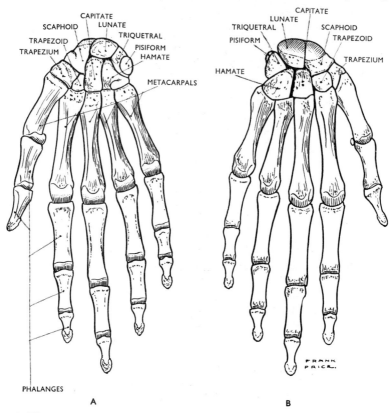

Fig. 56. The skeleton of the right hand seen A, from the front and B, from behind.

points downwards. The apex of the triangular cartilage is attached to the base of the styloid process.

The proximal half of the radius is surrounded by muscles, but the head can be felt, especially during movements of pronation and supination. The back of the lower end of the radius, and especially the styloid process are easily felt. The olecranon process of the ulna and the whole length of the shaft can be felt, together with the head and styloid process. The tip of the styloid process of the radius is lower than that of the ulna.

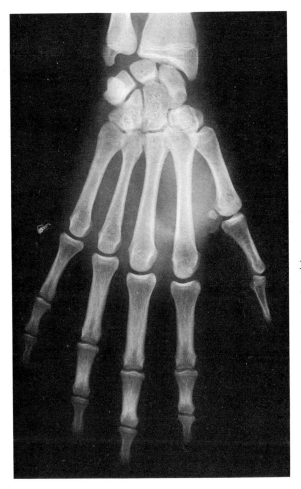

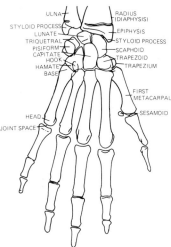

Fig. 57. A radiograph of the wrist and hand, almost adult. Notice the epiphysis for the head of the ulna which is partially fused.

The radius is the weight-bearing bone of the forearm. The hand articulates with it and not with the ulna. The shafts of the radius and ulna, with the interosseous membrane connecting them, form a wide area for attachment of the muscles of the forearm.

THE HAND: The hand consists of the carpus, or wrist, the metacarpus and the digits or fingers.

The **carpus** consists of eight small bones—short bones—arranged in two rows of four (Figs. 56 and 57). Named from lateral to medial side they are the **scaphoid, lunate, triquetral** and **pisiform** in the proximal row, and the

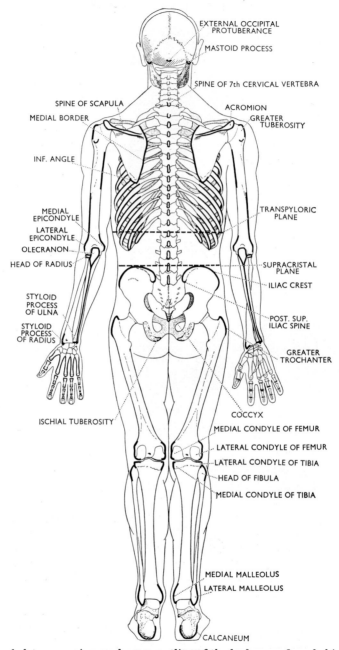

Fig. 58. The skeleton superimposed on an outline of the body seen from behind. The parts of the bones which can be easily felt are marked heavily.

trapezium, trapezoid, capitate and hamate in the distal row. Looked at from the front they form a hollow which the flexor retinaculum (see p. 193) converts into the carpal tunnel.

The five metacarpal bones, miniature long bones, articulate with the distal row of the carpus, and with each metacarpal bone one finger articulates.

The five digits are, named from the lateral side, the thumb, the index finger, the middle finger, the ring finger and the little finger. (To avoid mistakes it is preferable to use these names rather than to number the digits from one to five starting with the thumb.)

The bones of the digits are miniature long bones, the phalanges. The thumb has two and all the others have three.

The Skeleton of the Lower Limb

Pelvic girdle. The pelvic girdle (Fig. 59) connects the lower limbs with the trunk. It has to be strong and stable to carry the weight of the body, and so mobility of the girdle is restricted. This contrasts strongly with the shoulder girdle which is specialized for mobility.

The pelvic girdle is composed of the two hip bones and the sacrum (p. 132). The two hip bones articulate anteriorly in the midline at the symphysis pubis, and each articulates with the sacrum at the sacro-iliac joint. The incorporation of the sacral part of the vertebral column into the pelvic girdle adds to its strength and stability.

Hip bone. The hip bone (Fig. 59) is a large irregular bone formed of three bones, the ilium, the ischium and the pubis which are united in the region of the acetabulum.

The acetabulum, which is on the lateral aspect, is a deep cup-shaped socket for the head of the femur. The ilium forms the upper part of the bone and is wide and flat; medially it is thick and strong to transmit the body weight from the sacrum to the femur (Fig. 61); the medial surface forms the floor of the iliac fossa of the abdominal cavity and its posterior part carries the surface for articulation with the sacrum; the lateral surface gives origin to the gluteal muscles (p. 212); the upper border, the iliac crest is long and sinuous, ending anteriorly in the anterior superior iliac spine and posteriorly in the posterior superior iliac spine. The ischium is the lower posterior part of the bone; it carries the ischial spine, which points medially, and the ischial tuberosity which bears the weight of the body in the sitting position and gives origin to the hamstring muscles (p. 216). The pubis forms the anterior part of the bone and is flat and rectangular. Its upper border carries a rough ridge, the pubic crest which ends laterally in the pubic tubercle. From the pubis the

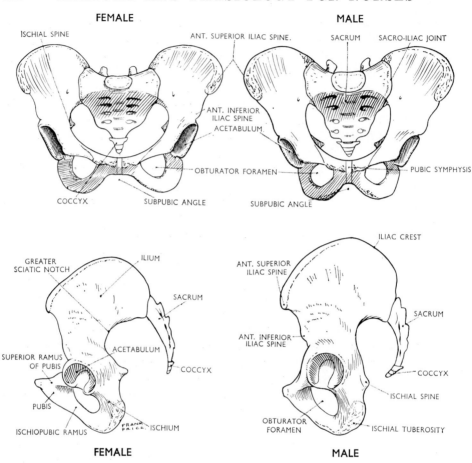

Fig. 59. The female pelvis and the male pelvis, seen from the front, and from the side.

superior ramus passes to the acetabulum and the **inferior ramus** joins the **ramus of the ischium** which extends forwards from the ischial tuberosity. This **ischiopubic ramus** gives origin to the adductor muscles (p. 216). Bounded by the ischium and pubis and the rami is a large oval foramen, the **obturator fora-men,** which in life is closed by the **obturator membrane,** except for a canal in its upper part which transmits the obturator nerve and vessels. On the pos-terior border of the hip bone, the **greater sciatic notch** lies between the ilium and the ischial spine and the **lesser sciatic notch** is between the ischial spine and the ischial tuberosity.

THE PELVIS AS A WHOLE: The bony pelvis has two parts, the **greater (false) pelvis** which consists of the two iliac fossæ and forms part of the boundaries of the abdominal cavity, and the **lesser (true) pelvis** which is the pudding-basin shaped lower part. The lesser pelvis is a short wide canal with an inlet or **pelvic brim,** bounded by the promontory of the sacrum, the arcuate line of the ilium, the pubic crest and the upper border of the symphysis pubis; and an **outlet** bounded by the coccyx, the sacrotuberous ligaments (p. 168), the ischio-pubic ramus and the lower border of the symphysis pubis. The cavity between inlet and outlet forms a curved passage with a short anterior wall, the symphysis pubis, and a long curved posterior wall, the sacrum and coccyx.

In the ordinary standing position, the pelvis is orientated so that the anterior superior iliac spine and the pubic tubercle are in the same vertical plane; the upper border of the symphysis pubis, the spine of the ischium and the tip of the coccyx are in the same horizontal plane. The plane of the inlet of the lesser pelvis, therefore, faces more forwards than upwards.

Several parts of the pelvis can be felt in the living subject and form useful landmarks. The crest of the ilium can be felt below the waist and traced throughout its length, forwards to the anterior superior spine and backwards to the posterior superior spine. The highest part of the iliac crest, well round to the back, is at the level of the fourth lumbar vertebra. The pubis, the pubic symphysis, pubic crest, pubic tubercle and ischio-pubic ramus can all be palpated easily. The sub-pubic angle can be estimated by feeling the two ischio-pubic rami. The ischial tuberosities (Figs. 51 and 58) are easily identified by hands placed under the buttocks when the subject is in the sitting position.

Femur. The femur is the bone of the thigh (Fig. 60). The upper end articulates with the hip bone at the hip joint and the lower end with the tibia at the knee joint. It is large and strong to enable it to help to carry the body weight.

The femur is a typical long bone. The upper end carries the spherical **head** which fits into the acetabulum of the hip bone. The head is joined to the shaft by a **neck,** some two inches long, which makes an angle of about 120° with the shaft. The **greater trochanter** is a massive prominence on the lateral side of the junction of the neck and shaft. It gives attachment to muscles including gluteus medius and minimus. The **lesser trochanter** is a smaller prominence on the posteromedial aspect. It is for the insertion of psoas. The shaft is smooth except for a wide rough line, the **linea aspera,** on the posterior aspect. The lower end of the femur consists of two rounded masses, the **medial** and **lateral condyles,** which are united in front, but separated behind by the deep **intercondylar notch.** The distal surfaces of the condyles are smooth for articulation with the tibia, and the articular surface which unites them in front is for the patella.

The femur is well clothed by muscles and most of it cannot be palpated in

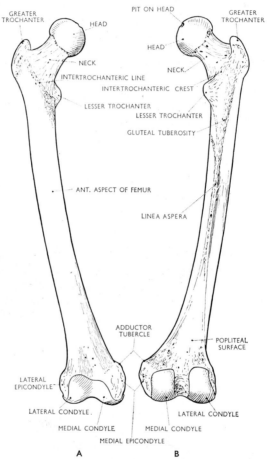

Fig. 60. The right femur: A, seen from the front; B, seen from behind.

the living subject. However, the greater trochanter and the outline of the condyles can be made out (Figs. 51 and 58).

Patella. The patella or knee cap is a **sesamoid bone** (a bone situated in a tendon where this plays on a bone) in the tendon of insertion of the quadriceps femoris (p. 214). It is round and flattened and articulates with the front of the

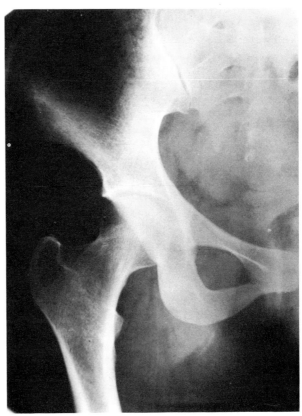

Fig. 61. A radiograph of the hip region.
The trabeculae in the spongy bone are
arranged along the lines of stress.

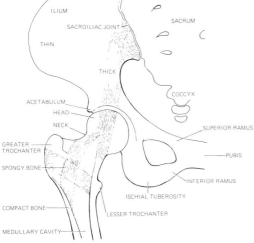

ILIUM

SACRUM

SACROILIAC JOINT

THIN

THICK

COCCYX

ACETABULUM

HEAD

NECK

SUPERIOR RAMUS

GREATER
TROCHANTER

PUBIS

SPONGY BONE

INFERIOR RAMUS

ISCHIAL TUBEROSITY

COMPACT BONE

LESSER TROCHANTER

MEDULLARY CAVITY

lower end of the femur. Its outline can be made out in the living subject and, when the quadriceps is relaxed, it can be moved from side to side.

Tibia. The tibia is the weight-bearing bone of the leg, i.e. the segment of

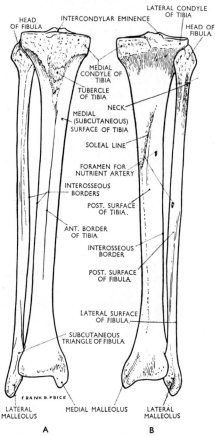

Fig. 62. The right tibia and fibula: A, seen from the front and B, seen from behind.

the lower limb between the knee and the ankle. It articulates above with the femoral condyles and below with the talus. It is a typical long bone (Fig. 62).

The massive upper end carries on its proximal surface for articulation with the femoral condyles, two oval, very slightly concave articular surfaces separated by a very rough **intercondylar eminence**. On the anterior aspect at the upper end of the shaft is the prominent rough **tuberosity** of the tibia for insertion of the patellar ligament. The shaft is strong and triangular in section. The medial surface is subcutaneous and the lateral border gives attachment to the interosseous membrane which connects it with the shaft of the fibula. The lower end is only slightly expanded. The medial part extends downwards as a pointed prominence, the **medial malleolus.** The distal surface of the lower end and the lateral surface of the medial malleolus, together with the lower end of the fibula, form the surface for articulation with the talus.

The outline of the upper end, the tuberosity, the subcutaneous surface and the medial malleolus are all easily palpated in the living limb (Figs. 51 and 58).

Fibula. The fibula is the second bone of the leg, and lies parallel with and postero-lateral to the tibia (Figs. 62 and 79). It is a long bone. The upper end, cubical in shape, articulates with the lateral part of the upper end of the tibia. The shaft, long and slender, is moulded by the attachment of many muscles and by the interosseous membrane by which it is connected with the shaft of the tibia. The pointed lower end forms the **lateral malleolus** and articulates with the talus.

The head and the lower end can be palpated in the living leg.

THE FOOT: The skeleton of the foot is basically similar to that of the hand, but is much modified to form a strong resilient arched structure (Figs. 63, 80 and 81) for weight bearing in the upright position.

The **tarsus** consists of seven bones as follows: The **talus,** which articulates with the tibia and fibula at the ankle joint, rests on the upper surface of the **calcaneum** whose posterior part forms the heel. The **cuboid** is in front of the calcaneum, and the **navicular** and **three cuneiform bones** are in front of the talus (Figs. 80 and 63). The five metatarsal bones articulate with the tarsus proximally, and distally with the five digits named from medial to lateral side, the great toe, the second, third, fourth and little toes.

The longitudinal arch of the foot has for its posterior pillar the posterior end of the calcaneum and for its anterior pillar the heads of the metatarsal bones. The transverse arch consists of the cuboid and cuneiform bones, together with the bases of the metatarsals.

SEX DIFFERENCES IN THE LOWER LIMB AND ITS GIRDLE: The female pelvis is modified for child bearing and the lesser pelvis is, therefore, roomy to allow the passage of the infant through it. The inlet is oval; the cavity is short and wide; and the outlet is as large as possible because of the wide sub-pubic angle (more than 90°), because the ischial spines point downwards rather than medially and because the mobile coccyx is well back owing to the straightness of the female sacrum (Fig. 59).

The male pelvis, although like other male bones it is large and massively built, has a small lesser pelvis. The inlet is heart-shaped because the sacral

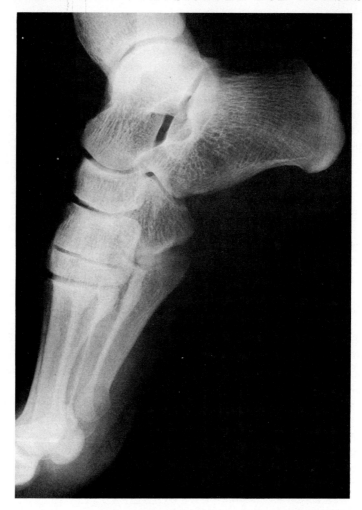

promontory projects more; the cavity is longer and narrower; and the outlet is restricted by the narrow sub-pubic angle (less than 90°), the medially pointing ischial spines and the forward curve of the coccyx and lower part of the sacrum (Fig. 59).

As for other bones, the female femur is smaller and lighter and has less prominent markings than the male bone. In addition the shaft is more oblique in the female and the angle between neck and shaft is smaller. This is because

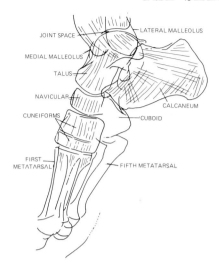

JOINT SPACE

LATERAL MALLEOLUS

MEDIAL MALLEOLUS

TALUS

NAVICULAR

CALCANEUM

CUNEIFORMS

CUBOID

FIRST METATARSAL

FIFTH METATARSAL

Fig. 63. A radiograph of the ankle and foot. Observe the trabeculae in the spongy bone, arranged along the lines of stress, and indicating the longitudinal arch.

of the extra width of the female pelvis (p. 151) and the relative shortness of the femur.

Because the upper ends of the femora are further apart in the female, there is increased angulation between the femur and the tibia in the region of the knee (Fig. 2). As the pull of the quadriceps muscle (p. 214) is along the axis of the femur, and that of the patellar ligament along the axis of the tibia, the increased angulation between those two bones in females results in women being more subject to dislocation (outwards) of the patella to which both the quadriceps muscle and patellar ligament are attached.

EPIPHYSES

The epiphyses of the different bones are indicated in Fig. 233. Typical long bones have an epiphysis (sometimes more than one) at each end. Short bones usually have no epiphyses. Flat and irregular bones have epiphyses round their margins and on prominences. (See also p. 109.)

JOINTS

A **joint** *is the union of two or more parts of the skeleton.* The nature of the union, that is the **structure of the joint,** depends on the requirements of **function.** A joint may be:

(*a*) movable (structure **synovial**)

(*b*) immovable (structure **fibrous**)

(*c*) partially movable (structure **cartilaginous**)

The different types of joint are illustrated in Fig. 64.

MOVABLE JOINTS

Most joints exist to allow adjacent rigid bones to move in relation to each other. These are the movable joints and, so that the movements may be really free, their complex structure includes a synovial membrane (q.v.) Hence these joints are called **synovial joints.**

Structure of a Synovial Joint

The articulating surfaces on the bones are smooth and are made even smoother by a layer of hyaline cartilage, so that they move on each other without friction. The bones are connected by a **joint capsule** or capsular ligament. This is a tube of fibrous tissue which encloses the ends of the bones and is attached to them near the edges of the articular surfaces. An interval, the **joint cavity,** is thus enclosed, bounded by the capsule and the bones. The capsule is lined by the thin **synovial membrane** which has a smooth shiny surface composed of a single layer of pavement epithelium. This synovial membrane extends from the inside of the capsule over every surface inside the joint, with the exception of the hyaline cartilage on the articular surfaces. Therefore, if one were able to stand inside the joint cavity everything in sight would be smooth and shining, being covered either by synovial membrane or by hyaline cartilage. The smoothness of these surfaces minimizes friction. Furthermore, the surfaces are lubricated by a small amount of **synovial fluid,** a clear liquid secretion of the synovial membrane.

It must be realized that the joint cavity in health is only a capillary interval, since the surfaces which bound it are in contact. The joint cavity becomes a real entity if it is filled with a pathological excess of fluid, e.g. in 'water on the knee' or with air when the capsule is opened at an operation.

A joint is made stronger by **ligaments** which are bands of fibrous tissue stretching from one bone to the other. Sometimes these ligaments are closely blended with the capsular ligament, e.g. the ilio-femoral ligament at the hip joint. In other cases, they are quite separate from the capsule, e.g. the lateral ligament of the knee joint. These ligaments are so situated as to withstand the special tensions at a given part of the joint.

Some synovial joints have an **articular disc,** made of fibrocartilage, interposed between the articulating surfaces of the bones, to help them to fit together

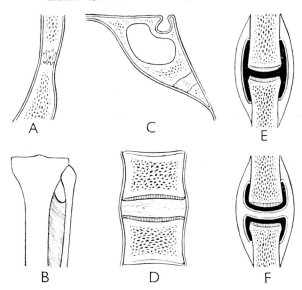

Fig. 64. Kinds of joints: A and B are fibrous joints (A, a suture; B, the interosseous membrane in the leg); C and D are cartilaginous joints (C, a temporary cartilaginous joint, between the body of the sphenoid and the occipital bone in the base of the skull; D, a permanent cartilaginous joint between the bodies of adjacent vertebræ); E and F are synovial joints (E is a typical synovial joint; in F the joint cavity is divided by an intra-articular disc).

better. The circumference of the disc is attached to the capsule, thus dividing the joint cavity into two parts. The temporomandibular joint contains such a disc, and the knee joint has two menisci which form an incomplete partition across the joint cavity.

Radiology of Joints

In radiographs of synovial joints the thin layer of compact bone covering the expanded end of one bone is separated from that of the other bone by a dark interval, the **radiological joint space** (Figs. 54, 57, 61, 63, 71 and 78). This represents the thickness of the hyaline cartilage covering the bony surfaces and any articular disc which may be present. It should be realized that the radiological joint space is **not** the joint cavity which is a capillary interval (see above).

Types of Synovial Joints (Fig. 65).

The shape of the articulating surfaces varies greatly from one joint to another, and is always closely related to the kind of movement which takes

Type of synovial joint	Examples	Movements allowed
Ball and socket	Hip Shoulder	'Universal joint' Flexion Extension Abduction Adduction Medial rotation Lateral rotation Circumduction
Condyloid	Wrist Metacarpophalangeal	Flexion Extension Abduction Adduction
Hinge	Elbow Knee Ankle Temporomandibular Interphalangeal	Flexion Extension
Pivot	Superior radio-ulnar Inferior radio-ulnar Odontoid process and atlas	Rotation in the long axis of one of the bones, i.e. pivoting
Plane	Intercarpal Intertarsal	Gliding

place at the joint. The types of synovial joint are named according to the shapes of the bones they join (see table above).

BALL AND SOCKET: At a 'ball and socket' joint, the spherical end of one bone fits into a cup-shaped socket on the other. At such a joint, movement can take place in any direction. Good examples are at the **shoulder** joint and the **hip** joint.

CONDYLOID: At a condyloid joint, which resembles a ball and socket joint, the ball is ovoid instead of spherical and the socket corresponds in shape. The **wrist** joint is one example. This modification in shape results in limitation of movement, so that only flexion and extension, abduction and adduction can be effected.

HINGE: A hinge joint allows only flexion and extension. One bone has a pulley-shaped surface to which the other corresponds. Good examples are the **elbow** and the **ankle** joints.

PIVOT: At a pivot joint one bone pivots on its own long axis, like the radius at the **superior radio-ulnar** joint.

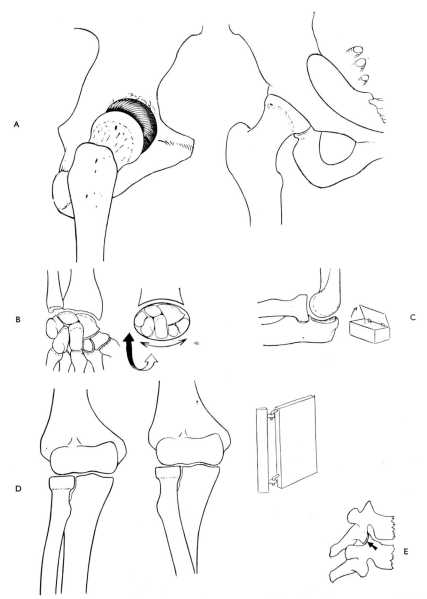

Fig. 65. Types of synovial joint: A, ball and socket joint (hip joint); B, condyloid joint (wrist joint); C, hinge joint (elbow joint;); D, pivot joint (superior radio-ulnar joint which allows the bones to pivot round each other as in the accompanying model; E, plane joint (joint between articular processes of vertebrae).

PLANE: A plane joint has two flat surfaces in articulation and allows gliding movements in any direction in that one plane. The joints between the bones of **carpus** and **tarsus** and between the articular processes of vertebrae are examples.

Movement

The possible movement at a synovial joint, whatever its type, may range from being very extensive to being very restricted. On the whole, the greater the range of movement, the less stable the joint (that is, the more likely it is to be dislocated), and vice versa. Mobility and stability are mutually incompatible.

It is important that the allowable range of movement at a joint should not be exceeded. Several kinds of **limiting factors** come into play. Firstly, and most important, **muscle tone** limits movements. For example, in flexion the tone of the extensor muscles eventually stops the movement. The muscles grouped around the capsule of the shoulder joint, by their tone, prevent movements from going too far.

Ligaments play an obvious important part in restricting movements. The ilio-femoral ligament of the hip joint effectively limits extension. **Apposition of soft tissues** may stop a movement, for example in flexion at the elbow joint, when the front of the forearm comes into contact with the front of the arm. Movement may be limited also by the **apposition of bony surfaces** as in extension at the elbow joint, when the olecranon process of the ulna comes into contact with the back of the humerus.

In people who are 'double jointed' the range of movement at the joints is greater than is usual. This is mainly due to a low level of tone in the muscles and laxity of the ligaments which usually restrict the movements. In acrobats an unusually wide range of movement is attained by long training and practice. The reverse happens if joints are not used regularly, for example in patients confined to bed for long periods without exercise. The muscles lose the ability to relax and movements become very restricted.

Immovable Joints

Most immovable joints are fibrous in structure. The bones are simply bound together by collagenous connective tissue. The joints between the bones of the vault of the skull, the **sutures,** are good examples.

Partially Movable Joints

Most partially movable joints are cartilaginous in structure. At some cartilaginous joints one bone is joined to the other by hyaline cartilage. In growing long bones (p. 109) the ossified ends are joined to the ossified shafts in this way. These joints are **temporary** and are obliterated by bone as the skeleton grows older.

At **permanent** cartilaginous joints the structure is a little more complex. The ends of the bones, covered by a layer of hyaline cartilage, are connected by a **disc of fibro-cartilage.** Ligaments of connective tissue support the joint on the outside. The most important joints of this kind are **between the bodies of the vertebræ** (p. 132). The **symphysis pubis** and the **manubriosternal** joint are other examples. It so happens that all permanent cartilaginous joints are situated in the midline of the body.

INDIVIDUAL JOINTS

THE TEMPOROMANDIBULAR JOINT: This joint is a synovial joint of the hinge variety. The ovoid head of the mandible articulates with the temporal bone of the skull (Fig. 66) at a surface which is concave behind and convex in

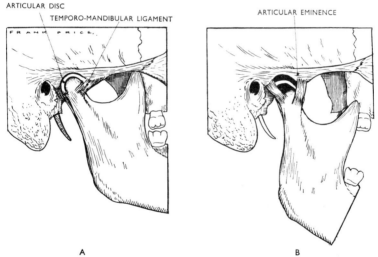

ARTICULAR DISC
TEMPORO-MANDIBULAR LIGAMENT
ARTICULAR EMINENCE

FRANK PRICE.

A   B

Fig. 66. The temporomandibular joint: A, mouth closed; B, mouth open.

front (p. 125). The joint is enclosed by a capsule and the cavity is divided into two parts by a disc of fibrocartilage, the surfaces of which are shaped to fit the incongruous bony surfaces of the joint.

During opening of the mouth, the head of the mandible is first drawn forwards on to the convexity of the temporal surface. This allows more room in front of the parotid gland for the ramus of the mandible to swing backwards during the simple hinge movement which follows. When the mouth is wide open, the head of the mandible is in an unstable position, and it is in these circumstances that dislocation occurs, for example in yawning. The mouth is opened by the action of gravity when the muscles of mastication (p. 183) relax (e.g. when students sleep during lectures). Gravity is aided by a group of muscles, relatively weak, which include digastric and the suprahyoid muscles. The mouth is closed by the powerful muscles of mastication. Side to side movements, used in chewing, also occur at this joint and are produced by the alternating action of the muscles of the two sides.

The Joints of the Vertebral Column

The bodies of the vertebræ articulate with adjacent bodies, by means of cartilaginous joints, to make a strong resilient column for carrying the weight of the trunk. The neural arches articulate at their articular processes by small plane synovial joints so that they form with the backs of the vertebral bodies a tunnel, the **vertebral canal,** in which lie protected the spinal cord and its membranes.

JOINTS OF THE VERTEBRAL BODIES: The cartilaginous joint between the bodies of adjacent vertebræ consists primarily of a flat round **intervertebral disc.** Each disc has an outer covering of fibrocartilage called the **anulus**

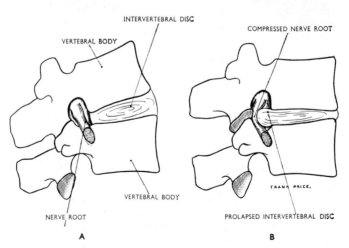

Fig. 67. A, normal relations of vertebral bodies, intervertebral disc and spinal nerve; B, 'slipped disc'. The vertebral column is flexed, and the disc is compressed so that it ruptures, bulges posteriorly and presses on the nerve.

fibrosus and a jelly-like centre called the **nucleus pulposus.** The disc is fixed to the surfaces of the vertebral bodies by a layer of hyaline cartilage and the joint is strengthened by fibrous ligaments in front and behind (Fig. 67).

Although the movement at any one joint is very small, the series of joints makes the column as a whole flexible and resilient.

Sometimes an intervertebral disc may be injured and this is most likely to happen in the lumbar region where the column is carrying considerable weight and where it is more movable than in the adjacent thoracic and sacral regions. The effort of lifting a weight, with the vertebral column flexed, causes the front part of the disc to be compressed and this may result in splitting of the posterior part of the anulus fibrosus, thus allowing the nucleus pulposus to protrude backwards. Very often this then presses on one of the nerve roots on its path from the spinal cord to the intervertebral foramen (Fig. 67), giving rise to great pain in the distribution of that nerve. This is the condition known as 'slipped disc'.

MOVEMENTS OF THE VERTEBRAL COLUMN: Flexion, extension and lateral bending can be carried out in the cervical and lumbar regions. Some rotation is possible in the lumbar region and is more extensive in the cervical region. Movements of the thoracic region are restricted by the ribs; only a little rotation is possible.

The force of gravity acts constantly to produce flexion of the vertebral column. This is counteracted by the tone of the extensor muscles of the back. People slump forwards when they fall asleep or faint, when the tone of these muscles is reduced.

ATLANTO-OCCIPITAL JOINTS: Each condyle of the occipital bone of the skull articulates with the lateral mass of the atlas at an atlanto-occipital joint (Fig. 68) which is a synovial joint of the condyloid variety. The movements which occur are nodding ('yes'), i.e. flexion and extension of the skull on the atlas, and sideways tilting of the head, i.e. abduction and adduction. No rotation can take place.

ATLANTO-AXIAL JOINTS: There are three atlanto-axial joints (Fig. 68). On each side a synovial joint of the plane variety connects the inferior aspect of the lateral mass of the atlas with the superior surface of the lateral mass of the axis. In addition, the column of the dens of the axis articulates with the back of the anterior arch of the atlas by means of a synovial pivot joint. The dens is held in position by means of an important **transverse ligament** which passes behind it, stretching from one lateral mass of the atlas to the other. Immediately behind this ligament is the spinal cord. If the ligament is torn the dens may be displaced backwards and injure the spinal cord. The movement which takes

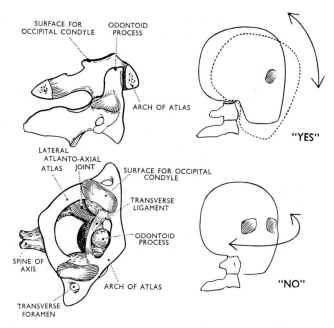

Fig. 68. The atlanto-axial joints for 'NO' movements. ('YES' movements occur at the atlanto-occipital joints.)

place simultaneously at these joints is rotation of the skull (with the atlas) on the axis ('no').

Joints of the Upper Limb

JOINTS OF THE SHOULDER GIRDLE

(a) STERNOCLAVICULAR JOINT: At the sternoclavicular joint the medial end of the clavicle articulates by means of a synovial joint of a modified ball and socket type with the upper lateral angle of the manubrium of the sternum. It is the only joint by which the shoulder girdle is connected with the skeleton of the trunk. This joint allows the clavicle to move so that its lateral end and the acromion which is joined to it (i.e. the point of the shoulder) can move upwards and downwards, forwards and backwards and in intermediate directions.

(b) ACROMIOCLAVICULAR JOINT: (Figs. 69 and 54). This is a synovial joint, of the plane variety, which allows the clavicle and scapula to move in relation to each other.

The scapula is attached to the skeleton of the trunk by muscles only.

The shoulder girdle, therefore, is almost independent of the skeleton of the trunk, and so has considerable freedom of movement. This promotes mobility of the upper limb as a whole. Movements at the shoulder joint are almost always associated with movements of the girdle.

SHOULDER JOINT: This joint is a synovial joint of the ball and socket variety. The large rounded head of the humerus fits into the much smaller shallow glenoid cavity of the scapula (Plate 5, A and Fig. 54). The size of the

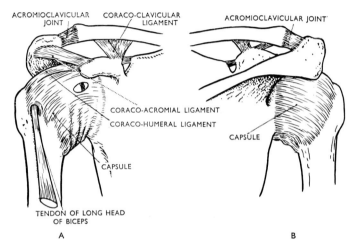

Fig. 69. The right shoulder joint, with the right acromioclavicular joint and the associated ligaments, A from the front and B from behind.

glenoid cavity is increased a little by a rim of fibrocartilage, the **glenoid labrum,** which is attached round its margin. Because of the large ball and the small socket the shoulder joint is inherently very mobile and also very unstable. The capsule is attached to the glenoid labrum and to the anatomical neck of the humerus, but extends down on to the shaft on the medial side. To allow free movement the capsule is lax, but its upper part is strengthened by the **coraco-humeral ligament** which stretches from the root of the coracoid process to the greater tuberosity and blends with the capsule.

The tendon of origin of the long head of the biceps arises from the upper part of the margin of the glenoid cavity within the capsule, and, covered by a sleeve of the synovial membrane passes through the joint cavity to enter the intertubercular groove (Plate 5). This tendon helps to prevent the head of the humerus from being displaced upwards.

The stability of this inherently unstable joint depends very largely on the

short muscles which stretch from the scapula to the humerus and closely surround the capsule (Fig. 90). These muscles act like ligaments, but with the
advantage that the tension exerted can be modified to meet the needs of the
moment. They are referred to collectively as the **'rotator cuff'**. This surrounds
the joint superiorly, anteriorly and posteriorly. Inferiorly the joint is relatively
unsupported. When the arm is abducted, therefore, dislocation is liable to occur
if pressure is applied to the humerus from above.

The great characteristic of the shoulder joint is the wide range of movements
which can be carried out, and this is enhanced by movements of the shoulder
girdle itself. At the shoulder joint the movements are classified as flexion (a
movement of the upper arm forwards), extension (the opposite of flexion),

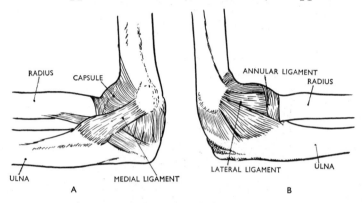

Fig. 70. The right elbow joint: A, from the medial side and B, from the lateral side.

abduction, adduction, medial rotation, lateral rotation and circumduction.
These movements are produced by the muscles which connect the shoulder
girdle and the trunk with the humerus.

ELBOW JOINT: This joint is a synovial joint of the hinge variety. The
capitulum and trochlea of the humerus articulate respectively with the head
of the radius and the trochlear notch of the ulna. The capsule is loose in front
and behind, and is strengthened at the sides by strong ligaments, the **medial
ligament** and **lateral ligament** (Plate 5 and Figs. 70, 71 and 72). The movements at the elbow joint are flexion, carried out by brachialis and biceps, and
extension, carried out by triceps.

WRIST JOINT: This joint is a synovial joint of the condyloid variety
(Fig. 73). The distal end of the radius articulates by means of its distal surface
with the proximal row of the carpal bones. The articular surface of the radius is
extended medially by a triangular plate of fibro-cartilage, the **triangular carti-**

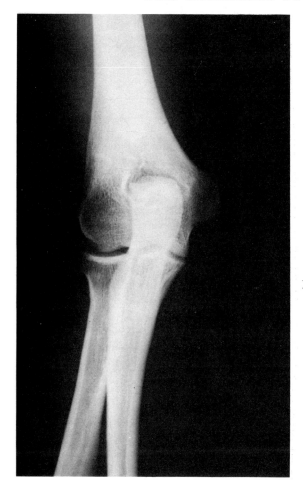

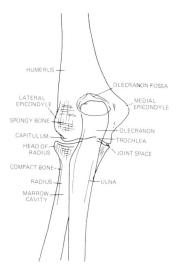

Fig. 71. A radiograph of the elbow
region, posterior view.

lage (Figs. 73 and pp. 140, 142). Of the carpal bones, the scaphoid and lunate articulate with the radius, and the triquetral with the triangular cartilage. The movements which take place are flexion and extension, adduction and abduction and some circumduction. The movements are produced by the muscles of the forearm whose tendons pass across the wrist joint to the wrist and fingers.

RADIO-ULNAR JOINTS: The superior and inferior radio-ulnar joints are both synovial joints of the pivot variety (Figs. 65, D and 74). At the superior radio-ulnar joint the sides of the head of the radius articulate with the radial notch of the ulna. The head of the radius is held in position by a fibrous brand,

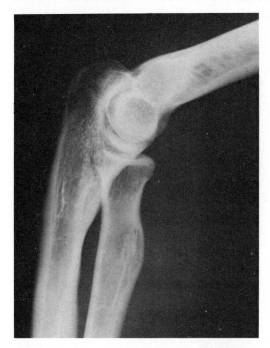

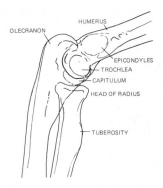

Fig. 72. A radiograph of the elbow region, lateral view.

the **annular ligament** the ends of which are attached to the ends of the radial notch. The capsule of this joint is continuous with that of the elbow joint and the joint spaces are, therefore, in continuity also. At the inferior radio-ulnar joint the head of the ulna articulates with the ulnar notch of the radius and with the upper surface of the triangular cartilage.

The movements, which always occur at both joints simultaneously, are pronation and supination. In **pronation** the bones of the forearm move so that the hand is rotated from the anatomical position until the palm faces backwards. **Supination** is the opposite movement which brings the hand back to the anatomical position, namely with the palm facing forwards. In these movements the ulna stays still and only the radius moves. In pronation the head of the radius rotates medially within the ring formed by the annular ligament and the radial notch, and the lower end of the radius passes round in front of the head of the ulna, carrying the hand with it. In full pronation the shaft of the radius lies across and in front of the shaft of the ulna. In supination the opposite occurs, and the shafts of the bones lie parallel.

The muscles which produce pronation are pronator teres and pronator

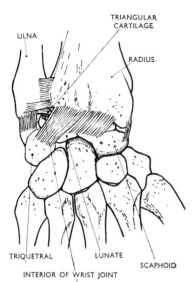

Fig. 73. The right wrist joint from behind, and the inferior radio-ulnar joint.

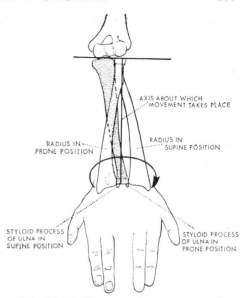

Fig. 74. To illustrate the movement of supination of the left forearm at the superior and inferior radio-ulnar joints.

quadratus, both specialized members of the flexor muscle group of the forearm. The muscles for supination are biceps (of the upper arm) and supinator which is a specialized muscle of the extensor group of the forearm. Supination is a much more powerful movement than pronation. (It is easier for a right-handed person to drive screws in than to take them out, or to screw up the cap of a bottle than to unscrew it.) Alone, pronation and supination allow the hand to be rotated through a semicircle. If, in addition, the humerus rotates, the hand turns through a full circle.

JOINTS OF THE HAND: Small gliding movements occur at the plane synovial joints between the carpal and metacarpal bones. Of special interest is the joint between the first metacarpal and the trapezium which has much more mobility, and allows flexion and extension, adduction and abduction, and a certain amount of pivoting. These movements give the thumb the all important facility of **opposition** to the other fingers. *Opposition is the bringing of the palmar aspect of the thumb into contact with the palmar aspect of the other fingers.* This makes grasping possible.

The metacarpals articulate by means of condyloid joints with the proximal phalanges, and the interphalangeal joints are hinge joints.

The Joints of the Lower Limb

SACRO-ILIAC JOINT: This joint is a synovial joint of the plane variety. The auricular surface of the sacrum articulates with the corresponding surface of the ilium (Fig. 75). The articular surfaces are not flat as in most plane joints but are irregularly undulating, so that the bones interlock to some extent. This restricts movement at the joint to a small amount of gliding. The joint transmits the body weight from the sacrum to the pelvis and is, therefore, strengthened by

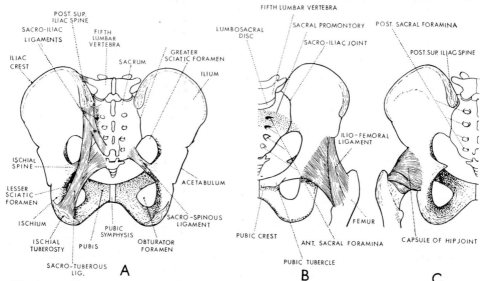

Fig. 75. A, The pelvis, showing the ligaments of the sacro-iliac joint; B, the left hip joint from the front; C, the left hip joint from behind.

thick strong **sacro-iliac ligaments,** which extend from the sacrum to the ilium mostly above and behind the articular surfaces. Strain of the ligaments of this joint is a common cause of backache.

Sacro-tuberous ligament (Fig. 75). This ligament, wide and strong, stretches from the back of the sacrum to the tuberosity of the ischium.

Sacro-spinous ligament (Fig. 75). This ligament passes from the sacrum and coccyx to the spine of the ischium.

These two ligaments are accessory ligaments of the sacro-iliac joint. They prevent rotation of the sacrum at the sacro-iliac joints under the influence of the body weight acting on the upper part of the sacrum.

SYMPHYSIS PUBIS: This is a permanent cartilaginous joint between the two pubic bones (Fig. 75).

HIP JOINT: The feature of the hip joint is its remarkable stability in spite of the great stresses it has to withstand in supporting the body weight in standing and in active movements. The hip joint is a synovial joint of the ball and socket variety (Fig. 76). The spherical head of the femur articulates with the deep cup-shaped acetabulum on the innominate bone. The acetabulum is further

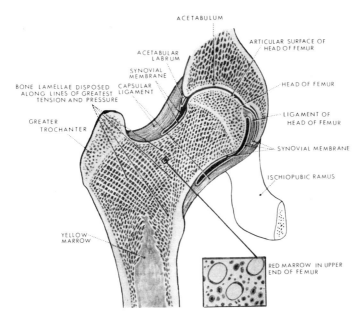

Fig. 76. A coronal section through the right hip joint and the upper end of the femur.

deepened by a rim of fibro-cartilage, the **acetabular labrum,** which fits closely round the distal part of the head, holding it in the socket.

The capsule is attached proximally round the margin of the acetabulum and distally it extends well down on to the neck. The synovial membrane lines the capsule and is reflected on to the intracapsular part of the neck (Fig. 76). A fold of synovial membrane, called the ligament of the head of the femur, stretches from the medial margin of the acetabulum to a rough pit in the middle of the head of the femur. It conveys blood vessels to the head but plays no part in maintaining stability. The front of the capsule is greatly strengthened by the **ilio-femoral ligament** or **Y-shaped ligament** which blends with it (Fig. 75B).

The movements at the hip joint are flexion carried out by iliopsoas; extension, a restricted movement, especially in women, but produced from the flexed position by gluteus maximus and the hamstrings; medial rotation by gluteus medius and minimus; lateral rotation by the small lateral rotator muscles; adduction by the adductors; abduction by gluteus medius and minimus; and circumduction which is a combination of all the movements.

The body weight falls behind the hip joints (Fig. 7); therefore, there is a constant tendency for the pelvis to roll backwards on the heads of the two femora, that is, for the hip joint to be over-extended. The strong ilio-femoral ligaments and the arrangement of the fibres at the back of the capsule, supported by tone in psoas prevent this. In the flexed position all these structures are relaxed, and it is in this position that the joint is liable to be dislocated.

Because of the deep socket which makes the hip joint so stable, movements are restricted in range. The effective range of movement of the lower end of the femur is increased however by the presence of the angulated neck which holds the shaft of the femur some distance lateral to the articulation.

KNEE JOINT: This joint is a synovial joint of the hinge variety (Figs. 77, 78, 79 and Plate 5). The medial and lateral femoral condyles articulate with the two oval surfaces on the proximal end of the tibia. The knee joint must be stable to withstand the body weight in motion; it also enjoys considerable mobility; combining as it does these incompatible attributes, it is structurally very complex. Because it is complicated it is easily damaged.

The convex femoral condyles are made to fit the almost flat tibial surfaces more closely because of the **medial** and **lateral menisci** (semilunar cartilages). These are crescents of fibrocartilage, wedge-shaped in section. They also act as shock absorbers and help to keep the joint lubricated. They may be damaged if they are nipped between the bones, but the lateral one, which is not attached to the lateral ligament, is more mobile and so less liable to be nipped and damaged.

The capsule of the joint is attached round the lower end of the femur and the upper end of the tibia; it is strengthened behind by fibres, reflected from the insertion of the hamstring muscles and in front it is replaced by the patella, fibres of insertion of the quadriceps, and the patellar tendon.

The posterior surface of the patella articulates with the front of the lower end of the femur between the condyles. The femur and tibia are held together mainly by the two **cruciate ligaments,** anterior and posterior, which pass from the intercondylar eminence of the tibia to the sides of the intercondylar notch of the femur, crossing each other as they go. They also prevent backwards and forwards movements between the bones, and are important for the stability of the joint.

Like all hinge joints the knee joint has strong ligaments at the sides. The

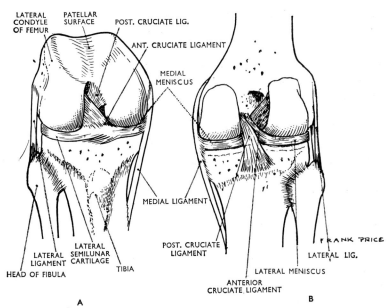

LATERAL CONDYLE OF FEMUR
PATELLAR SURFACE
POST. CRUCIATE LIG.
ANT. CRUCIATE LIGAMENT
MEDIAL MENISCUS
MEDIAL LIGAMENT
LATERAL LIGAMENT
LATERAL SEMILUNAR CARTILAGE
TIBIA
HEAD OF FIBULA
POST. CRUCIATE LIGAMENT
FRANK PRICE
LATERAL LIG.
LATERAL MENISCUS
ANTERIOR CRUCIATE LIGAMENT

A   B

Fig. 77. The right knee joint: A, from the front, with the limb flexed; B, from behind, with the limb extended. The semilunar cartilages are now called menisci.

medial ligament is a long wide flat band, blended with the capsule. The **lateral ligament** is a round cord quite separate from the capsule.

The synovial membrane of the knee joint (Plate 5) is extensive. It lines the capsule and covers the cruciate ligaments, excluding them from the joint cavity. It also extends upwards above the level of the patella between the quadriceps and the femur to form the **suprapatellar pouch.** There are several **synovial bursæ** between the soft tissue layers surrounding the knee. An inflamed pre-patellar bursa (between the skin and the patella and patellar ligament) (Plate 5) is called housemaid's knee.

The main movements at the knee joint are flexion produced by the hamstrings and extension produced by quadriceps femoris. In the last stages of full extension the femur rotates medially on the tibia. This is the 'locking' of the knee joint which enables it to be held rigidly in extension with a minimum of muscular effort. In relaxed standing, the patella can be moved freely from side to side showing that, though the knee is extended, the extensor muscle, quadriceps, is relaxed. It is important to emphasize that the stability of the knee joint is dependent, to a large extent, on the adequate support of the quadriceps muscle group.

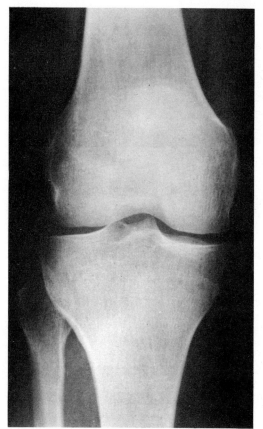

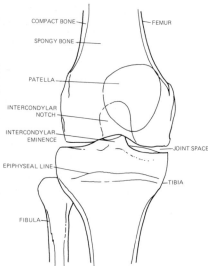

COMPACT BONE
SPONGY BONE
PATELLA
INTERCONDYLAR NOTCH
INTERCONDYLAR EMINENCE
EPIPHYSEAL LINE
FIBULA
FEMUR
JOINT SPACE
TIBIA

Fig. 78. A radiograph of the knee joint, posterior view.

ANKLE JOINT: This joint is a synovial joint of the hinge variety (Figs. 80 and 81). It is one of the most stable joints in the body, but movement is limited. The lower ends of the tibia and fibula form a socket into which the pulley-shaped upper surface of the talus fits. The capsule is loose in front and behind but is strengthened on the medial side by the **medial** or **deltoid ligament** and on the lateral side by the three bands of the **lateral ligament**. The movements are:

(a) Extension when the back of the foot is raised towards the front of the leg. This is called by some 'dorsiflexion'.

(b) Flexion, the opposite movement, called by some 'plantar-flexion'.

Thus the extensor muscles of the leg produce extension or 'dorsiflexion' and

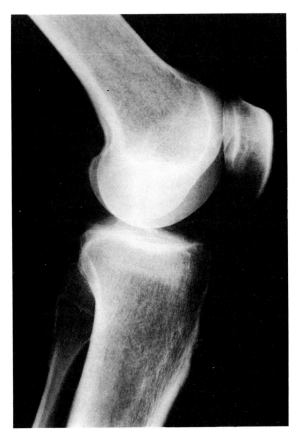

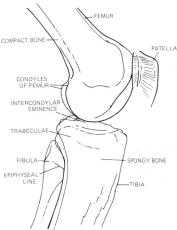

Fig. 79. A radiograph of the knee
joint, lateral view.

the flexor muscles of the calf produce flexion or, according to some, 'plantar-flexion'. Because of the wedge-shaped upper surface of the talus, the joint is more unstable when the foot is flexed, as in this position the narrow posterior part of the talus lies in the wide anterior part of the socket made by the tibia and fibula. It is in this position that injuries to this region occur.

SUBTALOID JOINTS: Between the talus and calcaneum are two joints, the subtaloid joints, at which twisting gliding movements occur in conjunction with the joint between the calcaneum and the cuboid (Fig. 81). As a result movements of the foot called inversion and eversion occur. These movements are associated with gliding between other joints of the tarsus. **Inversion** is a movement in which the sole of the foot is turned to face medially. **Eversion** is a movement in which the sole of the foot is turned to face laterally.

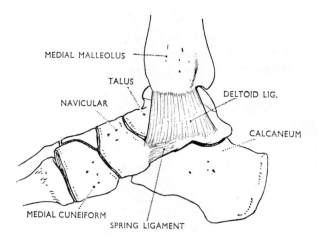

Fig. 80. The right ankle joint and the tarsus seen from the medial side.

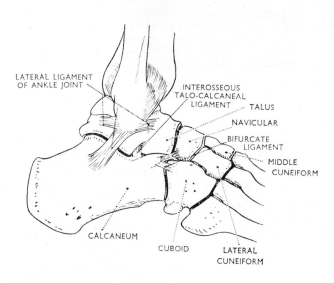

Fig. 81. The right ankle joint and the tarsus seen from the lateral side.

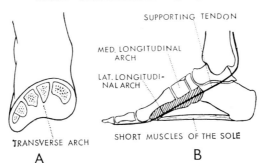

Fig. 82. The arches of the foot: A, the transverse arch; B, the longitudinal arches.

The Arches of the Foot

The arched form of the foot makes it strong and resilient for weight bearing, and makes it a strong lever for use in propelling the body forwards in locomotion.

The skeleton forms a longitudinal arch and a transverse arch (p. 151, Fig. 82), linking the three points of a tripod formed by the heel and the balls of the big and little toes. The arched form of the foot is maintained by muscles and ligaments (Fig. 82) which stretch from one segment of the arch to the next, or tie the two ends of the arch together like the string of a bow, or act as a sling passing under the arch. Ligaments very soon stretch if they are subjected to prolonged stress. Thus the muscles, or the tendons connected to the muscles, whose tension is due to the active contractile tone of the muscle cells, are the most important factor in maintaining the arches. In treating painful 'flat foot' where the arches have sagged, the muscles of the leg and foot are exercised to help them to regain their tone. When the toes are curled up or extended, tension increases in the ligaments acting like bowstrings, and the curvature of the arches is increased. The same effect is obtained by 'toe-raising' exercises

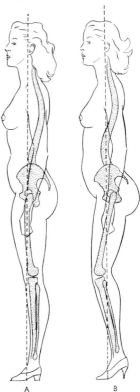

Fig. 83. To show the increased curvatures of the spine, the forward tilting of the pelvis and the bending of the lower limb which are necessary to maintain balance when wearing high heels.

or by wearing high heels, a fact well known to flat-footed people, who find it difficult to walk in low-heeled shoes or bare-footed.

Inter-relationship of joints

To maintain balance, the position of joints is controlled reflexly by the nervous system acting on the muscles. This means that the positions of the different joints of the vertebral column and lower limb are inter-related (Fig. 83). When the sole of the foot is flat on the ground, the tibia and femur are vertical, the knee is straight, the hip joint is not flexed and the vertebral column has its normal curves. However, if the heel is raised, for example by wearing high heels, the tibia is tilted forwards. The flexion at the knee restores the balance; this in turn causes flexion at the hip joint and a compensating increase in the lumbar curvature.

Similarly, if a joint is diseased so that its range of movement is restricted, unusual positions are adopted by other joints, and compensatory movements occur in them. For example, if a hip joint is relatively fixed in the adducted position, the pelvis tilts and the lumbar spine develops a lateral curvature to enable the foot to be placed flat on the ground in standing and walking.

CHAPTER VII

THE SYSTEM OF SKELETAL MUSCLES

SKELETAL muscles are built up of striped muscle fibres (p. 114) and are supplied by nerves from the central nervous system. Skeletal muscles are attached by their ends, to the skeleton; the proximal attachment, which is usually fixed, is the **origin,** the distal attachment, which usually moves, is the **insertion.** (Note that muscles often work from a fixed insertion, in which case the origin moves.)

Muscle fibres are connected together to form muscles by fibrous connective tissue. Each fibre is surrounded by a delicate sheath, the **endomysium,** the fibres are bound into bundles by the **perimysium** and the bundles form the muscle itself which is surrounded by the **epimysium** (Fig. 36, A). A muscle is sometimes attached directly to bone, but very often it is attached by means of a thick bundle of strong white shiny collagen fibres called a **tendon** (Fig. 37). Muscles may have tendons of origin and tendons of insertion. Flat muscles very often have wide flat tendons called **aponeuroses.**

DIFFERENT KINDS OF MUSCLES

Skeletal muscle fibres range in length from 1 mm to 30 cm. They are arranged in a number of different ways to form muscles of different kinds:

parallel (e.g. sartorius, Fig. 100)   unipennate (e.g. flexor pollicis longus)
fusiform (e.g. biceps brachii, Fig. 92)   bipennate (e.g. rectus femoris, Fig. 100)
triangular (e.g. temporalis, Fig. 84)   multipennate (e.g. deltoid, Fig. 91)

The structure of a muscle reflects its function because, when a muscle fibre contracts, it shortens to approximately half of its relaxed length. The longer the muscle fibres, the greater the range of movement the muscle produces; the parallel and fusiform types are most effective in this respect. The greater the number of muscle fibres in a muscle, the more power it can exert; the multipennate type is specialized in this direction.

NERVE SUPPLY

Skeletal muscles are supplied by cranial or spinal nerves. No muscle can contract unless its nerve supply is intact. A knowledge of the nerve supply of muscle groups is, therefore, important.

Not only do muscles receive efferent, motor fibres, but also afferent, sensory fibres for position sense. Thus, even if the eyes are shut, one knows if one's limbs have been moved passively to a new position by someone else.

BLOOD SUPPLY

Skeletal muscles, being at times very active tissues, need a good blood supply. The vessels are distributed throughout the muscles as a dense capillary plexus in the endomysium.

The blood vessels and nerves enter a muscle at one (or sometimes more) point, known as the **neurovascular hilum.**

FASCIÆ

Muscles are connected to each other and to the other soft tissues by areolar tissue which contains many collagen fibres. This we call **fascia.**

Superficial fascia. This connects the dermis of the skin with the underlying deep fascia. It is of a loose texture and often contains considerable quantities of stored fat, especially in women. This fat insulates the body against loss of heat.

Deep fascia is the membranous layer of fascia deep to the superficial fascia. It invests the muscles with a continuous covering and also forms the layers between them. Some parts of it are given special names if they are notably thick and strong, for example, the **fascia lata** of the thigh.

SYNOVIAL BURSÆ

When muscles move, the layers of fascia between them must necessarily move on each other. Where such movement is frequent or extensive, often near joints, **synovial bursæ** develop to minimize friction. A bursa is a closed sac of synovial membrane (p. 154), flattened so that two opposite sides are in contact. The simple squamous epithelium of the inside is very smooth, so the surfaces can move easily one on the other. Lubrication is provided by a film of synovial fluid. The prepatellar bursa (p. 171) is one example. Bursæ very close to the joints sometimes communicate with the joint cavity. Inflammation of a bursa is called **bursitis.**

SYNOVIAL SHEATHS

A **synovial sheath** *is a cylindrical bursa which surrounds a tendon*, especially where the tendon passes through a restricted space, for example, the carpal tunnel (p. 193). It facilitates the to and fro movement of the tendon as its muscle belly contracts and relaxes. Inflammation of such a synovial sheath is called **synovitis,** and is very painful.

Muscle Function

When a muscle contracts, it shortens the distance between its origin and insertion usually by moving the insertion nearer to the origin. In this way the parts of the skeleton are moved in relation to each other. If the positions of the origin and insertion are known, the action of the muscle on a given joint (or joints, if it passes over more than one) can be worked out.

GROUP ACTION OF MUSCLES

The muscles which contract to produce a given movement are called **prime movers.** Thus the flexors in the upper arm (brachialis and biceps) are the prime movers in flexion at the elbow joint. The muscles which could produce the opposite movement are the **antagonists,** in this case, the extensors in the upper arm (triceps). During the contraction of the prime movers the antagonists must relax to allow the movement to occur. *The controlled relaxation of the antagonists is important for producing smooth movement.* **Fixation muscles** hold the skeleton steady while other muscles act as prime movers; for example, in movements at the shoulder joint, the muscles connecting the shoulder girdle to the trunk contract as fixation muscles to keep the girdle steady.

Movements are complex. Even an apparently simple movement calls a number of muscles into play, to act as prime movers. A knowledge of muscle groups, rather than of individual muscles, is, therefore, sufficient to afford considerable understanding of the functioning of the system of skeletal muscles.

MUSCULAR INSUFFICIENCY

A muscle can contract to half of its relaxed length and no more. Effort to contract further only gives pain. A muscle may therefore not be able to contract enough to produce the full range of movement of the joints over which it passes. This is **active insufficiency.** The hamstrings can produce extension at the hip joint and flexion at the knee. Extend the hip joint; flex the knee; it will be found that as long as extension is maintained at the hip joint the knee can be flexed only partially.

A muscle relaxes to a given length. An attempt to stretch it further only tears the tissue. The muscle may not be able to relax enough to allow the full range of movement of the joints. This is **passive insufficiency.** Clench the fist; now bend the wrist as far as possible, keeping the fist clenched; the pain felt on the back of the hand is due to stretching of the extensor musculature; if further flexion at the wrist is attempted, the fingers cannot remain clenched.

DEMONSTRATION OF SUPERFICIAL MUSCLES

To observe any superficial muscle in the living subject, make it contract, especially against resistance, and watch for the swelling of the muscle under the skin, or feel it bulging with the flat of the hand.

CONTRACTION OF MUSCLES

When a muscle contracts it literally becomes shorter. Each individual muscle cell (fibre) can contract to about half of its relaxed length. When it contracts the protein molecules, which constitute the myofibrils in the sarcoplasm, come to overlap more extensively and make the whole fibre shorter. The energy needed to produce this change comes from the oxidation of food materials in the muscle cells (p. 181). Much of the energy so produced is wasted in the form of heat (p. 550). A skeletal muscle fibre contracts only when it receives a strong enough stimulus from the motor nerve which supplies it. When it contracts it contracts to the fullest extent possible. This is the **'all or none'** law. Of course, a *whole muscle* may at any given time have a larger or smaller number of its fibres in a state of contraction, that is, it may contract more powerfully or less powerfully as the occasion demands, depending on the number of muscle fibres stimulated by the nerve.

Fatigue

After repeated or sustained contractions a muscle fibre becomes fatigued and is no longer able to contract. This is due to lack of oxygen and to accumulation of metabolites, the waste products produced by the chemical reactions which have been taking place. Blood flow through the muscle is hampered by the contractions and is not sufficient to allow the necessary exchanges. With rest the oxygen debt (p. 181) is repaid and the metabolites are washed away.

Muscle Tone

In health all muscles, even when at rest, are in a continuous state of slight contraction. This is called muscle tone. A few motor units functioning in any one muscle at a given time are enough to produce muscle tone. The groups of motor units working change periodically, so that tone can be maintained without fatigue. Muscle tone is produced reflexly by afferent impulses coming from stretch receptors in the muscles themselves. If any part of the reflex arc is damaged (for example the nerve supplying the muscle, or the part of the spinal cord to which the nerve is connected), tone is lost and the muscle becomes flaccid. Muscle tone is lessened during sleep.

Chemistry of Muscular Contraction

Muscle fibres contain two proteins, myosin and actin, which, when the fibre contracts, unite to form actomyosin, shortening as they do so. This needs energy. The energy comes from the carbohydrates in the food (p. 550) but there are a great many stages in this complex process of oxidation.

The energy which produces actomyosin comes from the breaking down of adenosine triphosphate, A.T.P.

For the muscle to go on working, the A.T.P. must be reformed. Glycogen in the muscle fibre breaks down quickly without oxygen to provide the energy necessary to reform A.T.P. Pyruvic acid and lactic acid are produced in the process.

If plenty of oxygen is available, as it is during ordinary movements, the pyruvic acid is broken down in the muscle cells by stages to carbon dioxide and water, with the release, at each stage, of energy which is used to reform A.T.P. Some of the lactic acid, too, can be broken down, in the presence of oxygen, to release energy. This energy may then be used to reform glycogen from the remainder of the lactic acid. (See also p. 558.)

If insufficient oxygen is available, any pyruvic acid is reduced to lactic acid which accumulates and produces fatigue.

Oxygen Debt. During severe muscular exercise the physiological mechanisms involved in conveying oxygen to the muscles are stepped up to meet the increased demand (see below). Even so, and particularly at the start of the effort, not enough oxygen reaches the muscle cells. Although some of the pyruvic acid is fully oxidized, lactic acid accumulates. It diffuses into the tissue fluid and into the blood stream.

After the exercise is over, the rate and depth of respiration continue at an increased level, stimulated by the lactic acid in the blood acting on the respiratory centre. This continues until enough extra oxygen has been taken in to allow the muscle and liver cells to remove the lactic acid by oxidizing it completely or by converting it to glycogen.

The extra oxygen needed to remove the accumulated lactic acid after the cessation of severe exercise is known as the **'oxygen debt'**.

Heat Production. The chemical reactions which occur in the muscle cells during contraction result in the production of heat (p. 318). This is one of the important ways in which heat is produced to keep the body warm. Indeed, if the body cools down, involuntary contractions (shivering) start, to produce more heat.

During exercise more heat is produced than the body needs, and readjustments take place to increase heat loss (see below).

MUSCULAR EXERCISE

During muscular exercise considerable physiological readjustments take place. Extra oxygen must be supplied to the active muscles for the oxidation of glycogen, and the carbon dioxide and other waste products must be got rid of. Also, the heat generated must be dissipated.

Respiratory Changes

The **rate** and **depth** of respiration are increased (p. 343). The 'oxygen debt' (p. 181) must be repaid.

Circulatory Changes

Increased cardiac output (p. 381).
Rise in blood pressure (p. 381).
Redistribution of blood (p. 388).

Heat Loss

Heat loss is increased (p. 319). The arterioles in the skin, initially constricted for the redistribution of blood to the muscles, dilate again to facilitate heat loss, and sweating occurs.

THE PRINCIPAL GROUPS OF MUSCLES

MUSCLES OF FACIAL EXPRESSION

The muscles of facial expression (Fig. 84), unlike most skeletal muscles, are attached to skin, namely to the skin of the face. Their contraction moves the skin and so alters the expression. Circular fibres round the eyelids can screw the eye tightly shut, and similar fibres round the mouth purse the lips. Muscle in

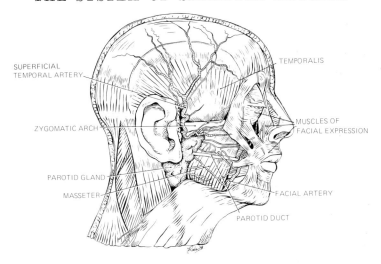

SUPERFICIAL
TEMPORAL ARTERY

TEMPORALIS

ZYGOMATIC ARCH

MUSCLES OF
FACIAL EXPRESSION

PAROTID GLAND

MASSETER

FACIAL ARTERY

PAROTID DUCT

Fig. 84. The muscles of the face.

the cheek presses food between the teeth during mastication. The muscles of
facial expression are supplied by the **facial nerve.** A lesion of the facial nerve
results in paralysis of these muscles—loss of expression on the affected side,
inability to close the eye, with irritation of and perhaps damage to the exposed
conjunctiva, dribbling of saliva from the imperfectly closed mouth, and difficulty
in mastication because the cheek cannot be pressed against the teeth.

MUSCLES OF MASTICATION

The muscles of mastication are powerful muscles which close the jaw, acting
on the temporomandibular joint. They can support the body weight, as is shown
by the acrobat hanging by his teeth. The **temporalis** and the **masseter** are the
largest (Fig. 84). All the muscles of mastication are supplied by the **mandibular division** of the **trigeminal nerve.**

Temporalis is a fan-shaped muscle which arises from the side of the skull. The
fibres converge on a tendon which passes medial to the zygomatic arch and is inserted
into the coronoid process of the mandible (Fig. 41).

The masseter arises from the zygomatic arch and is inserted into the lateral surface
of the ramus of the mandible (Fig. 41).

Both muscles can be seen and felt when the jaw is clenched.

THE EXTRINSIC MUSCLES OF THE EYE

The extrinsic muscles of the eye have their origin within the orbit from the bone round the optic foramen and are inserted into the sclera of the eyeball.

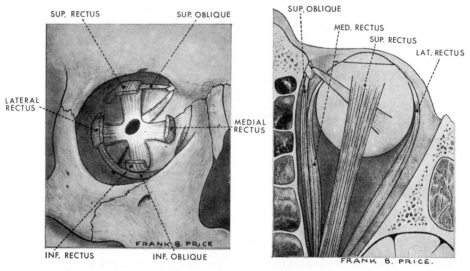

Fig. 85. The right orbit showing the origins of the extrinsic muscles of the eye.

Fig. 86. The extrinsic muscles of the eye in the right orbit, seen from above.

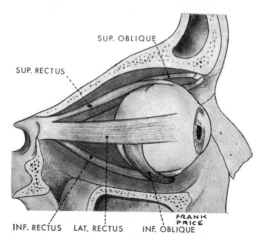

Fig. 87. The extrinsic muscles of the eye in the right orbit, seen from the right side.

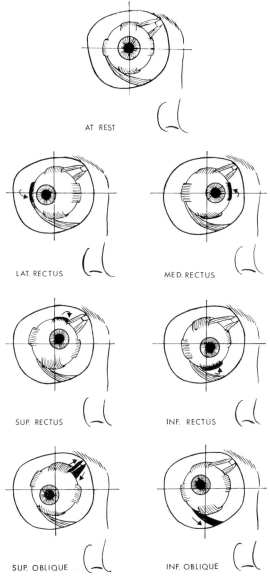

AT REST

LAT. RECTUS   MED. RECTUS

SUP. RECTUS   INF. RECTUS

SUP. OBLIQUE   INF. OBLIQUE

Fig. 88. A scheme to show the actions of the individual extrinsic muscles of the right eye.

They rotate the eyeball causing the pupil to face in different directions. (Figs. 85, 86, 87 and 88).

The **medial rectus** turns the eyeball so that the pupil faces **medially.**

The **lateral rectus** turns the eyeball so that the pupil faces **laterally.**

The **superior rectus** turns the eyeball so that the pupil faces **upwards and medially.** This is because the line of pull of the muscle, in the axis of the orbit, is not in direct line with the meridian of the eyeball.

The **inferior rectus** turns the eyeball so that the pupil faces **downwards and medially** for the same reason.

The **superior oblique** turns the eyeball so that the pupil faces **downwards and laterally.**

The **inferior oblique** turns the eyeball so that the pupil faces **upwards and laterally.**

Nerve Supply

The extrinsic muscles of the eyeball are supplied by the **oculomotor nerve** *except* for the **superior oblique** which is supplied by the **trochlear nerve** (sometimes called the pathetic nerve—action: down and out) and the **lateral rectus** supplied by the **abducent nerve.**

THE MUSCLES OF THE NECK

Sternomastoid

The sternomastoid (Figs. 89 and 91) is a large superficial muscle on the side of the neck. It arises from the medial third of the clavicle and from the front of the sternum and is inserted into the mastoid process of the skull and the bone behind it. It is supplied by the **accessory nerve.** Acting together, the muscles of the two sides tilt the head backwards and bend the neck forwards. One muscle acting alone bends the neck to its own side and turns the face towards the opposite side.

Trapezius

Trapezius is an extensive flat triangular muscle which arises from the back of the skull, from the spines of the cervical vertebræ (indirectly through a layer of fascia) and from all the thoracic spines. It is inserted into the lateral third of the clavicle, the acromion and the spine of the scapula (Fig. 90). It is supplied by the **accessory nerve.** Its upper fibres raise the tip of the shoulder in shrugging, the intermediate fibres draw the scapula towards the midline and its

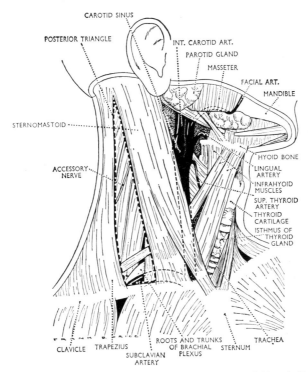

Fig. 89. The muscles of the neck. The heavy interrupted line indicates the posterior triangle.

lowest fibres, besides pulling the scapula downwards, help to rotate it so that the glenoid cavity faces upwards instead of laterally, as in full abduction of the arm.

The Triangles of the Neck

To make descriptions easier, the front and side of the neck is said to be divided into an **anterior triangle** in front of sternomastoid and a **posterior triangle** behind it. The anterior triangle is bounded medially by the midline and above by the mandible. It contains among other things, the carotid arteries and the internal jugular vein (Fig. 89). The posterior triangle is bounded posteriorly by trapezius and inferiorly by the clavicle. It contains the roots, trunks and divisions of the brachial plexus, and the upper part of the phrenic nerve (Fig. 89).

Suprahyoid Muscles. This group of small muscles connects the hyoid bone (p. 131) mainly with the mandible and the tongue (Fig. 89). Mylohyoid forms the oral diaphragm, that is, the floor of the mouth. The suprahyoid muscles assist in swallowing, raising the hyoid bone, and, indirectly, the larynx. If the hyoid bone is fixed by the infrahyoid muscles, they assist in opening the mouth.

Infrahyoid Muscles. This group of small strap-like muscles (Fig. 89) connects the hyoid bone with the larynx and the larynx with the sternum. The main action is to draw the hyoid bone downwards, or to anchor it during the action of the suprahyoid muscles.

Fascia of the Neck

Plate 6 shows the simple pattern in which the layers of fascia of the neck are arranged. The strong **investing layer** forms a roof for the two triangles and splits to enclose the sternomastoid and trapezius. The **prevertebral fascia** covers the front of the vertebræ and the muscles associated with the vertebral column. The **pretracheal fascia** covers the trachea and invests the thyroid gland. Laterally, it blends with the **carotid sheath** which encloses within a fascial tunnel the common and internal carotid arteries, the internal jugular vein and the vagus nerve. The pretracheal layer extends down into the thorax where it blends with the pericardium.

THE MUSCLES OF THE BACK

The **extensor muscles of the back** (Fig. 90) comprise a group of powerful muscles which lie along the whole length of the back of the vertebral column, from the back of the skull to the sacrum. The superficial muscles are long, extending over many segments, the deep ones being short, from one segment to the next. These muscles are supplied by the **posterior primary rami of the spinal nerves.** They are very important **postural muscles,** that is, by their tone they maintain the upright posture by acting constantly against gravity which tends to flex the head on the neck, and to flex the vertebral column. (See also pp. 22 and 156).

Lumbar Fascia

The superficial surface of the extensor muscles is covered by a layer of fascia which is thick and strong in the lumbar region. At the lateral margin of the lumbar part of the extensor muscles it is joined by two more layers of fascia from between deeper muscle layers. These three layers and the single layer formed by their fusion, are called the lumbar fascia (Fig. 90).

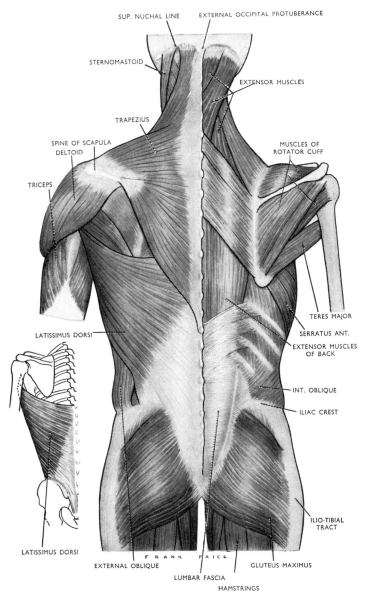

SUP. NUCHAL LINE

EXTERNAL OCCIPITAL PROTUBERANCE

STERNOMASTOID

EXTENSOR MUSCLES

TRAPEZIUS

SPINE OF SCAPULA
DELTOID

MUSCLES OF
ROTATOR CUFF

TRICEPS

TERES MAJOR

LATISSIMUS DORSI

SERRATUS ANT.

EXTENSOR MUSCLES
OF BACK

INT. OBLIQUE

ILIAC CREST

ILIO-TIBIAL
TRACT

LATISSIMUS DORSI

FRANK PRICE

EXTERNAL OBLIQUE

GLUTEUS MAXIMUS

LUMBAR FASCIA

HAMSTRINGS

Fig. 90. Muscles of the trunk and shoulder girdle seen from behind. On the right side of the body, the trapezius and latissimus dorsi have been removed. The inset shows the attachments of latissimus dorsi.

MUSCLES CONNECTING THE UPPER LIMB WITH THE TRUNK

Several large muscles connect the shoulder girdle and humerus with the trunk. They are the principal means of connexion since there is only the one small joint, the sternoclavicular, connecting the girdle with the trunk. These muscles, illustrated in Figs. 90 and 91, are the trapezius, latissimus dorsi, serratus anterior, pectoralis major and pectoralis minor. They produce the movements of the shoulder girdle on the trunk and some of the movements at the shoulder joint. In addition, the latissimus dorsi, serratus anterior and pectoralis major are **accessory muscles of respiration** (p. 341). When the upper limb is fixed they exert their effect on their thoracic attachments, serratus anterior and pectoralis major pulling the ribs outwards in inspiration and latissimus dorsi compressing the thorax on expiration. (To test this, place the hands over latissimus dorsi and cough.)

AXILLA OR ARMPIT

The axilla is the space between the upper arm and the side of the chest wall (Fig. 121). The space is shaped like a pyramid with a base and four sides. The base is formed by the skin. The medial wall is formed by the upper ribs covered by the serratus anterior muscle. The narrow lateral wall is the shaft of the humerus. The posterior wall is the scapula, with the subscapularis, teres major and latissimus dorsi muscles. The anterior wall is formed mainly by the pectoralis major muscle. The apex of the axilla, a small triangular space bounded by the first rib, the clavicle and the upper border of the scapula, communicates with the root of the neck. Through it blood vessels and nerves pass from the neck into the axilla on the way to supply the upper limb.

The axilla contains (1) the axillary artery and vein which lie close to the humerus, (2) the nerves to the upper limb, namely the cords of the brachial plexus and their branches, the radial, musculocutaneous, median and ulnar nerves, all lying close to the axillary artery and (3) the axillary lymph nodes (p. 416).

MUSCLES ROUND THE SHOULDER JOINT

Several small muscles close to the shoulder joint capsule are important in maintaining its stability (p. 164 and Fig. 90). They are called the 'rotator cuff'.

Deltoid (Figs. 90 and 91) covers the shoulder joint in front, behind and at

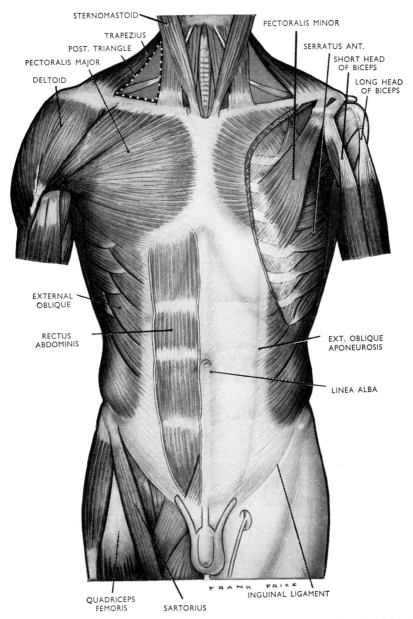

STERNOMASTOID

TRAPEZIUS

POST. TRIANGLE

PECTORALIS MAJOR

DELTOID

PECTORALIS MINOR

SERRATUS ANT.

SHORT HEAD OF BICEPS

LONG HEAD OF BICEPS

EXTERNAL OBLIQUE

RECTUS ABDOMINIS

EXT. OBLIQUE APONEUROSIS

LINEA ALBA

FRANK PRICE

QUADRICEPS FEMORIS

SARTORIUS

INGUINAL LIGAMENT

Fig. 91. Muscles of the trunk and shoulder girdle seen from the front. On the right side of the body the anterior wall of the rectus sheath has been removed. On the left side part of the pectoralis major and of the external oblique muscles have been cut away.

the side, arising from the lateral third of the clavicle, from the acromion and from the spine of the scapula, and being inserted into the deltoid tuberosity of the humerus (Fig. 52). It is supplied by the axillary (circumflex) nerve. Depending on which part contracts it produces flexion, extension or abduction at the shoulder joint.

To perform abduction, the deltoid needs the assistance of **supraspinatus,** one of the muscles of the 'rotator cuff' (Fig. 90). It is a small muscle extending from the supraspinous fossa of the scapula (Fig. 53) to the greater tuberosity of the humerus. Its tendon passes between the acromion and the head of the humerus and is here subject to wear and tear. Inflammation in and round this tendon is common and makes raising the arm painful.

FLEXORS AND EXTENSORS IN THE UPPER LIMB

As explained on pp. 271-272 the muscles developed on the ventral aspect of the limb are **flexors** and are supplied by the **anterior divisions** (which in the brachial plexus form the medial and lateral cords) **of the anterior primary rami of the spinal nerves;** the muscles developed on the dorsal aspect of the limb are **extensors** and are supplied by the **posterior divisions** (in the brachial plexus these form the posterior cord) **of the anterior primary rami** (Fig. 120).

MUSCLES OF THE UPPER ARM

Flexors. The muscles on the front of the upper arm are flexors at the elbow joint, and are supplied by the musculocutaneous nerve from the lateral cord of the brachial plexus. They are **brachialis** and **biceps** (Fig. 92). Biceps has two heads, the long head which arises above the glenoid fossa within the shoulder joint and the short head from the coracoid process. The bellies unite and the tendon, which can be felt in the bend of the elbow, is inserted into the radial tuberosity. Besides producing flexion at the elbow joint, biceps is an important supinator of the forearm (p. 166) and helps to produce flexion at the shoulder joint.

Extensors. The muscle on the back of the upper arm is **triceps** (Fig. 92), with three heads. It is the extensor at the elbow joint. It is supplied by the radial nerve from the posterior cord of the brachial plexus.

MUSCLES OF THE FOREARM

Flexors. The muscles on the front of the forearm (Fig. 93) are flexors of the wrist and fingers. They are supplied by the **median nerve** derived from the medial and lateral cords of the brachial plexus. The flexors are divided into a **superficial group** which takes origin from the medial epicondyle of the humerus, known therefore as the **common flexor origin;** and a **deep group** which arises from the front of the radius, of the ulna and of the interosseus

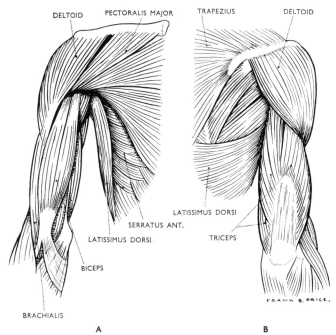

Fig. 92. The muscles of the right shoulder and upper arm, seen A, from the front, and B, from behind.

membrane. The fleshy bellies of these flexor muscles are in the forearm and they all have long tendons which pass to the bones of the carpus or to the fingers, producing flexion at the wrist joint and at the joints of the hand and fingers. The tendons pass through the **carpal tunnel.** kept in place there by the strong fibrous band, the **flexor retinaculum** (Fig. 94). This keeps them from springing away from the wrist during flexion. Similar wide fibrous bands, the fibrous flexor sheaths (Fig. 94), keep the flexor tendons in position on the fingers. Where the tendons pass through these constricted tunnels they are surrounded by **synovial sheaths** (p. 178).

Two small muscles of this flexor group in the forearm, **pronator teres** and **pronator quadratus** are specialized to perform pronation of the forearm (p. 166). They too are supplied by the **median nerve**.

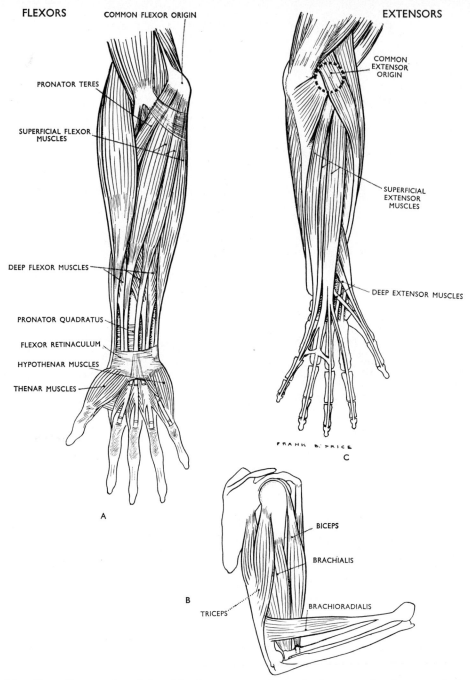

FLEXORS

COMMON FLEXOR ORIGIN

PRONATOR TERES

SUPERFICIAL FLEXOR
MUSCLES

DEEP FLEXOR MUSCLES

PRONATOR QUADRATUS

FLEXOR RETINACULUM

HYPOTHENAR MUSCLES

THENAR MUSCLES

A

EXTENSORS

COMMON
EXTENSOR
ORIGIN

SUPERFICIAL
EXTENSOR
MUSCLES

DEEP EXTENSOR MUSCLES

FRANK B. PRICE

C

BICEPS

BRACHIALIS

BRACHIORADIALIS

TRICEPS

B

Fig. 93. A, the muscles of the right forearm seen from the front; B, the flexors and the extensors acting on the right elbow joint; C, the muscles of the right forearm, seen from behind.

Extensors. The muscles of the back of the forearm (Fig. 93 c) are the extensors of the wrist and fingers. They are supplied by the deep branch (posterior interosseous nerve), of the radial nerve from the posterior cord. They too are divided into a superficial group and a deep group. The **superficial group** takes origin from the lateral epicondyle of the humerus, the **common extensor origin,** and the **deep group** from the back of the radius, ulna and interosseous

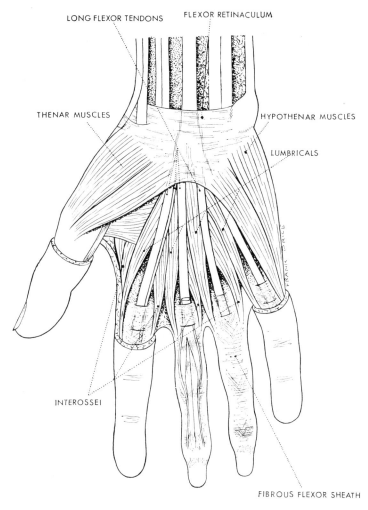

LONG FLEXOR TENDONS   FLEXOR RETINACULUM

THENAR MUSCLES   HYPOTHENAR MUSCLES

                                  LUMBRICALS

INTEROSSEI

FIBROUS FLEXOR SHEATH

Fig. 94. The muscles and tendons in the right hand.

membrane. Their fleshy bellies are on the back of the forearm and the long tendons pass to the bones of the carpus and fingers. They are held in close contact with the lower end of the radius by a fibrous band, the **extensor retinaculum** and are surrounded by **synovial sheaths.**

One small muscle of this extensor group, **supinator,** is specialized to perform, along with biceps, supination of the forearm. Supinator is supplied, like the extensors by the deep (posterior interosseous) branch of the **radial nerve.**

Cubital Fossa

The cubital fossa is the hollow in front of the elbow joint. It is triangular in outline, bounded above by a line joining the medial and lateral epicondyles of the humerus, bounded medially by the flexor muscle group (pronator teres) and laterally by the extensor muscle group. It contains the superficial veins, cephalic, basilic and median cubital (p. 376, Plate 30) often used for injections and transfusions. More deeply, and separated from the veins by a thickening of the deep fascia, the **bicipital aponeurosis,** lie the tendon of the biceps, the median nerve and the termination of the brachial artery.

THE MUSCLES OF THE HAND

In addition to the long flexor and extensor tendons, the hand contains a number of small muscles which give the thumb and fingers extra movements. The fleshy ball of the thumb, called the **thenar eminence,** contains three small thenar muscles for flexion, abduction and opposition (pp. 23 and 167) of the thumb; the **hypothenar eminence** at the base of the little finger contains three hypothenar muscles. In addition, between the metacarpal bones are **interosseous muscles** some of which spread out the fingers and others which bring them together again. These small muscles of the hand are supplied by the **ulnar nerve** (except for the thenar muscles which are supplied by the median nerve).

The flexor tendons are inserted into the phalanges as shown in Fig. 94. The superficial flexor tendon to each finger divides to allow the deep tendon to pass through it, and is then inserted into the middle phalanx. The deep tendon continues, and is inserted into the base of the terminal phalanx.

As each extensor tendon approaches its finger, it broadens out to form the **extensor expansion.** The middle part of the expansion is inserted into the middle phalanx and the two side parts go to the base of the terminal phalanx. The interosseous muscles and the lumbrical muscles (which take origin from the deep flexor tendons in the palm, Fig. 94) are attached to the sides of the extensor expansions.

They can therefore produce extension at the interphalangeal joints as well as flexion at the metacarpophalangeal joints, the 'writing' position.

Finger Tips. The 'fleshy' part of the finger tip is composed of fibrous adipose tissue, the **digital pulp** (Fig. 95), which is contained in a number of compartments separated by tough fibrous septa. To ensure free drainage in an infected finger tip, it is essential to break down these septa by passing a drain right through the pulp from one side of the finger to the other. If free drainage is not established, pressure rises in the pulp, and the arteries supplying the bone may be obliterated so that the bone dies and sloughs off. The epiphysis (Fig. 95), to which the tendons are attached, usually

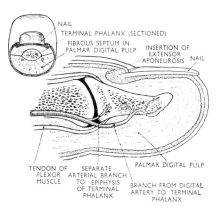

Fig. 95. A finger tip seen in transverse and in longitudinal section, to show the arrangement of the septa, digital pulp, and arteries.

escapes in such a case, because it is supplied by arteries which arise before the main vessels enter the digital pulp.

THE THORACIC WALL

The thoracic wall is formed largely by the skeleton of the thorax (p. 133). The intervals between the ribs, known as intercostal spaces, are filled by the intercostal muscles, of which, as in the abdominal wall, there are three layers. The innermost layer is not well developed.

In each intercostal space then, there is an **external intercostal muscle** and an **internal intercostal muscle.** The external intercostal has fibres which pass obliquely downwards and forwards from the rib above to the rib below. The internal intercostal fibres pass, at right angles to them, obliquely upwards and forwards from the rib below to the rib above. The intercostal muscles are supplied by the **intercostal nerves.** They are important and powerful muscles of respiration. The external intercostals and the anterior parts of the internal intercostals raise the ribs in inspiration, thus increasing the antero-posterior and transverse diameters of the thorax (p. 339). The posterior parts of the internal intercostals assist in expiration by pulling the ribs down.

The wall of the thoracic cage, formed by the vertebræ, ribs, sternum and intercostal muscles, is lined by a layer of fascia, the **thoracic fascia.** Attached to this is the innermost layer of the wall, the **parietal pleura** (p. 331).

The thoracic wall is supplied by the **intercostal nerves** which lie on the internal aspect of the lower borders of the ribs as they pass round the chest wall (Plate 13). They supply motor branches to the intercostal muscles and sensory branches to the skin and to the parietal pleura. (The lower five intercostal nerves and the subcostal nerve supply also the muscles, skin and parietal peritoneum of the anterior abdominal wall.)

The **intercostal arteries** and **veins** travel with the nerves and supply the same structures.

The external surface of the thoracic cage is covered by large flat muscles which belong to the upper limb (latissimus dorsi, serratus anterior, pectoralis major) and to the abdomen (external oblique). These muscles influence its movements, acting as accessory muscles of respiration.

Surface Anatomy p. 136 and p. 332.

DIAPHRAGM

The diaphragm (Fig. 111) is a thin musculotendinous sheet which separates the thoracic cavity from the abdominal cavity. It is a very important muscle of respiration. It is composed of **striated skeletal muscle** and is supplied by the **phrenic nerve.** The phrenic nerve comes mainly from the fourth cervical nerve and has a long course through the neck and down the side of the mediastinum to reach the diaphragm.

The diaphragm has a continuous circular origin from the internal aspect of the inferior boundary of the thoracic cage (Fig. 39), and is inserted into a central tendon. It takes origin from the back of the xiphisternum, from each of the lower six costal cartilages, and from the twelfth rib; from the **lateral arcuate ligament,** a fibrous band which arches across quadratus lumborum from the twelfth rib to the first lumbar transverse process; from the **medial arcuate ligament,** a fibrous band which arches across psoas from the first lumber transverse process to the body of the first lumbar vertebra; from the right side of the bodies of the first three lumbar vertebræ by means of the **right crus;** from the **left crus** by means of which it arises from the left side of the bodies of the first and second lumbar vertebræ; and from the **median arcuate ligament** which arches across the aorta from the right crus to the left crus. The attachment to the xiphisternum, costal cartilages and twelfth rib is sometimes called the **costal origin** of the diaphragm; the attachment by the crura and arcuate ligaments is the **vertebral origin.** The fibres arch upwards to form a highly domed shape as they are inserted into the **central tendon**

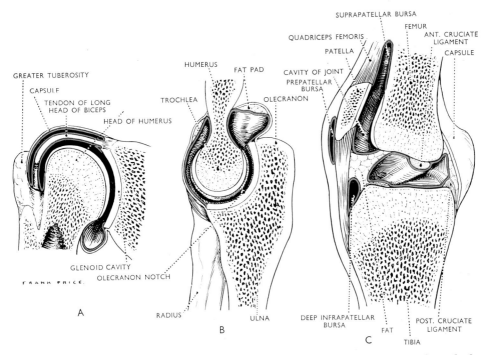

Plate 5. A, a coronal section through the shoulder joint; B, a sagittal section through the elbow joint; C, a sagittal section through the knee joint. Cut edges of the synovial membrane are shown in blue.

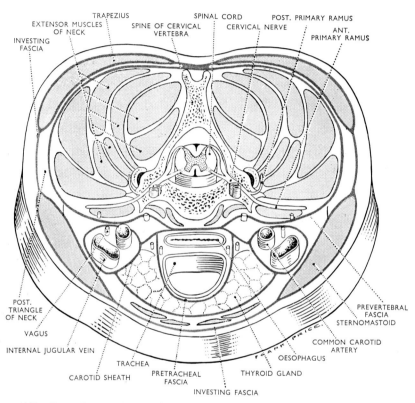

TRAPEZIUS

EXTENSOR MUSCLES
OF NECK

SPINE OF CERVICAL
VERTEBRA

SPINAL CORD

CERVICAL NERVE

POST. PRIMARY RAMUS

ANT.
PRIMARY RAMUS

INVESTING
FASCIA

POST.
TRIANGLE
OF NECK

VAGUS

INTERNAL JUGULAR VEIN

TRACHEA

CAROTID SHEATH

PRETRACHEAL
FASCIA

INVESTING FASCIA

THYROID GLAND

OESOPHAGUS

COMMON CAROTID
ARTERY

STERNOMASTOID

PREVERTEBRAL
FASCIA

Plate 6. A horizontal section of the neck, showing, in red, the arrangement of the fascial layers.

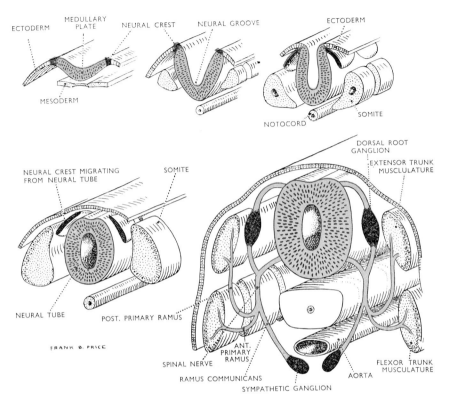

Plate 7. A scheme to show the development of the spinal cord from the medullary plate and nerve ganglia from the neural crest, the development of the main muscle masses from the mesodermal somites and the relationship between the nerves and the muscle masses.

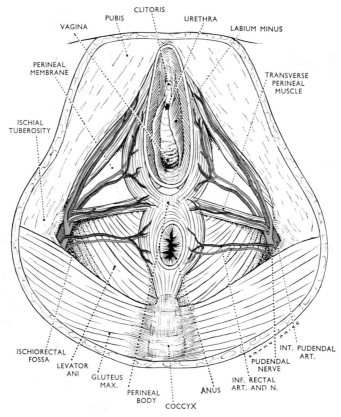

CLITORIS

VAGINA   PUBIS   URETHRA   LABIUM MINUS

PERINEAL
MEMBRANE

TRANSVERSE
PERINEAL
MUSCLE

ISCHIAL
TUBEROSITY

ISCHIORECTAL
FOSSA

LEVATOR
ANI

GLUTEUS
MAX.

PERINEAL
BODY

COCCYX

ANUS

INT. PUDENDAL
ART.

PUDENDAL
NERVE

INF. RECTAL
ART. AND N.

Plate 8. The female perineum: muscles, nerves and arteries. The external sphincter surrounds the anal canal.

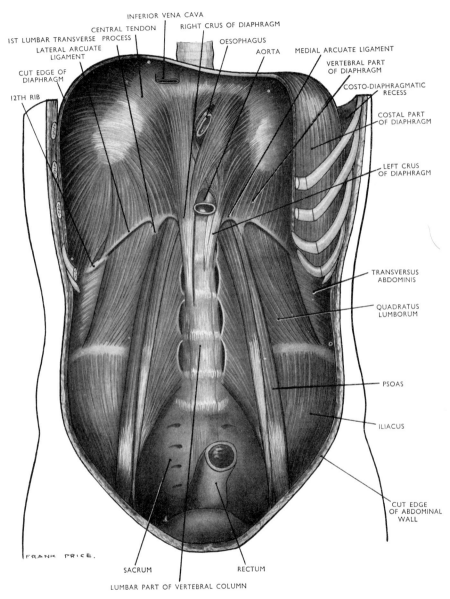

INFERIOR VENA CAVA

CENTRAL TENDON

RIGHT CRUS OF DIAPHRAGM

1ST LUMBAR TRANSVERSE PROCESS

OESOPHAGUS

LATERAL ARCUATE
LIGAMENT

AORTA

MEDIAL ARCUATE LIGAMENT

CUT EDGE OF
DIAPHRAGM

VERTEBRAL PART
OF DIAPHRAGM

12TH RIB

COSTO-DIAPHRAGMATIC
RECESS

COSTAL PART
OF DIAPHRAGM

LEFT CRUS
OF DIAPHRAGM

TRANSVERSUS
ABDOMINIS

QUADRATUS
LUMBORUM

PSOAS

ILIACUS

CUT EDGE
OF ABDOMINAL
WALL

FRANK PRICE.

SACRUM

RECTUM

LUMBAR PART OF VERTEBRAL COLUMN

Fig. 96. The muscles of the posterior abdominal wall and the diaphragm.

which is shaped like a clover leaf, one small leaflet pointing forwards and one larger leaflet extending to each side. The muscle fibres arising from the xiphisternum are very short, those from the lower costal cartilages, arcuate ligaments and crura are long. The central tendon is at the level of the xiphisternal joint, slightly lower than the parts of the diaphragm on each side, so that we talk of a **right dome** and a **left dome** of the diaphragm. The right dome is a little higher than the left because of the size of the liver.

As the diaphragm arches upwards from its origin, a very acute angle is formed between the origin and the thoracic wall. This is known as the **costodiaphragmatic recess,** and is very deep at the sides and deeper still posteriorly.

Openings

There are a number of openings in the diaphragm, the most important of which are those for the inferior vena cava, the œsophagus and the aorta. The **opening for the inferior vena cava** is in the central tendon at the level of the xiphisternal joint. When the muscle fibres of the diaphragm contract in inspiration they pull on the edges of the central tendon and hold the opening widely open. The negative intrapleural pressure of inspiration at the same time sucks blood into the thorax, that is, into the heart, and so the venous return is aided. The **opening for the œsophagus is in** the muscular part of the diaphragm, to the left of the midline, and behind the central tendon, opposite the tip of the eighth left costal cartilage. When the diaphragm contracts, it constricts the opening, thus preventing regurgitation of stomach contents into the thoracic part of the œsophagus during inspiration. The **opening for the aorta** is between the body of the twelfth thoracic vertebra and the median arcuate ligament, that is, it is an interval in the attachment of the diaphragm to the vertebral column.

Function

When the diaphragm contracts in inspiration it pulls the central tendon **downwards.** In addition the right and left domes are flattened. This enlarges the volume of the thoracic cavity by increasing the vertical height. When the diaphragm relaxes in expiration it returns to its domed shape (see also p. 339).

THE ANTERIOR ABDOMINAL WALL

The anterior abdominal wall (Fig. 91) is composed, on each side, of three large flat muscles and one long wide strap-like muscle, the **rectus abdominis,** close to the midline. The three flat muscles are the **external oblique,** the outer layer; the **internal oblique,** the intermediate layer; and the **transversus abdominis** the inner layer. These muscles form a continuous anterior wall for the abdominal cavity, stretching from the costal margin above to the pelvis (iliac crest and pubis) below, and round to the lumbar fascia at the sides (p. 188 and Fig. 91).

This muscular anterior abdominal wall is covered by skin and superficial fascia which often contains a thick layer of fat. The deep part of the superficial fascia is membranous and extends downwards over the inguinal ligament to be attached to the fascia lata, and over the pubis to be attached to the medial edges of the ischiopubic rami and to the posterior edge of the perineal membrane (p. 210, Plate 8).

The muscular wall is lined by fascia, the **transversalis fascia,** and this in turn is lined by the **parietal peritoneum.**

External Oblique

The fibres of the external oblique are directed downwards and medially. This muscle takes origin by digitations from the lower eight ribs. The muscle soon forms a wide aponeurosis (Fig. 91). The posterior muscular fibres are inserted into the anterior half of the iliac crest. The greater part of the aponeurosis meets that of the other side in the midline and is inserted by intermingling with it to form a dense band of white collagenous tissue, the **linea alba,** which stretches from the xiphisternum to the symphysis pubis. The aponeurosis is also attached to the pubic crest and to the pubic tubercle. The lower edge of the aponeurosis is turned under on itself to form the **inguinal ligament** which stretches from the anterior superior iliac spine to the pubic tubercle.

Internal Oblique

The fibres of the internal oblique are directed at right angles to those of the external oblique, that is upwards and medially. The internal oblique takes origin from the lateral two thirds of the inguinal ligament, from the anterior two thirds of the iliac crest and from the lumbar fascia (p. 188). It too forms a wide aponeurosis, and is inserted into the costal margin, into the **linea alba,** and, together with part of the transversus abdominis, as the **conjoined tendon** into the pubic crest and superior ramus of the pubis.

Transversus Abdominis

The fibres of the transversus abdominis are directed in the main, horizontally. This muscle takes origin from the lateral one third of the inguinal ligament, from the anterior two thirds of the iliac crest, from the lumbar fascia and from the internal aspect of the costal margin, interdigitating with the origin of the diaphragm. The aponeurosis is inserted into the **linea alba,** and with part of the internal oblique, as the **conjoint tendon.**

Rectus Abdominis

This is a broad strap-like muscle which takes origin from the front of the pubis and from the pubic crest, and is inserted into the seventh, sixth and fifth costal cartilages (Fig. 91).

Rectus Sheath

The three flat muscles, as they pass medially to the linea alba, form a sheath for the rectus muscle. The aponeurosis of the internal oblique splits into two layers, one going in front of rectus, the other behind. Thus the anterior wall of the rectus sheath is made up of the aponeurosis of the external oblique and the anterior layer of the internal oblique aponeurosis, and the posterior wall is made up of the posterior layer of the internal oblique aponeurosis and the aponeurosis of the transversus abdominis. The lower quarter of the sheath is deficient posteriorly, because, in this part, all three aponeuroses pass in front of the rectus.

The arrangement of the muscles adds strength to the abdominal wall. The different directions of the fibres of the three flat muscles is something like the plan of the wood grain in plywood. The rectus sheath supports the rectus, especially in the lower part, where all three aponeuroses pass in front. Effective support here is advantageous because it is here that the weight of the viscera mainly impinges in the upright posture.

The Inguinal Canal (Fig. 97)

The inguinal canal is an oblique tunnel through the abdominal wall. It is about two inches long and lies above the medial half of the inguinal ligament. The internal end, the **internal ring,** which is an opening in the transversalis fascia, is opposite a point half an inch above the midpoint of the inguinal ligament. The external end, the **external ring,** is a triangular opening in the external oblique aponeurosis just above and lateral to the pubic tubercle. The anterior wall of the canal is made up of the aponeurosis of the external oblique, reinforced in its lateral half by the most medial fibres of origin of the internal oblique. The posterior wall is transversalis fascia, reinforced in its medial half by the conjoined tendon. The floor is the inguinal ligament and the roof is the

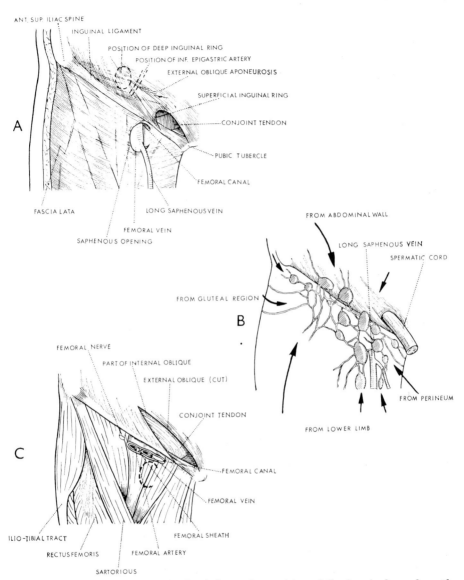

Fig. 97. The inguinal region: A, the fascia lata: the position of the inguinal canal; B, the superficial inguinal lymph nodes: the spermatic cord emerging from the inguinal canal; C, the inguinal canal: the external oblique aponeurosis has been split to show the internal oblique muscle where it forms the 'roof' and posterior wall of the canal. The femoral triangle (p. 216): the femoral nerve and femoral sheath (cut); the position of the saphenous opening (dotted outline).

lowest fibres of the internal oblique arching over from the anterior wall to the conjoint tendon in the posterior wall.

The inguinal canal transmits the spermatic cord in the male and the round ligament of the uterus in the female. In the male, during the eighth month of intra-uterine life, the testis descends through the canal from the abdominal cavity to the scrotum.

INGUINAL HERNIA: A hernia is the protrusion of a viscus through an opening in the abdominal wall. The inguinal canal is a potential weakness in the abdominal wall and herniation of part of the greater omentum or of a loop of gut through it is common. The hernia appears as a bulge through the external inguinal ring. Because the canal is temporarily opened up in the male by the descent of the testis, the male is much more subject to inguinal hernia than the female.

Nerve Supply and Blood Supply of the Abdominal Wall

The muscles, the skin and the parietal peritoneum are supplied by the **lower five intercostal nerves,** the **subcostal nerve** and the **first lumbar nerve** (iliohypogastric and ilioinguinal). The **intercostal** and **subcostal arteries** supply it together with the **superior epigastric artery** (a branch of the anterior thoracic artery) and the **inferior epigastric artery,** from the external iliac artery.

Umbilicus

The umbilicus is a knot of scar tissue left by the umbilical cord. It is situated in the linea alba at about the level of the fourth lumbar vertebra. (The level varies from one person to another.) If the anterior abdominal wall is examined from the inside, through the peritoneum there can be seen leading to the umbilicus from below, three fibrous cords, the median and the two lateral umbilical ligaments (p. 391). A fold of peritoneum, the falciform ligament, stretches from the liver to the abdominal wall above the level of the umbilicus. In its free edge is the round ligament of the liver, connecting the liver with the umbilicus (p. 391).

Functions of the Anterior Abdominal Muscles

SUPPORT: The muscle tone of the abdominal wall supports the weight of the viscera and prevents them from sagging.

RESPIRATORY ACTION: In inspiration when the diaphragm contracts, it descends, pushing the viscera downwards. A lowering of the muscle tone of the abdominal wall allows it to bulge, making room for the viscera. In expiration, renewed firm tone in the musculature presses on the viscera and through them on the relaxed diaphragm, driving it upwards. The excursion of the diaphragm and the associated movement of the abdominal wall is known as 'abdominal respiration' in contrast to 'thoracic respiration' which involves movements of the ribs (p. 339). In forced expiration and in coughing the abdominal muscles contract powerfully.

EXPULSIVE ACTION: If the abdominal muscles contract at the same time as the diaphragm, the intra-abdominal pressure is raised. This raised pressure can expel the contents of the viscera for example in defaecation, micturition, parturition and vomiting.

PROTECTION: Contraction of the muscles makes the wall taut and strong, for example to withstand an expected blow. In addition, the muscles contract reflexly if the peritoneum is irritated—this is called 'rigidity'; it immobilizes the viscera.

MOVEMENTS OF THE TRUNK: Rectus abdominis effects flexion of the vertebral column. The oblique muscles produce lateral bending of the trunk and also effect twisting movements.

Surface Anatomy of Abdominal Wall

The **skeletal landmarks** surrounding the abdominal wall are the costal margin, the iliac crests, the pubic crests and the pubic tubercles (Fig. 51).

Regions of the abdominal wall are given the names illustrated in Fig. 183, namely the **epigastrium,** the **umbilical region,** the **hypogastrium,** the **right** and **left hypochondria,** the right and left lumbar regions and the right and left iliac regions or **iliac fossæ.**

Abdominal planes are described for convenience.

The **transpyloric plane** (Fig. 51) is a horizontal plane which passes through the first lumbar vertebra, the middle of the costal margin at the tips of the ninth costal cartilages, the fundus of the gall bladder, the hilum of each of the kidneys (although there is a difference in level, see p. 483) and the origin of the superior mesenteric artery. (The transpyloric plane passes through the pylorus in a cadaver but not in a living person, in whom the pylorus lies at a lower level.)

The **supracristal plane** is a horizontal plane which passes through the highest part of the iliac crests (p. 147 and Fig. 58), the fourth lumbar vertebra, the bifurcation of the aorta and often through the umbilicus.

EXAMINATION OF THE ABDOMINAL WALL follows the routine of inspection, palpation, percussion and auscultation.

Inspection reveals the normal contours, with the umbilicus near the middle at the level of the fourth lumbar vertebra. Its level is variable, however, and it is always lower in children, in whom the pelvis is not yet fully developed. The abdominal wall moves gently with every respiration, bulging a little on inspiration and falling back on expiration. The outline of the rectus abdominis muscles can be seen easily if they are made to contract, for example, by a subject lying on his back lifting his legs in the air.

Palpation. Provided that the subject is relaxed and that the examiner's hand is warm, the abdominal wall feels soft and yielding. The descending colon can often be felt, and sometimes the right kidney (p. 483).

Percussion. The method is the same as for percussion of the thorax (p. 6). A dull note can be elicited over the liver and a resonant note over the stomach and intestines which contain a varying amount of air.

An overdistended bladder gives a dull note in the midline above the symphysis pubis.

Auscultation. Normal bowel sounds can always be heard with a stethoscope. They sound like faint 'tummy rumbling' and are due to the normal movements of the gut (p. 448).

POSITION OF THE VISCERA: The surface projection of some of the viscera is shown in Fig. 183, and is described as follows: liver, p. 472; gall bladder, p. 479; stomach, p. 451; intestines, pp. 455 and 461–466; and kidneys, p. 464.

THE POSTERIOR ABDOMINAL WALL

In the midline of the posterior abdominal wall the bodies of the five lumbar vertebræ project forwards, the more so because of the forward convexity of this part of the vertebral column. To the sides of the vertebral bodies and to their transverse processes is attached the **psoas** muscle (Fig. 96). The rounded belly passes downwards and laterally, passing along the inlet of the lesser pelvis to leave the abdominal cavity by entering the thigh behind the inguinal ligament. Lateral to the upper part of the psoas is the **quadratus lumborum** which stretches from the posterior part of the iliac crest to the twelfth rib. It helps to steady this rib for the pull of the diaphragm during inspiration. The three layers of the **lumbar fascia** (p. 188) blend at the lateral margin of this muscle, and give attachment to transversus abdominis and internal oblique muscles (Fig. 96). The lower lateral part of the posterior abdominal wall is formed by the iliac fossæ. **Iliacus** arises from this part of the ilium and blends with the lateral side of psoas as it enters the thigh.

The posterior abdominal wall is far from flat although some illustrations make it look as if it were. The lumbar vertebral bodies project forwards leaving a deep hollow on each side.

THE ABDOMINO-PELVIC CAVITY

This cavity can be divided into a large upper part, the abdomen, and a small lower part, the **lesser** (true) **pelvis.** The two parts are continuous at the **brim** of the lesser pelvis. Apart from the lumbar part of the vertebral column posteriorly and the iliac bones at the sides, the walls of the abdominal cavity are composed of muscles which allow the capacity to be adapted to changes in the size of the viscera—for example, the stomach after a large meal, or the pregnant uterus. The lesser pelvis is a much smaller cavity, and with rigid bony walls it cannot alter its capacity.

Because of the domed shape of the diaphragm the abdominal cavity extends upwards under shelter of the rib cage. The upper limit (Fig. 96) is at about the level of the fifth rib and the xiphisternal joint. The shape of the abdominal cavity is indicated in Fig. 178. The bodies of the vertebræ encroach greatly in the midline leaving a deep hollow on each side. The upper part, under the diaphragm, is deep and roomy. The lower part in the region of the iliac fossæ is very shallow. The region of the umbilicus is separated by a relatively small interval from the front of the vertebral bodies. This means that the lower part of the abdominal aorta is close to the anterior abdominal wall.

The abdominal cavity is bounded above by the diaphragm (p. 198), in front and at the sides by the anterior abdominal wall, behind by the posterior abdominal wall, and below it is continuous with the lesser pelvis.

THE LESSER PELVIS

The bony walls of the lesser pelvis are described on p. 147. Two small muscles of the lower limb are attached to the interior: posteriorly piriformis, which leaves the lesser pelvis through the greater sciatic foramen and, laterally, obturator internus which leaves through the lesser sciatic foramen.

THE PELVIC FLOOR

The lesser pelvis is closed inferiorly by a muscular sheet called the **pelvic floor** or **pelvic diaphragm**. If the lesser pelvis is like a pudding basin (tilted forwards, p. 147), the pelvic floor is the bottom of the basin. It obviously has to support the pelvic viscera to prevent them from falling through. It has openings in the midline to transmit the urethra in front, the rectum behind and,

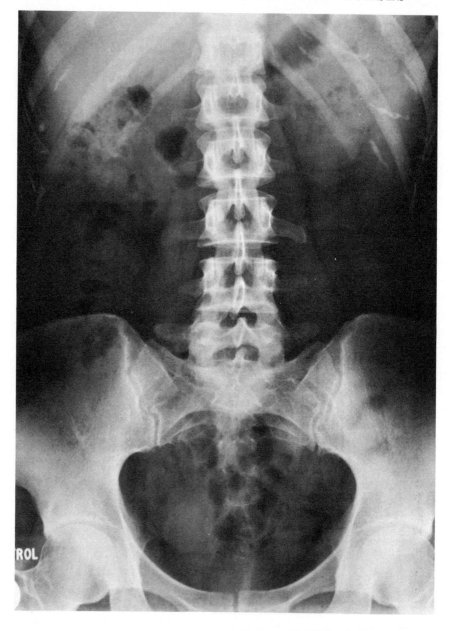

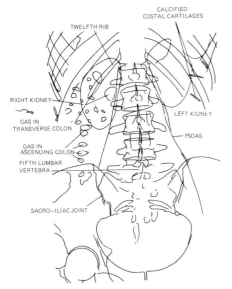

CALCIFIED
COSTAL CARTILAGES
TWELFTH RIB
RIGHT KIDNEY
LEFT KIDNEY
GAS IN
TRANSVERSE COLON
PSOAS
GAS IN
ASCENDING COLON
FIFTH LUMBAR
VERTEBRA
SACRO—ILIAC JOINT

Fig. 98. A radiograph of the abdomen.

in the female, the vagina between the other two. The pelvic floor consists of two thin flat muscles, **levator ani** and **coccygeus**.

The **levator ani** arises fom the back of the **pubis** and from the **fascia** lining the side wall of the pelvis round as far as the **spine of the ischium.** The fibres sweep to their insertion in the midline. The most posterior fibres from the spine reach the side of the **coccyx** (Plate 8). Those a little further forward are inserted into a mass of connective tissue, the **anococcygeal body** placed between the tip of the coccyx and the anal canal. Further forwards the fibres reach a knot of connective tissue, the **perineal body,** which is in front of the anal canal and blends with the middle of the posterior border of the perineal membrane (p. 210). In the female the perineal body is between the vagina and the anal canal. The most anterior fibres of the levator ani sweep backwards rather than medially, above the fibres just described. Those near the midline sweep round the sides of the prostate (levator prostatæ) or the vagina (sphincter vaginæ) to reach the perineal body. Those a little more lateral pass round behind the junction of the rectum and anal canal, some of them finding insertion into the anococcygeal body, but most uniting with those of the other side to form a sling (**puborectalis**) which blends with the external sphincter of the anal canal. By contracting, these sling-like fibres increase the angulation of the junction of the rectum with the anal canal and prevent the untimely descent of fæces.

The levator ani is supplied by fibres from the **third** and **fourth sacral nerves.**

The **coccygeus** which completes the pelvic floor posteriorly, stretches from the spine of the ischium to the side of the coccyx and lower part of the sacrum.

Functions of the Levator Ani

SUPPORT: First and foremost, levator ani supports the pelvic viscera, preventing them from falling through the pelvic outlet. (This is necessary because of the upright posture of Man. In four-footed animals this muscle wags the tail.) Levator ani, therefore, supports the rectum and the bladder and, most important, the uterus (see also p. 538).

SPHINCTERIC ACTION: The pubo-rectalis fibres, described above, play an important part as a sphincter of the anal canal. The fibres which circle the vagina compress its walls.

Clearly, good tone in the levator ani is important if it is to perform these functions adequately. During childbirth, the muscle is stretched and, especially after repeated deliveries, the tone may be poor. In such a case prolapse of the rectum, or of the bladder and urethra, or of both may occur because of inadequate support. The uterus too may prolapse, the cervical ligaments (p. 538) being deprived of the assistance of the levator ani in supporting the organ. During delivery the muscle may be torn, especially where it is inserted into the perineal body. If such a tear is not properly repaired prolapse is likely to develop.

THE PERINEUM

The perineum is the region bounded above by the levator ani and below by the pelvic outlet. In outline it is diamond shaped. The part in front of the ischial tuberosities is the **urogenital triangle:** the part behind is the **anal triangle.**

Urogenital Triangle

In the urogenital triangle (Plate 8) the **perineal membrane,** triangular in shape, stretches across between the ischiopubic rami. On its deep surface is a fascial space, the **deep perineal space** through which the urethra passes. Surrounding this part of the urethra in the deep pouch is the **sphincter urethræ** muscle, a voluntary skeletal muscle, supplied by the **pudendal nerve.** On the superficial aspect of the perineal membrane is the **superficial perineal space** which is formed by the attachment of the membranous layer of the superficial fascia of the abdominal wall (p. 201) to the ischiopubic rami and the posterior edge of the perineal membrane.

In the male, the superficial space contains the roots of the penis, namely the two corpora cavernosa penis, one on each side, and the corpus spongiosum penis in the midline (Plate 37). The urethra passes through the perineal membrane and enters the corpus spongiosum. The superficial space contains the small perineal muscles of the roots of the penis. The transverse perineal muscles (Plate 8) stretch from the ramus of the ischium on each side along the posterior border of the perineal membrane to be inserted into the perineal body. They are important in anchoring the perineal body which plays such a notable part as one of the insertions of levator ani. If they are torn during childbirth, they must be repaired so that the levator ani can function from a properly fixed insertion.

In the female the urogenital triangle is modified by the passage of the vagina which passes through both deep and superficial spaces and divides the perineal membrane almost completely. The posterior border, with the transverse perineal muscles, anchors the perineal body immediately behind the vagina. The superficial space contains the roots of the clitoris which are much smaller than the roots of the penis and the **greater vestibular glands (Bartholin's glands).** The urethra passes through both deep and superficial spaces and opens directly in front of the vagina. (Fig. 219.)

Anal Triangle

The anal triangle contains the **anal canal** which points downwards and backwards in the midline and on each side an **ischiorectal fossa** (Plate 8). This is a deep, wedge-shaped space between the anal canal medially and the ischium laterally. The base of the wedge is the skin and the thin edge of the wedge is the origin of the lateral part of levator ani from the side wall of the lesser pelvis. The ischiorectal fossa is filled with loose fatty tissue. Because of its proximity to the anal canal and the fact that fat has a poor blood supply, the contents of the fossa are prone to infection which produces an ischiorectal abscess.

Nerve Supply

The structures in the perineum are supplied by branches of the **pudendal nerve** which leaves the lesser pelvis through the greater sciatic foramen and enters the ischiorectal fossa through the lesser sciatic foramen. Branches cross the fossa to reach the anal canal and the contents of the perineal spaces (pouches) (Plate 8).

Blood Supply

The **internal pudendal artery,** a branch of the internal iliac, follows the course of the pudendal nerve from the lesser pelvis.

Lymphatic Drainage

Most of the lymph vessels of the perineum, including those of the skin of the anal canal and of the lowest third of the vagina, pass to the medial group of **superficial inguinal lymph nodes.**

THE MUSCLES OF THE LOWER LIMB

In considering the classical actions of the muscles of the lower limb, like flexion and extension, we usually think of the proximal origin as being fixed and the distal insertion moving. However, when the limb is used for walking the muscles usually work from fixed insertions, causing the origin to be moved. A foot firmly planted on the ground is fixed. The body is moved in relation to the foot and to the ground on which it stands. Many examples will follow.

MUSCLES ROUND THE HIP-JOINT

Psoas

Psoas, arising from the lumbar vertebræ, forms part of the posterior wall of the abdomen (p. 206), enters the thigh by passing behind the medial part of the inguinal ligament and is inserted into the lesser trochanter of the femur. It is joined by iliacus, the combined muscle sometimes being called iliopsoas. Psoas is supplied by branches from the lumbar plexus and is a powerful flexor at the hip joint.

Gluteal Muscles

The gluteal muscles are the large fleshy muscles of the buttock. **Gluteus maximus** (Figs. 90 and 99) is superficial and under cover of it lie **gluteus medius** and **gluteus minimus.** Lower down and somewhat medial to gluteus medius and minimus is the greater sciatic foramen through which comes the **sciatic nerve,** many other nerves and the gluteal arteries. This area must not be injured. **If intramuscular injections are given into the buttock, they must be given into the upper outer quadrant where they can do no damage.**

Gluteus Maximus

This is a large muscle which takes origin from the posterior part of the crest of the ilium and from the back of the sacrum. It is inserted into the shaft of the femur just below the greater trochanter and into the **iliotibial tract** (p. 217). It is supplied by a **nerve from the sacral plexus** and is an extensor at the hip joint. If one is standing and bending down to touch the toes, gluteus maximus acting from its fixed insertion, raises the trunk to the upright position. It also acts in walking up stairs and in rising from a sitting position.

Gluteus Medius and Gluteus Minimus

These two muscles arise from the outer surface of the ilium and are inserted into the front of the greater trochanter. They are abductors and medial rotators at the hip joint. If one stands on one leg, the gluteus medius and gluteus

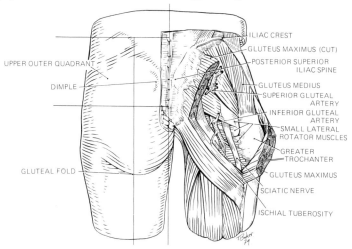

ILIAC CREST
GLUTEUS MAXIMUS (CUT)
POSTERIOR SUPERIOR ILIAC SPINE
UPPER OUTER QUADRANT
GLUTEUS MEDIUS
SUPERIOR GLUTEAL ARTERY
DIMPLE
INFERIOR GLUTEAL ARTERY
SMALL LATERAL ROTATOR MUSCLES
GREATER TROCHANTER
GLUTEAL FOLD
GLUTEUS MAXIMUS
SCIATIC NERVE
ISCHIAL TUBEROSITY

Fig. 99. The gluteal region.

minimus on that side contract, tilting the pelvis over to the supporting side and up on the other side, thus giving the opposite leg room to swing clear. Furthermore, at the same time these muscles rotate the pelvis on the femur so that the opposite side swings forwards; this lengthens the stride. They are supplied by a **nerve from the sacral plexus.**

Small Lateral Rotators

A group of small muscles from the pelvis to the greater trochanter produce lateral rotation at the hip joint and protect the back of the joint where the capsule is relatively weak.

FLEXORS AND EXTENSORS IN THE LOWER LIMB

It has been shown (pp. 217–272) that **flexor muscles** which are formed on the developmentally ventral surface of a limb are supplied by the **anterior**

divisions of the anterior primary rami of the spinal nerves. The **flexor muscles** of the lower limb are supplied, therefore, by the **tibial nerve** (medial popliteal), and by the **obturator nerve** (p. 277), both derived from the anterior divisions of the roots of the lumbar and sacral plexuses (Plate 16). The **extensor muscles,** which are formed on the developmentally dorsal surface of the limb, are supplied by the **femoral** and **common peroneal** (lateral popliteal) nerves derived from the posterior divisions of the roots of the lumbar and sacral plexuses.

However, the lower limb has undergone a rotation during development (p. 20) so that the developmentally ventral surface is behind and the developmentally dorsal surface is in front. The flexor muscles are, therefore, on the back of the limb and the extensor muscles on the front.

THE MUSCLES OF THE THIGH

The thigh is the segment between the hip joint and the knee joint. There are three main groups of muscles: extensors, flexors and adductors.

Extensor Group of Muscles

The large extensor muscle group occupying the front of the thigh is the **quadriceps femoris** (Fig. 100). It takes origin from the front and sides of the shaft of the femur, except for one head, the **rectus femoris,** which is attached to the ilium above the acetabulum. It is inserted into the patella and, through the **patellar ligament** (tendon) and fibres passing on each side of the patella, into the tuberosity of the tibia. It is a powerful extensor at the knee joint and, because its apparatus of insertion, namely the patella, the patellar ligament and associated fibres, replaces the capsule of the knee joint, it exercises close control of the joint. It is supplied by the **femoral nerve.**

Sartorius is a long strap-like muscle stretching from the anterior end of the iliac crest to the medial side of the upper end of the tibia. Its action is to pull the lower limb into the position for sitting cross-legged, hence its name: *sartor* means tailor. During walking sartorius produces flexion simultaneously at the hip joint and at the knee joint. It is supplied by the femoral nerve.

Sartorius belongs to the extensor group, even though in fact it flexes the limb. It develops from the extensor muscle mass, but, during evolution, its attachments to the skeleton have gradually altered in relation to the joints so that its action has become to flex. It retains its original nerve supply.

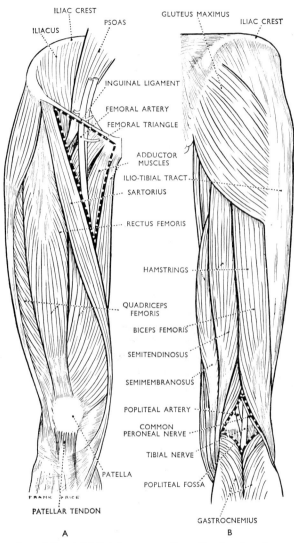

ILIAC CREST

ILIACUS

PSOAS

GLUTEUS MAXIMUS

ILIAC CREST

INGUINAL LIGAMENT

FEMORAL ARTERY

FEMORAL TRIANGLE

ADDUCTOR
MUSCLES

ILIO-TIBIAL TRACT

SARTORIUS

RECTUS FEMORIS

HAMSTRINGS

QUADRICEPS
FEMORIS

BICEPS FEMORIS

SEMITENDINOSUS

SEMIMEMBRANOSUS

POPLITEAL ARTERY

COMMON
PERONEAL NERVE

TIBIAL NERVE

PATELLA

POPLITEAL FOSSA

FRANK PRICE

PATELLAR TENDON

GASTROCNEMIUS

A

B

Fig. 100. The muscles of the right thigh: A, seen from the front and B, seen from the back.
The femoral triangle and the popliteal fossa are outlined by interrupted lines.

FEMORAL TRIANGLE

The femoral triangle is a shallow hollow bounded above by the inguinal ligament, medially by the adductor muscles (adductor longus) and laterally by the sartorius muscle (Figs. 100 and 97). It contains (1) the superficial inguinal lymph nodes; (2) the end of the long saphenous vein which goes through the saphenous opening in the fascia lata to join the femoral vein and (3) the femoral artery and vein which pass through it from the middle of the inguinal ligament to its apex. The proximal inch of the femoral artery and vein are enclosed in the **femoral sheath,** a funnel-shaped prolongation of the fascia lining the abdominal cavity. This fascia is drawn down behind the inguinal ligament to clothe the artery and vein. The empty medial part of the femoral sheath is the **femoral canal** (Fig. 97).

SUBSARTORIAL CANAL

This is a narrow space behind the sartorius muscle, and between the quadriceps femoris and the adductor muscles. It contains the femoral artery (and vein) after it leaves the femoral triangle until it goes through the adductor magnus to become the popliteal artery.

Flexor Group of Muscles

The flexor muscles in the thigh are known as 'hamstrings'. They take origin from the ischial tuberosity and are inserted just below the knee joint, some on the medial side into the tibia, and one (biceps femoris) into the head of the fibula on the lateral side. They are supplied by the **tibial part of the sciatic nerve.** They produce flexion at the knee joint and also extension at the hip joint. They can be used to demonstrate active insufficiency (p. 179). They also demonstrate passive insufficiency. Lie on the back and flex the thigh on the trunk, keeping the knee straight. At a certain point no more flexion at the hip is possible because of pain in the hamstrings—they are relaxed to the limit and are passively insufficient to allow both full extension at the knee and full flexion at the hip.

The Adductor Muscles of the Thigh

The adductor muscles arise from the ischiopubic ramus of the hip bone and are inserted into the linea aspera of the femur. The largest, the **adductor magnus,** arises partly from the ischial tuberosity. They are powerful adductors, of the thigh at the hip joint. The group is supplied by the **obturator nerve** and is a subdivision of the flexor muscle mass.

POPLITEAL FOSSA

The popliteal fossa (Fig. 100) is the diamond-shaped hollow behind the knee joint. It is deep, especially when the knee is bent, being bounded above by the hamstring muscles and below by gastrocnemius. It contains the popliteal artery and vein, the popliteal lymph nodes, and the tibial (medial popliteal) and common peroneal (lateral popliteal) nerves. When the knee is bent the popliteal artery can be compressed against the lower end of the femur.

THE FASCIA OF THE THIGH

The deep fascia of the thigh forms a tense firm sheath for the muscles, and is called the **fascia lata** (Fig. 97). Below, it is attached to the upper end of the tibia and above it is attached round the root of the limb, that is to the inguinal ligament, to the crest of the ilium, to the ischial tuberosity and to the ischio-pubic ramus. This fascia, and the similar strong investing fascia of the leg, play an important part in the functioning of the **'muscle pump'** on the veins (p. 383). A thickened band of the fascia lata extending from the iliac crest to the tibia is called the **iliotibial tract** (Fig. 100). On the front of the upper part of the thigh 4 cms below and lateral to the pubic tubercle there is an oval opening in the fascia lata, the **saphenous opening** (Fig. 97). It lies in front of a funnel-shaped sheath of fascia which has three compartments, one for the femoral artery, one for the femoral vein medial to the artery, and medial to the vein, a compartment containing fat, the **femoral canal,** which leads from the abdominal cavity into the thigh and allows for expansion of the neighbouring vein. A femoral hernia may push its way down the femoral canal and then through the saphenous opening to bulge under the skin. Femoral hernia is commoner in the female, because the extra width of the pelvis and the slighter development of muscles leaves more room for a larger canal.

THE MUSCLES OF THE LEG

The leg is the segment of the limb between the knee and the ankle.

Flexor Muscles

The flexor muscles on the back of the calf (Fig. 101) are arranged in three groups. All are supplied by the **tibial nerve.** The superficial group, the **flexors**

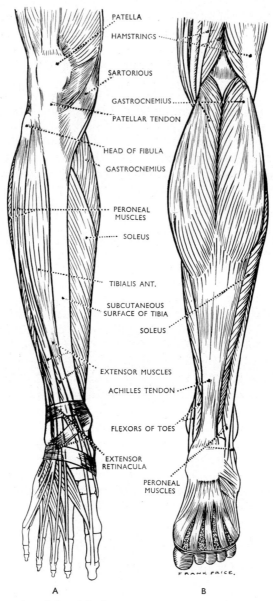

PATELLA

HAMSTRINGS

SARTORIOUS

GASTROCNEMIUS

PATELLAR TENDON

HEAD OF FIBULA

GASTROCNEMIUS

PERONEAL
MUSCLES

SOLEUS

TIBIALIS ANT.

SUBCUTANEOUS
SURFACE OF TIBIA

SOLEUS

EXTENSOR MUSCLES

ACHILLES TENDON

FLEXORS OF TOES

EXTENSOR
RETINACULA

PERONEAL
MUSCLES

FRANK PRICE.

A   B

Fig. 101. The muscles of the right leg, seen A, from the front and B, from behind.

at the ankle joint (plantar-flexors), consist of **gastrocnemius** and **soleus.** They take origin from the back of the lower end of the femur and from the tibia and fibula respectively, and combine to form the **Achilles tendon** which is inserted into the back of the calcaneum. They plantar-flex the foot at the ankle joint. In standing, when the foot is fixed, soleus acts as a postural muscle, preventing the leg from falling forwards over the foot under the action of gravity, which falls in front of the ankle joint (Fig. 7). Gastrocnemius provides the motive power in walking, the foot being used as a lever applied to the ground at the balls of the toes.

The second layer is composed of the (plantar) **flexors of the toes.** The fleshy bellies are in the leg, and the long tendons, surrounded by synovial sheaths, reach the toes. Their main functions are to help to maintain the longitudinal arches of the foot and to assist gastrocnemius in producing motive power.

The deepest layer is **tibialis posterior,** which is specialized for inversion of the foot (p. 173).

Extensor Muscles of the Leg

The extensor muscles on the front of the leg (Fig. 101) produce extension (dorsiflexion) of the foot at the ankle joint, and of the toes. They are supplied by a branch of the **common peroneal (lateral popliteal) nerve.** The deepest muscle of the group, tibialis anterior, is specialized for inversion (p. 173).

A subdivision of the extensor group on the lateral side of the leg, the **peroneal muscles** (Fig. 101) produce eversion of the foot. They too are supplied by a branch of the **common peroneal nerve.**

MUSCLES OF THE FOOT

There are a number of short muscles of the foot (Fig. 102), arranged similarly to those in the hand. They are supplied by the **tibial nerve.** Their main function is to assist the ligaments in maintaining the longitudinal and transverse arches of the foot.

POSTURE AND BALANCE

The posture of the body depends on the tone of its muscles.

In standing upright, the head must be carefully balanced on the trunk, the trunk on the lower limbs and the lower limbs on the feet. This is at first far

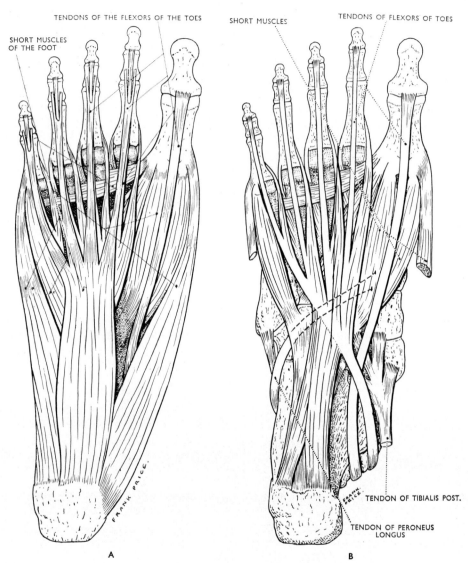

Fig. 102. The sole of the right foot: A, superficial short muscles of the foot; B, deeper tendons and muscles.

from easy, and it takes an infant many months to learn to stand unsupported. The force of gravity tends constantly to cause the body to fall forwards. Tone in the muscles on the back of the body prevents this. Muscles which act against gravity in this way are called antigravity or postural muscles. The extensor muscles of the back are an important group of postural muscles.

The tone in the different groups of muscles which control balance varies according to the needs of the moment. The tone is regulated reflexly by afferent nervous impulses coming from stretch receptors in the muscles themselves, from the eyes, from the semicircular canals, and from pressure receptors in the skin, especially the skin of the soles of the feet.

'Good posture' means holding the body in such a position that the muscles, particularly the postural muscles, can maintain it with the minimum of contraction. For example, the head should be held up, shoulders back, back straight and 'tail tucked in'. Any other position results in harder work for the muscles and therefore in fatigue.

CHAPTER VIII

THE NERVOUS SYSTEM

N ERVOUS tissue is structurally specialized for the expression of two of the basic properties of protoplasm (p. 89), namely irritability and conductivity. The basic functions of nervous tissue are, firstly to act as a tissue which is receptive to the stimuli arising either outside or inside the body, and secondly, when stimulated, to conduct nervous impulses rapidly and often over great distances to muscle or glandular tissue.

Superimposed on these basic functions, there are other more complex ones. The environment of the individual provides so many stimuli, that he would be in a chronic state of convulsion and his glands would never stop secreting, if all stimuli were automatically and immediately translated into responses. There must, therefore, be a mechanism within the nervous system, which permits the sorting out of impulses set up by the stimuli of the environment, and for permitting only some of them to reach the muscles and glands. In such a complex organism as Man, there are also mechanisms that permit a delayed response to stimuli and which subserve memory, the initiation of voluntary activity, consciousness and the appreciation of different sensations.

SUBDIVISIONS OF THE NERVOUS SYSTEM

Nervous tissue extends to almost every part of the body, yet every portion of nervous tissue in the organism is linked to some other portion, so that a structural and functional unit is formed—it is termed **the nervous system.**

Nervous tissue is not, however, equally distributed within the body. It is concentrated within the skull as the brain and within the canal of the backbone, or spine, as the spinal cord. This concentration in the midline of the body—**the brain and spinal cord**—constitutes **the central nervous system.** The remainder of the nervous tissue constitutes the **peripheral nervous system** and consists of cord-like nerves, which emerge through holes (foramina) in the skull and between the vertebræ of the spine. These nerves are known respectively as **cranial nerves,** and **spinal** or **peripheral segmental nerves.** The peripheral nervous system also includes small collections of nerve cells outside the central nervous system known as **ganglia.**

The **autonomic nervous system** controls the viscera, glands and **all the** smooth muscle in the body. As its name implies, it is to some extent independent of the higher centres in the central nervous system and of the will. Components of the autonomic nervous system are to be found in both the central nervous system and in the peripheral nervous system.

SOME BASIC UNITS AND FUNCTIONAL CONSIDERATIONS

The nervous system is made up of nerve cells or **neurones** and a special type of connective tissue cells called **neuroglia,** which provide a supporting network for the neurones. Attention has already been drawn, on p. 116, to the fact that the majority of tumours in the central nervous system arise from this neuroglia and that such a tumour is known as a **glioma.**

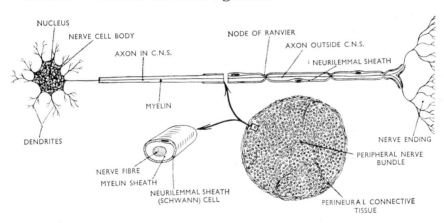

Fig. 103. Scheme to show the components of a neurone and the relations of its axon.

THE NEURONE

A neurone *consists of a nerve cell and all its processes* (Fig. 103).

The Cell Body of the Neurone

The cell bodies of neurones vary in size from small to large and the larger ones, about 120 μm in diameter, are amongst the largest cells in the body. Their shape varies from round, or oval, to pyramidal. Within the cell body, there is a nucleus which is generally placed centrally, is usually large and spherical, and contains a prominent nucleolus. The cytoplasm of nerve cells contains small blocks of basophilic material, known as **Nissl substance,** which tends to break up and disappear when the cell is exhausted or damaged—a phenomenon known as **chromatolysis.**

In general (with the exception of sensory ganglia of cranial nerves, dorsal root ganglia and autonomic ganglia), the cell bodies of neurones are located within the central nervous system.

The Processes of the Neurone

From the cell body, there may extend several short processes which convey impulses towards the cell body; these are **dendrites.** From the cell body, there usually extends one long process which conveys impulses away from the cell body; this is the **axon.** Axons are the **nerve fibres** found both within the central nervous system and in peripheral nerves. They vary considerably in diameter, the thicker ones conducting impulses more rapidly than the thinner ones. Axons often branch.

Axons are surrounded by **myelin sheaths,** myelin being a fatty substance. The amount of myelin varies considerably; in fact some small fibres have so little as to appear 'unmyelinated'. Within the central nervous system, the myelin is produced by the neuroglia which surround the nerve fibres.

Outside the central nervous system, nerve fibres have an additional covering —the **neurilemmal sheath**—which is made up of **neurilemmal** (Schwann) **cells.** These cells play an important rôle in nerve fibre regeneration, a process which is thus possible only outside the central nervous system (p. 600).

Outside the central nervous system where neurilemmal cells and sheaths are present, the neurilemmal cells lay down the myelin around the fibres. This myelin, laid down by neurilemmal cells, is notched at regular intervals, the notches being called **nodes** (of Ranvier).

The Synapse

Where part of one neurone links up with an adjoining one, the link is known as a synapse, but although neurones are in contact with one another at a synapse, there is no cytoplasmic continuity between them.

NERVE ENDINGS

Afferent or Sensory Nerve Endings

Nerve endings may be afferent to the central nervous system, i.e. structures which are adapted to setting up an impulse when stimulated by a particular stimulus. The impulse is then conveyed to the central nervous system along afferent (sensory) nerve fibres.

The receptors concerned with smell, taste, sight and hearing and appreciation of movement in relation to gravity will be considered in the chapter dealing with the special sense organs.

The afferent receptor nerve endings described in this section are concerned with the appreciation of **touch, pressure, pain** and **temperature.**

The sense of touch may be subserved by a **tactile** (Meissner's) **corpuscle,** a tangle of curved nerve endings within a capsule, or by **tactile** (Merkel's) **discs,** expanded discs on the terminal twigs of a branched nerve ending. In addition, **hair follicles** are surrounded by a basket-like arrangement of nerve fibres, so that hairs act as sense organs for touch.

A sensory nerve fibre may also end peripherally in an ovoid structure made up of layers of cells, called a **lamellated** (Pacinian) **corpuscle,** which responds to pressure. Special encapsulated end-organs have been described as the receptor organs for heat and cold.

Another important peripheral nerve ending to be considered is the **free** or **naked nerve ending,** which consists of very fine branching nerve fibres that end in fine beaded terminals between the cells of the deeper layers of the epidermis. These are pain receptors, which are protective in function, and do not distinguish the specific nature of the stimulation, but respond to a mechanical, chemical or thermal stimulus, provided it is intense enough. (Some sensory nerve endings are illustrated in Plate 20.)

The endings so far described tend to be located in the skin, but in addition there are afferent (sensory) nerve endings which respond to changes in **tension** or **pressure** in muscles (**neuromuscular spindles**), in tendons (**neurotendinous organs**) and in joints. All these receptors consist of branching nerve fibres which end within a capsule of connective tissue. The neuromuscular spindle also contains some attenuated striated muscle fibres. The nervous impulses set up by these encapsulated endings enable an individual to appreciate changes of position, even with the eyes closed.

Efferent or Motor Nerve Endings

Efferent or motor nerve fibres end in relation to striated muscle fibres at structures known as **motor end-plates** (Fig. 110). As the nerve fibre approaches the muscle fibre, it loses its myelin sheath and ends in terminal branches which have club-like ends in contact with the cell membrane of the muscle fibre. The part of the muscle fibre in the immediate vicinity of the nerve ending is devoid of striations. It must, however, be realized that the axon from one effector (motor) neurone branches repeatedly, and so, is connected to a number of motor end-plates on different muscle fibres. Motor impulses conveyed by that axon will, therefore, be transmitted to several muscle fibres. These muscle fibres and the axon which supplies them constitute what is known as a **motor unit.**

Nerve Conduction

The response of a nerve cell is always the same whatever the stimulus, and the resulting **impulse** is conducted over the whole extent of the neurone and travels along the axon at a speed of up to 100 metres per second.

The change of state taking place in a nerve and its fibre, when an impulse is being conducted, is highly complicated. It involves changes in the electrical state and oxygen consumption with the liberation of heat and carbon dioxide.

Chemical Transmitters

Neurones link up by the contact of their processes at a **synapse** (p. 224). As there is no protoplasmic continuity between neurones at a synapse, an impulse is conveyed from one neurone to another, when the first neurone liberates a chemical substance which excites a fresh nerve impulse in the next neurone. The chemical substance is called a **chemical transmitter.** Different chemical transmitters are known, for example **acetyl choline** and **adrenaline.**

As well as being found at every synapse in the central nervous system and in the nerve ganglia (p. 229 and p. 280) of the peripheral nervous system, a chemical transmitter is liberated by sensory receptors to stimulate impulses in the axons of sensory, afferent neurones; similarly, an impulse in the axon of a motor, efferent neurone liberates a chemical transmitter at its motor end-plate in order to stimulate the muscle fibre.

Muscle relaxant drugs act by interfering with the action of the chemical transmitter at the motor end-plate.

STRUCTURAL BASIS OF FUNCTION WITHIN THE NERVOUS SYSTEM

It has already been explained how the central nervous system is made up of **neurones** and their processes with supporting cells or **neuroglia** (pp. 116 and 223). Neurones connect with one another at **synapses** (p. 224), the nerve cell bodies being located in **grey matter** (p. 228), whereas fibres tend to be collected up into bundles or **tracts,** which run in **white matter** (p. 228). **Afferent (receptor** or **sensory) neurones** (p. 228) convey impulses coming into the central nervous system, and interruption of this path may lead to loss of sensation or anæsthesia; **efferent (effector** or **motor) neurones** convey impulses out of the nervous system to effector structures, usually muscle or gland tissue, and interruption of this pathway to a muscle leads to its paralysis. Thus, the simplest **reflex arc** consists of a **receptor** or sensory nerve ending (p. 224), an **afferent neurone,** a **synapse** with an **efferent neurone** and an **effector organ.** Very often the afferent and efferent neurones are separated and linked indirectly by an intermediate, intercalated or **connector neurone,** which is joined to the other two neurones by means of synapses (Plate 9, A).

Such a connector neurone may have synaptic links with a number of efferent and afferent neurones, and so can spread the impulse to a number of efferent neurones, or can concentrate the impulses coming in from a number of afferent neurones on to a limited number of efferent neurones.

The greatest delay in the transmission of a nerve impulse occurs at the synapse, and the number of synapses an impulse has to pass through, before reaching an effector neurone, plays an important rôle in determining the timing and sequence of arrival of impulses at a particular neurone. Although a given impulse may not be sufficient to trigger off a neurone (**a subliminal stimulus**), it may be sufficient to sensitize the neurone to subsequent subliminal stimuli which may now trigger off the neurone. This sensitization process, whereby a neurone is sensitized to a subliminal stimulus by another subliminal stimulus from another source, is termed **facilitation.**

Another process in which synapses play an important rôle is **inhibition,** whereby a neurone fails to respond to a stimulus which is strong enough to make it respond in other circumstances. This may be associated with the fact that, after a neurone has responded to stimulation, it enters a recovery, or **refractory phase,** during which it 'recovers' and during which it cannot respond to further stimulation.

GENERAL FORM AND STRUCTURE OF THE NERVOUS SYSTEM

As stated above, the nervous system is made up of neurones, that is, of nerve cells together with their processes, the short dendrites and the long axons which are called nerve fibres. The nervous system is subdivided into the central nervous system (C.N.S.) and the peripheral nervous system (P.N.S.).

Central Nervous System

The central nervous system, which consists of the **brain** and the **spinal cord,** contains nearly all the nerve cells present in the body together with their dendrites and part at least, but often the whole, of their axons. The naked eye can make out within the central nervous system, **grey matter** which is made up of greyish jelly-like nerve cell bodies, and **white matter** which is made up of nerve fibres (axons). These nerve fibres are surrounded by fatty myelin sheaths which make them look white. Some of these fibres run the whole of their course within the central nervous system. Others run part of their course in the white matter and then leave the central nervous system to continue their course within peripheral nerves (see below).

In the spinal cord, the grey matter is placed centrally and is surrounded by white matter. In the brain, however, some of the grey matter is spread out as a layer covering the surface of some areas; this is known as **cortex.** In addition, there is a considerable amount of grey matter interspersed among the white matter nearer the centre of the brain.

Within the central nervous system, any small mass of grey matter, that is, a circumscribed group of nerve cells, is called a **nucleus,** or if it is larger, a **nuclear mass.** Nerve fibres are grouped in bundles in the white matter. Such bundles are called **tracts.**

Peripheral Nervous System

The peripheral nervous system comprises the parts of the nervous system outside the brain and spinal cord. These are the **peripheral nerves** and some small collections of nerve cells known as **ganglia.**

A nerve is a bundle of nerve fibres. Some of these fibres, the motor or efferent fibres, have their cell bodies within the central nervous system. Other fibres, the sensory or afferent fibres, have their cell bodies in a sensory ganglion (see below). Thus the peripheral nerves are usually **mixed nerves,** that is, they contain both (*a*) **motor fibres,** which are efferent and carry impulses to muscles to cause them to contract, and (*b*) **sensory fibres** which are afferent and carry impulses to the central nervous system, thus conveying information of different kinds (p. 224). If a peripheral nerve is cut, impulses cannot pass in either direction. The muscles supplied by that nerve are paralysed and the skin supplied by it loses its sensation.

Some of the cranial nerves are purely motor, for example, the hypoglossal nerve (p. 268) or purely sensory, for example, the vestibulocochlear or auditory nerve; others are mixed nerves, for example, the trigeminal nerve.

Spinal peripheral nerves are mixed nerves and are connected to the spinal cord by means of two roots: one posteriorly placed, termed the **dorsal root,** which carries the **dorsal root (sensory) ganglion** and conveys afferent sensory fibres; and another anteriorly placed, termed the **ventral root,** which conveys efferent motor fibres.

A **ganglion** *is a collection of nerve cells* **outside** *the central nervous system.* There are two kinds, (*a*) sensory and (*b*) autonomic. A **sensory ganglion** has nerve cells whose *axons are T-shaped*. The stem of the T is attached to the cell; one end of the crossbar, very long, is connected with the sensory receptor at the periphery, for example in the skin; the other end of the crossbar, shorter, is connected with the central nervous system. All sensory nerve fibres are the axons of cells situated in a sensory ganglion, and all sensory nerves, therefore, have a sensory ganglion attached to them, usually close to the connection with the central nervous system. **Autonomic ganglia** are found in association with the autonomic nervous system (p. 280). *An autonomic ganglion consists of* **motor nerve cells** *and is a* **relay** station.

THE CENTRAL NERVOUS SYSTEM

OUTLINE OF DEVELOPMENT

As was described on p. 78 the notochord induces the overlying ectoderm to form a **neural plate** from which the nervous system develops. Where the lateral edge of the neural plate is continuous with the ectoderm, there is a raised margin, the **neural crest,** from which a great variety of cells develop, including sensory ganglion cells, autonomic ganglion cells, the suprarenal medulla, neurilemmal sheath cells, cells of the pia and arachnoid layers of the meninges and some of the mesenchymal cells of the head region. The pigment cells, melanoblasts, of the body are also developed from the neural crest.

The neural plate has a simple medio-lateral localization of cells, which is related to function (see Plate 9, A). The lateral margin of the neural plate, as already explained, is continuous with the ectoderm along the neural crest, and, because this ectoderm becomes the epidermis of the skin, it is understandable that this marginal region acquires a sensory function and that neurones developed from the neural crest become, therefore, **sensory** or **receptor neurones.** At the other extreme, the neurones developed in the most medial part of the neural plate establish connections with muscle and so become **motor** or **effector neurones.** The intermediately situated neurones link together the sensory and motor neurones, and are known as intermediate or **connector neurones.** Thus, a simple reflex arc (p. 262) is established, which provides the means for muscle to be induced to contract as a result of stimulation of the epidermis, i.e. the basis of a simple withdrawal reflex from an injurious environment.

As development proceeds, the neural plate folds in (Plate 9, c) to form first a groove and, when this groove closes in, a tube—the **neural tube,** which sinks below the dorsal surface of the embryo and loses direct contact with it (Plate 9, D and E).

As the tube closes, the neural crest, which has hitherto made up the margins of the groove, separates from the tube, and the part of the neural crest which gives rise to the dorsal root sensory ganglia migrates to occupy a dorsolateral relation to the tube, while the rest of the neural crest migrates further afield (Plate 9, E, F and G). As a result of these movements the three basic neurones come to lie in a different spatial relationship to one another. The sensory neurone is now outside the neural tube or central nervous system, the intermediate or connector neurone lies in the dorsal part of the tube, and the motor neurone lies in the ventral part of the tube.

To start with, the neural tube is made up of a single layer of cells, but they multiply and soon are arranged in three distinct layers:

i. An inner single layer of epithelium lining the lumen of the neural tube; this layer is called **ependyma.**

ii. A middle cellular layer, made up of connector and motor neurones, which becomes the **grey matter** of the central nervous system.

iii. An outer marginal layer consisting of axons (i.e. nerve fibres) arranged in bundles, known as **tracts** or **fasciculi,** which run up and down the wall of the tube. This outer layer becomes the **white matter** of the central nervous system.

Arrangement of Nerve Nuclear Components

Because the basic types of neurones have a definite spatial relationship to one another (Plate 9, G) the grey matter develops into two parts, **a dorsal column** or **horn** containing connector neurones which receive the terminations of receptor or sensory neurones, and mainly concerned with receiving sensory impulses, and a **ventral column** or **horn** containing the effector or motor neurones.

Within these horns, the cells are grouped into six columns of nuclei, three sensory or afferent in the dorsal horn, and three motor or efferent in the ventral horn. Three kinds of organs are supplied by nerves:

1. Somatic structures (i.e. the body wall and the limbs).
2. Visceral structures (i.e. organs like the gut, the lungs and the heart).
3. Structures developed from the branchial (gill) region of the early embryo (i.e. the muscles of the jaw and face, the soft palate, the pharynx and the structures in the middle ear).

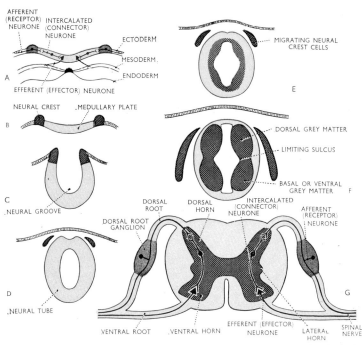

Plate 9. Schemes to show the development of the medullary (neural) plate to form the spinal cord.

[facing page 230

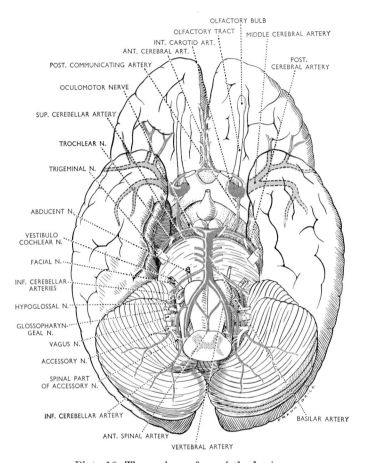

OLFACTORY BULB

OLFACTORY TRACT

MIDDLE CEREBRAL ARTERY

INT. CAROTID ART.

ANT. CEREBRAL ART.

POST.
CEREBRAL ARTERY

POST. COMMUNICATING ARTERY

OCULOMOTOR NERVE

SUP. CEREBELLAR ARTERY

TROCHLEAR N.

TRIGEMINAL N.

ABDUCENT N.

VESTIBULO
COCHLEAR N.

FACIAL N.

INF. CEREBELLAR
ARTERIES

HYPOGLOSSAL N.

GLOSSOPHARYN-
GEAL N.

VAGUS N.

ACCESSORY N.

SPINAL PART
OF ACCESSORY N.

INF. CEREBELLAR ARTERY

BASILAR ARTERY

ANT. SPINAL ARTERY

VERTEBRAL ARTERY

Plate 10. The undersurface of the brain.

[between pages 230/231 facing Pl. 11

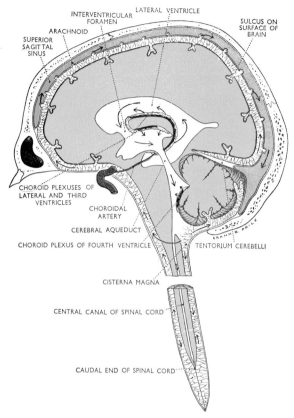

INTERVENTRICULAR
FORAMEN

LATERAL VENTRICLE

SULCUS ON
SURFACE OF
BRAIN

ARACHNOID

SUPERIOR
SAGITTAL
SINUS

CHOROID PLEXUSES OF
LATERAL AND THIRD
VENTRICLES

CHOROIDAL
ARTERY

CEREBRAL AQUEDUCT

CHOROID PLEXUS OF FOURTH VENTRICLE

TENTORIUM CEREBELLI

CISTERNA MAGNA

CENTRAL CANAL OF SPINAL CORD

CAUDAL END OF SPINAL CORD

Plate 11. Scheme illustrating the circulation of cerebrospinal fluid. The arrows indicate the direction of the flow.

[between pages 230/231 facing Pl. 10

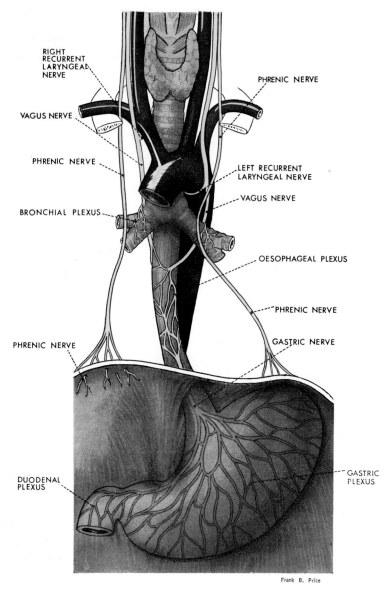

RIGHT
RECURRENT
LARYNGEAL
NERVE

PHRENIC NERVE

VAGUS NERVE

PHRENIC NERVE

LEFT RECURRENT
LARYNGEAL NERVE

VAGUS NERVE

BRONCHIAL PLEXUS

OESOPHAGEAL PLEXUS

PHRENIC NERVE

PHRENIC NERVE

GASTRIC NERVE

GASTRIC
PLEXUS

DUODENAL
PLEXUS

Frank B. Price

Plate 12. The vagus and phrenic nerves in the lower neck, thorax and upper abdomen

[facing page 231

The six columns of nerve nuclei provide motor (efferent) neurones to these three types of organ and connector neurones to receive sensory (afferent) impulses from them. (Fig. 104 indicates the relationship of these six columns to one another.) Their order in a dorsoventral sequence is:

1. Somatic sensory or general afferent.
2. Branchiosensory or special visceral afferent.
3. Viscerosensory or general visceral afferent.
4. Visceromotor or general visceral efferent.
5. Branchiomotor or special visceral efferent.
6. Somatic motor or general efferent.

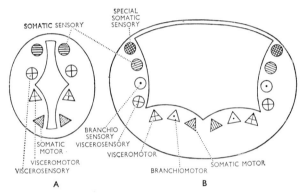

Fig. 104. Drawings showing the relative positions of the components of nerve nuclei. A, in the spinal cord; B, in the medulla.

Nuclear columns 2 and 5 are present in the brain stem and not in the spinal cord. All the structures developed from the branchial region are supplied by cranial nerves which originate in the brain stem. Thus, in the spinal cord only general somatic motor and sensory columns and general visceral motor and sensory columns are represented. The general visceral motor and sensory columns contain the cells associated with the innervation of the viscera.

Some Defects in Development

Varying degrees of malformation may result from failure of closure of the neural groove, or from failure of separation of the neural tube from the dorsal surface of the embryo, with consequent failure of completion of the neural arches of the vertebræ. The general term for these malformations is **spina bifida.** A new-born child may have, in the middle of the back, a red area in which the central neural canal opens, discharging cerebrospinal fluid on to the surface— a malformation known as **myelocoele;** on the other hand the neural tube may have been formed completely, but the surrounding meninges may form a cystic swelling protruding from the back of the baby—a malformation known as **meningocoele.**

There may be even more severe defects of development in the central nervous system, when the brain fails to develop properly from the cranial end of the neural plate. The general term for these malformations is **anencephaly.**

FORM AND GROSS STRUCTURE OF THE CENTRAL NERVOUS SYSTEM

The Form of the Spinal Cord

The spinal cord is a part of the neural tube that preserves its original more or less tubular shape. It lies protected within the vertebral canal of the vertebral column (p. 132), but it is considerably shorter than the vertebral canal in an adult. It extends from the foramen magnum in the base of the skull only to the upper border of the second lumbar vertebral body, or to the lower border of the first. Thus, the lower three lumbar vertebræ and the sacrum are not related to the spinal cord, but only to the lower nerve roots. In a new-born baby, however, the cord reaches a somewhat lower level, the caudal end being opposite the lower border of the second or upper border of the third vertebral body. In the fetus the spinal cord extends right to the lower end of the vertebral canal (Fig. 229).

Although it has been said that the spinal cord is more or less tubular in shape, the tube varies in diameter, being thicker in the regions to which the large nerves of the cervical, lumbar and sacral plexuses are attached. These regions, known respectively as the **cervical** and **lumbar enlargements,** contain more grey matter, more neurones being needed to form nerves and their connexions for the limbs, which are supplied from these regions of the spinal cord.

At its lower end, the spinal cord tapers down to a cone, the **conus medullaris,** which is continuous at its apex with a thread-like structure, the **filum terminale,** which tethers it to the coccyx.

Although the spinal cord is shorter than the vertebral column, the spinal nerves still leave the vertebral canal through their appropriate intervertebral foramina (Fig. 118), so that the lower nerve roots run down a considerable distance within the vertebral canal before they reach the proper foramina. These lower nerve roots are arranged round the filum terminale, where they form a leash which has been likened to a horse's tail and is called the **cauda equina** (Fig. 118).

The spinal cord is about 10–15 mm in diameter. It is wider from side to side than from front to back. The spinal cord is considerably narrower than the vertebral canal, so that there is a space round the spinal cord. This space contains the meninges, blood vessels and the cerebrospinal fluid. This arrangement allows movement of the vertebral column to take place without damaging the spinal cord.

The Structure of the Spinal Cord (see Plate 9 and Fig. 104)

In transverse sections, the **grey matter** is seen to be disposed as a band across the midline around the central canal, and from this band extend in each lateral half a dorsal and ventral horn. The **dorsal horn,** which is capped posteriorly by the jelly-like band called the **substantia gelatinosa,** contains the cell bodies of connector neurones and the termination of the afferent neurones about them; the **ventral horns** contain the motor efferent neurones. In the thoracic region, there is a **lateral horn** to accommodate the visceromotor neurones for the sympathetic outflow. Around the grey matter, is the **white matter** divided into three **columns** termed posterior (dorsomedial to the dorsal grey horn), lateral (lateral to the grey matter) and anterior (anteromedial to the ventral grey horns). The **posterior** or **dorsal white columns** contain mainly ascending sensory tracts.

The general pattern of the **lateral** and **anterior columns** is such, that intersegmental fibres lie close to the grey matter, descending motor tracts in the intermediate position, and ascending sensory tracts nearest the surface. The exception is the ventral cortico-spinal tract lying along the wall of the **anteromedian fissure,** which extends the whole length of the ventral aspect of the cord.

VENTRAL AND DORSAL ROOTS OF NERVES: Each segmental peripheral nerve is connected to the spinal cord by means of a **dorsal** and a **ventral root** (Plate 9, G). The former possesses a swelling—the **dorsal root ganglion** which contains the cells of the receptor neurones, the peripheral processes of which are the sensory fibres of peripheral nerves, whereas their central processes enter the spinal cord. The **ventral root** consists of the axons of motor neurones situated in the ventral horn of grey matter (also see p. 227).

The Form of the Brain and its Subdivisions (Figs. 105 and 106)

The cranial end of the neural tube expands into three main vesicles called, forebrain, midbrain and hindbrain, arranged in cranio-caudal sequence. The **forebrain** expands to such an extent that it overshadows the rest of the brain; it contains the highest centres for the control and integration of the activities

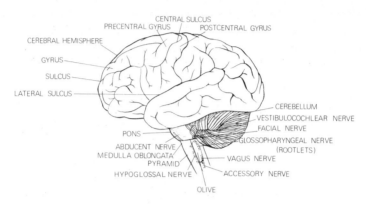

Fig. 105. The lateral aspect of the brain.

of the nervous system. At this level, sensory impulses 'reach consciousness' and motor impulses are initiated by the will. The **midbrain,** which as its name implies, connects the forebrain to the hindbrain, contains among other things, visual and auditory reflex centres and other centres affecting motor activity. The **hindbrain** is connected to the midbrain above, and to the spinal cord below. It contains centres for the control of balance and motor activity, and centres controlling the vital activities of the body such as respiration, circulation of the blood and digestion.

The Forebrain

The forebrain is made up of two expanded cerebral hemispheres, one on each side, and a midline part called the diencephalon to which the cerebral hemispheres are attached.

Each cerebral hemisphere has, on the outside, a thin layer of grey matter, the **cerebral cortex**; inside this is the white matter. Within the white matter is a central mass of grey matter, the **corpus striatum** or **basal ganglia.** Each cerebral hemisphere is traversed by a fanned-out band of fibres ascending to, and descending from the cerebral cortex. This band, called the **internal capsule,** is bent so that when the brain is cut horizontally it appears almost L-shaped and consists of an **anterior** and a **posterior limb** (Fig. 115) joined by a region called the **genu.** The internal capsule is situated lateral to the thalamus and in between the basal ganglia (Fig. 116).

The two hemispheres are connected to one another by a broad bridge of transverse fibres which pass across the midline above the third ventricle (p. 106). This bridge is called the **corpus callosum** (Plate 36 and Fig. 000).

The cerebral cortex forms a very convoluted covering for each cerebral hemisphere. The ridges are termed **gyri** and the grooves **sulci.**

The two main sulci (Plate 19 and Fig. 105) are the **lateral sulcus** (of Sylvius) and the **central sulcus** (of Rolando). The part of the hemisphere in front of the

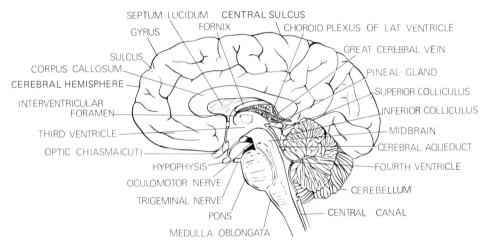

Fig. 106. A median sagittal section of the brain.

central sulcus and above the lateral sulcus is the **frontal lobe.** The part below the lateral sulcus is the **temporal lobe.** The **occipital lobe** is at the posterior pole of the hemisphere, and the part between the occipital lobe and the frontal lobe is called the **parietal lobe.** If the margins of the lateral sulcus are pulled apart, a buried portion of cortex related to the lateral aspect of the corpus striatum is revealed. This buried island of cortical tissue is called the **insula** (Fig. 115).

The ridge immediately in front of the central sulcus is known as the **precentral gyrus** and consists of motor cortex (p. 252); the ridge immediately behind the central sulcus is the **postcentral gyrus** and consists of sensory cortex (p. 252).

The diencephalon is made up of several parts, the principal being the **two thalami** (Fig. 115), which are large ovoid masses of grey matter lying, one on each side of the midline, in the lateral wall of the third ventricle (p. 238). Below the thalami in the floor of the third ventricle, lies the **hypothalamus** to which the **hypophysis** (pituitary gland) is attached (Plate 36).

The Midbrain

The midbrain (Fig. 107) is made up of a dorsal roof plate (**tectum**) consisting of four hillocks of grey matter—the **superior** and **inferior colliculi;** a middle segment (**tegmentum**) containing two nuclear masses, one on each side—the **red nuclei,** and an interlacing system of fibres and nuclei—the **reticular formation,** and the fibres from the superior cerebellar peduncle (Fig. 112); and ventrally two columns, one on each side, called the **crura cerebri** or **cerebral peduncles** (Fig. 107), which are separated from the tegmentum by a strip of grey matter (the **substantia nigra**)(Fig. 112). Each crus cerebri is made up of fibres that are continuous above with the internal capsule (Fig. 116).

The Hindbrain

The hindbrain (Fig. 107) is made up of three interconnected parts, the pons, the cerebellum and the medulla.

The **pons is** continuous above with the midbrain. As well as containing a **reticular formation,** it contains **pontine nuclei** (Figs. 110, 112 and 113) ventral to it. Between the pontine nuclei, there pass fibres which are continuous above with those of the crura cerebri. The **cerebellum** (Fig. 107) lies dorsal to the pons and is made up of two lateral hemispheres on each side of the median **vermis.**

Like the cerebral hemisphere, the cerebellum is made up of an outer layer of grey matter, the **cerebellar cortex,** and a central core of white matter in which is set a bilateral collection of central nuclei. The principal central nucleus of the cerebellum is known as the **dentate nucleus** (because of its indented outline) (Figs. 110 and 113). The cerebellum is joined to the rest of the brain by three pairs of peduncles. The **superior cerebellar peduncles** join it to the midbrain; the **middle cerebellar peduncles** join it to the pons, the **inferior cerebellar peduncles** join it to the medulla (Fig. 107, B).

The **medulla oblongata** is the lowest part of the hindbrain, being continuous above with the pons and below, through the foramen magnum, with the spinal cord. Whereas the medulla's lower part has the same general shape as the spinal cord with a centrally placed central canal (Fig. 112), the upper part's shape is much modified because the lateral walls of the neural tube, especially

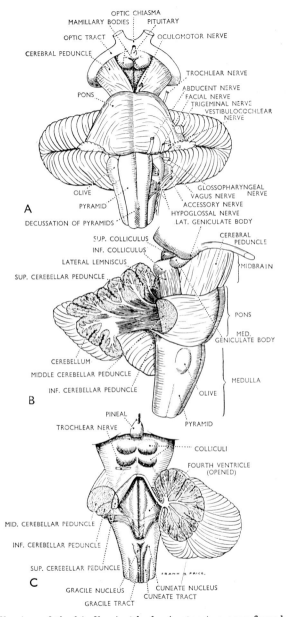

Fig. 107. The midbrain and the hindbrain (the brain stem). A, seen from below; B, seen from the right side (part of the cerebellum and middle cerebellar peduncle have been cut away); C, seen from above (most of the cerebellum and the roof of the fourth ventricle have been removed).

the dorsal parts, have been displaced laterally with consequent extreme thinning of the roof of the tube (Figs. 107 and 112). In this way, the dorsal (sensory function) parts of the neural tube come to lie lateral to the ventral (motor function) part of the tube.

The medulla has a complicated structure but, in general terms, the most ventral part is made up of bilateral, longitudinal columns of fibres, the **pyramids** (Figs. 107 and 112), which are continuous above, through the pons, with the fibres of the cerebral peduncles. Most of the fibres of the pyramids cross over to the other side in the lower part of the medulla. This is known as the **motor decussation** (Fig. 112, D). Dorsal to the pyramids is the medullary part of the **reticular formation,** and in the most lateral portion of the upper expanded part is a nuclear mass of grey matter which causes a bulge in the surface and which is called the **olive** (Figs. 107 and 112). This is concerned with motor function, and is linked both to the spinal cord and to the cerebellum.

THE VENTRICLES OF THE BRAIN (Figs. 107, 115 and Plate 11): Within the brain, the original central canal of the neural tube is expanded into chambers which are situated inside certain parts of the brain. These are known as the **ventricles** of the brain and they are linked to one another by a system of narrow connexions. Inside each cerebral hemisphere there is a chamber of curved shape, a **lateral ventricle,** which communicates near its anterior end through the narrow **interventricular foramen** (of Monro) with the **third ventricle.** This third ventricle is a narrow midline chamber, situated between the two thalami, and its posterior end is continuous with the narrow cerebral **aqueduct** (of Sylvius), which passes through the midbrain. The **fourth ventricle** is a space, diamond shaped in outline, which has the pons and upper part of the medulla in its floor and the cerebellum covering its roof. The anterior end of the fourth ventricle is continuous with the aqueduct of Sylvius, and its posterior end is continuous with the central canal in the lower part of the medulla and in the spinal cord.

THE CHOROID PLEXUSES (Plate 11): In relation to each ventricle there is a **choroid plexus.** This consists of a network of capillaries in a fold of pia mater (p. 259), which has been invaginated, or pushed into the ventricle from outside the brain, in such a way that the brain substance has been thinned out to a layer of ependyma one cell thick. The ependyma covers the choroid plexus, which lies within the ventricular cavity having been pushed in, either from the side wall of the lateral ventricles, or from the roof of the third and fourth ventricles. The choroid plexuses secrete **cerebrospinal fluid** which fills the ventricular system and the subarachnoid space (p. 259).

THE STRUCTURE AND FUNCTION OF THE
CENTRAL NERVOUS SYSTEM

The Main Ascending Sensory Tracts (Fig. 108)

On p. 224 the different types of peripheral nerve endings have been described and attention was drawn to the way the different endings respond to specific stimuli. Afferent fibres convey these impulses, and as the **dorsal root** approaches the cord it divides into a **large medial division,** made up of thick fibres, and a **small lateral division** made up of fine fibres.

All types or **modalities** of sensation travel in the mixed (motor and sensory) peripheral nerves, but, once the fibres reach the cord, they are accurately segregated into separate tracts according to the type of sensation they convey.

There are always at least three neurones concerned with conveying an impulse to the sensory area of the cerebral cortex, and impulses from one side of the body are invariably conveyed to the cortex of the other side of the brain.

FINE TOUCH: The sense of **fine touch** is conveyed by large heavily myelinated fibres that enter the posterior or dorsal column by way of the large medial division of the dorsal nerve root. They ascend to the medulla in the **gracile** and **cuneate tracts** of the dorsal column (Fig. 108) and terminate in the **gracile** and **cuneate nuclei** of the dorsal part of the lower medulla. Here they relay, and the fibre of the **second sensory neurone** crosses the midline in the **sensory decussation** and then ascends in the **medial lemniscus** to the posterior part of the **thalamus,** where it relays. The **third sensory neurone,** whose cell body is in the thalamus, sends its axon through the **posterior limb of the internal capsule** to the strip of sensory cortex on the **post-central gyrus.**

CRUDE TOUCH: The other pathway for tactile impulses (**crude touch**) is through the central process of the **first sensory neurone.** This ascends for a few segments of the cord in the **posterior column,** as previously described, and then relays in **cells in the posterior horn.** The axon of this **second sensory neurone** then crosses the midline near the central canal to reach the **anterior spinothalamic tract** in the anterior column of white matter. The fibres then turn up in this tract and ascend through the medulla, pons and midbrain in the **spinal lemniscus,** which joins the lateral aspect of the **medial lemniscus,** and its fibres terminate by relaying in the posterior part of the thalamus, from which the **third sensory neurone** passes through the internal capsule to reach the **sensory cortex.**

The essential features of both these sensory pathways are that the first sensory neurone ascends for a varying number of segments before relaying, and

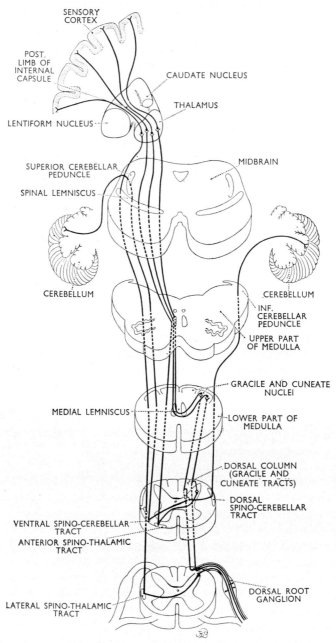

Fig. 108. Scheme to show the dispositions of the sensory pathways in the central nervous system.

that, as it ascends in the dorsal column, it gives off collaterals (or branches). In other words, the incoming impulse is scattered over several segments before it is conveyed to sensory neurones of the second order, which convey the impulse to the thalamus.

PAIN AND TEMPERATURE: Sensation of pain and temperature is conveyed in the dorsal nerve root by fine, poorly myelinated fibres, which enter the cord by way of the small lateral division. They relay at the same level of the cord as the one at which they entered it, by synapsing with neurones situated at the apex or dorsal extremity of the posterior horn, called the **substantia gelatinosa.** This **second neurone's** axon crosses the midline at once to reach the **lateral spinothalamic tract** in the lateral column of white matter. In this, it ascends to the brain stem, where the lateral spinothalamic tract joins the anterior spinothalamic tract to form the **spinal lemniscus,** in which it ascends to the posterior part of the thalamus. There, it synapses with the **third sensory neurone** which ascends via the **posterior limb of the internal capsule** to reach the **sensory cortex.**

PROPRIOCEPTION: The types of sensation so far described all concern the reception of information about the external environment of the body. The remaining sensory pathway to be described is one that conveys impulses bringing information to the brain about the position of the limbs and tension in muscles, so that it is possible to know the spatial relationships of the various parts of the body without needing to look at them. This is referred to as **proprioceptive sensation.** The axons of the first sensory neurones conveying this type of sensation are of the large myelinated variety and they enter the cord by the large medial division of the sensory root. They ascend in the dorsal columns, where they reach one of two destinations. Either the impulse is destined for the sensory cerebral cortex, at which level it reaches consciousness with other sensory impulses, or it is destined for the cortex of the cerebellum so as to play a part in the control of balance-maintaining mechanisms.

In the case of those impulses destined for the cerebral cortex, the pathway is **identical with that conveying fine touch.**

Impulses destined for the cerebellum travel along fibres that soon synapse with neurones, the cell bodies of which are situated in the **posterior horn** of grey matter. The axon of this **second sensory neurone** then ascends either in the **dorsal spinocerebellar tract** of the same side, or in the **ventral spinocerebellar tract** of the opposite side, to the **cerebellar cortex.** The former reach the cerebellum via the inferior cerebellar peduncle and the latter via the superior cerebellar peduncle (Fig. 126).

SOME DISORDERS OF SENSATION: **Herpes zoster** or **shingles** is an inflammation of dorsal root ganglia, manifested by a vesicular eruption on the skin of the corresponding dermatomes (p. 83). It is associated with pain (**neuralgia**) in these segments, and this may persist long after the vesicles have disappeared.

Tabes dorsalis is a late manifestation of syphilis affecting the dorsal white columns. Consequently, not only is the sense of fine touch impaired, but proprioceptive sense is abolished, so that when the patients close their eyes they lose their balance, or when walking in the dark they have to shine a light on their feet to know 'where they are'.

Syringomyelia is a localized degeneration affecting the substance of the spinal cord in the vicinity of the central canal. It therefore affects those sensory fibres which cross close to the central canal, that is, those conveying crude touch, pain and temperature. However, as the tactile impulses are spread over several segments, no alteration in tactile sensation is noticed, but pain and temperature sensation, which is conveyed by fibres that cross over at the level at which the impulses entered the cord, is abolished over the affected segments.

SURGICAL RELIEF OF PAIN: Advantage may be taken of the fact that the different types of sensation are carried along different pathways in cases of incurable pain. Local division of the lateral spinothalamic tract abolishes pain and temperature sense, while leaving the appreciation of other modalities of sensation intact.

REFERRED PAIN: Irritation of an internal organ sometimes results in pain being felt, not in the organ itself, but in a particular area of the skin. This is called a referred pain. It occurs when the nerve to the internal organ and the nerve to the skin come from the same part of the central nervous system, for example, from the same segment of the spinal cord. The brain is accustomed to receiving pain impulses from the skin, but not from the viscera, so that pain stimulation of that given segment, even if it comes from a viscus, is interpreted as if it came from the skin. A good example is the referred pain felt on the tip of the shoulder when either the upper or the lower surface of the diaphragm is irritated (p. 271).

The Main Descending (Motor) Pathways (Fig. 109)

There are always at least two neurones concerned with conveying an impulse from the motor area of the cerebral cortex to a muscle.

Essentially, the main motor pathways within the central nervous system consist of **upper motor neurones,** whose cell bodies are **giant pyramidal cells** (of Betz), situated in the precentral gyrus in the motor cortex, and **lower motor neurones,** whose cell bodies are situated in cranial nerve nuclei or in the

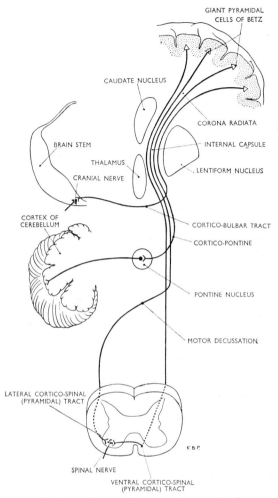

Fig. 109. Scheme to show the dispositions of motor pathways in the central nervous system.

anterior horn of the spinal cord. The axon of such a Betz cell descends through the **genu of the internal capsule** and then the **cerebral peduncle** as a **cortico-spinal fibre** (or cortico-bulbar if going to synapse with a cell in a cranial nerve motor nucleus). It descends through the pons between the pontine nuclei and enters the **pyramid** (hence its synonymous name of **pyramidal fibre**). In the pyramid, it usually crosses over to the other side at the level of the lower medulla, in what is known as the **motor descussation,** to reach the **lateral cortico-spinal tract** of the spinal cord. When it reaches its appropriate level in the cord, it synapses with a cell in the anterior horn of the grey matter. If the fibre did not cross in the medulla, it descends in the **ventral cortico-spinal tract** and crosses over just before terminating in the anterior horn.

The axon of the lower motor neurone leaves the brain stem in the motor root of a cranial nerve, or leaves the spinal cord via the ventral or anterior nerve root. This neurone is also known as the **final common pathway** for, as Fig. 110 illustrates, it is in synaptic relation with many neurones besides the upper motor neurone. The influence of the upper motor neurone on the lower motor neurone is thus modified by impulses coming to it from the basal ganglia, the substantia nigra and tectal nuclei of the midbrain, the cerebellum via the red nucleus and reticular formation (see later), the vestibular nuclei associated with the eighth nerve, the olive and impulses coming in through the dorsal root of the spinal nerves. Only the main influences are illustrated in Fig. 10.

The **reticular formation** needs special mention at this stage as, though it is ill-defined and its functions are not wholly understood, it obviously plays a very important rôle in motor activity in the central nervous system, and plays an important rôle in the conduction of impulses upwards through the brain stem. It is situated ventrolateral to the neural canal and consists of dispersed nuclear masses with many interconnecting fibres and synapses; it extends from the subthalamic region to the spinal cord. It plays a very important rôle in **facilitating** and **inhibiting** (see p. 227) impulses coming down from or travelling up to the cortex. In this way, it affects the wakefulness and consciousness of the individual (see p. 257).

SOME DISORDERS OF MOTOR FUNCTION: If the final common pathway is damaged, i.e. in a **lower motor neurone lesion,** flaccid paralysis ensues because the outflow from the central nervous system to that muscle is completely interrupted. If the anterior horn cell itself is damaged, as in poliomyelitis, there is flaccid paralysis of the muscle supplied by it and the damage is permanent, but if the axon is damaged outside the central nervous system, it is capable of regeneration (see p. 600) and the paralysis may be only temporary.

In an **upper motor neurone (pyramidal) lesion,** which may occur if a cerebral hæmorrhage in the region of the internal capsule interrupts the axon, the ensuing paralysis is rigid because impulses from other (extra-pyramidal) higher centres still reach the lower motor neurone, and permanent because fibres within the central nervous system do not regenerate (see p. 600).

Damage to the other fibre systems (**extra-pyramidal**), which are in

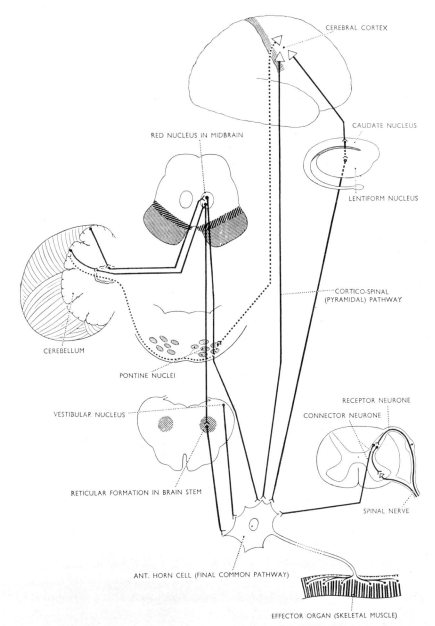

CEREBRAL CORTEX

CAUDATE NUCLEUS

RED NUCLEUS IN MIDBRAIN

LENTIFORM NUCLEUS

CORTICO-SPINAL
(PYRAMIDAL) PATHWAY

CEREBELLUM

PONTINE NUCLEI

RECEPTOR NEURONE

VESTIBULAR NUCLEUS

CONNECTOR NEURONE

RETICULAR FORMATION IN BRAIN STEM

SPINAL NERVE

ANT. HORN CELL (FINAL COMMON PATHWAY)

EFFECTOR ORGAN (SKELETAL MUSCLE)

Fig. 110. Scheme to show the routes by which impulses reach an anterior horn cell, the final common pathway to skeletal muscle.

synaptic relation with the final common pathway, gives rise to disorders of muscular control, rigidity and tremors e.g. **Parkinsonism** (see also p. 252).

The Brain Stem

The brain stem is a term which includes the medulla, pons and midbrain.

In order to understand the structure of the brain stem, it is necessary to appreciate that, as well as important ascending and descending tracts, it contains the **nuclei of the cranial nerves** and, in addition, to have some idea of what structures they supply and which functions they subserve.

The cranial nerves (Fig. 111) consist of twelve pairs which are known by both a number and a name as follows:

I—**Olfactory:** conveys olfactory impulses from the mucous membrane of the nose.

II—**Optic:** is not a true peripheral nerve, but a tract of the brain which conveys visual impulses from the retina.

III—**Oculomotor:** conveys motor impulses to all the extrinsic muscles of the eye, except superior oblique and lateral rectus, and to the sphincter pupillæ and ciliary muscle.

IV—**Trochlear:** conveys motor impulses to an extrinsic muscle of the eye the superior oblique.

V—**Trigeminal:** conveys sensory impulses from the face and tongue and motor impulses to the muscles of mastication.

VI—**Abducent:** conveys motor impulses to an extrinsic muscle of the eye the lateral rectus.

VII—**Facial:** conveys motor impulses to the muscles of facial expression, secretomotor impulses to salivary glands and impulses of taste from the tongue. Where the facial nerve emerges from the brain stem its secretomotor fibres and taste fibres form a separate bundle called the nervus intermedius.

VIII—**Vestibulocochlear or Auditory:** conveys impulses from the vestibule of the inner ear, concerned with sensations of motion and balance, and auditory impulses from the cochlea of the inner ear.

IX—**Glossopharyngeal:** conveys sensory impulses from the tongue, pharynx and carotid sinus and body, and secretomotor fibres to salivary glands.

X—**Vagus:** conveys sensory and motor impulses to and from 'branchial' (see p. 230) and visceral structures in the neck, thorax and abdomen.

XI—Accessory: Its **cranial** part is distributed with the vagus to 'branchial' structures: its **spinal** part conveys motor impulses to the sterno-mastoid and trapezius muscles.

XII—Hypoglossal: conveys motor impulses to the muscles of the tongue.

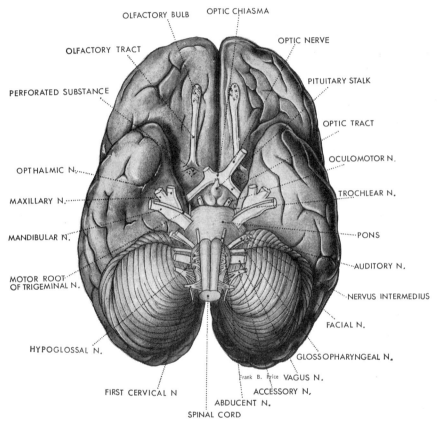

OLFACTORY BULB — OPTIC CHIASMA

OLFACTORY TRACT

OPTIC NERVE

PERFORATED SUBSTANCE

PITUITARY STALK

OPTIC TRACT

OPTHALMIC N.

OCULOMOTOR N.

MAXILLARY N.

TROCHLEAR N.

MANDIBULAR N.

PONS

MOTOR ROOT OF TRIGEMINAL N.

AUDITORY N.

NERVUS INTERMEDIUS

FACIAL N.

HYPOGLOSSAL N.

GLOSSOPHARYNGEAL N.

Frank B. Price VAGUS N.

FIRST CERVICAL N

ACCESSORY N,

ABDUCENT N.

SPINAL CORD

Fig. 111. The base of the brain showing the cranial nerves.

THE MEDULLA: STRUCTURE, MAIN CONNEXIONS AND FUNCTIONS: The structure of the **lower medulla** is similar to that of the spinal cord but modified (see Fig. 112) by the **sensory** and **motor decussations,** which break up the grey matter and lead to the formation of the **medial lemniscus** near the midline ventral to the central canal, and the **pyramids** along the ventral aspect of the medulla.

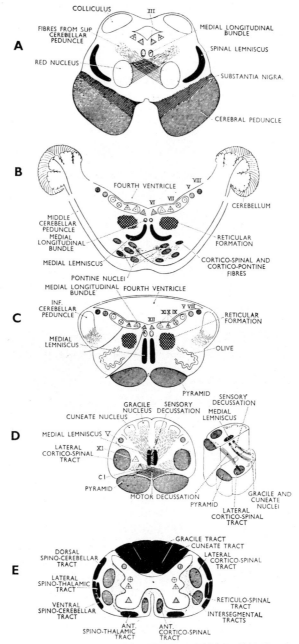

Fig. 112. Diagrams of transverse sections at different levels of the brain stem and of the spinal cord. The symbols for the components of nerve nuclei are the same as those used in Fig. 104. The number of a cranial nerve is indicated by the appropriate roman numeral.

A, midbrain; B, pons; C, upper medulla; D, lower medulla; E, spinal cord.

The **substantia gelatinosa** is continued up as the **spinal nucleus of the fifth** or **trigeminal nerve,** which represents the somatic sensory column (see p. 231) at this level. The dorsal columns are replaced by grey matter in the form of the **gracile** and **cuneate nuclei.**

The branchiomotor column (see p. 231) is represented by the **nucleus of the accessory nerve** and the somatic motor column by the **nucleus of the hypoglossal nerve.**

The **upper part of the medulla** is further modified by the fact that the central canal has been widened out to form the fourth ventricle, so that the sensory nerve components come to lie lateral to the motor (see Fig. 104). A mass of grey matter, **the olive,** is present dorsolateral to the pyramid and is connected to higher motor centres, such as the cerebral cortex and basal ganglia, and to the cerebellum and spinal cord.

Just dorsal to the medial lemniscus is a bundle, the **medial longitudinal bundle,** which links the various cranial nerve nuclei, but especially those governing eye movements (III, IV and VI) and the spinal accessory nerve (XI) which is concerned with head turning movements. The most lateral and dorsal part of the medulla is occupied by the **inferior cerebellar peduncle,** and medial to it are cranial nerve nuclei. The somatic sensory column (p. 231) is represented by **nuclei of the trigeminal and vestibulocochlear nerves;** the branchio- and viscerosensory and motor columns (p. 231) are represented by the **nuclei of the glossopharyngeal, vagus** and **accessory nerves,** and most medially of all the somatic motor column (see p. 231) is represented by the **nucleus of the hypoglossal nerve.** Situated between the cranial nerve nuclei and the olive, and lateral to the medial lemniscus, is the **reticular formation.**

THE PONS: STRUCTURE, MAIN CONNEXIONS AND FUNCTIONS: The pons (bridge) (Figs. 107 and 112) is so called because it contains transverse fibres which travel by way of the middle cerebellar peduncle to the cerebellar cortex. These fibres have their cells of origin in the ventrally placed **pontine nuclei,** and go to the middle cerebellar peduncle of the other side. The pons is in fact continuous with a middle peduncle at each side, the junction being marked by the attachment of the trigeminal nerve.

Cortico-spinal fibres descend between the pontine nuclei, as do the **cortico-pontine fibres** before they relay in the pontine nuclei. Situated between the transverse pontine fibres ventrally and the **reticular formation** dorsally, is another transverse system of fibres, the **trapezoid body.** This is made up of secondary acoustic neurones crossing over to the **lateral lemniscus** of the other side to ascend to the inferior colliculus and medial geniculate body.

As regards cranial nerve nuclei, the somatic sensory column (p. 231) is represented by the **trigeminal** and **vestibulocochlear nerve nuclei,** the branchiosensory, viscerosensory, visceromotor and branchiomotor columns (p. 000) are represented by the **nuclei of the facial nerve** and the somatic motor column is represented by the **nucleus of the abducent nerve.**

THE MIDBRAIN: STRUCTURE, MAIN CONNEXIONS AND FUNCTIONS: The Midbrain (Figs. 107 and 112) consists of a roof plate or **tectum** made up of four hillocks of grey matter—the **colliculi**—the upper pair being centres for visual reflexes and the lower for auditory reflexes.

The **tegmentum,** which is situated ventral to the level of the cerebral **aqueduct** (of Sylvius) and dorsal to the cerebral peduncles or crura cerebri, contains the **lateral, spinal and medial lemnisci** in its lateral portion. The **decussation of the superior cerebellar peduncles** and the **red nucleus** are nearer the midline and related to the reticular formation. The **medial longitudinal bundle** is near the midline close to the nuclei of the **oculomotor** and **trochlear nerves,** which represent the somatic motor column (see p. 231), at this level of the brain stem.

A strip of grey matter—the **substantia nigra**—associated with motor function, separates the tegmentum from the **cerebral peduncle** which contains fibres descending from the cerebral cortex to lower levels of the nervous system.

THE CEREBELLUM: STRUCTURE, MAIN CONNEXIONS AND FUNCTIONS: The cerebellum consists of a core of white matter, which contains nuclear masses of grey matter such as the **dentate nucleus** (also see p. 236), and a superficial covering of grey matter, the **cerebellar cortex.**

The cerebellum is connected by **three peduncles** on each side to the rest of the brain (Fig. 107).

In general, the reflex arc within the cerebellum consists of an incoming fibre ascending to the cerebellar cortex, where it synapses with another neurone which sends its axon down to the central nuclei. There another synapse takes place before a fibre emerges from the cerebellum.

Its connexions, which are illustrated in Fig. 113, may be summarized in terms of **incoming fibres arising at lower levels of the central nervous system,** e.g. dorsal spino-cerebellar fibres, olivo-cerebellar fibres, vestibulo-cerebellar fibres, which enter by way of the inferior cerebellar peduncles, and the ventral spino-cerebellar fibres which enter by way of the superior peduncles; **incoming fibres arising at higher levels of the central nervous system,** e.g. cortical fibres which relay in pontine nuclei from which fibres enter by way of the middle peduncles; and **outgoing fibres** arising in the cells of the central nuclei, such as the dentate nucleus, which emerge by way of the superior peduncle to reach the **red nucleus** of the midbrain. Here they relay to give rise to **rubro-spinal** fibres, which descend to the spinal cord, or **rubro-reticulo-spinal fibres,** which relay in the reticular formation from which another axon descends to the spinal cord.

The cerebellum, as its connexions make clear, is concerned with the co-ordination of muscular movements and with the reflexes which maintain

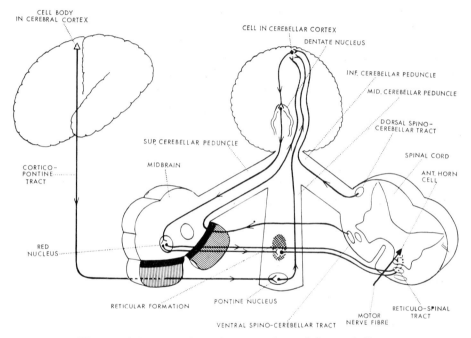

Fig. 113. Scheme to show the connexions of the cerebellum.

balance. **Lesions of the cerebellum** are associated with **ataxia** and other inco-ordinations of movement, with interference in **postural reflexes** and sense of **balance.**

SUMMARY OF FUNCTIONS OF THE BRAIN STEM: From the descriptions of the cranial nerve nuclei in the brain stem, it will be appreciated that this part of the brain contains important centres for controlling the vital activities of the body such as respiration, circulation of the blood and digestion, in addition to its provision of centres for visual and auditory reflexes, and for the control of balance and motor activity.

The Forebrain

THE DIENCEPHALON: This is made up of a number of constituents which include the thalamus, hypothalamus and, connected to it, the neurohypophysis. It also contains the third ventricle the roof of which lies the pineal.

The **thalamus** is important, not only as an important relay station on the ascending sensory pathways (p. 241) but also because it has important connexions with the hypothalamus and with the basal ganglia. By means of the latter connexions, it plays a part in the control of muscular activity and disorders of motor muscular activity, such as **Parkinsonism,** may be treated by surgical operations on parts of the thalamus.

The **neurohypophysis** is described on p. 519.

The **hypothalamus** controls the activity of the **hypophysis** (p. 517) and also contains centres which control the **autonomic nervous system.** It is concerned with the regulation of feeding responses, of adiposity and emaciation, of water balance and of temperature control.

It is important as a relay centre for pathways concerned with the **expression of emotion,** evidence of emotion being provided, not only by changes in facial expression and pallor, but by changes in the heart-rate, in the blood pressure, in the peristaltic acitivity of the gut, by sweating and by hyperglycæmia, which may result in glycosuria.

There is considerable evidence that the hypothalamus, particularly its posterior part, is concerned with the **mechanism of sleep** (p. 256).

THE STRUCTURE AND FUNCTION OF THE CEREBRAL HEMISPHERE: As described above, the cerebral hemisphere consists of a central core of white matter, in which the grey matter of the corpus striatum is embedded. The white matter is covered by the cerebral cortex which is convoluted into ridges (**gyri**) and grooves (**sulci**) to provide a greater surface area.

The **cerebral cortex** is a stratified layer of cells, those which receive the termination of the sensory pathways being **rounded** or **granular** cells, whereas those that initiate motor impulses are **pyramidal** in shape. There is quite well-established functional localization within the cortex (Plate 19) and this is reflected in the histology of the region, granular cells preponderating in areas concerned with sensory activity, and pyramidal cells in areas concerned with motor activity.

The **precentral gyrus,** situated immediately in front of the central sulcus, is concerned with the initiation of **voluntary movements** on the opposite side of the body, whereas the **postcentral gyrus** is concerned with the conscious appreciation of **sensation** originating on the opposite side of the body. In both instances the body is represented upside down in these strips, with the feet uppermost and the face lowermost.

The upper part of the **temporal lobe** is concerned with the appreciation of **hearing,** whereas the front part of the undersurface of this lobe and the adjoining part of the frontal lobe are associated with the appreciation of the **sense of smell.** The medial aspect of the **occipital lobe** is concerned with the conscious appreciation of **visual** impulses originating from the fields of vision on the opposite side of the body (see p. 300 and Plate 18).

Just anterior to the lower part of the motor area, there is a **motor speech centre** on each side, but there is evidence that normally only one of these is used; the left one in right-handed individuals and the right in left-handed people.

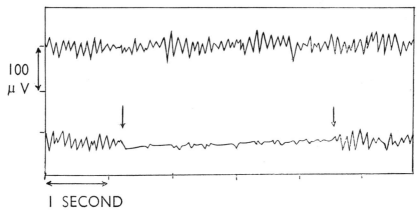

Fig. 114. An electroencephalogram (E.E.G.). The upper tracing represents a normal record taken with the eyes of the subject closed. The part of the lower tracing between the arrows shows the alteration in the record of the same subject when the eyes are opened.

In between these areas, there are some whose functions are not so clearly defined. These are **association areas,** which, among other things, integrate the functions described above. Thus, in the parietal region there are areas which integrate tactile sensation with vision and vision with hearing, i.e. they enable the individual to appreciate the written word as well as the spoken word, etc. In the **frontal lobe,** anterior to the precentral sulcus, are association areas that affect motor activity and send fibres to the thalamus and to the corpus striatum, but they are also instrumental in the manifestation of the **personality** of the individual. Damage in this part of the brain is often associated with disorders in the manifestation of personality, i.e. character changes.

ELECTRICAL ACTIVITY IN THE CEREBRAL CORTEX: Activity of the

cortical cells is associated with electrical activity. Even at rest and during sleep, electrical activity is detectable; it is increased or altered during mental and physical activity; it is increased and the pattern of 'resting' activity is altered in certain diseases, e.g. epilepsy. Tracings of such electrical activity in the brain are called **electroencephalograms** (see Fig. 114).

The **internal capsule** (Figs. 115 and 116; see also p. 234) has its constituent

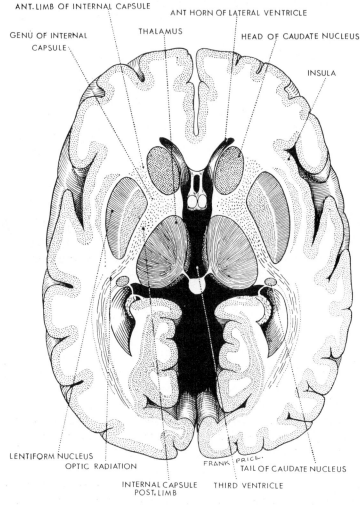

Fig. 115. A horizontal section through the cerebral hemispheres.

fibres arranged in a definite order, the **anterior limb** containing fibres from the frontal lobes to the corpus striatum, thalamus and pons. In its **genu** and **anterior part of the posterior limb,** the cortico-bulbar and cortico-spinal fibres are arranged with the fibres controlling head, arm, trunk and leg movements in a corresponding anteroposterior order. The **posterior part of the posterior**

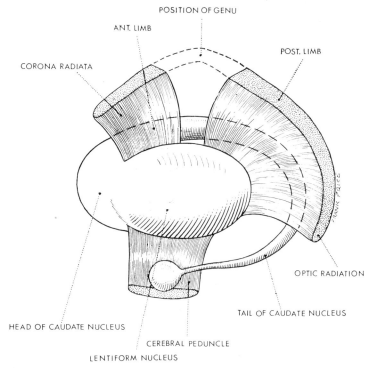

Fig. 116. Diagram showing the relations of the internal capsule to the basal ganglia the region of the genu of the internal capsule has been removed).

limb consists mainly of fibres ascending to the sensory areas of the cortex. It will be appreciated that, as all the cortico-bulbar and cortico-spinal fibres are crowded into a part of the internal capsule around the genu and anterior part of the posterior limb (Fig.116), a relatively small lesion may interrupt all of them and cause complete paralysis of the other side of the body (**hemiplegia**).

The **corpus striatum** (Figs. 115 and 116) consists of a comma-shaped **caudate nucleus,** which receives fibres from the cerebral cortex and elsewhere, and the **lentiform nucleus,** whose outer **putamen** also receives incoming fibres, but whose inner **globus pallidus** give rise to fibres leaving the corpus striatum. The caudate nucleus and the lentiform nucleus are separated from each other (except in front) by the internal capsule. Attached to the tip of the 'tail' of the caudate nucleus, is the small rounded **amygdaloid nucleus,** which functions as part of the limbic system (see below). The corpus striatum influences the function of the final common pathway and is concerned with the regulation of muscle tone. When it 'overacts', it causes involuntary movements and rigidity.

The Limbic System

Whereas the olfactory components (see p. 309 for olfactory system) dominate the cerebral hemispheres in lower animals, in Man a large part of the 'smell brain' has lost its direct relation to the olfactory system. Instead, this part has become incorporated into what is termed the limbic system.

Strips of **cerebral cortex** on the medial and inferior aspects of the cerebral hemispheres (Plate 19), the **hippocampus** with its associated structures, the amygdaloid nucleus, parts of the **hypothalamus** (especially the mamillary bodies), and the anterior portion of the **thalamus** constitute the grey matter of the system.

The **mamillothalamic tract** and the **fornix,** which arches below the corpus callosum (Fig. 106), are fibre tracts of the system.

The functioning of the limbic system is exceedingly complex but, in general terms, it may be said to be associated, in the first place, with the emotional aspects of behaviour concerned with survival, both of the individual and of the species, together with the visceral responses accompanying these emotions. Secondly, the system, particularly the hippocampus inside the temporal lobe, provides the brain with mechanisms for memory. The limbic system is sometimes referred to as the **'visceral brain'** and the investigation of its structure and function is very relevant to the study of certain types of mental illness. This will be readily understood when realizing that, not only is it concerned with memory, but also with such emotions as fear, anger, appetite and those associated with sexual behaviour.

SLEEP

Sleep is a reversible, periodically recurring state, when muscular activity and sensory reactivity are reduced. It is an important part of the normal circadian rhythm (p. 562).

Little is known about why sleep is necessary and about how much is needed. Some eight hours seems to be the usual adult requirement, but individuals vary widely in their needs. Young children clearly need more than adults. Irritability, inattention and slowness of thought are some of the consequences of insufficient sleep.

Besides changes in the functioning of the nervous system, sleep is associated with physiological changes in other systems. There is a distinct fall in blood pressure and in body temperature; the pulse rate, respiration rate and urine production are reduced; the pupils are contracted.

There is evidence that wakefulness depends to some extent on sensory impulses reaching the cerebral cortex (see also p. 239), and that physiological conditions favouring a decrease in these impulses, resulting in a decrease in cortical activity predispose to sleep. This explains why comfort, warmth, quiet and darkness are well-known aids to sleeping.

The reticular formation of the spinal cord (p. 244), the hypothalamus (p. 252) and the thalamus (p. 252) all play some part in regulating the transmission of impulses to the cerebral cortex, and are involved in the mechanism of sleep.

What happens in the brain during sleep is not understood. That spontaneous activity does not stop is shown by encephalograms. When sleep begins, the normal pattern of the waves in wakefulness (Fig. 114) changes. They become slower and larger. After about an hour, **paradoxical sleep** supervenes. During this, though the waves become smaller, they continue and other characteristics appear. Muscle tone varies, but is reduced in the main, and rapid eye movements occur behind the closed lids. The sleeper is harder to waken and dreams occur. Dreams, even though the sleeper may remember nothing of them, seem to be necessary for refreshing sleep. Paradoxical sleep alternates with ordinary sleep during the sleeping period. It seems that drugs used to induce sleep are not wholly successful, because they interfere with the normal cycles of paradoxical sleep.

THE MENINGES AND THE BLOOD SUPPLY TO THE CENTRAL NERVOUS SYSTEM

The brain, spinal cord and nerve roots attached to them are covered by three membranes (the **meninges**), the dura mater, the arachnoid mater and the pia mater (Fig. 117).

THE DURA MATER

The dura mater is the outer covering and it is tough and fibrous. Where it lines the inside of the skull, it consists of two layers: an outer layer and an inner layer. The **outer layer** of the dura is really the periosteum (or endosteum) of the inner aspect of the skull bones, and of course it follows every detail of the bony surface. The **inner layer** of the dura has a smooth surface facing towards

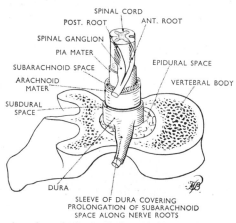

Fig. 117. Diagram showing the relations of the spinal cord and of the nerve roots to the meninges and to a vertebra.

the brain, and does not follow the outer layer exactly. In places, it sweeps away from the skull and back again to form large folds of the inner layer, which support the brain substance. One such fold, attached along the line of the sagittal suture, is the **falx cerebri.** It separates the two cerebral hemispheres. The **tentorium cerebelli** is a similar fold, which is horizontal and forms a roof for the posterior cranial fossa, separating the occipital lobes of the cerebral hemispheres above from the cerebellum in the fossa below. The posterior end of the falx cerebri is attached to the tentorium cerebelli (Plate 29).

The **venous sinuses of the skull** (p. 376) are channels between the layers of the dura (Plate 29), lined with the endothelium characteristic of blood vessels (p. 351).

In the vertebral canal, surrounding the spinal cord, the dura consists of a single layer continuous with the inner layer of the dura in the skull.

The inner layer of the dura in the skull and the dura surrounding the spinal cord send out short prolongations, like sleeves, round the roots of the cranial and spinal nerves, clothing them until they emerge through the foramina of the skull or the intervertebral foramina of the vertebral column (Fig. 117). The subarachnoid space (see below) is thus continued for a short distance along the nerve roots.

THE PIA MATER AND THE ARACHNOID MATER

These two meninges are most easily considered together. The **pia**, or innermost layer, consists of interlacing bundles of collagen, reticulin and elastic fibres covered by a continuous layer of flattened squamous cells. It follows every contour of the brain and spinal cord. The **arachnoid** on the other hand forms a delicate cobweb-like spongework which joins the pia to the dura. Its interstices contain cerebrospinal fluid, and constitute what is known as the **subarachnoid space.** The pia is a very vascular layer and the **blood vessels** supplying it and the brain substance run within the subarachnoid space. If such a vessel bursts, it gives rise to a **subarachnoid hæmorrhage** which, as it increases in size, may press on the subjacent nervous tissue.

BLOOD SUPPLY TO THE BRAIN

The brain substance, which is so vulnerable to oxygen-lack (p. 116), is supplied by two sets of vessels derived from branches from the **cerebral arterial circle of Willis,** which is itself made up by the terminations of the **internal carotid** and **vertebral arteries** (Plate 10).

The **cerebral arteries** are of two types: superficial and central. The **superficial** arteries run on the surface of the brain, while the **central** arteries enter the substance of the hemispheres through the base of the brain. These two sets do not anastomose with one another, except by capillaries, thus they constitute what are known as **end arteries.** If one of them is blocked, its linkage with an artery of the other set is inadequate to maintain the blood supply to the part which was supplied by the blocked vessel. This part therefore dies. Such a blockage is known as a **cerebral thrombosis.** On the other hand, one of the central arteries supplying the interior of a hemisphere may burst; this is a **cerebral hæmorrhage.** The artery supplying the internal capsule seems to be particularly prone to this type of 'cerebrovascular accident'.

It should be noted that the walls of cerebral arteries are particularly liable to give way under the stress of a varied blood pressure, because their walls are thinner than those of arteries elsewhere in the body.

CEREBROSPINAL FLUID (C.S.F.): ITS PRODUCTION AND CIRCULATION

The **cerebrospinal fluid** (C.S.F.) is a clear watery fluid which fills the sub-arachnoid space, the ventricular system of the brain and the central canal of the spinal cord. It is **secreted** by the choroid plexuses of the ventricles and fills the ventricular system. It passes into the subarachnoid space by way of holes in the roof of the fourth ventricle (Plate 11) called the **median aperture** (of Magendie) and the two **lateral apertures** (of Lushka). Thence it spreads over the surface of the brain and spinal cord and is reabsorbed into the venous sinuses by means of **arachnoid granulations** and **arachnoid villi** which project into venous sinuses.

Functions of Cerebrospinal Fluid

Cerebrospinal fluid acts as a tissue fluid for the central nervous system, and also serves as support for the jelly-like, semi-liquid brain substance, providing it with a cushion of fluid which prevents it from being injured when the head moves violently. By increasing or diminishing its production, the intracranial contents are maintained at even pressure and the intracranial volume is kept constant, even if the volume of the brain itself changes, e.g. by the appearance of a growth.

The cerebrospinal fluid is said to be a secretion rather than a simple filtrate of plasma, because energy is utilized in its production and certain substances, such as bile-pigments and penicillin, do not pass from the choroid plexus capillaries into cerebrospinal fluid. Radioactive ions pass only very slowly.

Lumbar Puncture and Cisternal Puncture

In clinical medicine, it is often necessary to measure the pressure of the cerebrospinal fluid and to analyse its chemical composition, which is changed in certain diseases.

Access to the subarachnoid space is possible because, although the spinal cord reaches down only to the upper two lumbar vertebræ, the subarachnoid space is continued around the cauda equina down to the second piece of the sacrum. **Lumbar puncture** consists of inserting a long hollow needle into the subarachnoid space, by passing it through the interval between the neural arches of the third and fourth lumbar vertebræ.

It may be necessary to obtain C.S.F. from inside the skull, e.g. to compare it with that obtained by lumbar puncture in cases of blockage of the vertebral canal. This is done by inserting the same type of needle in the back of the upper part of the neck, passing it into the foramen magnum through the interval between the altas vertebra and base of the skull, and so tapping an expanded portion of the subarachnoid space in the cerebello-medullary angle, called the **cisterna magna** (Plate 11). Hence the name of the procedure—a **cisternal puncture.**

Derangements of the Circulation of Cerebrospinal fluid

Attention has already been drawn to the fact that certain parts of the ventricular system are particularly narrow, e.g. the aqueduct of Sylvius. At these sites, the circulation of cerebrospinal fluid may become blocked by, for example, a tumour; alternatively the holes in the roof of the fourth ventricle may become blocked as a result of meningitis around them.

Although the outlets towards the arachnoid granulations and villi are blocked, the choroid plexuses still produce cerebrospinal fluid against the mounting pressure within the ventricular system, so that the ventricles tend to expand. If this condition occurs in a child, this expansion is possible because the skull is still growing and can allow the ventricles to expand, stretching the brain substance as they do so. The condition is known as **hydrocephalus** or 'water on the brain'. The stretching of the brain substance damages it and usually affects the intelligence of the child.

In an adult, however, the bones of the skull have fused and so form a rigid container for the brain which consequently cannot expand. Thus, the only possible result is **increased intracranial tension** with compression of brain substance which, if unrelieved, will ultimately lead to coma and death.

THE PERIPHERAL NERVOUS SYSTEM

The constituents of this subdivision of the nervous system are described on p. 222 and on p. 228.

SOME BASIC STRUCTURAL AND FUNCTIONAL CONSIDERATIONS

Reflex Action

Reflex action is the **involuntary** production of a **response,** such as activity in muscles or glands, resulting from the **stimulation of afferent nerve fibres.** It always involves part of the **central nervous system.** It occurs without the necessary intervention of consciousness. It is inborn and occurs in every member of the species.

Reflex Arc

A reflex arc is the chain of structures which is concerned in the production of a reflex action.

The **afferent path** consists of a **sensory end organ** or **receptor,** where the stimulus is received, and the **sensory neurone** which conducts it to the central nervous system.

The **reflex centre** is in the central nervous system, and connects the afferent and efferent paths. It consists of one or more **intercalated** or **connector neurones,** and may be in the spinal cord or in the brain stem.

The **efferent path** consists of a **motor neurone** and an **effector organ,** which may be a muscle or a gland.

The reflex mechanism becomes fatigued quickly.

Spinal Reflexes

A spinal reflex is one example of reflex action. The **'knee jerk'** is a spinal reflex. To demonstrate the knee jerk, the knee is supported and the leg is allowed to hang loosely in a partially flexed position. The patellar tendon is tapped with a hammer (the **stimulus**), the quadriceps muscle then contracts (the **response**), causing the foot to kick forwards as the quadriceps extends the leg on the thigh at the knee joint. The sensory receptor is a stretch receptor in the quadriceps muscle. The afferent neurone is a sensory nerve fibre in the femoral nerve with the cell body in the posterior root ganglion of the third or fourth lumbar nerves. The centre is in the spinal cord. The central process of the afferent neurone in this case transmits the impulse direct to the motor nerve cell in the anterior horn of the spinal cord. The axon of this cell, the motor nerve fibre, emerges in the anterior root of the third or fourth lumbar nerve and travels in the femoral nerve to the quadriceps, where it ends in motor end-plates and causes the muscle to contract. This kind of spinal reflex is a 'stretch reflex' because tapping the tendons has the effect of stretching the muscles concerned, which react by contracting. Other similar reflexes, which can be demonstrated easily, are the **'biceps jerk'** (p. 275) the **'triceps jerk'** (p. 275) and the **'ankle jerk'** (p. 279). A normal response to the stretch stimulus indicates that every part of the reflex arc is functioning normally. No response shows that some part of the reflex arc is damaged. An exaggerated response shows that the upper motor neurone is not exercising its proper inhibitory control on the anterior horn cell (p. 244).

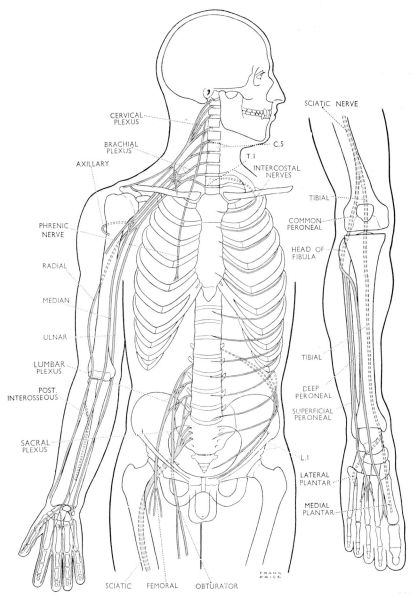

Plate 13. The principal peripheral nerves, shown in relation to the skeleton.

[facing page 262

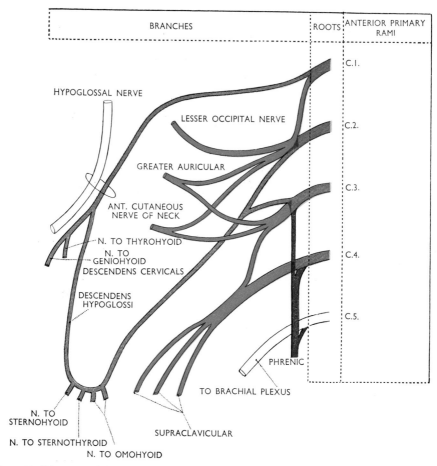

Plate 14. Diagram of the cervical plexus; the roots of the plexus are orange; the phrenic nerve is red; branches to the infrahyoid muscles are purple and cutaneous branches are green.

[between pages 262/3 facing Pl. 15

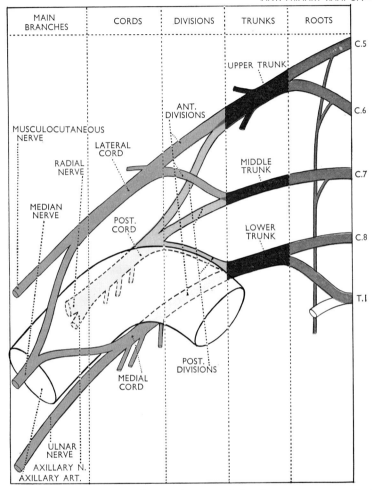

Plate 15. Diagram of the brachial plexus; the roots of the plexus are orange; the trunks are red; anterior divisions and their branches are yellow; posterior divisions and their branches are blue.

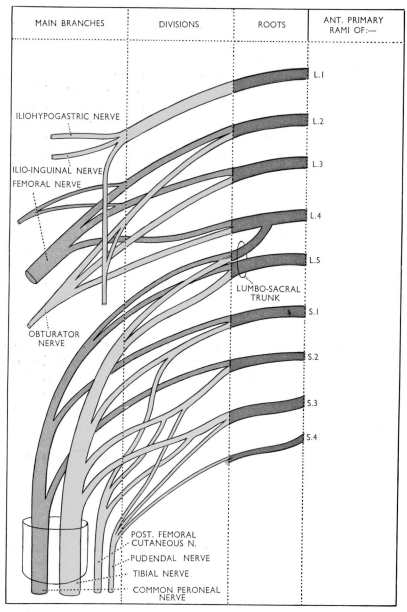

MAIN BRANCHES	DIVISIONS	ROOTS	ANT. PRIMARY RAMI OF:—

L.1

ILIOHYPOGASTRIC NERVE

L.2

ILIO-INGUINAL NERVE
FEMORAL NERVE

L.3

L.4

LUMBO-SACRAL
TRUNK

L.5

S.1

OBTURATOR
NERVE

S.2

S.3

S.4

POST. FEMORAL
CUTANEOUS N.
PUDENDAL NERVE
TIBIAL NERVE
COMMON PERONEAL
NERVE

Plate 16.Diagram of lumbar and sacral plexuses; the roots of the plexuses are orange; the anterior divisions are yellow; posterior divisions are blue.

The **abdominal reflexes** (p. 271) and the **plantar response** or **reflex** (p. 279) are cerebral reflexes—they involve pathways to the brain.

Many other examples of reflex action can be shown in the functioning of the body. The **respiratory** and **cardiovascular** systems are controlled by reflex action (pp. 342 and 385). The **pupillary light** and **accommodation reflexes** (p. 301) adjust the eye for vision in different circumstances. Normally the bladder and rectum are under control of the will. In **infants,** in whom voluntary control has not been learned, and in injured adults, where the spinal cord has been damaged, cutting off control from the higher centres, the **bladder** and **rectum** are emptied reflexly in response to the stimulus of stretching when they fill up.

Inhibition

A nervous impulse acting on a motor neurone may, instead of stimulating it to send an impulse along its axon, prevent any such impulse from being transmitted. Those neurones, which send inhibiting impulses of this kind, are called inhibitory neurones and several of these act on the anterior horn cells of the spinal cord (Fig. 110).

Reciprocal Innervation

The nerve supply of opposing groups of muscles is closely related, so that if the prime movers (p. 179) contract, the antagonists (p. 179) relax. This is part of the spinal reflex mechanism. The sensory neurone of the reflex arc, besides stimulating the anterior horn cells supplying the prime movers, also sends inhibitory impulses to the anterior horn cells supplying the antagonists and so causes them to relax. The inhibitory impulses stop the flow of impulses which maintains the muscle tone of the antagonists. This mechanism for simultaneous control of the opposing muscle groups is called **reciprocal innervation.**

THE PERIPHERAL NERVES

The peripheral nerves are divided into two groups, the cranial nerves, connected with the brain, and the spinal nerves connected with the spinal cord.

THE CRANIAL NERVES

The cranial nerves are the twelve pairs of peripheral nerves which come from the brain. Each pair is known both by its number and by its name.

I	Olfactory	VII	Facial
II	Optic	VIII	Vestibulocochlear
III	Oculomotor	IX	Glossopharyngeal
IV	Trochlear	X	Vagus
V	Trigeminal	XI	Accessory
VI	Abducent	XII	Hypoglossal

Unlike spinal nerves, which all contain both motor and sensory fibres, the cranial nerves differ in the kinds of fibres they contain, some being sensory, some motor, some mixed and some containing fibres of the parasympathetic system. They may contain only one or several of the nerve components (p. 231).

I. Olfactory Nerve

The olfactory nerve is a **nerve of special sense,** the sense of smell. The cell bodies are situated between the columnar epithelial cells of the mucous membrane in the roof of the nose. Each cell has dendrites (**olfactory hairs**) which project on the surface and are stimulated by odours in the inspired air; each cell also has an axon connected with the brain. Bundles of axons form olfactory nerve fibres, which pass through the cribriform plate and synapse in the **olfactory bulb** (Fig. 111), part of the brain which lies on the cribriform plate. Fractures of the skull often involve the cribriform plate, which is thin and easily broken. This damages the olfactory nerve fibres, so that the sense of smell is lost. Much of what we consider the sense of taste is in fact appreciated through the olfactory organs (p. 310).

II. Optic Nerve

The optic nerve is a **nerve of special sense,** the sense of sight. It is really a tract of the brain, and not a true peripheral nerve (p. 288). The nerve fibres from the **retina** (p. 294) converge on the **optic disc,** and pass through it, to form the thick optic nerve which leads from the back of the eyeball, through the optic foramen at the back of the orbit, to meet the optic nerve from the other side at the **optic chiasma** (Fig. 111). This lies on the base of the brain, immediately in front of the hypophyseal stalk. In the optic chiasma, the nerve fibres from the medial half of each retina cross to the opposite side to join with the fibres from the lateral half of the retina of that side, forming in this way the **optic tract.** This passes to a relay station, called the **lateral geniculate body,** just below the thalamus. From there, the **geniculocalcarine tract** passes to the **visual cortex** on the occipital lobe.

The optic nerve, optic chiamsa, optic tract, lateral geniculate body, geniculocalcarine tract and visual cortex constitute the **visual pathway.**

III. Oculomotor Nerve

The oculomotor nerve contains **somatic motor fibres** for all the extrinsic muscles of the eye (p. 184), except the superior oblique and the lateral rectus. It also contains **parasympathetic fibres,** which relay in the **ciliary ganglion,** and supply the sphincter pupillæ muscle and the ciliary muscle which controls accommodation. The oculomotor nerve arises from the midbrain (Fig. 111) and leaves the cranium through the superior orbital fissure. In the orbit, it gives off its branches to the extrinsic muscles and to the eyeball.

IV. Trochlear Nerve

The trochlear nerve contains motor fibres (**somatic motor**) for the superior oblique muscle of the eye. It arises from the back of the midbrain, winds round to the front and passes forwards into the orbit through the superior orbital fissure.

V. Trigeminal Nerve

The trigeminal nerve is the large sensory nerve (**somatic sensory**) to the face and to the mouth, nose and paranasal sinuses. It also conveys motor fibres (**branchiomotor**) to the muscles of mastication. Being mainly a sensory nerve, it has a large ganglion, the **trigeminal ganglion,** which lies in a pocket of the dura mater on the apex of the petrous temporal bone, just behind and lateral to the hypophyseal fossa (Fig. 43). From the ganglion, the root passes medially to enter the pons. From the other side of the ganglion, arise the three large divisions of the nerve, the ophthalmic nerve, the maxillary nerve and the mandibular nerve.

(a) THE OPHTHALMIC NERVE: This nerve passes forwards into the orbit through the superior orbital fissure. Sensory branches (**somatic sensory**) are distributed to the skin of the nose, upper eyelid and forehead, to the conjunctiva and cornea, to the mucous membrane of the nose and of the frontal ethmoidal and sphenoidal sinuses, and to the eyeball.

(b) THE MAXILLARY NERVE: This nerve passes forwards through the foramen rotundum and along a canal in the floor of the orbit, its terminal branches emerging on the face. It gives sensory branches to the skin of the cheek, lower eyelid, nose and upper lip, to all the upper teeth and to the mucous membrane of the nose and maxillary sinus.

(c) THE MANDIBULAR NERVE: This nerve passes downwards through the foramen ovale. It contains **all the motor fibres** of the trigeminal nerve; these are distributed to the muscles of mastication. The **sensory fibres** are distributed to the skin over the mandible, to all the lower teeth and, by means of the lingual nerve, to the anterior two thirds of the tongue. The lingual nerve is joined by the **chorda tympani branch of the facial nerve** and this conveys fibres for the special sense of **taste (branchiosensory)** to the anterior two thirds of the tongue.

Sometimes intractable pain, **trigeminal neuralgia,** occurs in the distribution of one or more of the three divisions of the trigeminal nerve. Division of the nerve involved, or destruction of the trigeminal ganglion, is sometimes carried out for relief.

If the ophthalmic nerve is destroyed in this way, a shield must be worn to protect the eye, because sensation from the normally highly sensitive cornea and conjunctiva is lost. This means that the presence of foreign bodies on the surface of the eye may not be noticed by the patient, and the cornea may therefore be damaged.

VI. The Abducent Nerve

The abducent nerve contains motor fibres (**somatic motor**) for the lateral rectus muscle of the eye. It leaves the brain at the lower border of the pons (Fig. 111) and enters the orbit through the superior orbital fissure.

VII. Facial Nerve

The facial nerve carries motor fibres (**branchiomotor**) to the muscles of facial expression. It also conveys parasympathetic fibres (**visceromotor**) for the lacrimal, parotid, submandibular and sublingual glands, and sensory fibres for taste (**branchiosensory**) for the anterior two thirds of the tongue. The facial nerve leaves the brain at the lateral edge of the lower border of the pons (Fig. 111) and enters the internal auditory meatus in the petrous temporal bone. As it traverses a canal through the petrous temporal, it gives off the **chorda tympani,** a nerve which, carrying the taste fibres and some parasympathetic fibres, passes through the middle ear and eventually joins the lingual nerve (see above). The facial nerve emerges from the canal through the stylomastoid foramen. Finally, it divides into branches for the musculature of all parts of the face; these branches pass through the parotid gland as they travel to the surface.

VIII. Vestibulocochlear Nerve

This is a nerve of **special sense** and consists of two parts: the **vestibular nerve,** which supplies the saccule, utricle and semicircular canals, and is for the sense of balance; and the **cochlear nerve,** which supplies the spiral organ in the cochlea, and is for the sense of hearing. Both parts leave the brain close to the facial nerve (Fig. 111) and enter the internal auditory meatus. The vestibular ganglion lies on the vestibular nerve in the meatus and its peripheral fibres enter the petrous temporal bone to reach the semicircular canals, utricle and saccule. The cochlear nerve travels through the bone to reach the spiral ganglion in the cochlea. The short peripheral fibres from the ganglion cells go to the spiral organ (p. 306).

IX. Glossopharyngeal Nerve

The glossopharyngeal nerve carries motor fibres (**branchiomotor**) to the palate and pharynx; sensory fibres including taste (**branchiosensory**) to the tongue and palate; and sensory fibres (**branchiosensory**) to the carotid sinus and carotid body. The glossopharyngeal nerve arises from the lateral part of the front of the medulla oblongata, and leaves the skull through the jugular foramen. In the neck, it runs a short course, past the internal carotid artery to the pharynx.

X. Vagus Nerve

The vagus nerve carries motor fibres (**branchiomotor**) and sensory fibres (**branchiosensory**) to the pharynx and larynx; it also carries parasympathetic motor fibres (**visceromotor**) and sensory fibres (**viscerosensory**) to widely scattered viscera, namely to the heart and lungs and to the œsophagus, stomach, pancreas, liver, small intestine and large intestine. There is a small sensory branch (**somatic sensory**) supplying the external auditory meatus. This accounts for the nausea or vomiting, which may result reflexly from syringing the ear.

The vagus nerve arises from the medulla below the glossopharyngeal nerve (Fig. 111) and leaves through the jugular foramen. It travels through the neck and into the thorax in the carotid sheath (Plate 12). It crosses the lateral aspect of the subclavian artery on the right side, and the lateral aspect of the aortic arch on the left, and continues to the root of the lung which it supplies. The nerves from the two sides then form round the œsophagus a plexus, which is carried on again, as a nerve on each side, to the stomach and the rest of the gastro-intestinal tract. As it travels through the neck, the vagus gives off several branches, namely a pharyngeal branch, cardiac branches and the superior laryngeal nerve which supplies the mucous membrane of the larynx above the vocal cords (internal laryngeal nerve), and the cricothyroid muscle (external laryngeal nerve).

The **recurrent laryngeal nerve** is a most important branch which supplies the intrinsic muscles of the larynx. On the right side, it hooks under the sub-clavian artery, and on the left side, it hooks under the ligamentum arteriosum and aortic arch to travel back to the larynx in the groove between the trachea and œsophagus.

XI. Accessory Nerve

The **cranial part** of this nerve arises from the lateral aspect of the medulla and joins the vagus nerve. The **spinal part** of the accessory nerve carries motor fibres to the sternomastoid and trapezius. It arises from the lateral aspect of the upper segments of the spinal cord, in line with the vagus and glossopharyngeal nerves. It enters the skull through the foramen magnum and then leaves the skull through the jugular foramen. It supplies the sternomastoid and crosses the posterior triangle of the neck to reach trapezius.

XII. Hypoglossal Nerve

The hypoglossal nerve carries motor fibres (**somatic motor**) to the muscles of the tongue. It arises from the front of the medulla, near the midline, and leaves the skull through the anterior condylar canal. It then curves forwards lateral to the carotid sheath to reach the tongue.

THE SPINAL NERVES

Thirty-one pairs of spinal nerves are connected with the spinal cord, one for each segment of the body. There are eight pairs of cervical nerves, twelve thoracic, five lumbar, five sacral and one coccygeal. Each of these nerves is a mixed nerve arising from the spinal cord by two roots, a posterior sensory root on which is the sensory posterior root ganglion, and an anterior motor root. The roots join in the intervertebral foramen to form the spinal nerve (see also p. 228). There are eight pairs of cervical nerves, although there are only seven cervical vertebræ. The first cervical nerve emerges above the first vertebra, the atlas, coming out between it and the skull (Fig. 118). The other cervical nerves down to the seventh, emerge **above** the vertebra of corresponding number, like the first. The eighth cervical nerve emerges below the seventh cervical vertebra, that is, above the first thoracic vertebra; this foramen being occupied, the **first thoracic nerve** is the nerve which emerges **below** the first thoracic vertebra. All the succeeding nerves emerge through the intervertebral foramen **below** the vertebra of corresponding number (Fig. 118).

Anterior and Posterior Primary Rami

Each spinal nerve, as soon as it emerges from the intervertebral foramen, divides into an anterior primary ramus and a posterior primary ramus. The reason for this is explained on p. 19.

The posterior primary rami of all the spinal nerves go to supply the extensor muscles of the back, and the skin over them (Fig. 120). The anterior primary rami are much larger and, between themselves, they supply the rest of the trunk and the limbs. Except for the anterior primary rami of the thoracic nerves, which are distributed each to its own segment, adjacent anterior primary rami unite to a greater or lesser extent before they branch again to form the peripheral nerves. Four groups of anterior primary rami are linked in this way to form plexuses, namely the cervical plexus, the brachial plexus, the lumbar plexus and the sacral plexus. The branches of the brachial plexus supply the upper limb; the branches of the lumbar and sacral plexuses supply the lower limb.

The Thoracic Nerves

The distribution of the thoracic nerves illustrates most clearly the characteristic segmental pattern (see also p. 80 and

Fig. 118. A diagram, seen from the left side, to show the shortness of the spinal cord in relation to the vertebral column and the relation of the individual nerve roots to their corresponding vertebræ. For clarity, only one root is shown for each spinal nerve.

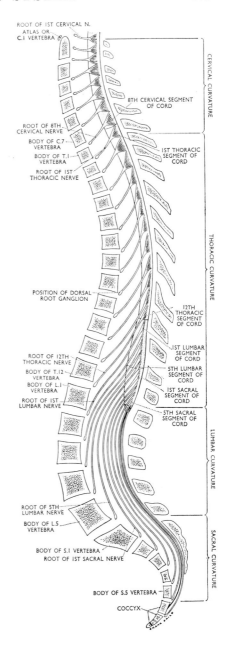

Figs. 119, B, and 120). Each pair of nerves supplied a band of the body wall, the motor fibres supplying the muscles and the sensory fibres the skin.

Each thoracic nerve, on emerging from the intervertebral foramen below the vertebra of its own number, divides into a **posterior primary ramus,** which supplies the **extensor** muscles of the back and the skin over them, and an

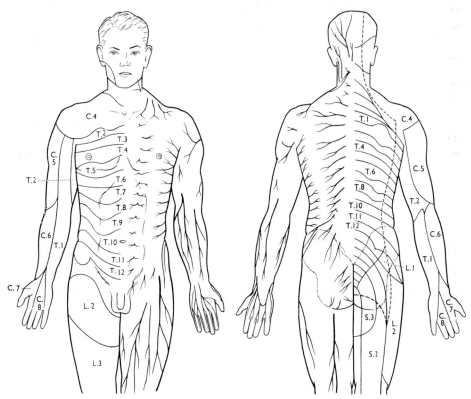

Fig. 119. The distribution of segmental nerves (numbered), and peripheral nerves to the skin of the trunk and upper limb, both front and back.

anterior primary ramus, much larger, which supplies the muscles and skin of the side and front of the body (Plate 13 and Fig. 119). The anterior primary rami of the first eleven thoracic nerves are called **intercostal nerves,** because they travel round the body wall between the ribs, supplying the muscles and skin. The twelfth, being below the last rib, is called the **subcostal nerve.** The lowest five intercostal nerves and the subcostal nerve also supply the anterior abdominal wall.

Besides supplying the **muscles** and **skin** of the thoracic and abdominal walls, the intercostal nerves supply the **serous membranes** lining these walls, that is, the costal part of the parietal pleura (p. 331) and the parietal peritoneum (p. 440).

Abdominal Reflex. If the skin of the abdominal wall is stroked towards the midline, a localized contraction of the abdominal muscles occurs, causing the wall to twitch. This normal response depends on the proper functioning of the pyramidal tracts, that is, it involves the cerebral cortex and is not a simple spinal reflex.

The Cervical Plexus

The cervical plexus is composed of the anterior primary rami of the first four cervical nerves (Plate 14). The most important branch is the **phrenic nerve** (Plate 12), which arises mainly from the fourth cervical nerve, with contributions from the third and fifth. It supplies the **diaphragm** with motor fibres and also with sensory fibres, which innervate the parietal pleura on the upper surface of the diaphragm and its parietal peritoneum on its lower surface.

A loop of nerve fibres from the first, second and third cervical nerves supplies the infrahyoid muscles.

A set of **cutaneous nerves** supplies the skin of the front and side of the neck. Another group of cutaneous nerves, the **supraclavicular nerves,** supplies the skin of the lower part of the neck and the tip of the shoulder.

Referred pain from the diaphragm is often felt on the tip of the shoulder. Such shoulder pain may be the result of diaphragmatic pleurisy (inflammation of the diaphragmatic pleura), or of irritation of the diaphragmatic part of the parietal peritoneum. The explanation is that the phrenic nerve, which supplies the diaphragm, and the supraclavicular nerves, which supply the tip of the shoulder, are both from the fourth cervical nerve (p. 242).

Innervation of the Limbs

Each limb is developed from the lateral and anterior parts of a number of segments of the body. Fig. 120, A, shows the tissues of one segment growing outwards to form a limb. In the axis of the limb, elements of the skeleton have already appeared. These bones have divided the muscle mass into two parts, one on the dorsal aspect of the limb and one on the ventral aspect. The dorsal muscles attached to the bones can straighten the limb, that is, they are extensors; the ventral muscles can bend the limb, that is, they are flexors. The anterior primary ramus of the spinal nerve, approaching the limb to supply muscles and skin, has to divide into a dorsal (posterior) division to supply the extensor muscles and the skin on the posterior aspect of the limb, and a ventral (anterior) division to supply the flexor muscles and the skin on the anterior aspect of the limb. No matter how complex the further development of the limb, the developmentally **dorsal aspect,** which contains the **extensor** muscles, is supplied by the **posterior divisions** of the anterior primary rami of the spinal nerves, and the developmentally **ventral aspect,** which contains the

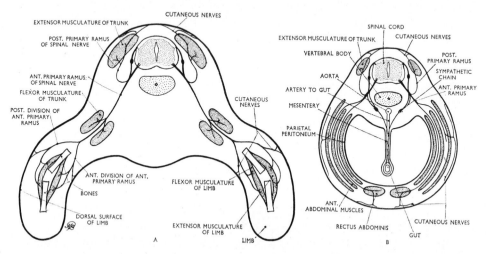

Fig. 120. A schematic representation of the nerve supply to muscles and skin, A, of limbs, and B, of the trunk.

flexor muscles, is supplied by the **anterior divisions** of the anterior primary rami.

Each limb is derived, not from one, but from several segments: the upper limb from five, the lower limb from seven. The anterior primary rami of the spinal nerves of these segments combine, to a greater or lesser extent, in the root of the limb to form the great limb plexuses, before breaking up again to form the peripheral nerves supplying the muscles and skin. Nevertheless, the simple basic pattern can still be discerned.

Because the lower limb has undergone a rotation during development (also see p. 20), the developmentally dorsal surface, the extensor surface, is on the anterior aspect of the limb, and the developmentally ventral surface, the flexor surface, is on the posterior aspect.

NERVES OF THE UPPER LIMB

The Brachial Plexus

The brachial plexus (Plate 15) is formed from the anterior primary rami of the fifth, sixth and seventh and eighth cervical and the first thoracic nerves. These are the **roots** of the plexus. The branches supply the muscles and skin of the upper limb. Fig. 119 shows the areas of skin supplied by each of the spinal nerves, as well as the cutaneous nerves from the plexus supplying the skin.

In forming the plexus (Plate 15), the roots unite to form the **trunks;** the fifth and sixth anterior primary rami unite to form the **upper trunk;** the seventh

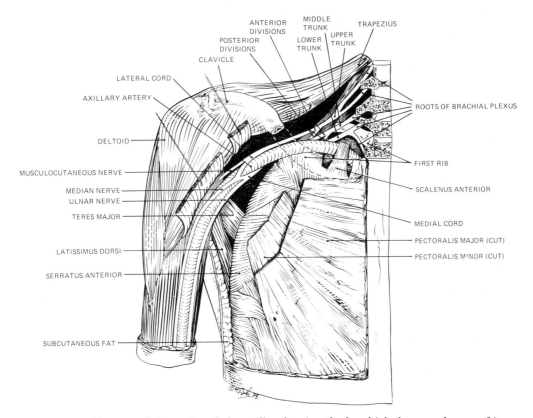

Fig. 121. The root of the neck and the axilla, showing the brachial plexus and some of its main branches.

continues as the **middle trunk**; and the eighth cervical and first thoracic form the **lower trunk**. Each trunk then divides into an **anterior division** and a **posterior division**. The anterior divisions will supply muscles and skin on the front of the limb, the posterior divisions the back.

The three posterior divisions unite to form the **posterior cord**. This divides into two main branches, the large **radial** (musculospiral) **nerve** and the smaller **axillary** (circumflex) **nerve**. The radial nerve, derived from the posterior cord, is the nerve which supplies the extensor muscles and the skin of the back of the upper arm and of the back of the forearm.

The anterior divisions of the trunks might unite in a similar way to supply the front of the limb. However, the axillary artery is in the way and prevents complete fusion. In fact, the anterior divisions of the upper and middle trunks unite to form the **lateral cord,** and the anterior division of the lower trunk continues as the **medial cord.** The branches of the lateral and medial cords, between them, supply the flexor muscles and the skin on the front of the limb.

The lateral cord divides into the **musculocutaneous nerve** and the **lateral** root of the **median nerve.** The medial cord divides into the **ulnar nerve** and the **medial** root of the **median nerve.** From the lateral and medial cord, therefore, three nerves for the front of the limb arise, the musculocutaneous, the median and the ulnar. The musculocutaneous supplies the flexor muscles in the upper arm (brachialis and biceps); the median nerve supplies the flexor muscles in the forearm; the ulnar nerve supplies the small muscles of the hand. In addition the cords and their branches supply the skin of the front of the limb.

Note that branches of the ulnar nerve supply the skin of the medial part of the hand, both front and back, and both surfaces of the little and ring fingers (Fig. 135). The median nerve supplies the skin of the palmar aspect of the lateral part of the hand and of the thumb, forefinger and middle finger. The back of these digits and of the lateral part of the hand is supplied by the radial nerve.

The roots, trunks, divisions and upper parts of the cords of the brachial plexus are in the posterior triangle of the neck (p. 187). The rest of the cords and the branches are in the axilla. The cords are grouped round the middle of the axillary artery in the positions indicated by their names. The main nerves arise from the cords in the axilla close to the axillary artery (Fig. 121).

The **radial nerve** (Plate 13) travels through the back of the upper arm, in contact with the **radial groove** of the humerus, spiralling downwards from the medial side to the lateral side. It gives branches to the extensor muscle on the back of the upper arm (triceps) and to the skin of the back of the upper arm and forearm. Near the elbow, it enters the lateral side of the cubital fossa. There it divides into a **superficial branch** and a **deep branch** (the posterior interosseus nerve). This deep branch winds laterally round the shaft of the radius to the posterior aspect of the forearm, where it supplies the extensor muscles. The superficial branch of the radial nerve continues through the front of the forearm to the wrist, where it passes backwards to supply the lateral part of the back of the hand and the back of the thumb, forefinger and middle finger (Fig. 135).

The **axillary nerve** passes backwards round the surgical neck of the humerus to supply the deltoid muscle.

The **musculocutaneous nerve** supplies the flexor muscles on the upper arm (biceps and brachialis) and continues to supply the skin of the lateral part of the forearm.

The **median nerve** (Plate 13) passes through the upper arm close to the brachial artery, and lies on its medial side in the cubital fossa. It travels through the forearm, between the superficial and deep layers of muscles, and enters the hand by passing with the flexor tendons through the carpal tunnel. It supplies the flexor muscles in the forearm, and in the hand it gives branches to the thenar muscles, to the skin of the lateral half of the palm and to the palmar surface of the thumb, index finger and middle finger.

The **ulnar nerve** (Plate 13) passes through the upper arm near the brachial artery, but near the elbow region, it winds backwards and medially to pass behind and directly in contact with the medial epicondyle. The nerve can be rolled under the skin on the back of the medial epicondyle; jarring of the nerve here gives the name **'funny bone'** to the region. The tingling, which this produces, illustrates the distribution of the cutaneous branches to the front and back of the medial part of the palm, and to the little and ring fingers. The ulnar nerve passes down the front of the forearm (supplying the two muscles not supplied by the median nerve) and enters the hand by passing in front of the flexor retinaculum (unlike the median nerve which goes through the carpal tunnel). In the hand, it supplies all the small muscles except those of the thenar eminence, and gives the branches to the skin described above.

REFLEXES: If the tendon of the biceps is tapped in the cubital fossa, the biceps contracts causing a momentary flexion at the elbow joint. This is the **biceps jerk,** which is a characteristic spinal stretch reflex (p. 262).

The **triceps jerk** is a similar reflex, elicited by supporting the forearm with the elbow joint at a right angle and tapping the tendon of insertion of triceps just above the olecranon process. Contraction of triceps produces a momentary extension of the elbow joint.

The muscles of a group which produce a given movement are supplied by the same spinal nerves. This is associated with the group action of muscles.

Muscle group			Nerve
Muscles producing	abduction at the shoulder		C.5
,,	,,	lateral rotation at the shoulder	C.5 and C.6
,,	,,	flexion at the elbow	C.5 and C.6
,,	,,	extension at the elbow	C.7 and C.8
,,	,,	extension at the wrist and fingers	C.6 and C.7
,,	,,	flexion at the wrist and fingers	C.8 and T.1
Small muscles of the hand			T.1

The results of injuries of the brachial plexus illustrates this.

Erbs Paralysis. Forcible widening of the angle between the head and shoulder, such as may be caused by traction on the arm during birth, often tears the upper trunk (the union of C.5 and C.6, Plate 15). Muscles supplied by C.5 and C.6 are paralysed, namely abductors and lateral rotators at the shoulder, flexors at the elbow and some of the extensors at the wrist and fingers. The opposing groups of muscles act unrestrained and the arm hangs at the side in the "back-handed" position, that is, medially rotated with extended elbow and flexed wrist and fingers.

Klumpkes Paralysis. If the lower trunk of the brachial plexus is damaged, as sometimes occurs during birth, muscles supplied by C.8 and T.1 are paralysed. They are the flexors of the wrist and fingers and the small muscles of the hand. 'Claw-hand' is the result.

'Wrist-drop'. In injuries of the radial nerve (above the origin of its deep branch) the extensors of the wrist and fingers are paralysed. The flexed position of the wrist and fingers which results, is known as 'wrist-drop'.

NERVES OF THE LOWER LIMB

The anterior primary rami of the seven nerves (L.2, L.3, L.4, L.5, S.1, S.2 and S.3), which supply the lower limb, unite to form two plexuses, the **lumbar plexus** which lies on the posterior abdominal wall and the **sacral plexus** which is on the wall of the lesser pelvis (Plate 28).

The areas of skin supplied by each of the spinal nerves, as well as the cutaneous branches from the plexuses are shown in Fig. 122.

The Lumbar Plexus

The lumbar plexus (Plate 16) is composed of the anterior primary rami of the first, second, third and part of the fourth lumbar nerve. The rest of the fourth lumbar nerve joins the sacral plexus. Apart from the first lumbar nerve, which supplies the lowest part of the abdominal wall, the lumbar plexus supplies branches to the lower limb for both muscles and skin.

The second, third and fourth nerves divide into anterior and posterior divisions (Plate 16). The three anterior divisions unite to form the **obturator**

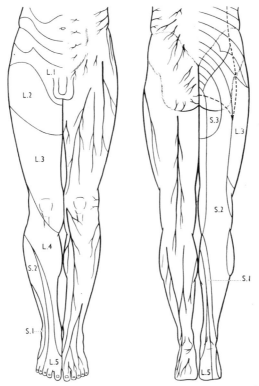

Fig. 122. The distribution of segmental nerves (numbered) and peripheral nerves to the skin of the lower limb, both front and back.

nerve (Plate 13) which supplies the adductor group of muscles of the thigh (specialized from the flexor mass). The three posterior divisions unite to form the **femoral nerve** (Plate 13) which supplies the extensor muscle, the quadriceps femoris (on the front of the thigh because of rotation of the limb), and the skin overlying it.

The lumbar plexus is surrounded by fibres of the psoas muscle. The obturator nerve emerges from the medial border of the muscle, travels along the side wall of the lesser pelvis and through the obturator canal to enter the adductor group of muscles. The femoral nerve emerges from the lateral border of psoas and leaves the abdominal cavity, to enter the thigh, by passing behind the inguinal ligament lateral to the femoral vessels. It divides at once into branches to the quadriceps muscle and to the skin of the front of the thigh. One very long branch, the **saphenous nerve,** supplies skin of the anteromedial surface of the limb as far as the instep.

The **knee jerk** is a spinal stretch reflex. It is described on p. 262.

The Sacral Plexus

The sacral plexus is formed by part of the anterior primary ramus of the fourth lumbar nerve and by the anterior primary rami of the fifth lumbar and of the first, second, third and fourth sacral nerves (Plate 16).

The contribution of the fourth lumbar nerve and the fifth lumbar nerve unite to form the **lumbosacral trunk,** which crosses the brim of the lesser pelvis to join the sacral nerves.

The sacral plexus lies on the posterior wall of the lesser pelvis, and its branches leave through the greater sciatic foramen to enter the gluteal region.

The roots of the plexus divide into anterior and posterior divisions. (The third and fourth sacral nerves have no posterior divisions.) The anterior divisions (of the fourth and fifth lumbar and the first, second and third sacral nerves) unite to form a very large nerve, the **tibial nerve,** which supplies the flexor muscles in the thigh (the hamstrings) and the flexor muscles in the calf. The posterior divisions (of the fourth and fifth lumbar and the first and second sacral nerves) unite to form the **common peroneal nerve** which supplies the extensor muscles in the leg. The tibial and common peroneal nerves are bound up in one fascial sheath to form the **sciatic nerve.**

The **sciatic nerve** (Plate 13 and Fig. 99) runs in the lower medial part of the gluteal region, under cover of gluteus maximus, emerging through the greater sciatic foramen. It passes down the back of the thigh under cover of the hamstrings, where its tibial part supplies the hamstrings, and just above the popliteal fossa it divides into the tibial nerve and the common peroneal nerve. The **tibial nerve** passes straight down through the popliteal fossa into the posterior compartment of the calf, where it supplies the flexor muscles including gastrocnemius and soleus. Its terminal branches enter the foot, by passing deep to the flexor retinaculum, and supply the small muscles of the foot and the skin of the sole.

The **common peroneal nerve** (Plate 13) passes to the lateral angle of the popliteal fossa (Fig. 100), where it can be rolled under the skin on the back of the

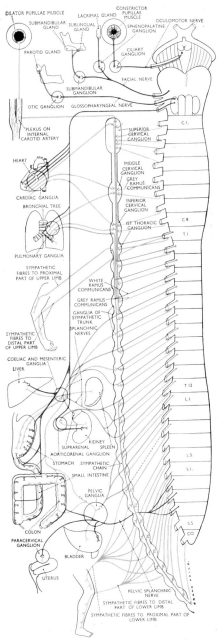

Plate 17. A diagram of the distribution of the autonomic nervous system. Sympathetic preganglionic fibres—blue. Sympathetic postganglionic fibres—yellow. Parasympathetic preganglionic fibres—red. Parasympathetic postganglionic fibres—green.

[facing page 278

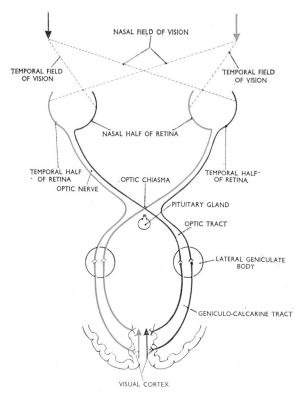

NASAL FIELD OF VISION

TEMPORAL FIELD
OF VISION

TEMPORAL FIELD
OF VISION

NASAL HALF OF RETINA

TEMPORAL HALF
OF RETINA

TEMPORAL HALF
OF RETINA

OPTIC CHIASMA

OPTIC NERVE

PITUITARY GLAND

OPTIC TRACT

LATERAL GENICULATE
BODY

GENICULO-CALCARINE TRACT

VISUAL CORTEX

Plate 18. A diagram of the visual pathway to show how impulses, set up by objects in the field of vision, reach the cerebral cortex.

head of the fibula. It is easily damaged here, for example, by the upper edge of a knee-length plaster cast. The nerve then winds round the neck of the fibula into the anterior compartment of the leg, where it supplies the extensor (dorsi-flexor) muscles, and the peroneal muscles, which are a subdivision of the extensor group. It also supplies the skin of the lateral part of the leg and the dorsum of the foot.

The **posterior femoral cutaneous nerve** arises from the anterior divisions of the first, second and third sacral nerves and supplies the skin of the back of the limb (the flexor surface). It leaves the pelvis through the greater sciatic foramen and passes down the back of the limb to the middle of the calf.

The **pudendal nerve** from the second, third and fourth sacral nerves leaves the pelvis through the medial part of the greater sciatic foramen and at once turns inwards again, through the lesser sciatic foramen, to enter the perineum. It travels forwards on the lateral wall of the ischiorectal fossa, giving off a branch which crosses to the medial wall of the fossa (Plate 8) to supply the striated muscle in the external sphincter and the skin of the anal canal. It ends by giving branches to the skin and muscles of the urogenital triangle, including the external sphincter of the bladder.

The **ankle jerk** is a spinal stretch reflex elicited by tapping the tendo calcaneus when the leg is flexed at the knee joint and the foot slightly extended (dorsiflexed) at the ankle. Contraction of the gastrocnemius and soleus flexes the foot momentarily on the leg.

The **plantar reflex.** This is a reflex action which involves both the spinal cord and the pyramidal tracts. The lateral border of the sole of the foot is firmly stroked with a blunt point. The normal **plantar response** is flexion of the great toe associated with flexion and crowding together of the other toes. The abnormal response is an extension (dorsiflexion) of the great toe and a spreading out of the other toes. Such an **extensor response** indicates interference with the normal function of the pyramidal tracts. In infants, in whom the pyramidal tracts are still without myelin sheaths and are not yet fully functional, an extensor response is normal.

Sciatica. Sciatica is pain in the distribution of the sciatic nerve and its branches often produced by a 'slipped disc' (p. 161) pressing on the nerve roots. Fig. 122) shows that if the fifth lumbar nerve is involved, pain will be felt on the front of the leg and on the medial border of the foot. If the roots of the first sacral nerve are compressed, the pain is felt on the lateral side of the foot.

'Drop-foot'. If the common peroneal nerve is damaged, for example where it is vulnerable near the head of the fibula, the muscles for extension of the foot are paralysed. Flexion (plantar flexion) is unopposed and causes the foot to 'drop' so that the toes trail on the ground during walking.

THE AUTONOMIC NERVOUS SYSTEM

The autonomic nervous system is the part of the nervous system which regulates the internal mechanisms of the body by controlling the smooth muscle in the viscera and the secretory activity of the glands. It is essentially motor. **Two neurones** (not one as in the cerebral and spinal nerves) form the path from the central nervous system to the organ; one has its cell body within the central nervous system and its axon, the **preganglionic nerve fibre,** goes to an autonomic ganglion (p. 229), where it ends in association with the second cell body, sometimes called the **ganglion cell,** whose axon, the **postganglionic nerve fibre,** goes to the smooth muscle or gland. Preganglionic nerve fibres are medullated (myelinated), and therefore look white. Postganglionic nerve fibres are non-medullated, or non-myelinated, and therefore look grey. An impulse, on its way from the central nervous system to the organ, must pass through the relay station, that is, must **synapse** in the ganglion. The impulse in the preganglionic fibre liberates **acetylcholine** at the synapse in all autonomic ganglia.

The autonomic nervous system consists of two distinct parts, the sympathetic and the parasympathetic systems, which differ both in structure and in function.

The **sympathetic system** is connected with the central nervous system by means of thoracic and first two lumbar segments of the spinal cord (the **thoraco-lumbar outflow**); it has a segmental system of ganglia, and relatively long postganglionic fibres. Stimulation of the sympathetic system sets the systems of the body in readiness for intense action—fright, flight or fight. **Noradrenaline** is released at the postganglionic nerve endings (except at sweat glands).

The **parasympathetic system** is connected with the central nervous system in the brain stem and in the third and fourth sacral segments of the spinal cord (the **craniosacral outflow**); the ganglia are tiny and widely scattered, often in the walls of the viscera; the postganglionic fibres are very short. Stimulation of the parasympathetic system promotes the vegetative functions of the body, like digestion. **Acetylcholine** is liberated at the postganglionic nerve endings.

Both the sympathetic and parasympathetic systems are under control of the central nervous system which has autonomic centres in the spinal cord, medulla and hypothalamus. In their functions, the sympathetic and parasympathetic systems are not antagonistic so much as complementary.

THE PARASYMPATHETIC SYSTEM

Distribution

The preganglionic fibres of the parasympathetic system leave the central nervous system in the oculomotor, facial, glossopharyngeal and vagus nerves from the brain stem, and in the pelvic splanchnic nerves from the third and fourth sacral segments of the spinal cord (Plate 17).

The fibres in the **oculomotor nerve** travel to the orbit and synapse there in a tiny ganglion, the **ciliary ganglion.** The postganglionic fibres enter the eye and supply the ciliary muscle, which is for accommodation (p. 297), and the sphincter pupillæ muscle, which constricts the pupil in bright light (p. 301).

The fibres in the **facial** and **glossopharyngeal nerves** supply secretomotor fibres to the lacrimal and salivary glands, after synapsing in small ganglia (**sphenopalatine, submandibular** and **otic**) near the glands.

The parasympathetic preganglionic fibres in the **vagus nerve** have a very wide distribution. The cell bodies are in the medulla, some of them forming the vital centres—the **cardiac centre** and the **respiratory centre.** The fibres are carried by branches of the vagus nerve (p. 267) to the heart, the lungs and parts of the gastro-intestinal tract, namely the œsophagus, stomach, the small intestine and the large intestine as far as the junction of the middle and distal thirds of the transverse colon.

The parasympathetic fibres from the **sacral nerves** form the **pelvic splanchnic nerves** which pass to the walls of the bladder and rectum, forming there the pelvic plexus which contains ganglion cells. The postganglionic fibres supply the distal third of the colon, the rectum, the bladder, the erectile tissue in the external genitalia and, in the female, the uterus. (To reach the colon, some of the fibres travel upwards in the hypogastric plexus to reach the inferior mesenteric artery and are then distributed with its branches.)

No parasympathetic fibres reach the body wall or the limbs.

Functions

Stimulation of the parasympathetic system promotes the vegetative functions of the body. The chemical transmission of the impulse to the effector organ (muscle or gland) is by means of **acetylcholine** released at the postganglionic nerve ending.

EYE: The parasympathetic constricts the pupil and accommodates the eye for near vision.

HEART: Stimulation of the vagus slows the heart rate and reduces the force of the contraction.

LUNGS: Stimulation of the vagus causes constriction of the bronchi and bronchioles.

GASTRO-INTESTINAL TRACT: Parasympathetic stimulation increases the secretion of digestive juices rich in enzymes, like saliva, gastric juice, pancreatic juice and intestinal juice. The muscle tone of the gut wall is raised and peristalsis is increased. Smooth muscle sphincters are relaxed. In this way, digestion is promoted. Defæcation may occur; parasympathetic impulses to the sphincter ani internus cause it to relax as the colon and rectum contract.

BLADDER: Stimulation of the parasympathetic nerves to the bladder produces voiding of urine. The smooth muscle sphincter (internal sphincter) relaxes and the bladder wall contracts.

ERECTILE TISSUE: Parasympathetic nerves cause dilatation of the arterioles of the penis and clitoris.

THE SYMPATHETIC SYSTEM

Distribution

The preganglionic cells of the sympathetic system lie in the lateral horn of the twelve thoracic segments and the first two lumbar segments of the spinal cord. Their axons, preganglionic medullated fibres, leave by way of the anterior roots of the spinal nerves of these segments. Soon after the nerve emerges through the intervertebral foramen, these sympathetic fibres are given off as **white rami communicantes** to the sympathetic trunk (Fig. 123).

The **sympathetic trunk** is a chain of sympathetic autonomic ganglia, connected by nerve fibres. It lies close to the vertebral bodies and stretches from the base of the skull to the lower end of the sacrum. Throughout most of the length of the sympathetic trunk, there is about one ganglion for every vertebra, but in the cervical region there are only three cervical sympathetic ganglia; the superior one is very large; the middle and inferior are small (Plate 34).

CONNEXIONS OF THE SYMPATHETIC TRUNK (Plate 17): The sympathetic trunk is connected to the central nervous system by the fourteen white rami communicantes of the twelve thoracic and first two lumbar nerves described above. It is also connected to **every spinal nerve** by means of a **grey ramus communicans,** which is composed of postganglionic non-medullated fibres. Branches, all postganglionic, are given to blood vessels and are distributed with

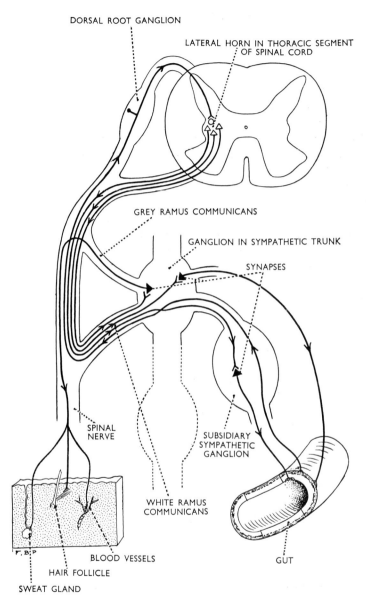

DORSAL ROOT GANGLION

LATERAL HORN IN THORACIC SEGMENT
OF SPINAL CORD

GREY RAMUS COMMUNICANS

GANGLION IN SYMPATHETIC TRUNK

SYNAPSES

SPINAL
NERVE

SUBSIDIARY
SYMPATHETIC
GANGLION

WHITE RAMUS
COMMUNICANS

BLOOD VESSELS

HAIR FOLLICLE

SWEAT GLAND

GUT

Fig. 123. A diagram of the distribution of sympathetic fibres from the lateral horn in the spinal cord. Three such fibres are shown. One relays in the sympathetic chain and the postganglionic fibre joins a spinal nerve to supply blood vessels, sweat glands and hair follicles in the skin. The other two supply viscera, one after synapsing in the sympathetic chain, the other after synapsing in a subsidiary sympathetic ganglion. An afferent fibre from a viscus is also indicated.

them. The external and internal carotid arteries, the subclavian arteries, the renal arteries, the cœliac artery, the superior and inferior mesenteric arteries and the common, external and internal iliac arteries all distribute postganglionic sympathetic fibres in this way.

In addition, the sympathetic trunk gives off **cardiac branches,** one from each of the cervical ganglia, to the heart. From the thoracic ganglia arise branches to the **pulmonary plexus** and three **sphlanchnic nerves,** containing both pre- and postganglionic fibres, which pierce the crura of the diaphragm to reach the front of the abdominal aorta. There they form a dense network of nerve fibres, which contains some ganglion cells, and is called the **cœliac plexus** (solar plexus). From it, postganglionic fibres are distributed with the cœliac artery. Many fibres are continued downwards over the aorta as the aortic plexus which is joined by new branches from the lumbar part of the sympathetic trunk. **Renal** and **mesenteric plexuses** are formed round the renal and mesenteric arteries. At the bifurcation of the aorta, the aortic plexus is continued downwards over the fifth lumbar vertebra and the promontory of the sacrum as the **superior hypogastric plexus** (presacral nerve), which is joined by preganglionic (parasympathetic) contributions from the sacral nerves, and then bifurcates to form the right and left **inferior hypogastric plexuses** (pelvic plexuses). Sympathetic ganglion cells are found in all these plexuses.

By means of all these branches of the sympathetic trunk, postganglionic sympathetic fibres are eventually distributed throughout the body, even though the sympathetic outflow is restricted to the thoraco-lumbar region. The preganglionic fibres synapse, either in the ganglia of the sympathetic chain itself, or with the ganglion cells in the sympathetic plexuses.

The following structures receive a sympathetic nerve supply:

SKIN: The sweat glands and arrector pili muscles of the hair follicles throughout the skin are supplied by the branches of the spinal nerves by way of the grey rami communicantes.

BLOOD VESSELS: The main blood vessels receive a sympathetic supply direct from the sympathetic trunk, from the aortic plexus, and in the limbs mainly from the peripheral nerves. Sympathetic nerves are distributed via the walls of blood vessels to many viscera.

EYE: Sympathetic fibres are carried to the dilator pupillæ muscle by the internal carotid artery and its ophthalmic branches.

HEART: The heart is supplied by the cardiac nerves.

LUNGS: The smooth muscle of the bronchi and bronchioles receives sympathetic fibres from the sympathetic trunk via the pulmonary plexus.

GASTRO-INTESTINAL TRACT: The stomach, small intestine and colon are supplied along the branches of their arteries. The rectum has branches from the inferior hypogastric plexus.

BLADDER: The trigone of the bladder and the internal sphincter are supplied from the inferior hypogastric plexus.

Functions

Stimulation of the sympathetic nervous system prepares the body for fright, flight or fight. The chemical transmission of the impulse to the effector organ (except the sweat glands) is by means of **noradrenaline** released at the post-ganglionic nerve ending. Secretion of noradrenaline and adrenaline by the adrenal medulla (p. 517) has the same effects as stimulation of the sympathetic system. The sympathetic nerve endings supplying the **sweat glands** are unusual in releasing **acetylcholine.**

EYE: Sympathetic fibres supply the dilator pupillæ, causing dilatation of the pupil. This happens in 'fright'.

HEART: Sympathetic stimulation increases the rate and force of the heart beat, to send more blood to active muscles in an emergency.

BLOOD VESSELS: In emergencies, blood vessels to the skin and to splanchnic viscera are constricted, but normal tone of vessels to skeletal muscle is relaxed. This gives skeletal muscle a better blood supply, the better to deal with the emergency in fight or flight.

LUNGS: The smooth muscle in the walls of bronchi and bronchioles is relaxed. This allows more air to enter in emergencies, and to permit better oxygenation of the blood.

GASTRO-INTESTINAL TRACT: The smooth muscle of the walls is inhibited, so that the tone is decreased and peristalsis stops. The sphincters are closed by increased tone. Digestion is therefore in abeyance during the emergency.

BLADDER: The muscle wall relaxes and the internal sphincter contracts. Voiding of urine must wait till the emergency is over.

SKIN: The arrector pili muscles makes the 'hair stand on end'. Sweating is increased.

AFFERENT FIBRES OF THE AUTONOMIC NERVOUS SYSTEM

Accompanying all the motor nerves of the autonomic system are the corresponding sensory nerves, which have the same relationship with the central nervous system as other sensory nerves. The cell body is in the posterior root ganglion, and the axon has its central connexion and its peripheral sensory nerve fibre. These peripheral fibres accompany the preganglionic and post-ganglionic fibres of both the sympathetic and parasympathetic systems to the viscera they innervate, passing through any ganglia without synapsing, of course.

The kinds of sensation transmitted by these visceral afferent fibres are different from those in spinal nerves. The sensations are dull and are badly localized. Distension of the stomach and intestines, and spasm of the muscle walls are painful, but cutting and burning are quite painless. Stretching of the ureter, for example by a urinary calculus, gives rise to severe pain. Heat and cold are appreciated in the oesophagus, but not in other viscera.

The visceral peritoneum is supplied by the sensory nerves of the viscera and has sensations like them. The parietal peritoneum, on the other hand, is supplied by the spinal nerves and has the more accurate sensations associated with them.

Many viscera, with irritated, exhibit the phenomenon of referred pain (p. 242). Pain from the ureter is referred to the groin. From the alimentary tract, parts developed from foregut (stomach, duodenum, see p. 427) refer pain to the epigastric region, parts developed from midgut (small intestine, ascending and transverse colon) refer pain to the umbilicus and parts developed from hindgut (descending colon, rectum and bladder) refer pain to the lower part of the abdominal wall. From the appendix (developed from midgut, p. 429), in the early stages of appendicitis pain is referred to the umbilicus, but later, when the parietal peritoneum is involved, the pain 'moves' to be felt in the abdominal wall over the side of the appendix in the right iliac fossa.

CHAPTER IX

THE SPECIAL SENSES

A **special sense** *is a sense whose receptors are aggregated into a single organ, which is called an organ of special sense.* (This contrasts with senses like those of pain, touch, temperature and the others described on p. 225. Their receptors are scattered over the body surface.)

The special senses are sight, hearing, the perception of movement and position in relation to gravity, olfaction (the sense of smell) and taste.

SIGHT

The sense of sight is the result of the stimulation by light rays of special nerve endings grouped together in the retina which is in the organ of sight, the eyeball. The impulses are carried to the brain by the optic nerve.

Light

Light is a form of energy which comes from the sun. During the day we use the light directly but at night we use light reflected from the moon or we produce artificial light from energy converted from other forms; or we may use the energy stored in combustible materials, such as coal (which gives us gas and is a source of electricity) and paraffin and the wax of candles.

Light is a form of energy that is transmitted at very great speed and is in the form of waves. (The speed of light is 300,000 km/sec or 186,300 miles/sec.) The human eye can detect light only within a certain range of wavelength, i.e. between infra-red light (long wavelength) and ultraviolet light (short wavelength).

THE EYE AND ITS ADNEXA

Development

Early in development the wall of part of the forebrain grows outwards to form a spherical **optic vesicle** which retains its connexion with the brain through the **optic stalk** (Fig. 124). Soon the outer half of the optic vesicle is invaginated so that a two-layered **optic cup** is formed. The optic cup develops into the retina, the inner layer containing the light-sensitive cells. From it are also derived the epithelium and the muscle of the ciliary body and of the iris. The optic stalk becomes the optic nerve, which is, therefore, not a typical nerve, but a tract of the brain. Its nerve fibres have no neurilemmal sheath and cannot regenerate (p. 600).

The pia and arachnoid mater, the nutritive vascular covering of the developing brain, cover the optic cup too. The developing dura mater of the brain is represented in the eyeball by its tough outer coat, the sclera.

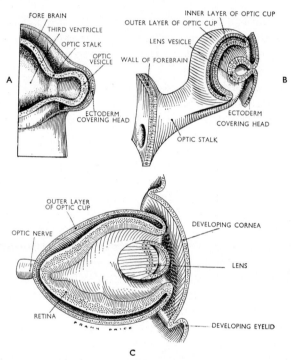

Fig. 124. Three stages in the development of the eye: A, the optic vesicle growing out of the forebrain; B, the optic vesicle has been invaginated to form the optic cup and the covering ectoderm has formed the lens vesicle; C, the inner layer of the optic cup is forming the light-sensitive retina and the lens is separate and further developed.

While the optic cup is developing, part of the skin overlying it grows inwards to form the **lens vesicle** whose cells form the lens. Later the skin of this region becomes the conjunctiva and the cornea (Fig. 124).

The eyeball is situated in the orbit suspended by a connective tissue sling from the side walls. It is protected in front by the upper and lower eyelids which are separated by the **palpebral fissure** and which have developed as specialized folds of skin.

The adnexa of the eye

EYELIDS: Each eyelid contains a **tarsal plate** of fibro-elastic tissue to support it, and part of the sphincter muscle of the eyelids (p. 182) which allows the lids to be closed. Relaxation of this sphincter, aided by a muscle which raises the upper lid, enables the lids to be opened. The outer surface is covered with thin skin and the inner surface is lined by a thin transparent stratified squamous epithelium, the **conjunctiva**. The conjunctiva is reflected from the attachments of the eyelids on to the front of the eyeball. From the margins of the lids grow hairs, the **eyelashes**, and associated with them are small sebaceous glands. In addition, between the tarsal plate and the conjunctiva there lies a row of larger sebaceous **tarsal glands** which open on the margin of the eyelids.

CONJUNCTIVAL SAC: When the eyelids are closed, the interval between the inner surfaces of the eyelids and the front of the eyeball is a closed space lined by conjunctiva. It is called the **conjunctival sac.** The conjunctiva is reflected from the eyelids on to the eyeball at the **upper** and **lower fornices.** The upper fornix is very deep, so deep indeed that the upper eyelid must be turned inside out if a foreign body lodged in it is to be located and removed.

LACRIMAL APPARATUS: When the eyelids are open, the conjunctiva and cornea are exposed to the drying action of the air. If their cells are to survive they must be kept moist and this is achieved by a continuous secretion of tears by the **lacrimal gland** which lies in the upper lateral angle of the orbit. The tears enter the lateral part of the upper fornix and are moved medially over the front of the eyeball by blinking of the eyelids. At the medial end of the palpebral fissure the tears are conveyed to the **lacrimal sac,** which lies in the lacrimal fossa (p. 130). The **nasolacrimal duct** leads from the sac to the front of the lower part of the nose.

If the secretion of the lacrimal gland is excessive, as it is in weeping, or if the nasolacrimal duct is blocked, the tears overflow through the palpebral fissure.

The Eyeball (Fig. 125)

The eyeball is almost spherical and consists of three coats. The innermost coat is the **retina,** derived from the brain. It contains the light-sensitive cells. The middle coat which is vascular to supply the eyeball with blood, is the **choroid coat.** The choroid with the iris and ciliary body constitute the **uveal tract.** (Inflammation of this coat of the eye is thus called uveitis.) The outer coat, which is tough and strong to protect the delicate structures inside, consists of the sclera and the cornea. Inside the eyeball are its contents, the **lens,** the **aqueous humour** and the **vitreous humour.**

MOVEMENTS OF THE EYEBALL: The eyeball is rotated within the orbit by its extrinsic muscles which are inserted into the sclera (p. 184) and Figs. 86 and 87).

THE CONSTITUENTS OF THE EYEBALL:

Sclera

The sclera is made of dense collagenous connective tissue. Its anterior part is

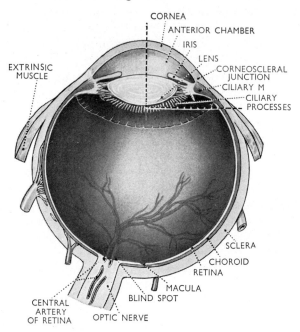

Fig. 125. A horizontal section through the eyeball; the part marked with interrupted lines is enlarged in Fig. 126.

the 'white' of the eye. In the middle of the front of the eyeball, however, the place of the sclera is taken by the transparent cornea.

Cornea

Like the sclera, the cornea is made up of fibrous connective tissue, but it is transparent because of the special nature of the intercellular substance, because of the regular arrangement of the fibres and because of its different water content. The cornea is covered by a layer of stratified squamous epithelium continuous with the conjunctiva. This is very sensitive, to protect the eye. The cornea contains no blood vessels, and maintains its metabolism by exchanges with the aqueous humour in contact with its deep surface, and with the tear fluid on its outer surface. As well as containing oxygen from the air in contact with the eye, tear fluid contains carbon dioxide given off by the corneal cells. Normally this is given off to the air in contact with the eye. If, however, it is trapped by contact lenses it makes the tear fluid acid and this irritates the cornea and the conjunctiva. It is because of this that buffer solutions (see p. 31) are used when contact lenses are fitted.

The cornea can be grafted successfully even to an unrelated recipient because there are no blood cells to stimulate the normal defensive response which casts off foreign cells. Also, the cornea does not need to be vascularized by the host's blood vessels in order to survive (see p. 598).

At the corneoscleral junction a process of scleral tissue, the **scleral spur,** projects inwards. Close to it lies the **venous sinus** of the sclera (canal of Schlemm). The periphery of the iris is attached to the scleral spur, so this region is often called the **iridocorneal angle** (Fig. 126).

Choroid

The choroid is a vascular membrane which lines the posterior two thirds of the sclera. It is dark blue because of the pigment cells it contains. The pigment makes this part of the eyeball opaque and prevents reflection of light inside the eye.

Ciliary Body

The ciliary body is a circle of tissue, joining the iris to the choroid. It projects inwards from its contact with the sclera just behind the corneoscleral junction. A cross section of the ciliary body is triangular, one side of the triangle being in contact with the sclera (Fig. 126).

On the posterior surface of the ciliary body (that is the surface facing towards the vitreous humour, q.v.) nearer the centre of the circle there are radial ridges separated by grooves—these ridges are the **ciliary processes** (Fig. 125). The smoother peripheral part of this surface is the **ciliary ring.** The ciliary processes and the ciliary ring are clothed on the inside by a layer of epithelium derived from the retina. To the ciliary processes is attached the **ciliary zonule** (the suspensory ligament of the lens). The substance of the ciliary body is the **ciliary muscle,** smooth muscle controlled by parasympathetic nerve fibres. It is concerned with accommodation (p. 297).

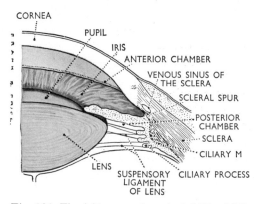

Fig. 126. The iridocorneal angle (cf. Fig. 125).

Iris

The choroid coat continues forwards in front of the ciliary body as the iris. This is a flat ring of tissue which is the coloured part of the eye seen through the cornea. Its posterior surface, which is covered by a layer of pigmented epithelium derived from the retina, rests against the front of the lens. The periphery is attached to the scleral spur and forms the iridocorneal angle with the cornea. The circular opening in the middle of the iris is the **pupil.** The pupil looks black because all the light which enters the eye through it is absorbed.

The iris regulates the amount of light entering the eye through the pupil, by means of the smooth muscle fibres it contains. Some of these, the **sphincter pupillæ,** are arranged round the pupil so that, by contracting, they make it smaller and let less light in. Others, the **dilator pupillæ,** are arranged radially, so that by contracting they make the pupil larger to let more light in. The sphincter pupillæ is supplied by parasympathetic nerves; the dilator pupillæ is supplied by sympathetic nerves.

The colour of the iris is due to the amount and position of the pigment it contains. The pigment always present at the back of the iris, seen through the tissues, looks blue. Any pigment nearer the front of the iris modifies the blue colour; the more there is, the darker and browner the iris.

Retina

The retina is the innermost coat of the eyeball. Its posterior two thirds, the retina proper, is light sensitive. The anterior third forms the pigmented epithelium of the ciliary body and iris.

The retina develops from the invaginated optic vesicle (p. 287) and consists of

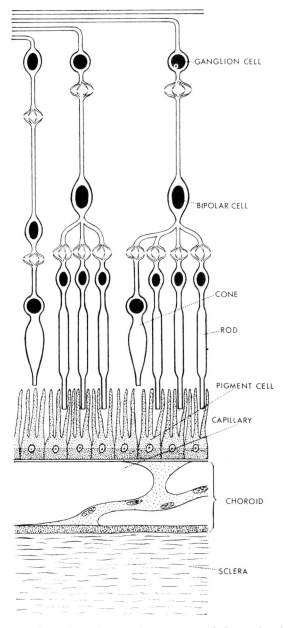

GANGLION CELL

BIPOLAR CELL

CONE

ROD

PIGMENT CELL

CAPILLARY

CHOROID

SCLERA

Fig. 127. A scheme to show the microscopic structure of the retina in relation to the choroid and sclera.

an outer heavily pigmented layer and an inner sensitive layer. This light-sensitive part consists of three layers of cells, the outermost being the layer of rod and cone cells which are the true light receptors. The rods and cones are in contact with the pigmented layer of the retina. Rods are stimulated by dim light and are useful in 'twilight'. They register only black and white images. The cones are stimulated only by fairly bright light, and come into play in the perception of colour and fine detail. From the rods and cones emerge nerve fibres which synapse with the next layer of cells in the retina, the **bipolar cells.** These in turn synapse with the third, innermost, layer of cells in the retina, the **ganglion cells.** The axons of the ganglion cells run over the internal surface of the retina to collect at the **optic disc** near the back of the eyeball where they pierce the choroid and the sclera to form the optic nerve. The optic disc is the 'blind spot' on the retina, because there are no rods and cones in this area. A small area of the retina on the back of the eyeball directly opposite the pupil is modified for especially acute vision. It is the **macula.** Only cones are found here and the other layers are thinned out so that light falls almost directly on them. The blind spot is medial to the macula.

The retina is supplied on its internal surface by the **central artery of the retina** (Fig. 125). This small artery is a branch of the ophthalmic artery. It enters the optic nerve behind the eyeball, and travels in it to reach the retina through the middle of the optic disc, from which its branches radiate. They supply the innermost layers of the retina. The rods and cones, however, are supplied by diffusion from the choroid.

Using an ophthalmoscope, it is possible to inspect the interior of the eyeball through the pupil. The macula, the blind spot and the retinal arteries and veins can be seen.

Detachment of the Retina. This is the reappearance of the gap between the two layers of the optic cup (p. 287) as a result of which the rods and cones which are in the inner layer, become separated from their oxygen supply, which is by diffusion from the choroid.

Lens

The lens is a biconvex disc which bulges more posteriorly than anteriorly. It is transparent and elastic and is composed of **lens fibres,** specialized epithelial cells which have lost their nuclei. The lens is surrounded by the **lens capsule** which is a thick elastic layer of homogeneous intercellular substance. The periphery of the lens capsule is connected to the ciliary processes by the **ciliary zonule** (suspensory ligament of the lens), which is a ring of fibrous intercellular substance. The ciliary zonule holds the lens with its capsule in position, but in addition it exerts a constant pull on the periphery of the lens capsule. This in turn flattens the elastic lens. In effect this means that in the resting eye (that is, when the ciliary muscle is relaxed) the lens is forced by the capsule and the ciliary zonule to assume a flatter shape than is natural to it. In accommodation (p. 297) the ciliary muscle contracts, stimulated by parasympathetic nerve fibres. This makes the circle formed by the ciliary processes (that is the peripheral attachment of the ciliary zonule) smaller, which means that the ciliary zonule is no longer tense and pulling on the lens capsule. The elastic lens, no longer held flat by the capsule, immediately assumes its natural more rounded shape.

Aqueous Humour

The **anterior chamber** of the eye is the space bounded in front by the cornea and behind by the iris. The **posterior chamber** is bounded in front by the iris and behind by the lens, the ciliary zonule and the ciliary body. The two chambers communicate through the pupil. They are filled with a watery fluid called the **aqueous humour** which is probably secreted by the epithelium of the ciliary processes. It circulates through the pupil into the anterior chamber and reaches the iridocorneal angle. There it seeps into spaces (of Fontana) related to the scleral spur and then into the venous sinus of the sclera, which takes it to the veins of the orbit. There is thus a continuous circulation of aqueous humour.

The functions of the aqueous humour are (a) to nourish the avascular cornea and lens and (b) to regulate the intra-ocular pressure by the balance of its secretion and absorption. The intra-ocular pressure must be carefully regulated because of the tough inelastic sclera. Even small increases in pressure have serious effects through compressing the blood vessels inside the eyeball. This compression in turn leads to an inadequate supply reaching the retina with resulting damage to its cells and possibly blindness.

Vitreous Humour

The vitreous humour is a transparent jelly-like mass which fills the eyeball behind the lens and ciliary processes.

Refractive Media

The complicated structure of the eyeball is the mechanism for allowing the light reflected from objects we look at to fall exactly on to the light-sensitive rods and cones.

Light from distant objects, said to be at infinity, travels in parallel lines.

Before they can fall on the retina such straight rays must be bent (Fig. 128, A) or **refracted**. Refraction occurs as light passes from one medium into another, for example from air into water or vice versa. A straight stick partly immersed in water looks bent at the surface of the water. In the same way light entering the eye is refracted at the anterior surface of the cornea, as it passes from air into the substance of the cornea.

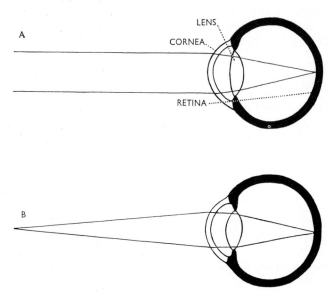

Fig. 128. To show how light is focused on the retina. A, the resting eye: parallel rays of light from infinity are brought to a focus on the retina by the refractive media; B, the eye in accommodation: diverging rays from a near object are also brought into focus on the retina. The lens is now more convex and so has more converging power.

The substances in the eye through which light must pass before it reaches the retina are called the **refractive media.** They are the cornea, the aqueous humour, the lens and the vitreous humour. Of these the cornea is by far the most important. The lens plays an important part too, because by changing shape, in accommodation, it can alter the extent of the bending. A normal eye, in which both far and near objects can be focused on the retina, is said to be **emmetropic.**

Fig. 128A shows how an object at infinity is brought into focus on the retina. The light is refracted at the cornea and focused by the relatively flat lens of the resting eye (p. 295).

Accommodation

Fig. 128, B shows what happens when a near object is looked at. The light rays are no longer parallel, but diverge as they approach the eye. Consequently they must be bent more than rays from infinity in order to be focused on the retina. This is brought about by **accommodation** which occurs reflexly. The ciliary muscles contract and slacken the ciliary zonule so that the lens bulges (p. 295). The more convex lens now focuses the light on the retina. Accommodation of the lens is associated with **reflex constriction of the pupil** to provide greater depth of focus and with **convergence** of the eyes. (Convergence consists of rotating the eyes inwards so that the pupils face the object being looked at.)

ERRORS OF REFRACTION: These are present when the object cannot be focused on the retina.

In **hypermetropia** (long sight) the eyeball is too short so that light from infinity is focused behind the retina (Fig. 129, B). Continuous tiring efforts at accommodation bring distant objects into focus, but near objects cannot be seen clearly. Hypermetropia is corrected (Fig. 129, C) by putting a biconvex lens in front of the eye.

In **myopia** (short sight—Fig 129, D) the eyeball is too long so that parallel light rays from infinity are focused in front of the retina and distant objects cannot be seen clearly. This can be corrected by putting a biconcave lens in front of the eye (Fig. 129, E).

Presbyopia is the longsightedness which develops in normal eyes about the age of forty-five. The lens loses its elasticity, so that during accommodation it is no longer able to spring into the necessary rounded shape. This is corrected by a convex lens for close work like reading.

Astigmatism is the inability to focus vertical and horizontal lines at the same time. It is usually due to unequal curvatures of the cornea in different planes. If the lens is focused correctly for the light coming through one plane it is wrong for that from other planes. Astigmatism is corrected by a lens which compensates for the differences in the curvatures of the cornea.

THE PHYSIOLOGY OF VISION

When light reaches the retina it passes through the internal layers (the axons of the ganglion cells, the ganglion cells themselves, and the bipolar cells (Fig. 127) before it reaches and stimulates the rods and cones. These light-sensitive cells differ, rods functioning in dim light, cones in bright light.

Cones

The **cones** are stimulated only by bright light and are used in the perception of colour and of fine detail. The **macula,** directly opposite the pupil, is composed of cones alone and is the part of the retina brought into use when the eye looks directly at an object.

Colour Vision. The perception of colour is a property of the **cones** which are sensitive to three different kinds of colour, namely red, yellow-green, and blue-violet. All the colours of the spectrum can be obtained by fusing different proportions of these, so that all colours can be perceived.

Colour blindness is due to an inherited defect in the cones. It is usually partial and most often affects the ability to distinguish between red and green. About eight in every hundred males are affected, but only one in two hundred females (see p. 59 for the explanation of this sex-linkage).

Rods

'Night Vision'. The **rods** respond to minimal light stimulation and are used in dim light for 'night vision'. They contain a pigment **visual purple** which is bleached by light. This is part of the process by which dim light stimulates the rods. Visual purple is formed from vitamin A; one of the results of vitamin A deficiency is lack of visual purple and resulting 'night blindness'.

DARK ADAPTATION: If a person passes from a brightly lit room into the dark, vision is at first poor, but it improves quite quickly during the first few minutes and more slowly over as long as an hour. In the absence of strong light the amount of visual purple in the rods increases during this process of dark adaptation so that they become very much more sensitive.

Visual Pathway

The optic nerve, optic chiasma, optic tract, lateral geniculate body, geniculo-calcarine tract and visual cortex constitute the visual pathway.

When the rods or cones of the retina are stimulated, the nervous impulses are relayed to the bipolar cells and then to the ganglion cells whose axons form the **optic nerve,** which passes from the eyeball to the **optic chiasma** (p. 264).

In the optic chiasma the nerve fibres from the medial half of each retina cross to the opposite side to join with the fibres from the lateral half of the

Fig. 129. Errors of refraction. A, a normal (emmetropic) resting eye in which parallel rays are brought to a focus on the retina; B, a hypermetropic eye; the eyeball is too short and the rays are focused behind the retina; C, hypermetropia corrected by a convex (converging), lens; D, a myopic eye; the eyeball is too long and the rays are focused in front of the retina; E, myopia corrected by a concave (diverging) lens.

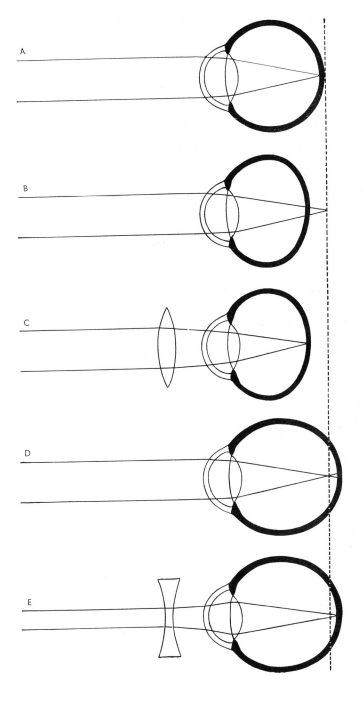

retina of that side, forming in this way the **optic tract.** This passes to a relay station called the **lateral geniculate body** just below the thalamus. From there the **geniculo-calcarine tract** passes to the **visual cortex** on the occipital lobe (p. 253). Impulses are also relayed from the lateral geniculate body to the **superior colliculus** in the roof plate of the midbrain and this arc plays an important part in the visual reflexes.

The way in which nerve impulses from the retina reach the brain is illustrated in Plate 18.

If a person looks at an object placed to his left, the image falls on the nasal (medial) half of the left retina and on the temporal (lateral) half of the right retina. The impulses from the nasal half of the left retina cross in the optic chiasma to join those from the temporal half of the right retina in the right optic tract and are transmitted to the visual cortex of the right occipital lobe. Destruction of the visual cortex of the right occipital lobe, therefore, would result in blindness involving the temporal half of the right retina and the nasal half of the left retina, thus affecting the temporal half of the field of vision of the left eye and the nasal half of the field of vision of the right eye (Plate 18).

It can be seen too that if the nerve fibres which cross in the optic chiasma are damaged (as they may be by pressure from a hypophyseal tumour) the nasal parts of both retinæ will fail to transmit impulses, so that blindness will occur in both temporal fields of vision.

The lens refracts the light in such a way that the image which falls on the retina is inverted. This inverted image is conveyed by nerve impulses to the visual cortex, which as a result of experience, reverses it so that we see things the right way up.

Binocular Vision

In binocular vision two eyes observe a single object. Normally the two eyes are rotated reflexly by the contraction of the appropriate extrinsic muscles (Figs. 85, 86, 87) so that both pupils point at the object. This is **convergence.** When it is achieved correctly the image falls on 'corresponding points' on the two retinæ. The image which falls on one retina is not exactly the same as the image which falls on the other. Both images are conveyed to the visual cortex which 'fuses' them so that only one object is seen. The fusing of the two different images produces a visual sensation which has depth and solidity. In other words, binocular vision is **stereoscopic.** If one eye alone is used, only one image reaches the cortex. Then objects seem flat and relative distances from the eye cannot be judged well.

Sometimes the movement of one eye is defective because of weakness of one or more of the extrinsic muscles (Fig. 88). The eye cannot then be made to converge correctly with the other in looking at an object. The image falls on points of the two retinæ which do not correspond. The visual cortex cannot fuse the images and two objects are seen where there really is only one. This is **diplopia.** In subjects who suffer from a squint or **strabismus,** the diplopia results in one of the images being suppressed in the cortex and one eye may become blind through 'lack of use'. Hence the importance of treating squints from early childhood.

Pupillary Reflexes

PUPILLARY LIGHT REFLEX: Increase in the intensity of light falling on the retina reflexly stimulates the parasympathetic fibres of the oculomotor nerve to cause the sphincter pupillæ to contract. This makes the pupil smaller so that less light can enter, and so protects the sensitive retina from the harmful effects of too much light.

CONSENSUAL LIGHT REFLEX: A light shone into one eye causes its pupil to contract as described above, but it also causes the pupil of the other eye to contract even though no light is allowed to enter it.

ACCOMMODATION REFLEX: When a near object is looked at, the pupil is constricted reflexly. This ensures that only the central, most effective part of the lens is used in close viewing and also provides a greater **depth of focus.** This phenomenon is made use of in photography, for, by reducing the aperture of the camera, it is possible to bring into focus on the plate or film objects which are at different distances from it. The pupillary accommodation reflex is associated with accommodation of the lens (p. 297) and convergence of the eyes (p. 300).

HEARING

The **ear** is the organ of hearing. It has three parts:

PARTS OF THE EAR

1. The **external ear** is the projecting flap or auricle and the short tunnel, called the external auditory meatus, which we can examine on the side of the head. It is closed at its inner end by the ear drum which separates it from the middle ear.
2. The **middle ear** is in the lateral part of the temporal bone and is a space, which is really an elongated extension from the pharynx, with which it communicates through the pharyngo-tympanic tube.

3. The **internal ear** is a delicate receptor organ which is embedded, for protection, in the petrous part of the temporal bone. Besides being the receptor organ for hearing, the internal ear is also the receptor organ for the perception of movement and position in relation to gravity.

OUTLINE OF DEVELOPMENT OF THE EAR

In lower vertebrates, for example in fish, the forerunner of the internal ear is concerned only with balancing mechanisms. In higher vertebrates the perception of sound is added to this, so that in Man we find a single organ concerned both with hearing, and with the perception of movement and position in relation to gravity. These functions are carried out by the internal ear. The external ear and the middle ear are extra structures developed to transmit the vibrations of sound travelling through air to the sensory internal ear.

Early in the development of the embryo a special area of the ectoderm on the side of the head sinks under the surface and forms a sac, the **otocyst.** From this the membranous labyrinth is formed. The bony labyrinth develops when the tissue round the membranous labyrinth ossifies to form the very hard, protecting petrous temporal bone.

The external ear and the middle ear are formed from the cranial end of the pharyngeal wall. Early in development the wall of the pharynx is made up of a series of six pharyngeal arches each with a cartilaginous skeleton, muscles, nerves and blood vessels. Between the arches are grooves lined with ectoderm on the outside of the pharynx, and pouches lined with endoderm on the inside. The ectoderm of a groove comes very close to the endoderm of the corresponding pouch. The wall of the pharynx at this stage resembles the series of gill clefts in fish, though there are no actual openings. The first pouch grows long and its end comes to lie lateral to the developing internal ear. This first pouch forms the cavity of the middle ear and of the pharyngotympanic tube. The corresponding first ectodermal groove forms the canal of the external ear. The apposition of the endoderm of the pouch to the ectoderm of the groove results in the formation of the ear drum. Parts of the cartilage of the first and second pharyngeal arches develop into the ossicles of the middle ear.

The External Ear

The external ear consists of two parts, the auricle and the external auditory meatus.

The projecting part of the external ear is the **auricle** or **pinna** which is supported by a moulded plate of hyaline cartilage covered on both sides by skin. The lowest part, the **lobe** is soft and contains no cartilage. It has a very rich capillary plexus and bleeds freely if it is cut or pricked. This makes it a convenient place from which to take small samples of blood.

The **external auditory meatus** is the S-shaped canal (Fig. 130) which leads towards the middle ear. It is two and a half centimetres long in the adult. In the outer third the wall is of cartilage, the rest of the canal being bony. The whole meatus points medially, but in addition, as its course is traced inwards, the direction in the outermost part is upwards and forwards, in the middle it is slightly backwards, and in the inner part it is forwards and downwards. In

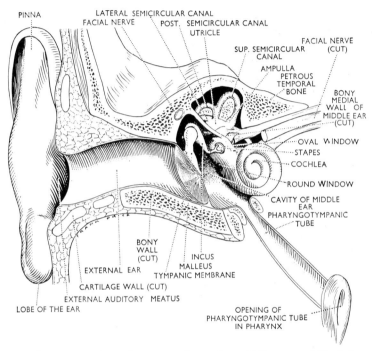

Fig. 130. A diagram to show the external ear, the middle ear and the internal ear.

order, therefore, to look along the canal to examine the tympanic membrane which closes its inner end, the canal must first be straightened as much as possible by pulling the cartilaginous part, which is fixed to the auricle, upwards and backwards.

In a young child the bony part of the canal has not yet developed, so the meatus is much shorter. The tympanic membrane is nearer the surface and is more easily seen. It is also more easily damaged by objects placed in the meatus. In a baby the ear drum is quite near the surface and this should be remembered when cleaning this region.

The external auditory meatus is lined with skin which, especially in men, carries hairs and sebaceous glands. The skin also contains specialized sweat glands, **ceruminous glands** which secrete the characteristic brownish wax. The hairs and the wax help to trap foreign particles. Sometimes an excess of wax blocks the canal and causes deafness.

THE EAR DRUM (TYMPANIC MEMBRANE): This is a thin circular membrane which is attached to the bony walls of the inner end of the external auditory meatus, completely separating it from the middle ear. It is made of fibrous connective tissue covered on its outer surface by skin and on its inner surface by the mucous membrane of the middle ear. The handle of the malleus (p. 305) is attached to it. The ear drum can be inspected with the help of an auriscope which directs a beam of light along the external auditory meatus. In health the ear drum is pearly grey in colour and the handle of the malleus can be seen stretching upwards and forwards from the centre.

The ear drum vibrates in response to the sound waves which reach it through the external ear.

The Middle Ear (Tympanic Cavity)

The middle ear is a narrow cavity in the lateral part of the temporal bone. It is the shape of a match box placed on its side and is about 15 mm from front to back, 15 mm from roof to floor and only 2 to 4 mm from lateral wall to medial wall.

The lateral wall of the middle ear is formed by the ear drum. The medial wall is formed by the lateral part of the petrous temporal bone which contains the internal ear. If a skull is examined, the ring-shaped groove which gave attachment to the ear drum can be seen at the bottom of the bony external auditory meatus. The ear drum is no longer present so that we can look into the middle ear and see its medial wall. The anterior part of this medial wall bulges (the **promontory**) and shows the position of the first turn of the cochlea. Above and behind this is an oval opening, the **vestibular window** (oval window), which leads into the internal ear. Below the oval window is another small opening, the **cochlear window** (round window).

From the anterior end of the cavity of the middle ear, the **pharyngotympanic tube** leads forwards and medially to the nasopharynx where it opens (Plate 34). In the upper part of the posterior wall of the cavity an opening leads into a space in the bone called the **tympanic antrum**. This in turn leads backwards into a network of small cavities, the **mastoid air cells**, which occupy the mastoid process of the petrous temporal bone (p. 125).

The mastoid air cells, the tympanic antrum, the middle ear and the pharyngotympanic tube are all lined by mucous membrane which is continuous with the mucous membrane of the nasopharynx. Under normal conditions, these cavities all contain air at atmospheric pressure. This means that the air pressure on both sides of the ear drum is the same and so the ear drum can vibrate easily in response to sound waves. If the atmospheric pressure is higher or lower than that in the middle ear, the ear drum bulges inwards or outwards causing severe pain and sometimes damage. Such differences of pressure develop in the ears of aeroplane passengers as the plane rapidly climbs or descends. The movements of swallowing help to open the pharyngo-tympanic tube and allow air to enter or leave the middle ear, thus equalizing the pressures inside and out. Air passengers are, therefore, given barley sugar or boiled sweets to suck during take-off and landing. Suckling infants should be given a feed on these occasions.

If the pharyngotympanic tube is blocked by swelling of its mucous membrane during a cold in the head, or by enlarged adenoids, air has no access. The air already in the middle ear is absorbed and is often replaced by exudate. The ear drum cannot vibrate and deafness results, until the tube is open again.

OSSICLES OF THE MIDDLE EAR: A chain of three tiny bones, the ossicles, stretches across the middle ear from the lateral wall to the medial wall. They are the **malleus** (hammer), the **incus** (anvil) and the **stapes** (stirrup), so named because of their shapes. The handle of the malleus is attached to the tympanic membrane, and its head articulates with the incus. The incus in turn articulates with the stapes. The footplate of the stapes fits into the oval window (Fig. 130).

When the ear drum vibrates the movements are transmitted from one bone to the next in such a way that the footplate of the stapes rocks in and out in the oval window. The vibrations are transmitted in this way to the internal ear.

The ossicles are covered by the mucous membrane which lines the middle ear.

The Internal Ear

The internal ear (Fig. 130) consists of a very delicate system of tubes called the **membranous labyrinth** because of its membranous walls. The membranous labyrinth is filled with a clear watery fluid called **endolymph**. The membranous labyrinth lies inside the petrous temporal bone in a space which has a complex shape, similar to that of the membranous labyrinth but wider. The wall of this space forms the **bony labyrinth.** The space between the outside of the membranous labyrinth and the wall of the bony labyrinth is filled with a fluid called **perilymph,** which is similar to the cerebrospinal fluid.

The membranous labyrinth consists of two connected parts: the **duct of the cochlea** which is the receptor organ for hearing, and the vestibular part, consisting of **three semicircular canals,** the **utricle** and the **saccule.** These constitute the receptor organ for the perception of movement and position in relation to gravity.

THE COCHLEA: This is the part of the bony labyrinth in which the cochlear duct lies.

The cochlea is a spiral tunnel which makes two and a half turns. It is like a snail's shell, laid on its side (Fig. 130). For ease of description, however, the cochlea can be imagined resting on its base (Fig. 131). The conical pillar in the centre, round which the tunnel spirals, is the **modiolus.** The tunnel itself is divided lengthwise into three separate tunnels by the two membranes forming the walls of the cochlear duct and stretching from the modiolus to the outer wall, the **basilar membrane** and the **vestibular membrane.** The

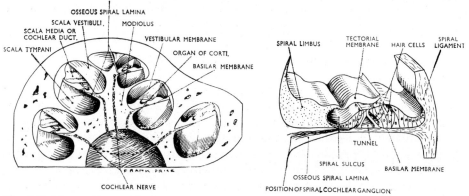

Fig. 131. The cochlea, with the cochlear duct.   Fig. 132. The spiral organ (of Corti).

middle tunnel, which is the cavity within the **cochlear duct,** has the basilar membrane in its floor and the vestibular membrane in its roof. It is part of the membranous labyrinth and is filled with endolymph. The other tunnels are the **scala vestibuli,** above the vestibular membrane, and the **scala tympani,** below the basilar membrane. They join at the top of the modiolus, and, being parts of the bony labyrinth, are filled with perilymph. The lower end of the scala vestibuli is close to the oval window in which lies the footplate of the stapes. The lower end of the scala tympani comes to the round window which is closed by a membrane.

Spiral Organ

In the cochlear duct, on the basilar membrane close to the modiolus, is a group of very specialized receptor cells which form the **spiral organ** (organ of Corti). Their central processes make contact with the sensory ganglion cells which lie in the modiolus and are called the **spiral ganglion.** Their axons unite to form the cochlear division of vestibulocochlear (auditory) nerve (p. 266).

The movements of the footplate of the stapes in the oval window (p. 305) transmit the vibrations to the perilymph in the scala vestibuli. These vibrations travel up the scala vestibuli and down the scala tympani, and are finally expended by causing the membrane in the round window to vibrate. As they pass up the scala vestibuli the vibrations are transmitted through the vestibular membrane to the endolymph in the cochlear duct and so move the basilar membrane. These movements stimulate the spiral organ. Different parts of the basilar membrane respond to vibrations of different frequencies and stimulate the corresponding part of the spiral organ. High pitched sounds are detected by the lower end of the spiral organ and low pitched sounds by the upper end. From the spiral organ nervous impulses are transmitted by the cochlear nerve to the junction of the medulla with the pons, and from there, after several synapses, to the auditory area of the cerebral cortex in the upper part of the temporal lobe (Plate 19) of the opposite side of the brain.

Some of the fibres of the cochlear nerve are connected with reflex centres which cause the head and eyes to be turned towards the origin of a sound.

Summary of the Mechanism of Hearing

Sound travels through air as a series of pressure waves. The more frequent the waves the higher the pitch of the sound. Sounds of low pitch have low frequencies which, if they are very low, can sometimes be felt as vibrations as well as being heard. The loudness of a sound depends on the size of the waves, that is on their amplitude.

In hearing, the sound waves are collected by the external ear and directed towards the ear drum which they cause to vibrate at a corresponding frequency and amplitude. These particular vibrations are transmitted by the ossicles to the perilymph in the scala vestibuli. This makes the appropriate part of the basilar membrane vibrate and stimulate the receptor cells of that part of the spiral organ. These cells send out corresponding nervous impulses which are carried to the brain by the cochlear division of the auditory nerve.

Deafness. Deafness can result from interference with any part of this complicated mechanism, as follows.

1. The sound waves may never reach the ear drum if the external meatus is blocked with wax.

2. The ear drum itself may have been perforated by injury or by infection of the middle ear cavity, and will, therefore, fail to vibrate properly. It may be prevented from vibrating because the air pressure in the middle ear is other than atmospheric (p. 305).

3. The ossicles may fail to transmit the vibrations effectively to the peri-lymph. One cause of this is otosclerosis, a condition in which the footplate of the stapes is fixed firmly in the oval window by fibrosis or even by ossification.

4. In nerve deafness the spiral organ is not able to respond to the vibrations of the basilar membrane.

SEMICIRCULAR DUCTS, UTRICLE AND SACCULE

This part of the membranous labyrinth is a very complicated shape, hence the name labyrinth.

The larger central part is the bag-like **utricle.** This is connected by a narrow channel to the smaller **saccule** which in turn is connected to the duct of the cochlea (the utricle and saccule lie together in the widest part of the bony laby-rinth, the **vestibule**). The **three semicircular ducts** are tubes, with openings at both ends into the utricle. The three ducts are arranged in planes at right angles to one another; the anterior (superior) semicircular duct is vertical in the sagittal plane (roughly), the posterior semicircular duct is vertical in the coronal plane (roughly) and the lateral semicircular duct is horizontal.

Each semicircular duct has a dilation, or **ampulla,** at one end. Some of the cells in the wall of each ampulla are special receptor cells.

The utricle and saccule too have each a small area of special receptor cells, called a **macula.** On the surface of each macula lies a gelatinous membrane, the **otolithic membrane,** which contains fine solid granules of calcium carbonate called **otoliths.**

The utricle, saccule and semicircular ducts are all filled with endolymph.

The Bony Labyrinth

The utricle and saccule lie in the widest part of the bony labyrinth, the **vestibule.** The oval window is in the wall of the vestibule. The semicircular ducts are contained in the corresponding **semicircular canals** of the bony labyrinth. The vestibule and semicircular canals contain perilymph.

FUNCTION OF THE UTRICLE AND SACCULE: When the head is upright the macula of the utricle is horizontal and the macula of the saccule is vertical. Tilting the head backwards and forwards stimulates the macula of the utricle. Side to side tilting of the head stimulates the macula of the saccule. In this way the position of the head in relation to gravity is recorded and transmitted to the brain by the vestibular nerve.

FUNCTION OF THE SEMICIRCULAR DUCTS: During movements of the head the endolymph in the semicircular ducts is set in motion less quickly than the head moves. The lagging of the endolymph stimulates the receptor cells in the ampullæ which, therefore, transmit impulses to the brain along the vestibular nerve. Since the semicircular canals are set in different planes, different movements stimulate different ampullæ. In this way the semicircular canals sense the movements of the head.

Prolonged or intense stimulation of the vestibular nerve gives rise to the unpleasant sensations of dizziness and nausea. This is how sea-sickness is caused. It is a point of practical importance, that the receptor organs of the vestibular apparatus respond least to the stimulation caused by the motion of a ship when the subject is lying down. Hence persons suffering from 'sea-sickness' obtain relief by lying down.

It is important to realize that only a very small part of the information about the position and movements of the head reaches consciousness. Most of the impulses from the utricle, saccule and semicircular canals go to reflex centres in the brain stem and cerebellum, as the afferent parts of important reflex arcs concerned with balance.

OLFACTION AND TASTE

OLFACTION OR THE SENSE OF SMELL

The mucous membrane in the highest part of the roof of the nasal cavity round the cribiform plate (p. 127) is called the **olfactory mucous membrane** because it contains sensory cells specialized to detect odours. These cells have fine hairs which project from the surface. Some of the air inspired through the nose is deflected in eddies by the conchæ (p. 129) to the vicinity of these receptor cells. Any odours in this air stimulate them. The axons of the sensory cells pass in groups through the cribriform plate as the **olfactory nerve,** and end in the **olfactory bulb** (Fig. 111) where they synapse. From the olfactory bulb fibres pass back in the **olfactory tract** to the centres for smell on the inferior surface of the cerebral cortex (Plate 19). Smell plays a large part in the appreciation of what we usually call taste. However, the sense of smell is rudimentary in Man, and is much better developed in many animals.

TASTE

The special sensory receptor cells for the sense of taste are found in the middle of the little barrel-shaped groups of cells called **taste buds.** Most of the taste buds are situated in the epithelium of the tongue, but some are found in the palate and on the epiglottis. The taste buds are buried in the stratified squamous epithelium of these regions, and, in the tongue, they are especially numerous on the fungiform and circumvallate papillæ (p. 432).

From the taste buds afferent fibres pass by two main routes to the medulla oblongata. From the anterior two thirds of the tongue they travel first in the **lingual nerve** and then by means of the **chorda tympani** to the **facial nerve.** From the posterior third of the tongue they travel in the **glossopharyngeal nerve.**

Physiology of Taste

To be tasted, substances must be in solution. The saliva ensures this. The fluid seeps into the taste buds where it stimulates the sensory cells. Only four kinds of taste can be distinguished, namely sweet, sour, salt and bitter. Other flavours are detected by the olfactory mucous membrane. This is why, when the nose is obstructed by a 'cold', the sense of taste is largely lost.

The taste and smell of food play a part in reflexly causing the secretion of saliva (watering of the mouth), gastric juice, pancreatic juice and intestinal juice.

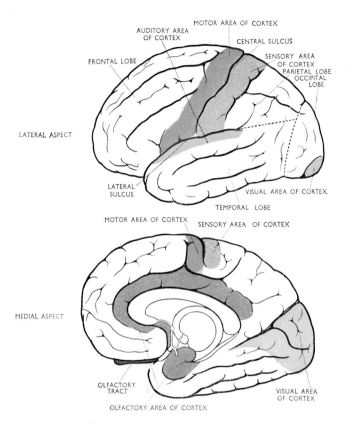

MOTOR AREA OF CORTEX

AUDITORY AREA
OF CORTEX

CENTRAL SULCUS

FRONTAL LOBE

SENSORY AREA
OF CORTEX
PARIETAL LOBE
OCCIPITAL
LOBE

LATERAL ASPECT

LATERAL
SULCUS

VISUAL AREA OF CORTEX

TEMPORAL LOBE

MOTOR AREA OF CORTEX

SENSORY AREA OF CORTEX

MEDIAL ASPECT

OLFACTORY
TRACT

VISUAL AREA
OF CORTEX

OLFACTORY AREA OF CORTEX

Plate 19. Drawings to show the main functional areas of the cerebral cortex. The purple areas labelled here 'olfactory area of cortex' form part of the limbic system (p. 256).

[facing page 310

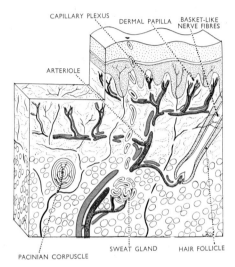

CAPILLARY PLEXUS　　DERMAL PAPILLA　　BASKET-LIKE
NERVE FIBRES

ARTERIOLE

PACINIAN CORPUSCLE　　SWEAT GLAND　　HAIR FOLLICLE

Plate 20. The microscopic structure of the skin. Pacinian corpuscles are now called
lamellated corpuscles.

[facing page 311

CHAPTER X

THE INTEGUMENTARY SYSTEM

THE skin is a very important organ; by means of it the body is brought into contact with the environment; its structure fits it for its main functions of protection, sensation and regulation of body temperature. Another important function, the production of vitamin D, is described on p. 567.

STRUCTURE OF THE SKIN

The skin consists of two parts, the **epidermis** which is the superficial epithelial layer derived from ectoderm, and the **dermis,** the deeper connective tissue layer derived from mesoderm.

EPIDERMIS

The epidermis (Plate 20) is a keratinized stratified squamous epithelium (p. 103). It consists of several layers (Fig. 133), the germinal layer, the prickle cell layer, the granular layer, the clear layer and the horny layer. The deepest layer called the **germinal layer** (Malpighian layer) consists of columnar cells, which are constantly dividing to produce the cells of the more superficial layers. The germinal cells contain granules of the dark brown pigment **melanin** which protects these cells and the underlying tissues from the ultraviolet light of the sun. Large amounts of melanin are found in the dark-skinned races and in white-skinned people melanin appears in response to exposure to sunlight—'tanning'. In the **prickle cell layer** the cells are connected closely by processes of cytoplasm. The cells of the **granular layer** contain granules which will become the horny material **keratin.** These cells are too far from the blood vessels of the dermis and are flattened and dying. In the **clear layer** this process has gone further; the cells are dead and their outline lost. The horny layer is quite dead and consists of layers of keratin which is tough, to protect the underlying layers, and waterproof, to prevent water from being lost from the skin as well as from entering. The keratin layer and the close packing of the cells of the other layers of the epidermis prevent entry into the tissues of foreign particles

311

and bacteria. The superficial layers are constantly being worn away and are replaced by cells pushed up from the germinal layer. The rapid regeneration of cells of the germinal layer allows the epidermis to heal quickly if it is damaged.

DERMIS

The dermis (Fig. 133) is composed of connective tissue. The surface is not flat but raised into **papillæ** with which the epidermis interlocks. Loose networks of **collagen fibres** are found in the papillæ, but, deeper in the dermis, the collagen forms a denser mesh which strengthens the skin. There are also many **elastic fibres** throughout the dermis; the elastic nature of the skin can easily be demonstrated by lifting the skin away from the back of the hand: as soon as it is released, it resumes the previous outline and disposition. If the skin is cut, retraction of the elastic fibres causes the wound to gape. The papillæ contain a rich network of **blood capillaries** and **nerve endings** (Plate 20). The blood capillaries are important for temperature regulation, and the nerve endings provide information, often protective, about the surroundings.

The deeper part of the dermis contains many **arterioles** by means of which the flow of blood through the capillary beds may be regulated. The dermis also contains networks of **lymphatic capillaries** and vessels.

SUBCUTANEOUS FAT

The dermis is separated from the underlying structures, e.g. muscles and bones, by a layer of loose areolar tissue (p. 105) called superficial fascia, in the interstices of which a varying amount of adipose tissue (p. 105) is found (Fig. 133).

In men, this subcutaneous fat is fairly evenly distributed over the whole body, but in women it tends to be collected in the region of the limb girdles and upper portions of the limbs as well as in the breasts. Also, women tend to have a relatively larger amount of subcutaneous fat. This fact is linked with a woman's greater need for reserves of food and energy, a need determined by her reproductive functions.

Subcutaneous fat acts as an insulating layer between the skin, through which heat is lost from the body (p. 318), and underlying structures, such as muscles, which produce the body's heat (p. 182). It also provides 'padding' which rounds off the outlines of the body and has a protective mechanical or 'cushioning' effect.

APPENDAGES OF THE SKIN

Specialized structures derived from the epidermis are known as skin appendages. They are hair follicles, sebaceous glands, sweat glands and nails. The mammary glands (p. 540) are also derived from the skin.

HAIR FOLLICLES (Fig. 133)

At a hair follicle the epidermis dips at an angle deeply into the dermis to form a narrow pit. The bottom of the pit is evaginated by a **connective tissue**

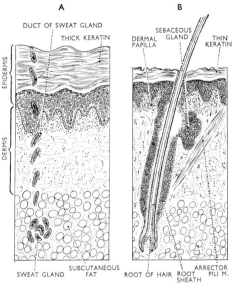

Fig. 133. A, thick skin showing a sweat gland; B, thin skin showing a hair follicle.

papilla which contains blood vessels and a nerve ending. The cells of the germinal layer over the papilla, the **germinal matrix** of the hair, multiply and the cells, as they are pushed further and further away, die and form the hair which is composed of keratin. The walls of the pit are the **root sheath** of the hair. To each hair follicle is attached a small **arrector pili** muscle (Fig. 133) made up of smooth muscle fibres under control of the sympathetic nervous system. When it contracts, the hair not only stands up straight but the muscle also pulls the whole follicle towards the surface and depresses the portion of skin to which it is attached with resulting dimpling. This gives the appearance of 'goose flesh'.

Development of Hair

The first hair of human fetuses begins to appear early in the third month of pregnancy, first in the eyebrows and on the upper lip and chin. At the end of the third month widely scattered fine hairs called **lanugo** appear. These tend to be shed before full term, so that the presence of much lanugo hair is a sign of prematurity. The lanugo is replaced by coarser hair.

At puberty, under the influence of sex hormones the pattern of hair growth characteristic for each sex becomes established (p. 11 and p. 530).

Hair Growth

Hair grows about 1·5 mm a week and faster in summer than in winter. There is no evidence that repeated cutting or shaving makes hair grow coarser or faster. Baldness appears to be determined by genetic factors, i.e. the tendency to baldness is inherited, but sex hormones also play a part. This is illustrated by the fact that women do not go bald, unless their hormonal balance is upset by the presence of masculinizing hormones in their blood stream.

Functions of Hair

Protection is obviously afforded by a layer of hair. Moreover, the slightest touch to a hair stimulates the nerve in its papilla and may give warning of danger. In animals like the cat the hair, when it stands on end, makes the creature look larger and fiercer to its enemies.

Hair can also **prevent heat loss**. This is not important in Man, but in animals the hair, especially when it stands up, traps a layer of still air next to the skin. Air conducts heat badly and so this layer is a good insulator, preventing loss of heat.

SEBACEOUS GLANDS

Near the neck of every hair follicle a sebaceous gland develops from the epithelium (Fig. 133). Sebaceous glands are holocrine (p. 104) and produce an oily secretion, **sebum,** which is discharged into the follicle when the hair stands up. Sebum lubricates the hair and the skin which it protects from drying and cracking. It may also help to kill bacteria. Large sebaceous glands are found in the absence of hair in some places, for example, on the nose.

SWEAT GLANDS

Sweat glands, derived from the epidermis, are coiled tubes which lie deep in the dermis (Plate 20). Each has a coiled duct which passes through the middle of a dermal papilla and through the epidermis to the surface. Under stimulation by sympathetic nerves (which liberate acetylcholine in this case (see p. 285)) the sweat glands secrete a watery fluid which contains sodium chloride, and a little urea and other waste products of metabolism. The sweat glands, therefore, act in a minor way as excretory organs. Their main function is to facilitate the loss of heat from the body by pouring on to the skin surface a watery fluid which can evaporate. The water, changing to water vapour, takes up a great deal of heat from the surface of the body as **latent heat of vaporization.** The surface of the body is thus cooled.

The ceruminous glands in the external ear (p. 304) are modified sweat glands.

NAILS

Nails are made of translucent keratin, like that of the clear layer of the epidermis, but the keratin of nails is harder. The nail is produced (Fig. 134) by multiplication of germinal cells which lie just proximal to the visible nail and under

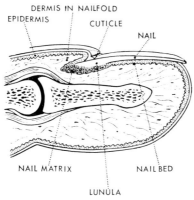

Fig. 134. A longitudinal section through the end of a finger to show the nail and related structures.

the **lunula,** the white semilune at the base of the nail. The nails protect the finger-tips and may be used as offensive weapons.

Nails grow about 0·5 mm a week; finger-nails grow faster than toe-nails, and both grow faster in summer than in winter.

Types of Skin

Skin is of two main types, thick and thin (Fig. 133).

Thick skin is found on the palms of the hands and on the soles of the feet. The epidermis is very thick, mainly because of a thick layer of keratin which effectively protects these surfaces which are exposed to wear and tear. The dermis in thick skin is thin, and has its papillæ arranged in parallel lines to form **papillary ridges.** The epidermis over these ridges reflects this pattern which can be observed easily in the living hand, and which is the basis of **finger-prints** (Fig. 135). The pattern is laid down for each individual in early embryonic life and is permanent and unique. No two people have the same pattern, hence the value of fingerprints in identification of individuals. The papillary ridges help to prevent the skin from slipping when smooth objects are grasped. Thick skin has very numerous **sweat glands** whose ducts open at the summit of the ridges. These minute openings can just be observed with the naked eye. Thick skin has no hair because of the absence of hair follicles.

Thin skin, on the other hand, has a thin epidermis and a thick dermis. It is found on all other parts of the body, being especially thin on the flexor surfaces. The dermal papillæ are arranged in a random pattern and there are numerous hair follicles. Even 'non-hairy' skin over most of the body carries very fine almost invisible hairs.

BODY TEMPERATURE

Cold-blooded creatures, like invertebrates, reptiles, fish and amphibians, have a temperature which varies directly with that of the surroundings. Warm-blooded creatures, the birds and mammals, have an almost constant temperature, quite independent of the environmental temperature, because of the heat regulating mechanism they possess.

The body temperature in Man, on an average in temperate climates, is about 36·8°C (98·4°F) in the closed mouth, about 0·5°C (1°F) more in the rectum and about 0·5°C (1°F) less in the axilla. The air is usually at a lower temperature than the body, so that the external surface, constantly cooled, registers a lower temperature than internal organs.

VARIATIONS IN TEMPERATURE

There is a **daily variation** of nearly 1°C (about 2°F) in the normal body temperature. It is highest in the early evening (when the muscular activity of the day has produced extra heat) and lowest in the early morning (when metabolism is at a minimum). In night workers the rhythm is reversed.

In the **tropics** the range is nearly 0·5°C (1°F) above that in temperate climates.

In women the temperature varies over a range of about 0·5°C (1°F) with the phases of the **menstrual cycle** (p. 545).

In **infants** the temperature varies considerably because the regulating

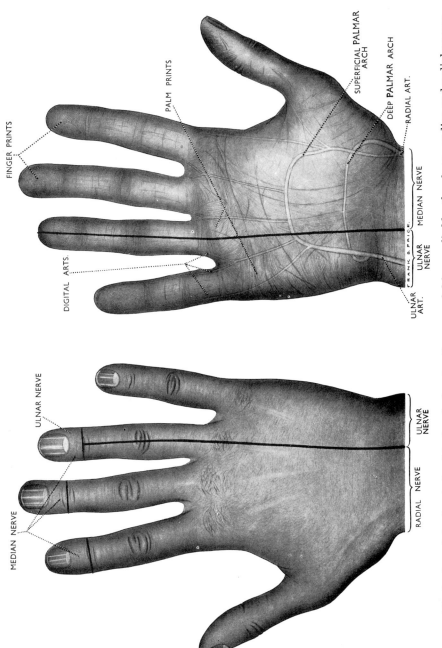

FINGER PRINTS

PALM PRINTS

SUPERFICIAL PALMAR ARCH

DEEP PALMAR ARCH

RADIAL ART.

MEDIAN NERVE

ULNAR NERVE

ULNAR ART.

DIGITAL ARTS.

FRANK D. PAIGE.

ULNAR NERVE

RADIAL NERVE

ULNAR NERVE

MEDIAN NERVE

Fig. 135. The back and the front of a right hand, showing the areas of skin supplied by the ulnar, median and radial nerves, finger and palm prints and the surface projection of the superficial and deep palmar arches.

mechanism is imperfectly developed. It is important, therefore, to adjust environmental conditions for them.

In the **elderly** the temperature tends to be lower than normal

REGULATION OF BODY TEMPERATURE

If the body temperature is to be kept constant, the amount of heat produced in the body must be equalled exactly by the amount of heat lost from the body.

Heat Production

Heat in the body is produced in the following ways:

Oxidation of foodstuffs in the cells of the body produces energy in the form of heat. This occurs in muscles, notably in the heart and in the skeletal muscles both in muscle tone and in exercise; the metabolic activities in the liver too produce considerable heat.

This heat production can be **increased** by:

1. Exercise.
2. Shivering (in which involuntary contractions of skeletal muscle occur to produce heat).
3. The ingestion of foodstuffs, especially protein, which stimulates metabolism.

Heat may also be **gained from the environment**:

1. By radiation from the sun (which is independent of the air temperature).
2. When the air temperature exceeds the skin temperature.
3. By a hot bath.
4. By ingesting hot food or fluids.

Heat Loss

Heat may be lost from the body:

1. By **radiation** from the skin.
2. By **conduction** of heat through the body tissues directly or in the blood stream, from the inside of the body to the skin, and **convection** in the air in contact with the skin.
3. By **evaporation** (see below).
4. By **excretion** of heat in warm urine and fæces.

Evaporation. Water changing into water vapour on the skin surface takes up a great deal of heat as latent heat of vaporization (see p. 36). There is a continuous small loss of heat in this way due to '**insensible perspiration**'. According to need, much larger amounts of heat can be lost by the **evaporation**

of sweat, produced by increased secretion by the sweat glands. This is accompanied by dilatation of the capillary plexus under the epidermis, so that more warm blood comes near the surface to be cooled.

Heat is also lost by evaporation during the warming and saturation with water vapour of the air passing through the upper respiratory tract on its way to the lungs (p. 322). The heat is lost to the body when this air is expired.

Heat-regulating Centres

The body temperature is regulated by nervous control exercised by two centres in the **hypothalamus.** The **anterior centre** prevents overheating; the **posterior centre** prevents chilling.

The centres are influenced in two ways:

1. By the temperature of the blood reaching them.
2. Reflexly by the stimulation of hot and cold nerve endings in the skin.

Loss of heat is promoted by stimulation of the anterior centre by warmer blood or by heat applied to the skin. This results in sweating and dilatation of the arterioles and capillaries in the skin through sympathetic impulses. Hot blood, coursing rapidly through the skin close to the surface, is cooled by radiation and by conduction and convection in the air in contact with the skin. The increased sweating associated with this increased blood flow through the skin results in heat loss by the evaporation of sweat.

Production of heat is promoted by stimulation of the posterior centre by cooler blood or by cold applied to the skin. This results in shivering caused by impulses in the cerebromotor system to the skeletal muscles. The oxidation of foodstuffs, associated with the contractions, produces the required heat.

Conservation of heat is promoted by the constriction of the arterioles in the skin which prevents much warm blood from reaching the surface.

When warm blood is thus prevented from reaching the surface of the skin, the subcutaneous fat acts as an insulating layer which helps the body conserve heat. Other things being equal, an individual who has a liberal amount of subcutaneous fat succumbs less readily to exposure to cold than one who possesses less subcutaneous fat.

In severe fevers and in prolonged exposure to high temperatures (heat stroke) the heat regulating centres become upset, the temperature rises uncontrolled, and death may occur. Extreme cold may also cause death.

HYPOTHERMIA: To reduce the oxygen demand of the tissues (p. 321) during operations which interrupt the blood circulation to them, the body temperature is deliberately lowered by cooling the external surface or by circulating the blood through a cooling system and returning it to the body. Shivering is prevented by anæsthesia and muscle-relaxing drugs.

ACCIDENTAL HYPOTHERMIA: Accidental hypothermia is likely to occur in infants and in the elderly, and may be fatal. The temperature of such patients must be taken with care, and, if necessary with a special low-reading thermometer. Exposure to cold is the main cause, but, in the elderly, endogenous factors such as immobility, illness and drugs (including alcohol) which promote loss of heat can precipitate the condition.

CHAPTER XI

THE RESPIRATORY SYSTEM

ALL living cells need a constant supply of oxygen to enable them to carry out the essential biochemical reactions of their metabolism. This oxygen supply is provided by the blood, which also removes the carbon dioxide and other waste products. Where does the blood get the oxygen, and what does it do with the carbon dioxide? The oxygen comes from the outside air into which also the carbon dioxide is discharged. The respiratory system provides the means of doing this. It consists of the nose, the pharynx, the larynx, the trachea and the lungs.

Development

The pharynx develops from the cranial part of the foregut. In the floor of the cranial part of the foregut there appears at an early stage a groove which will become the larynx. From the groove the trachea grows tailwards as a hollow bud of cells. This divides into the beginnings of the right and left main bronchus. Each of these then divides repeatedly to form the branching system of ducts which becomes the bronchial tree, the terminal branches eventually forming the alveoli. As these lung buds grow, they push out laterally, invaginating the pleural sac as they enlarge (p. 331).

In the early stages the lungs look like exocrine glands. At about the twenty-eighth week of intra-uterine life the bronchial tree begins to open up and the alveoli to expand a little. The fetus soon begins to make very small respiratory movements which draw in a small quantity of amniotic fluid. Nevertheless, right up to the time of birth at forty weeks, the lungs remain relatively collapsed.

With the baby's first breaths, however, the whole picture alters. Air is sucked into the lungs; all the bronchi fill with air which soon penetrates to all the alveoli, so that the lung expands. At the same time the ductus arteriosus contracts so that all the blood from the right ventricle of the heart now circulates through the lungs (p. 390).

For the lungs to expand normally at birth, a substance called **surfactant** must be present in the alveoli. It is secreted by special cells towards the end of pregnancy and reduces surface tension so that the walls of the still collapsed alveoli may lose contact easily and fill with air. In premature babies, surfactant may be deficient and this results in poor inflation of the lungs.

The lungs begin to develop high up in the cervical region of the embryo. As they grow and develop they come to lie more caudally, pushing the diaphragm tailwards before them. The diaphragm, which develops from the fourth cervical segment of the

321

embryo, is pushed down in this way until, when the lungs are fully developed and expanded, its central tendon is opposite the bottom of the eighth thoracic vertebra. This descent of the diaphragm explains the long course of the phrenic nerve, which retains its origin from the fourth cervical spinal nerve (Plates 12 and 13).

THE RESPIRATORY ORGANS

THE EXTERNAL NOSE

The external nose is the visible part of the nose. It is supported by the two small nasal bones (Fig. 44), but the rest of its skeleton is of cartilage. The skin covering it contains numerous large sebaceous glands, but only rudimentary hairs. The sebum helps to protect the skin on such an exposed prominence. The nostrils are lined by skin, which is very sensitive and which carries hairs to help to prevent entry of foreign particles.

The skin of the external nose is closely bound down to the underlying tissue. Any swelling, for example due to a boil, stretches the skin and causes much pain.

THE NASAL CAVITY

The skeleton of the nasal cavity is described on p. 129. The cavity is lined by **mucoperiosteum,** a mucous membrane whose lamina propria blends with the periosteum of the bones. The epithelium is of ciliated pseudostratified columnar cells (Fig. 34, c). The lamina propria contains small mucous and serous glands and a rich **capillary plexus,** especially where it covers the **conchæ** (Fig. 46). The conchæ by their shape present a large area to the incoming air and also create eddies which bring more of the air into direct contact with the mucous membrane. When the capillaries are dilated, the air passing over the epithelium on its way to the lungs is warmed by the warm blood. The mucus secreted by the glands moistens the air and prevents the epithelium from becoming dry and cracked, and it also traps some of the dust in the air. The cilia of the cells move the mucus backwards into the pharynx for swallowing or for expectoration.

Because the mucous membrane covering the conchæ is so vascular, it swells up readily when inflamed or irritated, to the extent of blocking the nasal cavity. This is why the nose is often blocked during a cold in the head. During a cold too, the secretions of the glands are excessive. The cilia are no longer able to move all the fluid back to the pharynx, partly because they may be temporarily inactivated by the infection; a 'running nose' is the result.

The epithelium of the mucous membrane in the uppermost part of the nasal cavity contains the olfactory cells for the sense of smell (p. 309). The conchæ divert some of the incoming air to the vicinity of these cells.

PARANASAL SINUSES (Figs. 46 and 47)

The paranasal sinuses are the maxillary sinus, the frontal sinus, the ethmoidal sinuses and the sphenoidal sinus. They are described on p. 129. They too are lined by mucoperiosteum, which is continuous with that of the nasal cavity where the sinuses open into it. The mucus secreted inside them is wafted into the nasal cavity by their ciliated epithelium. If the lining cells are infected by a cold the mucous membrane swells, sometimes blocking the outlet to the nose, the secretion is increased and the cilia are paralysed or perhaps destroyed. Fluid, therefore, accumulates in the sinuses to give the 'blocked up' feeling; the voice is altered too because there is now no air in the sinuses for resonance. As the infection subsides, the fluid drains away through the opening, at first helped by gravity, until the movements of the cilia begin again. The opening of the maxillary sinus, however, is high up on its medial wall, so that the drainage cannot be aided by gravity. The fluid remains stagnant in the sinus for longer, and this frequently leads to chronic maxillary sinusitis.

Nerve Supply

The mucous membrane of the nose is very sensitive. Even minor irritation reflexly causes sneezing, a violent expulsive effort, which protects the lungs from the inspiration of harmful substances. The mucous membrane of the nose and of the paranasal sinuses is supplied by branches of the trigeminal nerve.

NASOPHARYNX

The nasopharynx is the upper part of the pharynx (p. 437). It has back and side walls formed by the superior constrictor muscle, and an anterior wall which communicates through the posterior choanæ with the nasal cavity. Its roof is the base of the skull and its floor is the soft palate which, when raised to come into contact with the superior constrictor, completely shuts off the nasopharynx from the oropharynx below. It is lined by mucous membrane which has a columnar ciliated epithelium.

The **auditory tube** (pharyngotympanic tube) (p. 304) opens into the lower part of the lateral wall of the nasopharynx (Plate 34). On the posterior wall, behind the mucous membrane, is a mass of lymphoid tissue, the **pharyngeal** tonsil which, when enlarged by chronic infection, is called **adenoids**. Adenoids, which often occur in children, may block the auditory tube, and by preventing access of air to the middle ear (p. 305), cause deafness and recurrent infection there. If adenoids are very large they may project so much as to block the flow of air from the nose into the oropharynx in breathing. This results in persistent breathing through the mouth, which is undesirable because the air is then neither warmed nor moistened nor filtered before it goes to the lungs. Also, the nasal cavity does not grow properly, and the palate becomes excessively arched. This alteration in the shape of the bones of the face, together with a mouth constantly open for breathing, gives children suffering from adenoids a characteristic appearance.

THE LARYNX

The larynx is the 'voice box' which opens above into the pharynx and is continuous below with the trachea. From an evolutionary point of view it is a protective sphincter for preventing food from entering the air passages of the lung, and has subsequently developed into an organ which produces the voice sounds.

Skeleton of the Larynx

Its skeleton consists of a number of cartilages, three unpaired, the epiglottis, the thyroid cartilage and the cricoid cartilage, and one pair, the arytenoid cartilages.

The **thyroid cartilage** (Fig. 136) is made of two almost square plates of hyaline cartilage which are joined in front along adjacent edges in the midline. The posterior borders of the plates are widely separated posteriorly; each upper posterior angle forms a projection, the **superior horn;** each lower posterior angle forms the **inferior horn.** The thyroid cartilage makes the prominence in the living neck called the 'Adam's apple'. It is larger in the male than in the female.

The **cricoid cartilage** is made of hyaline cartilage and is shaped like a signet ring. The **ring** is in front and the thick four-sided plate or **lamina** is behind. The first ring of the trachea is joined to its lower border. The inferior horns of the thyroid cartilage articulate by means of synovial joints with small facets on its posterolateral aspect (Fig. 136).

The **epiglottis** is like a leaf, pear-shaped in outline, and is made of elastic cartilage. The stem of the leaf is fixed in the midline to the upper part of the back of the thyroid cartilage and above by the glosso-epiglottic fold to the back of

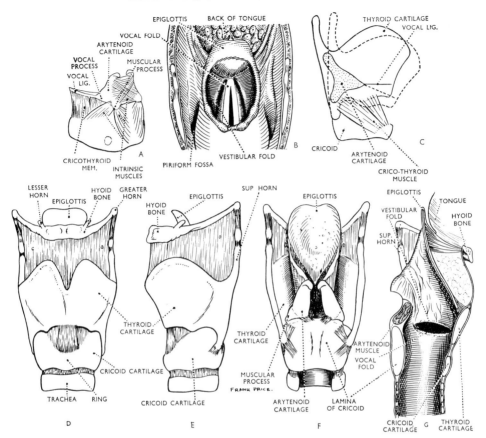

Fig. 136. The larynx: A, the cricoid and arytenoid cartilages with the cricothyroid membrane; B, the inlet of the larynx, seen from behind; C, the thyroid, cricoid and arytenoid cartilages—the interrupted outline shows the thyroid cartilage tilted forwards on the cricoid, to increase the tension of the vocal ligament; D, the cartilages and membranes of the larynx, from the front; E, the cartilages and membranes from the side; F, the cartilages and membranes from behind; G, a sagittal section of the larynx, showing the arrangement of the mucous membrane.

the tongue (Fig. 136). The rounded upper end of the epiglottis can be seen pointing upwards in the living pharynx, especially in a very young child, if the mouth is open and the tongue is depressed.

The **arytenoid cartilages** are a pair of small pyramids of hyaline cartilage. Each has a base and three sides. The apex points upwards. Of the three angles at the base, one points medially; another, the **vocal process**, points forwards and has the posterior end of the vocal ligament fixed to it; the third, the **muscular process,** points laterally and has several of the intrinsic muscles of the larynx inserted into it. The base of the arytenoid cartilage articulates by means of a synovial joint with the sloping 'shoulder' of the lamina of the cricoid cartilage.

Membranes and Ligaments of the Larynx

The walls of the larynx are completed by two fibro-elastic membranes, the thyrohyoid membrane and the cricothyroid membrane.

The **thyrohyoid membrane** is a thin sheet which stretches from the upper border of the thyroid cartilage to the hyoid bone (Fig. 136, D).

The **cricothyroid membrane** (conus elasticus) is attached below to the upper edge of the ring and lamina of the cricoid cartilage, and has a free upper margin. This upper margin is not circular like the lower edge but makes two parallel lines, running from front to back. The two parallel edges are the **vocal ligaments (cords).** (A rough model might be made by cutting out the top and bottom of a cylindrical food tin and then pushing in the upper part from two sides.) The anterior end of each vocal ligament is fixed to the thyroid cartilage in the midline; the posterior end is attached to the vocal process of the arytenoid cartilage (Fig. 136, A). It must be realized that the vocal ligament is not a true 'cord', but is the thickened upper edge of the cricothyroid membrane. It contains much elastic tissue. The interval between the two vocal ligaments is the **rima glottidis.**

The position of the vocal ligaments and, therefore, the size of the rima glottidis are altered by movements of the arytenoid cartilages; the length and tension of the ligaments is varied by movements of the thyroid cartilage on the cricoid cartilage (p. 328).

The **vestibular ligaments** are two thinner and weaker bands which stretch between the thyroid cartilage and the vocal processes of the arytenoid cartilages above the vocal ligaments.

Cavity of the Larynx

The cavity of the larynx extends from the inlet above to the lower border of the cricoid cartilage below. The inlet is very oblique, and is bounded above and in front by the epiglottis, below and behind by the apices of the arytenoid cartilages and, between these cartilages, by folds of mucous membrane containing muscles which by contracting can close the inlet during swallowing.

Mucous Membrane

The larynx is lined by mucous membrane which has a pseudostratified columnar ciliated epithelium. Where it covers the vestibular and vocal ligaments it is raised into folds called the **vestibular** and **vocal folds** respectively. On each side, between the vestibular and vocal folds, is a small pocket of mucous membrane, the **laryngeal sinus** (Fig. 137). The mucous membrane is very sensitive, and any foreign particle stimulates a violent cough reflex. The mucous membrane is tightly bound down over the vocal ligaments, but is very loosely attached to the walls of the larynx above them. Fluid may collect in the loose submucous tissue, for example in infections of the larynx, causing much swelling —œdema of the glottis. This may block the airway; if it does, tracheotomy is essential.

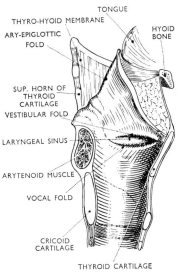

Fig. 137. A median sagittal section of the larynx.

Laryngoscopy

With the help of a laryngoscope, an instrument with a light and mirrors, the larynx can be inspected in the living subject. The aditus and the interior can be seen, including the vestibular folds and the vocal folds, but the sinus is out of sight.

Muscles of the Larynx

The **extrinsic muscles of the larynx,** also called the infrahyoid muscles, connect the cartilages of the larynx with the hyoid bone. Together with muscles which move the hyoid, they contract during swallowing to raise the larynx and pull it forwards.

The **intrinsic muscles of the larynx** move the laryngeal cartilages in relation to each other. They are supplied by the **recurrent laryngeal nerve,** a branch of the vagus, except for the cricothyroid muscle which is supplied by the external laryngeal nerve, also from the vagus.

Movements of the Larynx

The intrinsic muscles have three functions to perform:

1. To act as sphincters for the inlet of the larynx during swallowing (p. 324).
2. To open and close the rima glottidis.
3. To control the tension and the length of vocal ligaments.

When the vocal ligaments are close together in the midline, they are said to be adducted, and the rima glottidis is closed. When the posterior ends of the vocal ligaments and the arytenoid cartilages are apart, the ligaments are said to be abducted, and the rima glottidis is open.

Abduction and adduction of the vocal ligaments are produced by movements of the arytenoid cartilages on the shoulders of the lamina of the cricoid cartilage. The arytenoid cartilage can rotate round a vertical axis so that the vocal process points forwards in adduction of the vocal ligaments and anterolaterally in abduction. The arytenoid cartilage also glides downwards and laterally on the shoulder of the cricoid lamina in abduction of the vocal ligaments, and upwards and medially in adduction. These movements are produced by the intrinsic muscles inserted into the muscular process.

During quiet respiration the vocal ligaments are moderately abducted. In deeper respiration abduction is greater.

Adduction of the vocal ligaments is essential for the production of sound in

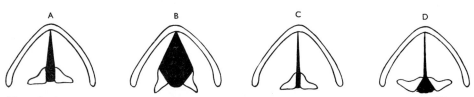

Fig. 138. Diagrams showing the vocal folds and arytenoid cartilages in different positions: A, at rest, during quiet respiration; B, the vocal folds and arytenoid cartilages widely abducted during **forced respiration;** C, the vocal folds and arytenoid cartilages adducted during **normal speech;** D, the vocal cords adducted, and the arytenoid cartilages abducted in **whispering.**

speech, that is for **phonation.** The rima glottidis is reduced to a narrow chink through which air being exhaled from the lungs is forced. The air makes the ligaments vibrate as it passes, and the vibrations of the ligaments produce sound waves. The more forceful the expiration the greater the amplitude of the vibrations and the louder the sound.

The length and tension of the vocal ligaments are altered by movements of the thyroid cartilage and the cricoid cartilage in relation to each other. If the thyroid cartilage is tilted forwards in relation to the cricoid cartilage by the cricothyroid muscle (Fig. 136, c) the vocal ligaments are lengthened and stretched at the same time. Tilting back again shortens and slackens the ligaments. The same effect is produced if the cricoid cartilage is tilted backwards. The pitch of the note made by the vibrating ligaments depends on the tension; the greater the tension the higher the pitch. (If the tension remained constant a longer ligament would emit a lower note, but in the larynx the accompanying increase in tension more than compensates for this.)

Speech

Speech is one of the most skilled and complicated activities of which Man is capable. It is hard to learn, and is easily upset.

Three main groups of muscles, respiratory, laryngeal and oral, are used, and their contractions must be controlled and co-ordinated very accurately by the central nervous system.

Respiratory Muscles

During speech the diaphragm is relaxed. The abdominal muscles contract, pushing the diaphragm upwards and driving air out through the larynx. The more forceful this is the louder the sound will be.

Laryngeal Muscles

The laryngeal muscles contract so as to adduct the vocal ligaments, making the rima glottidis a narrow slit. The air driven through makes the ligaments vibrate, producing the primary sound of the voice—phonation. The pitch of the sound is raised by increasing the tension in the vocal ligaments and lowered by slackening the ligaments. The ligaments are made to vibrate for only very short periods at a time in speech. Longer duration of the vibration makes a singing note.

Oral Muscles

The oral group of muscles includes the muscles of the tongue, floor of the mouth, jaws, palate, cheeks and lips. These muscles control the shape of the canal through which the sound passes, the shape of the opening through which it emerges, and the position and extent of obstruction to the sound during its passage.

Sounds are oral if the palate is raised and air escapes only through the mouth, nasal if the palate is lowered and the mouth shut, so that air escapes only through the nose as in humming.

Vowel sounds are phonated, that is the sound is produced in the larynx, and are oral, that is they come through the mouth. The different vowel sounds are made by altering the shape of the mouth, through which they emerge, by different positions of tongue and lips.

Obstruction to the flow of air at different places produces consonants. Thus if the lips are kept momentarily shut, the labial consonants M, P and B are formed. Lingual consonants are produced by pressing different parts of the tongue against the palate, for example tip alone gives L, tip and sides D and T, and dorsum G and K. Phonation may or may not occur simultaneously, thus altering the effect.

Nervous Control of Speech

The principal co-ordinating centre for the complex speech mechanism is the **motor speech centre** which is found on the left cerebral hemisphere in right-handed people (p. 253). Other areas of the cerebral cortex are associated with speech, for example parts of the auditory area and of the visual area. The cerebellum too is concerned with the accurate co-ordination of the different groups of muscles. The medulla shares in the control by giving origin to the hypoglossal nerve which supplies the tongue, and to the vagus which supplies the larynx.

THE TRACHEA

The trachea is the large air tube which begins at the lower end of the larynx and passes downwards in the midline in front of the œsophagus, to a point opposite the sternal angle, where it divides into the right main bronchus and the left main bronchus (Plate 21). The trachea can be felt in the lower part of the neck above the suprasternal notch. The wall of the trachea is made up of a series of horseshoe-shaped cartilages, the open part of the ring facing backwards, together with smooth muscle. The lining mucous membrane has a pseudo-stratified ciliated columnar epithelium.

Tracheotomy

The passage of air through the larynx may be blocked, for example by severe swelling of the mucous membrane. In these circumstances an artificial opening for a breathing tube can be made in the front of the trachea.

THE MEDIASTINUM

The thoracic cavity is the space above the diaphragm, enclosed by the ribs. It contains the two lungs, each enveloped by a pleural sac. Between the two pleural sacs lies the **mediastinum,** which is a thick partition separating completely one side of the thoracic cavity from the other. It stretches from the vertebral column behind to the sternum in front. The main constituent of the mediastinum is the heart, enclosed in the pericardium; also contained in the mediastinum are the great vessels (p. 358), the trachea (see above), the œsophagus (p. 449), the thoracic duct (p. 420) and the thymus gland (p. 412). The part of the mediastinum above the level of the sternal angle (p. 136), is called the

superior mediastinum. It contains, from front to back, the brachiocephalic veins, the arch of the aorta with its three large branches, the trachea down to its bifurcation at the level of the sternal angle, and part of the œsophagus.

THE PLEURAL CAVITIES

The pleura is a serous membrane (pp. 84 and 440) related to each lung. It forms a closed sac.

The pleura allows the lung to move freely and without friction within the thoracic cavity during the movements of respiration.

During development the closed pleural sac is at first lateral to the lung which grows outwards from the midline. As the lung grows it invaginates the **pleural sac** from the medial aspect and soon is enveloped on all sides (Fig. 139). One part of the pleura, the **visceral pleura,** covers the surface of the lung; the other part, the **parietal pleura,** lines the wall of the thoracic cavity. Both are parts of the same pleural sac; the parietal pleura is continuous with the visceral pleura round the hilum (root) of the lung. The parietal pleura is sometimes named according to the part of the thoracic wall with which it is in contact; the **costal pleura** against the ribs; the **diaphragmatic pleura** against the upper surface of the diaphragm; the **mediastinal pleura** against the mediastinum; and the **cervical pleura** in the root of the neck above the level of the first rib.

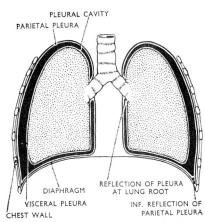

Fig. 139. A diagram of the relations of the pleura.

The diaphragm is dome-shaped. Consequently between the peripheral part of the diaphragm and the lower part of the rib cage there is a deep furrow. The corresponding deep recess of the pleura, where it passes from the ribs to the diaphragm, is the **costodiaphragmatic recess.** It is especially deep towards the back.

In health, the visceral pleura is everywhere in contact with the parietal pleura, separated by only a thin film of lubricating serous fluid. The pleural cavity is thus only a potential space. If air enters it (pneumothorax) either through a hole in the lung or through a hole in the chest wall, it becomes a real space. Similarly, if, as a result of disease, an excess of serous fluid accumulates (pleural effusion) the pleural cavity becomes a real space. The fluid collects in the lowest part of the space, that is, in the costodiaphragmatic recess.

Surface Anatomy

The outline of the pleural cavities in the living subject is indicated in Fig. 140. Notice that the lower border of the pleura passes round the chest from the

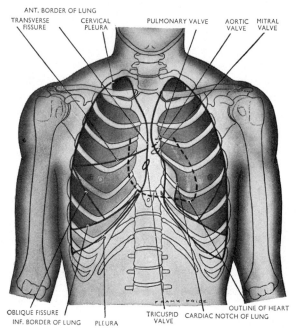

Fig. 140. The surface relations of the heart, lungs and pleura.

seventh costal cartilage, passing through a point two inches above the lowest part of the costal margin, to the spine of the first lumbar vertebra.

THE LUNGS

The lungs are a pair of large organs which are spongy in texture because they contain air. The lungs of people who have lived in the country are pinkish in colour, but those of people who have lived in the cities are greyish black because of the carbon particles from the inspired air which are trapped in the lymphatic vessels and lymph nodes of the lung. The lungs are somewhat conical in shape and are covered by the visceral pleura. On the medial side of each is an area, the **hilum** (root), through which the main bronchus and the pulmonary blood vessels enter and leave. Each lung is divided into **lobes.**

The **left lung** has two lobes, upper and lower, separated by the **oblique fissure** which extends from the surface to the hilum (Fig. 141). The **upper lobe** is mainly above and in front. Its **apex** extends above the first rib and the clavicle into the root of the neck (Fig. 140). The **lower lobe** is conical and lies mainly below and behind.

The **right lung** has three lobes, upper, middle and lower. The **lower lobe** is like that of the left lung, and is separated from the rest of the lung by a similar oblique fissure. The **transverse fissure** (Fig. 141) divides the rest of the lung into the **upper lobe** and the **middle lobe.**

The part of the upper lobe of the left lung which corresponds in position with the middle lobe of the right lung is called the **lingula** (little tongue) because of its shape (Fig. 140).

Surface Marking

The surface marking of the lungs and their fissures in a neutral phase of respiration is shown in Fig. 140. The lower border follows the sixth costal cartilage, crosses the eighth rib in the midaxillary line, the tenth rib in the scapular line and goes towards the eleventh thoracic spine. In deep inspiration the boundaries of the lung correspond with the boundaries of the pleural cavities.

Bronchial Tree

Each **main bronchus** enters the lung at the hilum and divides into branches, one for each lobe. Each of these then divides into the large named branches shown in Plate 21, namely, three for the upper lobe, two for the middle lobe or (for the lingula of the left lung) and five for the lower lobe (four in the left lung). Each of these divides again and again into smaller and smaller bronchi, and finally into tubes less than 1 mm in diameter, which are called **bronchioles.** This branching system of air tubes is called the **bronchial tree,** because the trachea is like the tree trunk, the right and left main bronchi are the limbs, the named bronchi are the large branches and finally the bronchioles represent the tiny twigs.

The bronchioles finally open into wider passages called **alveolar ducts** each of which ends in a spherical **alveolar sac.** From the walls of the alveolar ducts and sacs hemispherical **alveoli** bulge outwards (Plate 22). The walls of the alveolar ducts and sacs and of the alveoli are very thin and contain capillaries.

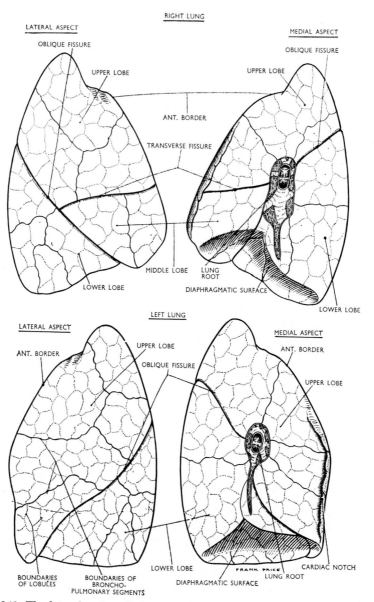

Fig. 141. The lateral and medial surfaces of the right lung and of the left lung.

It is here that the blood is able to take up oxygen from the air and discharge carbon dioxide into it.

Blood Vessels

At the hilum of the lung the large **pulmonary artery,** carrying deoxygenated blood, enters; and two large **pulmonary veins,** carrying oxygenated blood, emerge. The pulmonary artery follows the main bronchus very closely and divides in a similar way to the outer parts of the bronchial tree. There the blood enters the capillary plexus in the walls of the alveoli, and the gaseous exchange takes place. From the capillaries the blood drains into veins which follow a course through the lung tissue in the intervals between the arteries, and finally unite to form the pulmonary veins.

Lymphatic Drainage

The lungs contain a rich plexus of lymphatic capillaries. The lymph vessels follow the veins to the hilum of the lung. Large lymph nodes in the hilum filter this lymph, which finally enters the blood stream in the root of the neck (Fig. 169).

BRONCHOPULMONARY SEGMENTS

Each named bronchus (Plate 21) supplies a distinct segment of the lung tissue—a **bronchopulmonary segment** (Fig. 141) which also has its own large branch of the pulmonary artery and its own large tributary of the pulmonary vein. Each bronchopulmonary segment is separated from adjacent segments by a thin wall of connective tissue. Each segment is further subdivided into small units called **lobules.**

Microscopic Structure

Bronchi. The bronchi have walls very like the trachea (p. 330), except that plates of cartilage are arranged in an irregular pattern along their walls. This cartilage is necessary because when the lungs expand in inspiration, the lung tissue presses on them and would collapse them but for the cartilage. Inside the cartilage is a layer of circular smooth muscle fibres. The epithelium is columnar and ciliated, and is kept moist by mucus.

Bronchioles. Bronchioles have no cartilage in their walls, only a layer of smooth muscle, lined by a low columnar or cuboidal epithelium. There is no need for cartilage supports because they lie **inside** the lobules and when the lung tissue surrounding them expands in inspiration, it holds them open.

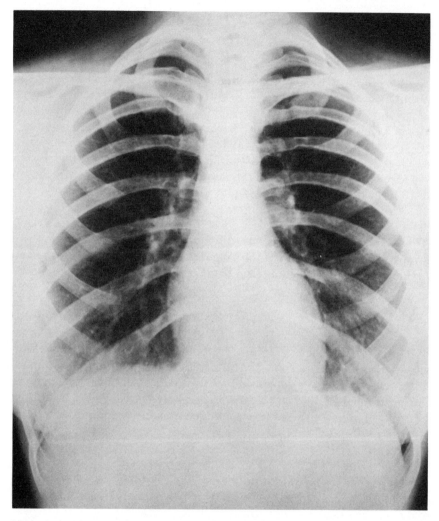

Alveolar ducts, alveolar sacs and **alveoli.** The walls consist of a single layer of simple squamous epithelium, the **respiratory epithelium,** covering the capillary plexus. Where one alveolus touches the next, the wall between them is a capillary plexus covered on both sides by respiratory epithelium. The gaseous exchange takes place easily through the thin barrier between blood and air— namely the endothelium of the capillary wall and the respiratory epithelium covering it.

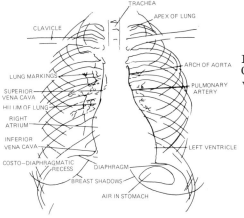

Fig. 142. A radiograph of a female thorax. Compare the outline of the heart shadow with Figure 151.

A small amount of connective tissue is found throughout the lung, supporting the blood vessels and the capillary plexus. It contains many elastic fibres. In inspiration when the lung is expanded, this elastic tissue is stretched. During expiration it recoils to its original size and is the principal means of driving air out of the lungs in quiet respiration.

RADIOLOGY OF THE RESPIRATORY SYSTEM

Air is more translucent to X-rays than the soft tissues of the body, so air filled spaces look dark on X-ray pictures. Many parts of the respiratory system can, therefore, be seen on 'straight' films, that is where no special technique has been used. The cavities of the nose, of the paranasal sinuses, of the mouth and of the pharynx, as well as the shape of the tongue and soft palate can be seen. In the neck and upper part of the thorax the lumen of the trachea is easily identified (Fig. 142). In anterior, lateral and oblique views of the thorax the air filled lungs look dark, contrasting well with the dense shadow cast by the heart. It should be noted that in the living subject the lungs extend into the neck and some way into the costodiaphragmatic recess. Throughout the lungs faint branching patterns, the **lung markings** can be traced; these are the shadows cast by the pulmonary blood vessels.

Bronchograms. A contrast medium like iodized oil can be introduced into the bronchial tree. Then the different branches of the bronchial tree can be identified.

THE PHYSIOLOGY OF RESPIRATION

External Respiration (Pulmonary Respiration) is the exchange of gases between the blood in the lung capillaries and the air in the alveoli of the lungs; the blood takes up oxygen from the air and gives out carbon dioxide.

Internal Respiration (Tissue Respiration) is the exchange of gases between the blood and the tissue cells; the cells take up oxygen from the blood to use in their metabolism, and give back to the blood the waste product, carbon dioxide.

VENTILATION OF THE LUNGS

For external respiration to continue, the air in the alveoli of the lungs must be exchanged regularly with the air outside so that new air, containing oxygen, is constantly reaching the alveoli. At the same time, the air from which oxygen has been taken and to which carbon dioxide has been added by the blood must be removed from the alveoli. This is achieved by the ventilation of the lungs by breathing.

Breathing consists of two phases, **inspiration** and **expiration.** During inspiration air is sucked into the lungs, which expand. During expiration air is expelled from the lungs. Inspiration followed by expiration is the **respiratory cycle.**

Age	Respiratory rate per minute
At birth	18–40
First year	25–35
2–4 years	20–30
5–14 years	20–25
Adult	16–20

The **respiration rate** *is the number of respiratory cycles per minute.* In the adult at rest it varies from sixteen to twenty per minute. In children it is more rapid (see table). The respiration rate is increased by exercise (p. 182) and by emotion.

RESPIRATORY MOVEMENTS

Inspiration

Inspiration is brought about by the **active contraction** of the respiratory muscles, that is of the **diaphragm** (p. 198) and of the **intercostal muscles** (p. 197); this increases the volume of the cavity of the thorax.

When the **diaphragm** contracts it pulls its central tendon downwards and flattens its domed shape; this increases the vertical measurement of the thorax by about 1·5 cm in normal quiet inspiration. In deep inspiration the

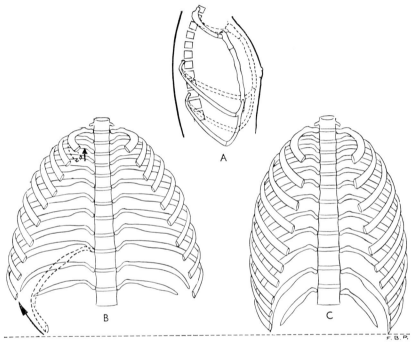

Fig. 143. The movements of the rib cage in external respiration. A, the chest seen from the side: the solid outline shows the ribs in expiration, the interrupted outline shows the position of the same ribs in inspiration and indicates the increase in the anteroposterior diameter of the thorax; B, the ribs seen from the front in inspiration, showing that the side diameter in the lower part of the chest is increased; C, the ribs seen from the front in expiration.

height of the thorax is increased by between 5 and 10 cm. The downward movement of the diaphragm presses the abdominal viscera downwards, and the muscles of the anterior abdominal wall relax their tone a little to make room for them.

When the **intercostal muscles** contract they rotate the ribs at their articulations with the vertebral column. The anterior ends of the ribs move forwards and laterally; the sternum is therefore lifted forwards, and each rib comes to the position previously occupied by the one above. This makes the thoracic cavity deeper from front to back and wider from side to side. During quiet respiration the circumference of the chest increases by 1·5 cm in inspiration; in deep inspiration it may increase by between 5 and 10 cm.

During inspiration the visceral pleura remains in contact with the parietal pleura because the pleural cavity is in effect a vacuum. As the volume of the interior of the thorax is increased by muscular contraction, the lung expands correspondingly to fill it as air enters through the bronchial tree.

Let us put it another way; air exerts a pressure, the atmospheric pressure, on every surface with which it comes into direct contact, for example on the outside of the chest and abdominal walls and on the inside of the walls of all parts of the bronchial tree. The atmospheric pressure is the same in all directions. During inspiration the chest walls tend to move outwards away from the outer surface of the lung, relieving this lung surface temporarily of the atmospheric pressure previously transmitted to it through the chest wall. The atmospheric pressure inside the bronchial tree and inside the whole of the lung is pressing as hard as before, and because the pressure on the outside of the lung is now reduced, the atmospheric pressure is able to push the surface of the lung outwards, that is, to make the lung expand.

To describe it in a third way, the movements of the chest wall and of the diaphragm in inspiration, create a negative intrapleural pressure which allows the atmospheric pressure to inflate the lungs.

Expiration

Expiration is **passive** in quiet respiration, that is, virtually no muscle contraction occurs.

The diaphragm relaxes and returns to its original domed shape. The tone of the abdominal muscles pushes the viscera against its lower surface and drives it up to its former level.

The intercostal muscles relax and the ribs fall back to their former positions assisted by the elastic recoil of the costal cartilages.

The thoracic cavity therefore grows smaller, its walls press on the lung surface and the negative intrapleural pressure disappears.

The lungs contain much elastic tissue (p. 337). In inspiration, when the lungs were inflated this was put on the stretch. The elastic tissue now recoils, making the lungs smaller and so driving air out through the bronchial tree. This elastic recoil of the lungs is the most important factor in driving the air out during expiration.

Types of Respiration

People differ in their ways of breathing. Some use the diaphragm much more than the chest wall; this is called **abdominal respiration** because movements of the abdominal viscera and abdominal wall always accompany movements of the diaphragm. Others use the chest wall more than the diaphragm; this is **costal** or **thoracic respiration.** The costal type of respiration usually predominates in women; this may be an adaptation for possible pregnancy, when the gravid uterus restricts movements of the diaphragm.

Accessory Muscles of Respiration

During deep breathing, and when breathing is difficult because of obstruction in the air passages, other skeletal muscles are brought into action to assist the diaphragm and intercostal muscles. These extra muscles are **accessory muscles of respiration.** Sternomastoid, serratus anterior and pectoralis major are accessory muscles of inspiration. If the parts of the skeleton into which they are inserted are held steady, their pulling on their origins on the chest wall helps to enlarge the thoracic cavity. The muscles of the anterior abdominal wall and latissimus dorsi are accessory muscles of expiration. They can be felt to contract during a forced expiration like coughing. A patient experiencing difficulty in breathing often sits gripping a table; this steadies the upper limbs giving some of the accessory muscles firmer attachments from which to act.

VOLUME OF AIR BREATHED

TIDAL VOLUME: During normal quiet respiration a relatively small volume of air, 500 ml, is breathed in and out in each respiratory cycle. This is the tidal volume.

INSPIRATORY CAPACITY: After a normal quiet expiration, a normal subject can take in, by a violent inspiratory effort, about 2500 ml of air. This is the inspiratory capacity. It includes, of course, the tidal volume.

EXPIRATORY RESERVE VOLUME: After a quiet expiration it is possible to blow out, by a violent effort, about 1300 ml of air. This is the expiratory reserve volume.

RESIDUAL VOLUME: Even after the deepest possible expiration, the lungs and respiratory passages still contain about 1600 ml of air. This is the residual volume.

FUNCTIONAL RESIDUAL CAPACITY: At the end of a quiet expiration the

lungs contain the expiratory reserve volume and the residual volume which together are called the functional reserve capacity, about 2900 ml of air.

VITAL CAPACITY: The vital capacity is the maximum volume of air which
a subject can breathe out after taking the deepest possible inspiration. It is
about 3800 ml. It is the sum of the inspiratory capacity and the expiratory
reserve volume.

The vital capacity is reduced in some diseases of the heart and lungs. If it
falls as low as 1500 ml the patient becomes breathless on moving even a little.

COMPOSITION OF INSPIRED AIR AND EXPIRED AIR

Inspired air is the atmospheric air and has a variable temperature and
humidity (degree of wetness or dryness). It contains approximately:

Oxygen	20% by volume
Carbon dioxide	0·04% by volume (i.e. a mere trace)
Nitrogen	80% by volume

Expired air is saturated with water vapour and has been raised to body
temperature. It contains less oxygen and more carbon dioxide, namely:

Oxygen	16% by volume
Carbon dioxide	4% by volume
Nitrogen	80% by volume

Alveolar Air

All the air in the lungs is not discharged at expiration and residual air is left
in the alveoli and bronchial tree. The fresh air of the next inspiration mixes
with the residual air, and it is with this mixture, the **alveolar air,** that the
blood comes into contact. It is saturated with water vapour and is at body temperature. It contains:

Oxygen	14% by volume
Carbon dioxide	6% by volume
Nitrogen	80% by volume

THE CONTROL OF RESPIRATION

Respiratory Centre

In the reticular formation of medulla oblongata (p. 249) there are groups of
nerve cells which constitute the respiratory centre. These cells send regular
impulses to the motor neurones in the anterior horn of the spinal cord, which

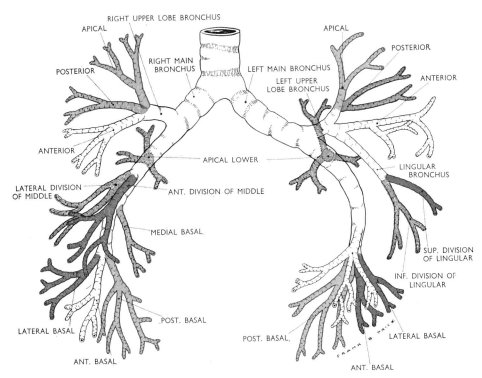

RIGHT UPPER LOBE BRONCHUS

APICAL

POSTERIOR

RIGHT MAIN
BRONCHUS

ANTERIOR

LATERAL DIVISION
OF MIDDLE

LATERAL BASAL

ANT. BASAL

MEDIAL BASAL.

ANT. DIVISION OF MIDDLE

APICAL LOWER

POST. BASAL

LEFT MAIN BRONCHUS

LEFT UPPER
LOBE BRONCHUS

APICAL

POSTERIOR

ANTERIOR

LINGULAR
BRONCHUS

SUP. DIVISION
OF LINGULAR

INF. DIVISION OF
LINGULAR

LATERAL BASAL

POST. BASAL.

ANT. BASAL

Plate 21. The principal bronchi of the bronchial tree.

[facing page 342

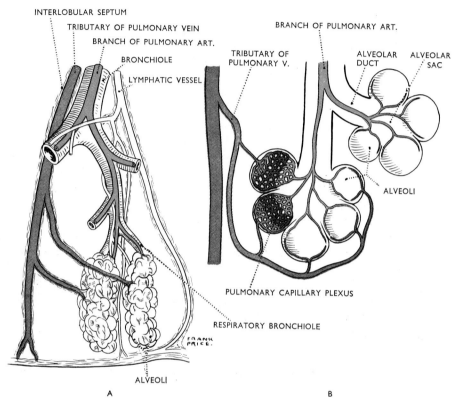

INTERLOBULAR SEPTUM

TRIBUTARY OF PULMONARY VEIN

BRANCH OF PULMONARY ART.

BRONCHIOLE

LYMPHATIC VESSEL

BRANCH OF PULMONARY ART.

TRIBUTARY OF PULMONARY V.

ALVEOLAR DUCT

ALVEOLAR SAC

ALVEOLI

PULMONARY CAPILLARY PLEXUS

RESPIRATORY BRONCHIOLE

FRANK PRICE.

ALVEOLI

A

B

Plate 22. The detailed structure of the lung: A, a lobule of the lung; B, a respiratory bronchiole leading to the respiratory epithelium which lines the alveolar ducts, the alveolar sacs and the alveoli. The circulation through the lung is also indicated; deoxygenated blood in the pulmonary arteries is blue, oxygenated blood in the pulmonary veins is red.

supply the diaphragm and the intercostal muscles. First the motor neurones are stimulated, the muscles contract and inspiration occurs. Then the motor neurones are inhibited, the muscles relax and expiration follows.

In this way the regular respiratory cycle is maintained.

The activity of the respiratory centre is regulated in two ways—(1) by chemical control and (2) by nervous control.

(1) CHEMICAL CONTROL: An **increase in the carbon dioxide in the blood** supplying the respiratory centre stimulates it so that breathing becomes **faster** and **deeper.** This is the most important factor in the regulation of respiration to meet the varying demands of the body. During **muscular exercise** much carbon dioxide is produced in the muscles by the oxidation of carbohydrate. The carbon dioxide in the blood, therefore, increases in amount and this directly stimulates the respiratory centre which increases the **rate** and **depth** of respiration. This makes available more oxygen in the alveoli for the blood to take up and carry to the muscles, and also eliminates more carbon dioxide. Besides carbon dioxide, any other substance which lowers the pH of the blood, can stimulate the respiratory centre.

(2) NERVOUS CONTROL: In inspiration the lung tissue is stretched. The stretching stimulates afferent fibres in the vagus nerve. These impulses reflexly stop inspiration so that expiration occurs.

Emotion, pain and any unusual sensation reflexly cause an increase in the respiratory rate. To record a subject's respiration rate accurately it is best to count the respirations without his knowledge.

COUGH REFLEX

Irritation of the laryngeal mucous membrane reflexly causes a cough, which is a violent explosive expiration. First the vocal ligaments are adducted to close the glottis. Then the abdominal muscles contract forcibly. This builds up pressure of air behind the closed glottis, which is opened suddenly, so that the air escapes with force. This is a protection against entry of foreign bodies into the larynx, and a means of getting rid of anything inside.

Sneezing is a similar action stimulated reflexly by irritation of the mucous membrane of the nose.

SWALLOWING REFLEX

Respiration is reflexly inhibited as soon as a swallowing movement is begun. This too is protective, because it lessens the chance of drawing food into the larynx with the inspired air.

SOME DISTURBANCES OF RESPIRATION

Hyperpnœa. This is an increase in the depth of respiration. It occurs in exercise and can be produced voluntarily for short periods. It also occurs in ketosis (p. 557) because the accompanying acidosis stimulates the respiratory centre (see above).

Apnœa. This means that breathing is suspended.

Dyspnœa is difficult breathing. The patient is conscious of the effort of breathing, and is uncomfortable or distressed. Rate or depth or both are increased.

Dyspnœic patients prefer sitting to lying down. This is because when they lie down the abdominal viscera push the diaphragm up, and this makes the ventilation of the lungs even more difficult.

Asthma is one cause of dyspnœa. In asthma, spasm of the smooth muscle in the walls of the bronchi and bronchioles narrows the lumen of these air tubes so that air passes through them less easily than before. Expiration is much more difficult than inspiration. Whereas in normal expiration the elastic recoil of chest and lungs by itself drives air out, this is no longer sufficient when the air tubes are narrow. The contractions of the muscles of inspiration overcome the difficulty more easily, because they are stronger than the muscles of expiration.

In asthma the accessory muscles of respiration (p. 341) are brought into play, especially latissimus dorsi and the abdominal muscles to assist in expiration.

Cyanosis is a violet or greyish colour of the skin. The colour of the skin, apart from any pigment it contains (p. 311), depends on the blood in the superficial capillaries. If this blood contains an excessive amount of reduced hæmoglobin its dark colour shows through and the skin accordingly looks violet or grey.

Hiccough is a spasmodic contraction of the diaphragm during which the glottis closes suddenly, preventing more air from entering. This produces the characteristic sensation and sound.

Snoring occurs during sleep which is deep enough to relax the soft palate. The air passing in and out during respiration, especially if the mouth is open, makes the flaccid soft palate vibrate, thus producing the characteristic noise.

Periodic Breathing

The respirations wax and wane, so that periods of hypernœa alternate with periods of apnœa. In Cheyne-Stokes respiration the patient is conscious during the hypernœa and confused or unconscious during the apnœa. This is a sign that the brain, including the respiratory centre, is not receiving enough oxygen from the blood.

ARTIFICIAL RESPIRATION

In emergencies like drowning, carbon monoxide poisoning and electric shock, respiratory failure occurs first, and heart failure only secondarily. If artificial respiration is started promptly enough, sufficient oxygen can be put into the patient's blood to maintain the heart and, therefore, the circulation until the respiratory centre recovers.

To be successful artificial respiration **must be started without any delay.** The heart fails very quickly after respiration stops and lack of oxygen does irreparable damage to the nerve cells of the cerebral cortex. If more than eight minutes elapse after the circulation stops, there is no hope of resuscitating the patient completely.

Artificial respiration **should be continued for at least two hours.**

METHODS

Whatever method is used, **always see that the airway is clear.** Remove foreign bodies, vomitus and water as quickly as possible. If the patient has been under water lay him face downwards, stand astride his hips, clasp your hands under his abdomen and lift him up until water stops running out of his mouth.

Mouth to Mouth Respiration (Fig. 144)

This should be started before clearing the mouth. Every fraction of a second counts.

1. Keep the airway open by extending the head on the neck and holding the lower jaw forwards with one hand.

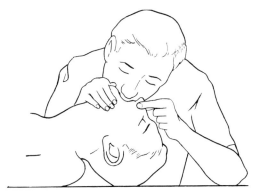

Fig. 144. The mouth to mouth method of artificial respiration.

2. Close the patient's nose firmly with your other hand by gripping the nostrils.
3. Place your lips over the patient's mouth, making sure of a close and air-tight fit.
   Alternatively the patient's mouth may be kept shut and one's lips placed over the patient's nose. In children the lips may be placed over both mouth and nose.
4. Breathe out strongly, so that your breath fills the patient's lungs and the chest can be seen to expand.
5. Remove your mouth. The elastic recoil of the patient's chest and lungs then drives the air out.

Breathe air into the patient's lungs in this way between twelve and twenty times a minute. If at first the chest does not expand, check the airway.

After the patient's lungs have been inflated a few times, it may be advantageous to clear the patient's mouth, to lay him on the back and to take up a more comfortable position, for example kneeling on his left side.

ADVANTAGES: This method can be used anywhere, at any time, by anybody. It can be carried out effectively in almost any situation. It is not tiring. It can be combined with **external cardiac massage** (p. 366).

Holger Nielsen Method

1. Lay the patient face downwards with the elbows bent so that one hand is on top of the other and one cheek rests on the uppermost hand (Fig. 145, A).
2. Kneel, facing the patient's feet with one knee near his head and the opposite foot near his elbow (Fig. 145, A).
3. Pull the tongue forwards and make sure the airway is clear.
4. Place your hands, with fingers spread out, on the back of the chest just below the shoulder blades. Rock forwards, keeping your elbows straight until your shoulders are directly above your hands (Fig. 145, B). Count (seconds), one, two.
5. Slide your hands under the patient's arms and grip them just above the elbow (Fig. 145, C). Count three.
6. Rock slowly backwards, lifting the patient's arms upwards and inwards until resistance is felt in the patient's shoulders (Fig. 145, C). Count four, five.
7. Lower the patient's arms and place your hands in the first position on the patient's back. Count six.

Repeat the movements, taking six seconds for each cycle. The rate of artificial respiration is then ten times per minute.

If natural respiration begins, time your movements to match the patient's respiratory movements.

ADVANTAGES: In the prone position, the toneless tongue falls forwards and

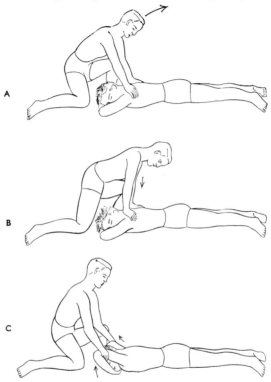

Fig. 145. The Holger Nielsen method of artificial respiration.

there is no danger of its blocking the pharynx (Fig. 177, c). Fluid, like water or vomitus, flows easily out of the mouth.

The forward swing compresses the chest and **actively** drives air out.

The backward swing allows the chest to recoil to its former position. Raising the arms **actively** pulls the chest wall outwards because of the passive insufficiency (p. 180) of the serratus anterior muscles. Both these factors contribute to the expansion of the chest which draws air into the lungs. Two or three times the normal tidal air can be made to enter in this way.

The movements can be kept up by one operator for long periods.

Rocking

This method is useful for infants.

1. Make sure the airway is clear.
2. Hold the infant face downwards in your arms.
3. Rock your arms to one side so that its head comes down to your waist and its feet are at your shoulder (Fig. 146, A).
4. Rock your arms to the other side so that its head comes up to your other shoulder (Fig. 146, B).

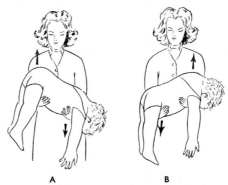

A   B

Fig. 146. The rocking method of artificial respiration.

Repeat the cycle, from one side to the other and back again, twenty times a minute.

When the head is down, the weight of the viscera falls on the diaphragm and pushes it into the chest, so driving air out. When the head is up the abdominal viscera slide down again pulling the diaphragm with them, and air is drawn into the lungs.

CHAPTER XII

THE CIRCULATORY SYSTEM

Introduction

ALL living cells must receive food materials and oxygen, and must be able to eliminate waste products. In small, simple organisms every cell is at, or close to, the surface and the exchange of these materials with the environment takes place directly. Larger, more complex organisms have evolved a system of transport, the circulatory system, which ensures the supply of every cell, no matter how far away from the surface of the body and from contact with the environment. A fluid, **the blood,** which carries the food materials, oxygen and waste products, is forced by a pump, **the heart,** through a system of tubes, **the blood vessels,** to the close vicinity of every cell and then on back to the heart to be pumped round again and again.

There are different kinds of blood vessels:

Arteries are blood vessels which carry blood away from the heart.

Veins are blood vessels which carry blood back to the heart.

Capillaries are very small thin-walled blood vessels which form networks round the cells of the body. Blood is brought to them by arteries and drained away by veins.

All breathing creatures need two circulations; one, the **pulmonary circulation,** carries blood through the lungs where oxygen is taken up and carbon dioxide given out; the other, the **systemic circulation,** circulates blood to the rest of the body, where the cells use up oxygen and return carbon dioxide as a waste product to the blood.

Outline of Development

During the first three weeks of intra-uterine life the human embryo effects the essential exchanges directly with its environment, and grows to a size at which this is no longer adequate (p. 69).

Networks of thin-walled blood vessels appear in the mesoderm and blood develops in them. Gradually some channels in the network develop thick walls and become arteries, other channels become veins and the parts of the networks persisting between them form the capillary beds.

349

Meanwhile, in the region ventral to the foregut, the heart begins to develop as two short parallel tubes which soon fuse to form a single blood vessel, the primitive heart. One end, the caudal end, is connected with the veins, the other, the cranial end, giving origin to the arteries (Fig. 147). By the beginning of the fourth week of intra-uterine life this primitive heart is already functioning as a pump. It soon develops from a simple tube into two chambers, one the atrium, to receive blood from the veins, the

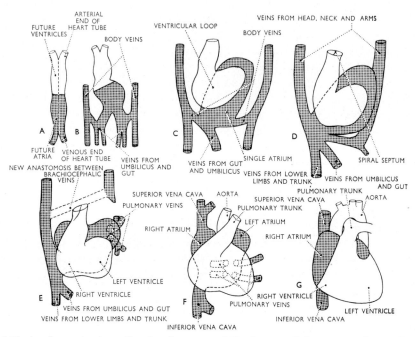

Fig. 147. A scheme to show the development of the heart, of the great veins, and of the aorta and pulmonary trunk. The veins and the atria are cross-hatched; the ventricles and the arteries are white.

other the ventricle to pump blood into the arteries (Fig. 147, c). In order to serve both the pulmonary and the systemic circulations, the whole heart is then divided into two. A septum, the **interatrial septum,** divides the atrium into a right atrium and a left atrium, and another, the **interventricular septum,** divides the ventricle into a right ventricle and a left ventricle (Fig. 148). At the same time the spiral septum divides the aortic sac, leading from the ventricle, into the aorta and the pulmonary artery (Fig. 147, D). The right atrium and right ventricle together form the 'right side' of the heart which is the pump for the pulmonary circulation, and the left atrium and left ventricle form the 'left side' of the heart which is the pump for the systemic circulation (Fig. 147 and Plate 24).

The interventricular septum separates the two ventricles completely at an early stage. During intra-uterine life the interatrial septum separates the two atria only partially. An opening, the **foramen ovale,** persists to the time of birth, and this allows blood to bypass the pulmonary circulation to the as yet non-functioning lungs, by flowing from the right atrium direct to the left atrium (p. 389, Fig. 148 and Plate 33).

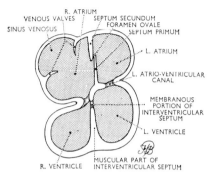

Fig. 148. A section through the developing heart, to show the separation into a right side and a left side, by the formation of an interatrial and an interventricular septum.

GENERAL STRUCTURE OF THE CARDIOVASCULAR SYSTEM

The structure of the walls of all the constituent parts of the circulatory system is essentially similar, and consists of three layers. The **inner layer** is the **endothelium.** This presents a very smooth surface to the blood which flows freely over it without clotting (p. 399). The **middle layer** is composed of smooth muscle and elastic tissue, except in the heart, where it is of cardiac muscle. The contraction of the muscle fibres in the heart produces, and in the blood vessels controls, the flow of blood. The **outer layer** is connective tissue which blends with adjacent connective tissue and anchors the blood vessels to surrounding structures.

THE HEART

The heart is the part of the circulatory system specialized to act as a pump to keep the blood flowing. The muscle coat is, therefore, highly modified for hard and continuous work. Not only is it a thick layer but the muscle fibres themselves are of a special kind known as cardiac muscle (p. 115). The lining endothelium is identical with that of other parts of the system, but is known as **endocardium.** The endocardium forms a covering for every structure in the interior of the heart. The connective tissue surrounding the heart is specially modified to form the **pericardium** (p. 358).

The Atria

The atria are collecting chambers for the blood returned to the heart. They then pump the blood into the adjacent ventricles. The cardiac muscle in their walls is a relatively thin layer, because the atria pump the blood only a short distance against minimal resistance.

The Ventricles

The ventricles supply the power to force the blood round the circulatory system, hence the cardiac muscle of their walls forms a thick layer. The right ventricle propels the blood only through the lungs, and its wall is thinner than that of the left ventricle, which has to maintain the circulation through the whole of the rest of the body.

THE BLOOD VESSELS

The endothelial lining of blood vessels and the connective tissue supporting it constitute the **tunica intima.** The middle coat is the **tunica media** and the outer connective tissue coat the **tunica adventitia** (Fig. 149).

The structure of the different kinds of blood vessels is related to the different functions they perform in a very striking way. The differences in structure are found mainly in the tunica media.

Arteries

Arteries are vessels which conduct the blood from the heart to the tissues. Starting with the aorta and pulmonary artery, which are over an inch in diameter in the adult, they become progressively smaller as they branch in their course to the periphery. Three kinds of arteries are described, the large arteries known as **elastic arteries,** the medium arteries known as **muscular or distributing arteries,** and the small arteries known as **arterioles.**

ELASTIC ARTERIES: These arteries are the large arteries which receive blood direct from the ventricles, that is the aorta and the pulmonary trunk, together with their largest branches. The principal feature of their structure is the great number of elastic fibres (p. 94) intermingled with the muscle fibres in the tunica media (Fig. 149). This allows the whole vessel wall to behave like a piece of elastic. It can be stretched and, after the stretching force is removed, it has a natural tendency to recoil to its original size and shape. This quality of the elastic arteries is important in that it converts the intermittent flow of blood coming from the rhythmically contracting ventricles into a continuous flow. Each ventricular contraction propels a volume of blood under pressure into the elastic arteries and stretches them. At the end of the contraction the propulsive force and the stretching stop, but the elastic recoil of the vessel walls allows them to press the blood onwards along the arteries until the next contraction

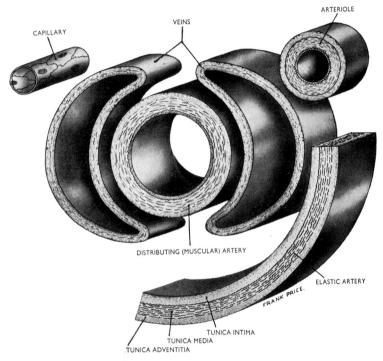

Fig. 149. The structure of the blood vessels.

begins. In this way a continuous, though pulsating, flow into the muscular arteries is maintained. The elastic recoil also propels blood into the coronary arteries which can deliver blood to the cardiac capillaries only when the cardiac muscle is relaxed in diastole (p. 364).

MUSCULAR ARTERIES: Muscular or distributing arteries are of medium size and the majority of the arteries described in regional anatomy are of this kind. Their walls are relatively thick because as their name suggests, there is considerable smooth muscle in the tunica media (Fig. 149).

The smooth muscle fibres are arranged round the lumen, so that by their contraction the lumen is reduced in size and less blood can flow through. In this way the volume of blood reaching a region is regulated by the distributing arteries.

ARTERIOLES: These are the smallest arteries, **half a millimetre or less in diameter.** They have walls which, in relation to the size of the lumen, are thick because of the thick layer of smooth muscle fibres in the tunica media (Fig. 149). Contraction of this muscle reduces the lumen which then allows less blood to pass. Damming back of blood by arterioles in this way reduces the pressure of the blood reaching the capillary bed (below and Plate 23), and raises the pressure in the systemic arteries. The arterioles play an important part in regulating the blood pressure.

Capillaries

Capillaries are the smallest blood vessels, the lumen being just large enough to allow red blood corpuscles to pass. The walls are very thin, consisting of only an endothelial layer, through which the oxygen and food materials diffuse into the body cells and the waste products return to the blood. Capillaries are arranged in networks round the cells of the body, the networks being fed at one end by arterioles and drained at the other by venules (Plate 23). These networks of capillaries are often called the **capillary bed.**

Veins

Compared with the corresponding arteries, veins have a larger lumen and thinner walls. Blood flows much more slowly through veins than through arteries although, in a given time, the same volume must be transmitted by both, hence the large lumen of veins. The pressure of the blood in the veins is low, therefore a thin wall containing very little muscle is adequate. In contrast, the blood pressure in the arteries is high and necessitates strong elastic or muscular walls. The thinness of the walls of veins renders them easily compressible and this is important in the consideration of venous circulation (p. 384).

The walls of veins have a tunica intima, a tunica media and a tunica adventitia. The tunica media consists mainly of fibrous tissue with only a few smooth muscle fibres. Superficial veins, however, have more muscle in their walls and this often goes into spasm if it is irritated, for example by an intravenous injection. **Valves** are found in most veins. Each is made up of two cup-shaped flaps of endothelium supported by connective tissue. These flaps allow blood to flow in one direction, over their convex surfaces, but prevent its passage in the opposite direction by filling out until the edges of the two flaps meet (Fig. 150).

VENULES: These are the smallest veins and they collect the blood from the capillary networks. Their walls consist of endothelium supported by a layer of fibrous tissue. They unite to form larger veins, and by the **joining of tributaries,** still larger veins are formed.

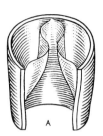

Lymphatic Vessels

The lymphatic vessels assist the veins in carrying back towards the heart, the fluid brought to the tissues by the arteries. They contain not blood but lymph, a fluid derived from the tissue fluid (p. 406). Lymphatic capillaries and lymphatic vessels are described.

The **lymphatic capillaries** are similar to the blood capillaries and their walls are formed of a single layer of endothelium. They have blind ends and form extensive lymphatic capillary networks in certain regions (p. 407). These networks are drained by **lymphatic vessels,** which are in structure like very small veins. Valves, however, are much more numerous in lymphatic vessels, and although lymphatic vessels do unite to form larger ones, they tend rather to run parallel to one another, and the largest is no bigger than a small vein.

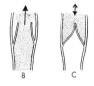

Fig. 150. A, a vein cut open to show the two cusps of a venous valve; B, a venous valve, open, to allow blood to flow towards the heart; C, the valve closed, preventing backflow.

GENERAL OUTLINE OF THE CIRCULATION

SYSTEMIC CIRCULATION

The systemic circulation is the circulation of blood through the whole of the body except the respiratory tissue of the lungs. It is maintained by the left side of the heart.

Blood enters the left atrium through two pairs of pulmonary veins which come from the lungs (Plate 24). Contraction of the left atrium drives the blood through the mitral valve (see below and Fig. 153) into the left ventricle. The left ventricle contracts powerfully and sends the blood under pressure through the aortic valve (see below and Fig. 153) into the aorta. The large branches of the aorta carry the blood to the main regions and organs of the body, and these arteries branch and branch again, and again, each branch being smaller than the parent stem, down to the arterioles which feed the capillary bed. The capillary bed is drained by venules which unite to form small veins, these in turn joining to form larger veins, all directed back towards the heart. A large vein emerges from each main region and organ, and these unite finally to form two large veins, the superior vena cava which receives blood from the head, neck, upper limb and thoracic wall, and the inferior vena cava which drains the lower limbs and the abdomen (Plate 24). The venæ cavæ return the blood to the right atrium of the heart.

THE PULMONARY CIRCULATION

The pulmonary circulation is the circulation of blood through the respiratory tissue of the lungs. It is maintained by the right side of the heart.

Blood depleted of oxygen and laden with carbon dioxide fills the right atrium. Contraction of the right atrium drives it through the tricuspid valve (see below and Fig. 153) into the right ventricle. This contracts and sends the blood through the pulmonary valve into the pulmonary trunk which conducts the blood by means of the right and left pulmonary arteries to the right and left lungs (Plate 24). After repeated branching these arteries feed the capillary bed in the lungs. The capillaries are in contact with the respiratory epithelium of the alveoli and oxygen is taken up by the blood while carbon dioxide is given off. The blood then drains into the tributaries of the pulmonary veins and is conveyed by two right and two left pulmonary veins to the left atrium of the heart (Plate 24). Thus the left atrium receives oxygenated blood for distribution to the systemic circulation.

It will be noted that the systemic circulation and the pulmonary circulation are quite separate, and that the blood circulates first through one and then through the other.

THE HEART AND PERICARDIUM

The heart is a hollow muscular organ about the size of the closed fist. It is something like a cone in shape and has, therefore, an apex and a base (Fig. 151). It lies in the mediastinum, to the left of the midline opposite the middle four thoracic vertebræ, with its base facing the vertebral column and its apex pointing downwards, forwards and to the left. The central tendon of the diaphragm is below it. The **surface projection** is shown in Fig. 140. *The 'apex beat' is defined as the lowest and most lateral point at which the heart beat can be felt* *distinctly*. It corresponds with the surface marking of the apex and is in the fifth intercostal space just medial to a perpendicular line drawn from the midpoint of the clavicle.

From the outside of the heart it can be observed that the thin-walled right and left atria form the base of the heart and that they lie above, behind and a

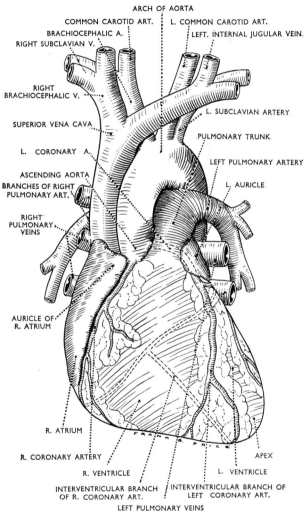

Fig. 151. The heart and great vessels, seen from the front. Compare this with the outline of the heart on the radiograph shown in Fig. 142.

little to the right of the thick-walled right and left ventricles. Projecting from the upper anterior part of each atrium is a small appendage—the (right or left) auricle. (Sometimes the term 'auricle' is used mistakenly for the whole atrium.) A groove, which separates the atria from the ventricles, can be traced right round the heart. It is the **coronary sulcus.**

THE GREAT VESSELS

At the upper border of the heart the **pulmonary artery** emerges from the right ventricle and, behind it, the **ascending aorta** leads from the left ventricle (Fig. 151). The **superior vena cava** enters the upper part of the right atrium and the **inferior vena cava** enters its lowest part. **Two right** and **two left pulmonary veins** open into the left atrium (Plate 25).

THE PERICARDIUM

The heart and the parts of the great vessels close to it are enclosed in a fibrous bag, the **fibrous pericardium.** Covering the exterior of the heart and lining the interior of the fibrous pericardium are the visceral and parietal layers respectively of a serous membrane, the **serous pericardium.** The visceral layer of the serous pericardium is also called the epicardium. The adjacent smooth surfaces of the serous pericardium allow the heart to move freely within the fibrous pericardium (Fig. 152).

THE INTERIOR OF THE HEART

All the surfaces in the interior of the heart are covered by **endocardium.** The right atrium has in its walls the openings of the superior vena cava, the inferior vena cava and the coronary sinus. It communicates with the right ventricle through a large opening, the **right atrioventricular foramen** which is guarded by the **tricuspid valve.** The left atrium has openings for the two right and the two left pulmonary veins and communicates with the left ventricle through the **left atrioventricular foramen** which is guarded by the **mitral valve.** The **interatrial septum** is a thin partition which separates the cavity of the right atrium from that of the left. It contains an ovoid depression—the **fossa ovalis** which is the site of the flap-valve for guarding the foramen ovale in the fetus (p. 389). Sometimes the foramen ovale persists after birth and is then one kind of 'hole in the heart'.

The cavities of the right and left ventricles are completely separated by a

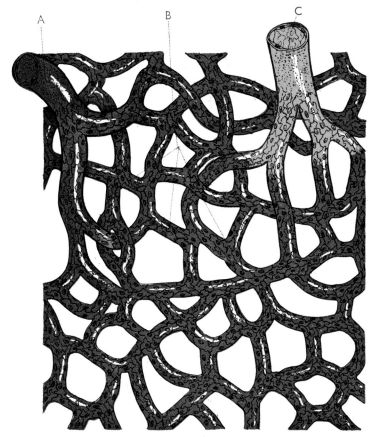

Plate 23. An arteriole, A; feeding a capillary plexus, B; drained by a venule, C.

[facing page 358

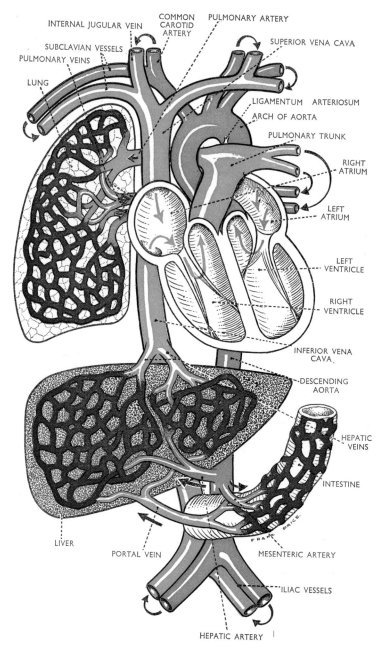

INTERNAL JUGULAR VEIN

COMMON
CAROTID
ARTERY

PULMONARY ARTERY

SUBCLAVIAN VESSELS

SUPERIOR VENA CAVA

PULMONARY VEINS

LUNG

LIGAMENTUM ARTERIOSUM

ARCH OF AORTA

PULMONARY TRUNK

RIGHT ATRIUM

LEFT ATRIUM

LEFT VENTRICLE

RIGHT VENTRICLE

INFERIOR VENA CAVA.

DESCENDING AORTA

HEPATIC VEINS

INTESTINE

LIVER

PORTAL VEIN

MESENTERIC ARTERY

ILIAC VESSELS

HEPATIC ARTERY

Plate 24. A diagram of the circulation of the blood. Oxygenated blood is red,
deoxygenated blood is blue.

[between pages 358/9 facing Pl. 25

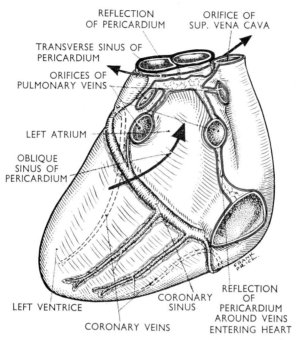

REFLECTION
OF PERICARDIUM

ORIFICE OF
SUP. VENA CAVA

TRANSVERSE SINUS OF
PERICARDIUM

ORIFICES OF
PULMONARY VEINS

LEFT ATRIUM

OBLIQUE
SINUS OF
PERICARDIUM

LEFT VENTRICE

CORONARY
SINUS

REFLECTION
OF
PERICARDIUM
AROUND VEINS
ENTERING HEART

CORONARY VEINS

Plate 25. The heart, seen from behind. The reflection of the serous pericardium round the arteries is shown in red; the reflection round the great veins is shown in blue.

[between pages 358/9 facing Pl. 24

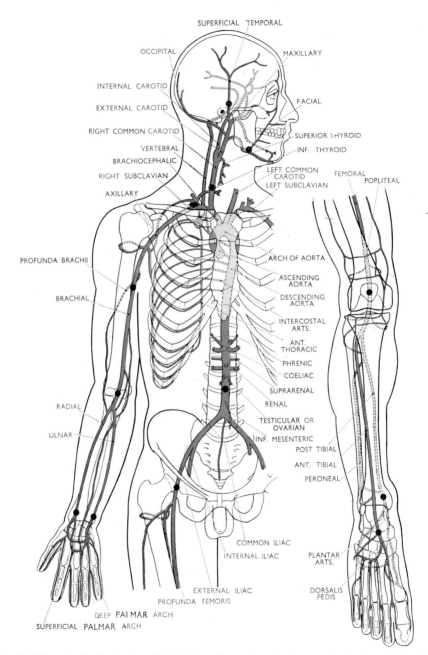

Plate 26. The principal arteries of the body, shown in relation to the skeleton. The black spots mark the pressure points.

[facing page 359

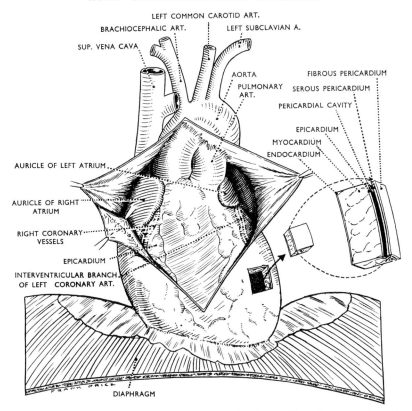

LEFT COMMON CAROTID ART.
BRACHIOCEPHALIC ART.
LEFT SUBCLAVIAN A.
SUP. VENA CAVA
AORTA
PULMONARY ART.
FIBROUS PERICARDIUM
SEROUS PERICARDIUM
PERICARDIAL CAVITY
EPICARDIUM
MYOCARDIUM
ENDOCARDIUM
AURICLE OF LEFT ATRIUM
AURICLE OF RIGHT ATRIUM
RIGHT CORONARY VESSELS
EPICARDIUM
INTERVENTRICULAR BRANCH OF LEFT CORONARY ART.
DIAPHRAGM

Fig. 152. The heart and pericardium seen from the front. The fibrous pericardium and the parietal layer of the serous pericardium have been opened to show the visceral layer of the serous pericardium, the epicardium. The inset shows the layers of the heart wall and pericardium.

thick wall of cardiac muscle, the **interventricular septum.** The right ventricle opens through the **pulmonary valve** into the pulmonary artery and the left ventricle opens through the **aortic valve** into the aorta.

The right and left atrioventricular foramina lie side by side (Fig. 153) and their margins are strengthened by fibrous connective tissue called the **fibrous rings** which are arranged like the figure eight (Fig. 155). This fibrous tissue separates completely the cardiac muscle of the atria from that of the ventricles.

The Valves of the Heart

The valves of the heart are made up of **cusps** which are thin flaps of fibrous tissue covered by endocardium. The cusps are arranged to allow blood to flow in one direction only.

The **tricuspid** and **mitral** valves have cusps which are triangular, with one side attached to the margin of the atrioventricular foramen and the other two sides anchored by **fibrous cords** (Chordæ tendinæ) to muscular processes projecting from the walls of the corresponding ventricle (Plate 24). These processes are called **papillary muscles.** The tricuspid valve has three cusps and the mitral valve has two (Fig. 153). When the atria contract, blood is easily pushed

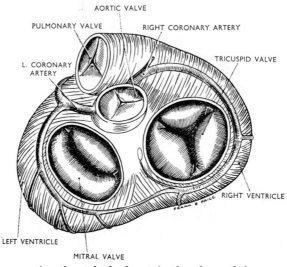

Fig. 153. An oblique section through the heart in the plane of the coronary sulcus, seen from above to show the coronary arteries and the valves of the heart.

between the cusps into the ventricles, but when the ventricles contract the cusps bulge towards the atria, their edges meet, are held in place by the cords which are taut because of the contracting papillary muscles (Fig. 155). Backflow of blood into the atria is prevented in this way.

The **aortic** and **pulmonary** valves are known as 'semilunar valves' because of the shape of their cusps (Fig. 153). Each has three cusps which are like 'half-moon' shaped pockets on the wall of the artery, and are similar to the cusps of venous valves (p. 354). When the ventricles contract blood flows into the aorta and pulmonary artery. When the ventricles relax the pressure exerted by the elastic walls of these arteries drives blood into the pockets, so that the edges of adjacent pockets meet and prevent the blood from flowing back into the ventricles. Sometimes one or more of the valves is damaged by disease. If a valve does not open fully, it does not let enough blood through and is said to be **stenosed.** If it does not shut properly, it allows some blood to flow in the wrong direction and is then said to be **incompetent.**

The Conducting System of the Heart

Conduction, a property of the protoplasm of all cells, is especially well developed in nerve cells. Cardiac muscle, too, is specialized for conduction and a part of it, more specialized in this way than the rest, is called the **conducting**

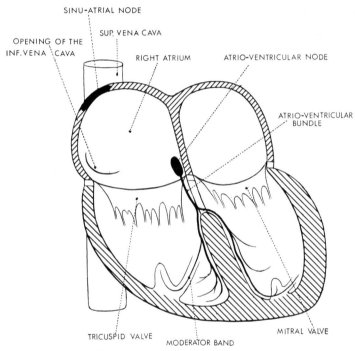

SINU-ATRIAL NODE

OPENING OF THE
INF. VENA CAVA

SUP. VENA CAVA

RIGHT ATRIUM

ATRIO-VENTRICULAR NODE

ATRIO-VENTRICULAR
BUNDLE

TRICUSPID VALVE

MODERATOR BAND

MITRAL VALVE

Fig. 154. A diagram of the conducting system of the heart.

system of the heart. This comprises the sinu-atrial node, the atrio-ventricular node and the atrio-ventricular bundle (Bundle of His) (Fig. 154).

All cardiac muscle has the unusual property of contracting rhythmically without stimulation by a nerve. The conducting system is necessary so that the contraction, once started, may spread through the heart muscle in such a way that the blood is pushed out of the atria into the ventricles, and then out of the ventricles into the aorta and pulmonary artery.

The **sinu-atrial node** (S.A. node) is an area in the wall of the right atrium near the opening of the superior vena cava. Although all cardiac muscle can contract rhythmically without nervous stimulation, the S.A. node is especially well developed in this respect. Each contraction of the heart starts at the S.A. node which is, therefore, often called the **'pacemaker'**. From there the contraction spreads in all directions through the cardiac muscle of the walls of the atria until it reaches the fibrous rings. In the wall of the right atrium, near the fibrous rings and close to the upper end of the interventricular septum, lies the **atrio-ventricular node** (A.V. node), from which the **atrio-ventricular** bundle (A.V. bundle) made up of special conducting fibres of cardiac muscle, passes across the fibrous rings into the interventricular septum. There it divides into a right branch, directed to the furthest part of the right ventricle, and a left branch to the apex of the left ventricle. The contraction passes rather slowly

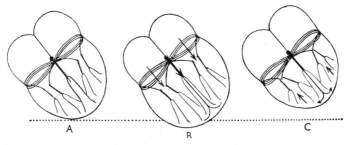

Fig. 155. A diagram to show the contracting atria and ventricles. The fibrous rings are shown as a figure of eight. A, the resting heart; B, atrial, systole driving blood downwards into the relaxed ventricles; C, ventricular systole, driving blood upwards into the aorta and pulmonary trunk while atrial filling starts.

across the A.V. node. This allows the contraction of both atria to be completed, As soon as the contraction reaches the A.V. bundle, it passes very rapidly to the furthest parts of the ventricles. These contract first at these distal parts, then nearer and nearer to the aorta and pulmonary artery, thus driving the blood into these great vessels.

The conducting system of the heart is so arranged that the contraction spreads in an orderly way through the heart to ensure the efficient emptying of the chambers, that is in a general downward direction in the atria and upwards in the ventricles (Fig. 155).

Other parts of the cardiac muscle besides the S.A. node can, in some circumstances, start the contraction. Indeed, if the A.V. bundle is interrupted by disease (a condition called heart-block), the ventricles, now cut off from the atria, begin to beat at their own slow inherent rate of about 40 per minute.

Blood Supply

The heart is supplied by the **right** and **left coronary arteries** (p. 370) and is drained by numerous veins of which the most important is the **coronary sinus** (p. 375 and Plate 25).

Nerve Supply

Although the heart beats rhythmically without nervous stimulation, it is supplied by sympathetic nerves from the cervical ganglia of the sympathetic trunk and by parasympathetic nerves which are branches of the vagus. These nerves regulate the heart rate and the force of the contraction (p. 385).

THE HEART BEAT

The heart beat is the contraction of the heart muscle. *Each* **beat** *consists of the simultaneous contraction of the two atria followed by the simultaneous contraction of the two ventricles.* The beat recurs regularly and rhythmically throughout life to maintain the circulation of the blood.

The **heart rate** *is the number of times the heart beats per minute,* and is **70 to 80** in an adult at rest. The rate is 140 in the newborn infant, and this gradually decreases until the age of puberty. An increase in the normal heart rate is called **tachycardia.** This occurs in exercise, when the heart has to pump more blood to the active muscles, and in some emotional states. It is associated too with fever. A decrease in the heart rate is **bradycardia.** It is found in athletes in training and in the elderly.

The heart rate usually corresponds with the pulse rate (p. 379). Occasionally in disease, some of the beats of the heart may be too weak to distend the peripheral arteries enough to make the distension palpable. Then the heart rate is greater than the pulse rate.

Control of the Heart Rate

The heart rate is controlled reflexly by the cardiac centre in the medulla. From it, parasympathetic impulses in the vagus nerve slow the heart rate. Sympathetic impulses, via the cardiac branches of the cervical sympathetic trunk, increase the heart rate.

The cardiac centre is stimulated to slow the heart rate by:

1. Stimulation of the stretch receptors in the carotid sinus (p. 386) by rising blood pressure.
2. Shock or fainting.

The cardiac centre is stimulated to increase the heart rate by:

1. Stimulation of chemoreceptors in the carotid body (p. 387) by a lowering in the oxygen tension of the blood.
2. Emotion or fright.
3. Pain impulses from most parts of the body.

Sinus Arrhythmia

The heart rate is often found, especially in children, to be faster during inspiration than during expiration. This is called sinus arrhythmia. Part of the explanation is that the increased venous return during inspiration (p. 384) reflexly causes an increase in the heart rate (p. 363). Reflexes which influence the respiratory and cardiac centres simultaneously are also involved.

The Cardiac Cycle

The cardiac cycle is the series of events which occur during one complete beat of the heart.

Contraction of the two atria is simultaneous and is called **atrial systole:** relaxation of the atria is called **atrial diastole:** similarly **ventricular systole** is the simultaneous contraction of the two ventricles, **ventricular diastole** is their relaxation.

If the heart is beating at the rate of 75 beats per minute, each cardiac cycle is lasting 0·8 second. Atrial systole takes 0·1 second, ventricular systole takes 0·3 second and during the remaining 0·4 second both atria and ventricles are resting, that is they are in diastole. When the heart rate quickens, for example in muscular exercise, the duration of atrial and ventricular systole remains the same, but diastole is shortened.

Because the changes occur simultaneously and in the same way in both the left and right sides of the heart, it will be enough to consider the changes in one side only, for example, in the left side.

Before the beginning of a contraction, the left atrium and the left ventricle are both in diastole. Blood is flowing into the atrium from the pulmonary veins and also from the left atrium into the left ventricle. Atrial systole then occurs and completes the filling of the ventricles. Ventricular systole follows immediately. Pressure of the blood in the contracting ventricle forces shut the mitral valve, pushes open the aortic valve and drives the blood out into the aorta. Meanwhile atrial diastole has begun, and the atrium is filling from the veins. Ventricular systole over, ventricular diastole begins, and the pressure inside the ventricle drops. The elastic wall of the aorta, stretched by the blood forced into it under high pressure by the contraction of the left ventricle now recoils and, as well as driving the blood onwards into the systemic circulation, fills the cusps of the aortic valve and snaps it shut. Since the pressure inside the left ventricle has fallen the mitral valve can now be opened by the blood which has collected in the left atrium and so the left ventricle begins to fill again. Conditions are now the same as when the cycle started, ready for the next to begin.

Heart Sounds

During the cardiac cycle certain sounds are produced. These can be heard by the ear placed in contact with the chest wall, or, more conveniently, through a stethoscope. Two sounds are heard with each heart beat—the **first sound** is a booming 'lubb' separated by a very short pause from the **second sound**, a shorter and more staccato 'dup'. A longer pause follows before the sequence is repeated. The first sound is produced by the contraction of the ventricles and the closing of the atrioventricular valves; the second is produced by the closing of the semilunar valves. Unusual extra sounds, known as **mumurs**, are sometimes heard. Stenosed or incompetent valves are a common cause.

ELECTROCARDIOGRAM

When any muscle contracts, electrical changes occur. The heart is no exception, and the electrical changes associated with each beat of the heart can be

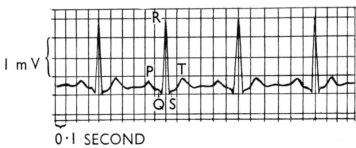

Fig. 156. An electrocardiogram (E.C.G.), showing the electrical record of four normal cardiac cycles.

recorded. Such a record, or **electrocardiogram,** is shown in Fig. 156. The wave marked 'P' is due to activity in the atria, 'Q.R.S.' is associated with the contraction in the ventricles and 'T' with the end of ventricular activity.

EXTERNAL CARDIAC MASSAGE

When the heart stops beating as a result of respiratory failure, it is sometimes possible to start it again by means of external cardiac massage. The technique is not without danger, and must not be attempted unless it is certain that the heart has stopped.

During mouth to mouth resuscitation (p. 345), ten or twelve breaths should bring about an improvement in the colour of skin and lips. If it does not, feel for the pulse at the carotid pressure point. If there is no pulse there, external cardiac massage should be started (Fig. 157).

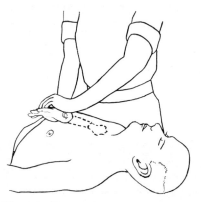

Fig. 157. External cardiac massage.

Continuing mouth to mouth resuscitation, place the patient on a firm surface like the ground or a table. Find the lower half of the sternum by palpating the chest. In an adult, place the palm of one hand over the lower half of the sternum and place the second hand on top of the first. After each inflation of the lungs, apply six to eight sharp presses, at the rate of one per second. In an infant or young child, place two fingers on the lower half of the sternum and apply six to eight sharp, but not violent, presses, one per second.

Check the pulse frequently, and stop cardiac massage as soon as the normal beat returns.

Mouth to mouth resuscitation and external cardiac massage can be carried out by one person. It is easier if two are present, one to do the mouth to mouth resuscitation and check the pulse, the other to perform the external cardiac massage.

THE CIRCULATION

THE BLOOD VESSELS

The description always follows the direction of the blood flow. **Arteries** *carry oxygenated blood, begin nearer the heart and give off branches.* **Veins** *carry deoxygenated blood, begin further away from the heart and receive tributaries.* The pulmonary vessels are exceptions to this general rule, in that the pulmonary artery contains deoxygenated blood and the pulmonary vein contains oxygenated blood.

THE ARTERIES

Aorta

The aorta is the main artery of the systemic circulation. It is about 2·5 cms in diameter and arises from the left ventricle. The first 5 cms, the **ascending aorta,** is directed upwards and to the right. The **arch of the aorta** then bends to the left and backwards, arching in front of the trachea and above the root of the left lung. At the end of the curve, the **descending thoracic aorta** begins, and passes downwards through the thorax in the mediastinum close to the vertebral column. It pierces the diaphragm at the level of the twelfth thoracic vertebra and becomes the **abdominal aorta.** This descends as far as the fourth lumbar vertebra where it divides into its two terminal branches, the left and right common iliac arteries.

Pressure Point. The **aorta** can be felt beating through a relaxed abdominal wall. It can be compressed by pressing firmly backwards against the bodies of the lumbar vertebræ.

MAIN BRANCHES OF THE AORTA:

Ascending Aorta	Right and left coronary arteries
Arch of Aorta	Brachiocephalic trunk (innominate)
	Left common carotid
	Left subclavian
Descending thoracic aorta	Posterior intercostal arteries (8 pairs)

Abdominal Aorta:

Unpaired	*Paired*
Cœliac	Suprarenal
Superior mesenteric	Renal
Inferior mesenteric	Ovarian or testicular
	Lumbar (4 pairs)
	Common iliac

THE ARTERIES OF THE HEAD AND NECK

The head and neck are supplied by the right and left **common carotid arteries** assisted by several branches of the subclavian arteries, the most important of which are the right and left **vertebral arteries.**

The **left common carotid** arises from the arch of the aorta (Plate 26). The **right common carotid** arises from the **brachiocephalic trunk** (innominate artery) behind the right sternoclavicular joint. Each common carotid artery ascends lateral to the trachea to the level of the upper border of the thyroid cartilage where it divides into the **external carotid artery** (distributed to the face and to the skull) and the **internal carotid artery** (distributed inside the skull, mainly to the cerebral cortex). The common carotid and internal carotid arteries are accompanied throughout their course by the internal jugular vein and the vagus nerve, all enclosed in a tube of fascia called the **carotid sheath** (Plate 6). The common carotid artery can be compressed against the transverse process of the sixth cervical vertebra, which is at the level of the cricoid cartilage. The beginning of the internal carotid artery is slightly dilated to form the **carotid sinus** (Fig. 89), which is sensitive to changes in the blood pressure. Near the carotid sinus lies a small ovoid mass of special cells called the **carotid body.** The cells are sensitive to a lowering of the oxygen tension and to a raising of the carbon dioxide tension of the blood. Afferent nerve fibres travel from the carotid sinus and the carotid body to the medulla of the brain in the glosso-pharyngeal nerve. The internal carotid artery enters the skull. Then it gives off the **ophthalmic artery** for the structures in the orbit, as well as the **anterior and middle cerebral arteries** which supply the greater part of the cerebral hemisphere. Branches of the internal carotid artery join on the base of the brain with those of the opposite side and with the **posterior cerebral arteries** derived from the vertebral arteries, to form an important anastomosis called the **cerebral arterial circle** (circle of Willis) (Plate 10).

The cerebral arteries have thinner walls than other arteries and therefore rupture more easily than other arteries, for example when the blood pressure is pathologically high.

The **external carotid artery** has several branches. The **superior thyroid artery** helps to supply the thyroid gland. The **lingual artery** goes to the tongue. The **facial artery** supplies the face and can be felt pulsating at the lower border of the mandible in front of the masseter muscle. The **superficial temporal artery,** which supplies part of the scalp, can be felt in front of the external auditory meatus (Plate 26). The **maxillary artery** which supplies the deep parts of the face, has an important branch, the **middle meningeal artery.**

This enters the skull through the small foramen spinosum in the base of the skull and occupies a deep groove, sometimes a tunnel, in the wall of the middle cranial fossa (Fig. 43). Thus anchored, it is liable to be torn if the skull is injured or if the head is hit or rocked violently, and severe extradural intra-cranial hæmorrhage results.

The **vertebral artery** arises from the subclavian artery, courses upwards through the foramina in the transverse processes of the upper six cervical verte-bræ and enters the skull through the foramen magnum. The two vertebral arteries unite to form the **basilar artery,** and from it branches supply the medulla, the pons, the cerebellum and, by means of the **posterior cerebral artery,** the posterior part of the cerebral hemisphere. The posterior cerebral arteries form the posterior part of the cerebral arterial circle.

PRESSURE POINTS

A **pressure point** *is a site where an artery can be compressed against a bone.* Its pulsation can be felt there. Also, the lumen can be obliterated by firm pres-sure to stop the blood flow through it. In this way hæmorrhage from the artery may be controlled.

The pressure points for the whole body are illustrated in Plate 26 and are described as follows:

Head and neck, *vide infra*
Upper limb, p. 370
Abdomen, p. 367
Lower limb, p. 374

Pressure Points in the Head and Neck (Plate 26)

The **subclavian artery** can be compressed against the first rib, behind the medial third of the clavicle.

The **common carotid artery** can be compressed against the transverse process of the sixth cervical vertebra, lateral to the ring of the cricoid cartilage.

The **facial artery** can be compressed against the lower border of the mandible in front of the masseter muscle (Fig. 84).

The **superficial temporal artery** can be compressed against the skull just above the external auditory meatus (Fig. 84).

ARTERIES OF THE UPPER LIMB

The **subclavian artery** (Plate 26) is the main channel of supply to the upper limb. It also sends several branches to other parts, notably the **vertebral** artery to the brain stem, to the cerebellum and to the posterior part of the cerebral hemisphere, the **anterior thoracic artery** (internal mammary) to the front of the chest wall, and the **inferior thyroid artery** to the thyroid gland. On the left side the subclavian artery arises from the arch of the aorta and on the right side from the brachiocephalic trunk. Each subclavian artery then arches laterally over the apex of the lung across the first rib and behind the clavicle to enter the apex of the axilla, where it is called the **axillary artery.** As it leaves the axilla it becomes the **brachial artery** which traverses the upper arm, at first medial to and then in front of the shaft of the humerus. It can be felt and compressed against the humerus. Just below the elbow joint in the cubital fossa (p. 196) it divides into the **radial artery** and the **ulnar artery** which descend to the wrist, the radial artery on the lateral side of the forearm, the ulnar artery on the medial side. The radial artery can be felt pulsating where it lies just under the skin in front of the lower end of the radius. Here the 'pulse' is usually 'taken'. The radial and ulnar arteries end by joining in the formation of two arches, the **superficial palmar arch** and the **deep palmar arch** which lie in the palm of the hand (Fig. 135).

Branches from these main arteries supply all the structures in the limb.

Pressure Points (Plate 26)

The **subclavian artery** can be pressed downwards against the first rib, behind the middle third of the clavicle.

The **brachial artery** can be compressed against the humerus by pressing laterally on the medial side of the upper part of the shaft, and also by pressing backwards against the lower end in the cubital fossa.

The **radial artery** can be compressed against the front of the lower end of the radius.

The **ulnar artery** can be compressed with difficulty against the lower end of the ulna.

THE ARTERIES OF THE THORAX

1. ARTERIES OF THE THORACIC WALLS (PARIETAL ARTERIES): The intercostal spaces are supplied by **posterior intercostal arteries,** most of which are branches of the thoracic aorta, and **anterior intercostal arteries** from the **anterior thoracic artery** (internal mammary) which comes from the subclavian artery (Plate 26).

2. ARTERIES OF THE THORACIC VISCERA (VISCERAL ARTERIES): The **right** and **left coronary arteries** (Fig. 151), branches of the ascending aorta, supply the heart. They arise just beyond the aortic valve. The right coronary

artery runs to the right in the coronary sulcus, and the left one to the left for a short distance. The left coronary artery then divides into the anterior interventricular artery and the circumflex artery which continues in the coronary sulcus to anastomose with the right coronary artery. The right coronary artery also gives an interventricular branch on the inferior aspect of the heart.

Small branches from the descending thoracic aorta supply the roots of the lungs and the œsophagus.

The Pulmonary Trunk

The **pulmonary trunk** (Fig. 151) is the main artery of the pulmonary circulation. It arises from the right ventricle of the heart and is directed upwards, backwards and to the left. It is 5 cm long, and ends by dividing into the right and left pulmonary arteries which go to the right and left lungs respectively. The **ligamentum arteriosum** connects the pulmonary trunk with the arch of the aorta distal to the origin of the left subclavian artery (Plate 24).

It should be noted that the arteries of the pulmonary circulation carry **deoxygenated blood** from the heart to the lungs.

Development of the Arteries

In the early embryo six pairs of arterial arches, one for each branchial arch (p. 428), lead from the single ventral aorta to the twin dorsal aortæ (Fig. 158, A).

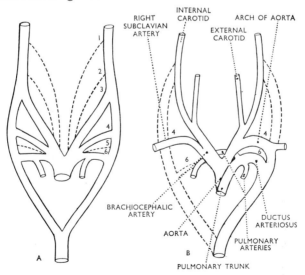

Fig. 158. The development of the branchial arch arteries. A, the early pattern; B, the final pattern; vessels which disappear during development are indicated by interrupted lines.

As development proceeds, the vessels are rearranged so that blood from the left ventricle reaches the aorta and blood from the right ventricle reaches the pulmonary arteries (Fig. 158, B). The fourth arch arteries form the subclavian artery on the right and the aortic arch on the left. The sixth arch arteries form the pulmonary arteries and, in addition, on the left, the ductus arteriosus.

ARTERIES OF THE ABDOMEN AND PELVIS

Arteries are distributed to the abdomen from the abdominal aorta. The aorta ends by dividing into **right and left common iliac arteries.** Opposite the sacro-iliac joint, on the brim of the lesser pelvis, the common iliac artery divides into the **external iliac** and the **internal iliac** arteries. The external iliac artery follows the brim of the pelvis, and passes behind the inguinal ligament to enter the lower limb as the femoral artery. The internal iliac artery supplies the walls and most of the viscera of the lesser pelvis.

ARTERIES OF THE ABDOMINAL WALLS: The posterior abdominal wall is supplied by **lumbar arteries,** branches of the abdominal aorta (corresponding with the posterior intercostal arteries in the thorax). The anterior abdominal wall, however, is also supplied by arteries from other sources. The **lowest posterior intercostal arteries** supply the lateral part, branches from the **anterior thoracic artery** the upper part, and a branch from the external iliac artery, the **inferior epigastric artery,** supplies the lower part.

ARTERIES OF THE ABDOMINAL VISCERA:

Branches of Abdominal Aorta

1. Unpaired Branches

The abdominal aorta has three large unpaired branches which supply the alimentary tract and the organs associated with it. They are:

(a) The cœliac trunk (which supplies the foregut and its derivatives, p. 428).
(b) The superior mesenteric artery (which supplies the midgut, p. 429).
(c) The inferior mesenteric artery (which supplies the hindgut, p. 429).

(a) The **cœliac trunk** (Fig. 159 and Plate 27) is very short and divides at once into three important branches; the **left gastric artery** runs to the left and supplies part of the stomach; the **splenic artery** travels to the left to reach the spleen, and also gives branches to the pancreas and to the stomach: the **hepatic artery** goes to the right to supply the liver with oxygenated blood, and it also gives branches to the stomach and to the gall bladder.

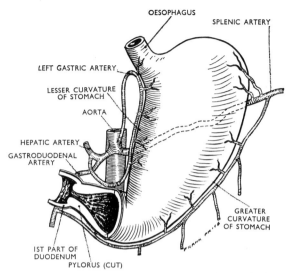

OESOPHAGUS

SPLENIC ARTERY

LEFT GASTRIC ARTERY

LESSER CURVATURE
OF STOMACH

AORTA

HEPATIC ARTERY

GASTRODUODENAL
ARTERY

GREATER
CURVATURE
OF STOMACH

IST PART OF
DUODENUM

PYLORUS (CUT)

Fig. 159. The stomach, showing its blood supply derived from the branches of the cœliac artery. Part of the pylorus has been cut away to show the pyloric sphincter.

(b) The **superior mesenteric artery** (Plate 27 and Fig. 188) supplies the whole of the small intestine and the large intestine from the appendix to the junction of the middle and distal thirds of the transverse colon. The branches to the small intestine reach it through the mesentery, and those to the large intestine travel over the posterior abdominal wall, or in the transverse meso-colon.

(c) The **inferior mesenteric artery** (Plate 27 and Fig. 188) supplies the large intestine from the left colic flexure onwards, including the rectum, which lies in the lesser pelvis.

2. Paired Branches

There are three sets of paired visceral branches (Plate 27), the suprarenal arteries, the renal arteries and the testicular or ovarian arteries.

(a) The **suprarenal arteries** are small and supply the suprarenal gland.

(b) The **renal arteries** are large vessels which arise from the sides of the aorta at the level of the second lumbar vertebra. They supply the kidneys with a large volume of blood under high pressure.

(c) The **ovarian** or **testicular arteries** arise just below the renal arteries. In the female, the ovarian artery has a long course down the posterior abdominal wall to the ovary in the lesser pelvis. In the male, the testicular artery has a similar course, but it is even longer because it traverses the inguinal canal to reach the testis in the scrotum.

ARTERIES OF THE LESSER PELVIS: The **internal iliac artery** (Plate 28) supplies the lesser pelvis.

Branches of Internal Iliac Artery

Parietal Branches

In addition to **branches to the pelvic walls,** the internal iliac artery gives off the **gluteal arteries** to the gluteal muscles, the **obturator artery** to the adductor muscles and the **internal pudendal artery** to the perineum.

Visceral Branches

The most important visceral branches of the internal iliac artery (Plate 28) are the **vesical arteries** and, in the female, the **uterine arteries.** In the adult the superior vesical artery (umbilical artery of fetus) can be traced beyond the bladder as a fibrous cord, the lateral umbilical ligament, upwards over the internal aspect of the abdominal wall to the umbilicus (see p. 391).

ARTERIES OF THE LOWER LIMB

The **femoral artery** (Plate 26) is the main artery of the lower limb. It begins as the continuation of the external iliac artery where it passes behind the inguinal ligament. The femoral artery travels down the front of the thigh, passing through the femoral triangle (p. 216), then through the subsartorial canal (p. 216). It then passes through an opening in the lower part of the adductor magnus to reach the popliteal fossa at the back of the knee. Here it is called the **popliteal artery** (Fig. 100). This passes downwards through the popliteal fossa, and at its lower end divides into the **posterior tibial artery** and the **anterior tibial artery.** The posterior tibial artery continues downwards between the flexor muscles on the back of the leg and at the ankle joint, as it passes behind the medial malleolus, it divides into the **medial** and **lateral plantar arteries,** which form the **plantar arch** and supply the sole of the foot. The anterior tibial artery pierces the interosseous membrane to reach the front of the leg and descends between the extensor muscles to the ankle joint. From there it continues on to the dorsum of the foot, as the **dorsalis pedis** artery.

THE PRESSURE POINTS in the lower limb are as follows:

The femoral artery can be compressed against the front of the hip joint just below the inguinal ligament.

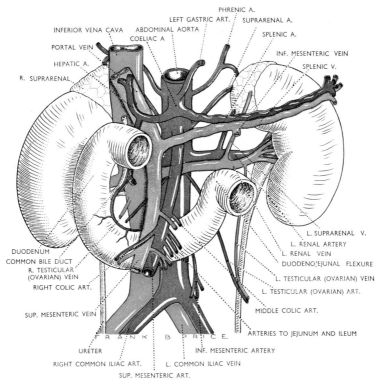

PHRENIC A.

LEFT GASTRIC ART.   SUPRARENAL A.

INFERIOR VENA CAVA   ABDOMINAL AORTA   SPLENIC A.
                     COELIAC A

PORTAL VEIN   INF. MESENTERIC VEIN

HEPATIC A.   SPLENIC V.

R. SUPRARENAL

                                           L. SUPRARENAL V.
                                           L. RENAL ARTERY
                                           L. RENAL VEIN
DUODENUM   DUODENOJEJUNAL FLEXURE
COMMON BILE DUCT
R. TESTICULAR   L. TESTICULAR (OVARIAN) VEIN
(OVARIAN) VEIN
RIGHT COLIC ART.   L. TESTICULAR (OVARIAN) ART.

                                           MIDDLE COLIC ART.
SUP. MESENTERIC VEIN

                                           ARTERIES TO JEJUNUM AND ILEUM
FRANK B PRICE

URETER   INF. MESENTERIC ARTERY

RIGHT COMMON ILIAC ART.   L. COMMON ILIAC VEIN

SUP. MESENTERIC ART.

Plate 27. The principal arteries and veins of the abdomen. The portal vein and its tributaries
are coloured mauve, to distinguish them from the systemic veins.

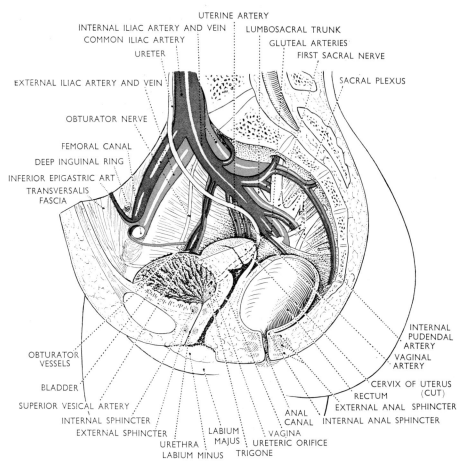

UTERINE ARTERY

INTERNAL ILIAC ARTERY AND VEIN

COMMON ILIAC ARTERY

URETER

LUMBOSACRAL TRUNK

GLUTEAL ARTERIES

FIRST SACRAL NERVE

EXTERNAL ILIAC ARTERY AND VEIN

SACRAL PLEXUS

OBTURATOR NERVE

FEMORAL CANAL

DEEP INGUINAL RING

INFERIOR EPIGASTRIC ART

TRANSVERSALIS
FASCIA

INTERNAL
PUDENDAL
ARTERY

VAGINAL
ARTERY

OBTURATOR
VESSELS

BLADDER

SUPERIOR VESICAL ARTERY

INTERNAL SPHINCTER

EXTERNAL SPHINCTER

URETHRA

LABIUM MINUS

LABIUM
MAJUS

TRIGONE

VAGINA

URETERIC ORIFICE

ANAL
CANAL

RECTUM

INTERNAL ANAL SPHINCTER

CERVIX OF UTERUS
(CUT)

EXTERNAL ANAL SPHINCTER

Plate 28. A sagittal section through the female pelvis to show the arteries and veins of the lesser pelvis, together with the sacral plexus and parts of the viscera.

[facing page 375

The popliteal artery is accessible in the popliteal fossa, if the knee is bent.

The posterior tibial artery can be compressed against the back of the medial malleolus and the dorsalis pedis can be felt on the proximal part of the dorsum of the foot, lateral to the tendon of the extensor of the great toe.

THE VEINS

Veins begin by the union of tributaries and, in the systemic circulation, carry deoxygenated blood from the capillary bed back towards the heart.

PULMONARY VEINS

The veins of the pulmonary circulation are the four **pulmonary veins,** two from the right lung and two from the left. They open into the left atrium of the heart. Note that the pulmonary veins carry **oxygenated blood** from the lungs to the heart.

SYSTEMIC VEINS

The veins of the systemic circulation form three large trunks which open into the right atrium of the heart. They are:

1. The **superior vena cava** which drains the head and neck, the upper limbs and the thoracic wall.
2. The **inferior vena cava** which drains the abdominal walls, the abdominal viscera and the lower limbs, and
3. The **coronary sinus** which drains the heart wall. (Plate 25)

General Arrangement of the Systemic Veins

Veins in every region are arranged in two sets:

(*a*) superficial and (*b*) deep.

The **superficial veins** lie in the connective tissue just under the skin. They are numerous, anastomose freely, communicate with the deep veins and finally empty into the deep veins as they leave their territory of drainage. The majority are not associated with arteries. Their walls are thicker and more muscular than the deep veins and they have more numerous valves.

The **deep veins** follow the arteries of a region closely. The smaller arteries are accompanied by two **venæ comitantes** and the large arteries are accompanied by one large vein.

THE VEINS OF THE HEAD AND NECK

Superficial Veins

These drain the face and scalp and some of them unite to form the **external jugular vein.** This vein is readily observed where it crosses the sternomastoid muscle before entering the subclavian vein. It stands out particularly well when a person coughs or strains.

The Deep Veins

The veins of the brain drain into the **venous sinuses of the skull** (Plate 29) which are channels between two layers of the dura mater (p. 258). They are lined with endothelium. The largest are the **cavernous sinus,** the **superior sagittal sinus,** the **transverse sinus** and the **sigmoid sinus** (Plate 29). The sigmoid sinus, towards which all the sinuses converge, is continuous with the **internal jugular vein** at the jugular foramen in the base of the skull. The internal jugular vein, therefore, drains the blood from the brain. It descends in the neck (Plate 34), inside the carotid sheath (p. 188), receiving tributaries from the structures in the neck, and ends on both right and left sides, by uniting with the subclavian vein behind the medial end of the clavicle to form the brachio-cephalic vein (innominate vein) of that side (Fig. 169).

THE VEINS OF THE UPPER LIMB

The **superficial veins** (Plate 30) are numerous and those in the cubital fossa, forearm and hand are used frequently for intravenous injections. On the back of the hand an irregular arch of veins can be seen. From its lateral end emerges the **cephalic vein** and from its medial end the **basilic vein.** The cephalic vein travels upwards along the lateral border of the limb, until it dips into the deep tissues just below the clavicle to join the axillary vein. The basilic vein follows the medial border of the limb to the middle of the upper arm, where it becomes deep, and joins the venæ comitantes of the brachial artery. The **median cubital vein** connects the cephalic and basilic veins in the cubital fossa. The sites of the valves (p. 354) in these veins can be demonstrated by milking the blood along the vein away from the heart with a finger-tip. Short sections of a vein can be emptied in this way, but blood cannot be forced through a valve in the wrong direction. The distended part of the vein proximal to the valve contrasts with the emptied section distal to the valve.

The **deep veins** of the upper limb accompany the arteries. The venæ comitantes of the brachial artery unite with the basilic vein at the lower border of the axilla to form the large **axillary vein,** which traverses the axilla and becomes the **subclavian vein** as it crosses the first rib. The subclavian vein, therefore, drains the whole upper limb. It ends by uniting with the internal jugular vein to form the **brachiocephalic vein** (Fig. 151).

THE VEINS OF THE THORAX

The **right** and **left brachiocephalic veins** unite behind the manubrium of the sternum to form the **superior vena cava** which descends to empty into the right atrium (Fig. 151).

The walls of the thorax are drained by **anterior intercostal veins,** which travel back along branches of the anterior thoracic artery and end in the subclavian vein, and by **posterior intercostal veins** which drain into the **vena azygos** (Fig. 169). The vena azygos ascends along the right side of the thoracic vertebral column, arches forwards above the root of the right lung and ends in the superior vena cava.

VEINS OF THE ABDOMEN AND PELVIS

Venous blood from the abdomen and pelvis reaches the heart through the **inferior vena cava** (Plate 27) which begins at the level of the fifth lumbar vertebra by the union of the **right** and **left common iliac veins.** It ascends along the right side of the abdominal aorta, passes behind the liver, and pierces the central tendon of the diaphragm to enter the right atrium of the heart.

Its tributaries correspond with the **paired** branches of the abdominal aorta and drain the posterior abdominal wall, the kidneys, the suprarenal glands and the ovaries or testes. In addition, just before it pierces the diaphragm the inferior vena cava receives the **right** and **left hepatic veins** from the liver (p. 475).

The veins from the walls of the lesser pelvis and from the pelvic viscera (apart from the intestine and the ovaries) drain mainly into the internal iliac veins, thence to the common iliac veins and inferior vena cava.

THE PORTAL SYSTEM OF THE LIVER

The veins which drain the blood from the intestines and related organs are unusual in that, *after collecting the blood from the capillary bed they do not return it direct to the heart like the other veins, but pour it into another capillary bed* in the liver. The system of veins leading from the capillaries in the intestine to the capillaries in the liver is called the hepatic portal system, and its main large vein is the **portal vein** (Plate 27). Through its tributaries the portal vein drains the blood from the alimentary canal between the lower end of the œsophagus and the upper end of the anal canal, that is, from the stomach, the small intestine and the large intestine. It also receives venous blood from organs which develop in association with the intestine, that is from the pancreas, the spleen and the gall bladder. The tributaries of the portal vein follow closely, and are named after, the arteries which supply these organs. The portal vein itself begins behind the pancreas by union of the **superior mesenteric vein** and the **splenic vein.** It travels upwards behind the duodenum, then in the free edge of the lesser omentum to reach the porta hepatis where it divides into **right** and **left branches** to distribute the blood to the corresponding lobes of the liver (see also p. 475). The blood in the portal vein contains food materials absorbed from the intestine, insulin from the pancreas and iron and bile pigments from the breaking down of red blood cells in the spleen. These materials are carried by the portal system direct to the liver, where the cells are specialized to met-abolize them (p. 478).

Communications between Systemic Veins and Portal Veins

In certain situations, for example, at the lower end of the œsophagus, in the anal canal and round the umbilicus, small veins of the portal system anastomose with small veins of the systemic system. If the blood pressure in the portal veins is higher than normal, these anastomoses become distended or 'varicose'. **Œsophageal varices** may develop in this way. Similar distended veins in the anal canal are called **hæmorrhoids** or 'piles', and distended veins radiating from the umbilicus form a striking pattern called a **'caput Medusæ'.**

VEINS OF THE LOWER LIMB

Superficial Veins (Plates 31 and 32)

The **great saphenous vein** begins on the medial side of the foot. It passes upwards in front of the medial malleolus, where it can always be located for an intravenous infusion. After crossing the subcutaneous surface of the tibia, where it is vulnerable because it lies directly between skin and bone, it reaches the posteromedial aspect of the knee. It then continues upwards across the medial aspect of the thigh to the **saphenous opening** (Fig. 97) where it pierces the deep fascia to enter the femoral vein. The **small saphenous vein** begins on the lateral side of the foot, passes behind the lateral malleolus and upwards over the middle of the calf. It pierces the popliteal fascia and ends in the **popliteal vein.**

Deep Veins (Plates 31 and 32)

The deep veins accompany the arteries. In the popliteal fossa they unite to form the **popliteal vein** which accompanies the popliteal artery and passes through the opening in adductor magnus to become the **femoral vein.** This vein traverses the thigh with the femoral artery and ends by becoming the external iliac vein as it passes behind the inguinal ligament.

There are many communications between the superficial veins and the deep veins to allow blood to drain from the superficial veins into the deep veins (p. 384, Fig. 160). All the veins in the lower limb, especially the superficial veins, have numerous valves (p. 354).

PHYSIOLOGY OF THE CIRCULATION

THE FLOW OF BLOOD IN ARTERIES

The blood in the arteries of the systemic circulation is bright red because it is oxygenated. The pumping action of the left side of the heart produces an intermittent flow, which is converted to a continuous but pulsating flow by the elastic arteries (p. 351). If an artery is cut, the bright red blood escapes in spurts which correspond with the contractions of the left ventricle.

The **velocity of the blood flow** in the blood vessels varies inversely with the total cross sectional area of the vascular bed. The total cross sectional area of all the distributing arteries is very much greater than that of the aorta. Therefore, the blood flows progressively more slowly in these arteries as they are traced away from the heart. In the same way, the blood flow is slower in the arterioles than in the distributing arteries, and slower still in the capillaries.

The **arterial pulse** is the recurring distension of an artery by the rise in blood pressure produced by each contraction of the ventricle. The powerful contraction of the left ventricle discharges blood under high pressure into the aorta. This blood pushes onwards the blood already in the aorta and that in turn pushes on the blood further away. In this way a pressure wave, the **pulse wave,** is transmitted all through the arterial system. It must be noted that the pulse wave is independent of the blood flow and that it travels much more rapidly. The arterial pulse can be felt, in any region where an artery lies between a bone and the skin. It is usually examined in the radial artery near the wrist.

The **pulse rate** is the number of beats of the pulse per minute. The normal adult pulse rate is between 70 and 80 per minute. It is much more rapid in children and diminishes with age as the following table shows:

Fetus in utero	150 per minute
New born	140
1st year	120
2nd year	110
5 years	100
10 years	90
Adult	70–80
Old age	60

The pulse rate usually corresponds exactly with the heart rate (p. 363). Occasionally in disease, some of the beats of the heart may be too weak to distend the peripheral arteries enough to make the distension palpable. Then the heart rate (counted by listening to the heart sounds with a stethoscope) is greater than the pulse rate.

BLOOD PRESSURE

By 'blood pressure' we usually mean the systemic arterial blood pressure, which is the pressure exerted on the walls of the arteries by the blood ejected from the left ventricle. The pressure is naturally greater during ventricular systole. This is the **systolic pressure.** During ventricular diastole the pressure falls, but is maintained to some extent by the recoil of the elastic arteries. This is the **diastolic pressure.** The usual systolic pressure is about 120 mm of mercury and the diastolic pressure 80 mm of mercury. This is written:

Blood pressure = 120/80.

(SI units are not used for measurements of blood pressure as yet.)

Measuring the Blood Pressure

The blood pressure is measured by an instrument called a **sphygmomano-meter.** An inflatable cuff is connected with a column of mercury. The cuff is placed round the upper arm and is inflated until the pressure is well above the systolic blood pressure. This stops the blood flow in the brachial artery. The bell of a stethoscope is placed over the brachial artery in the cubital fossa and the pressure in the cuff is allowed to fall slowly. A sudden clear tapping sound is heard when blood begins to flow again. The height of the mercury in the sphygmomanometer at this point is the systolic pressure. As the pressure is allowed to drop further, the sounds become louder and more muffled and suddenly die away. The reading at this point is the diastolic pressure.

Variations in Blood Pressure

In a given individual the blood pressure varies over a narrow range according to the needs of the body. The blood pressure is lowest when a person is at rest, and a measurement, taken when the subject has been sitting or lying quietly in a warm room for at least half an hour, is known as the **resting blood pressure.** Increased activity, such as muscular exercise, and emotion, such as excitement and anxiety, cause the blood pressure to rise. The systolic pressure rises more than the diastolic pressure.

The blood pressure alters with age. It is low in childhood and rises slowly as the years pass. This is associated with the gradual loss of elasticity in the arteries (p. 604). The blood pressure also varies considerably from one normal person to another, even at the same age. Average values for the resting blood pressure at different ages are given in the table.

Age	6 months	4 years	16 years	20 years	40 years	60 years
Blood Pressure .	90/60	100/62	120/65	120/70	130/80	135/85

Maintenance of Blood Pressure

The blood pressure is maintained at a level sufficient to ensure a blood flow adequate for the metabolic needs of the tissues, and, in particular to ensure an adequate supply of blood to the brain and an adequate filtration pressure in the kidneys.

The blood pressure depends on two main factors:

(*a*) The cardiac output.
(*b*) The peripheral resistance.

CARDIAC OUTPUT: The cardiac output is the volume of blood ejected by each ventricle in one minute. An average figure for a subject at rest is 5 litres per minute. It varies according to the needs of the body. The cardiac output increases greatly in exercise—in trained athletes it may reach 35 litres per minute. It also increases after a meal and in pregnancy.

The cardiac output depends upon:

1. The venous return.
2. The force of the contraction of the heart.
3. The heart rate.

Venous return. If the heart is to eject an adequate volume of blood, it is clear that sufficient blood must reach it from the veins. The factors which influence the flow of blood in the veins back to the heart are discussed on p. 383. They are the capillary and venous blood pressure, the contraction of skeletal muscle, and the intrathoracic negative pressure.

In addition, the total blood volume must be adequate. The average total blood volume is about 5 litres. A severe hæmorrhage or the loss of fluid from the blood into injured tissues reduces the blood volume, so that the venous return becomes inadequate, the cardiac output falls and therefore the blood pressure falls too.

Force of the heart. The volume of blood ejected depends on the power with which the heart muscle contracts.

Heart rate. Within limits, the faster the heart beats the greater its output.

Stimulation of the sympathetic nerves to the heart increases both the force of the contraction and the rate, that is, increases the cardiac output. By contrast, stimulation of the parasympathetic nerves to the heart, branches of the vagus nerves, decreases the force and the rate, and therefore decreases the cardiac output.

PERIPHERAL RESISTANCE: The peripheral resistance is the degree of obstruction offered to the blood as it tries to escape from the arteries. It is controlled mainly by the arterioles, by the tone of the smooth muscle in their walls. If the arterioles are relaxed their lumen is wide, escape is easy and the blood pressure is lower. If they contract, stimulated by the sympathetic vasoconstrictor nerves (p. 285), the lumen is narrow, escape is difficult and the blood pressure rises. Tone in the walls of the capillaries (p. 383) also contributes to the peripheral resistance.

Control of the Blood Pressure (see also pp. 385–388)

The blood pressure is controlled reflexly through the cardiac and vasomotor centres in the medulla of the brain. Stimulation of the carotid sinus by a rise in blood pressure reflexly causes it to fall. Stimulation of the carotid body by a fall in oxygen tension of the blood, reflexly causes the blood pressure to rise.

BLOOD FLOW IN THE PULMONARY ARTERIES

The blood flow in the pulmonary circulation is maintained by the pumping of the right ventricle of the heart. Note that the volume of blood which passes through the lungs in a given time, must be the same as that which goes through the systemic circulation during that same time.

The pressure in the pulmonary arteries, about 15 mm of mercury, is much less than that in the systemic arteries.

THE FLOW OF BLOOD IN CAPILLARIES

The total cross section of the capillary bed is very large and the blood flow is correspondingly very slow. This allows time for the exchanges between the blood and the tissue cells. The capillary blood pressure, reduced by the arteriole through which it has come (p. 382), is relatively low—about 30 mm of mercury at the arterial end and about 10 mm at the venous end. No pulsation is ordinarily discernible in capillaries, but if the arterioles supplying them are dilated, for example in inflammation, pulsation may be seen.

Capillary tone. Capillaries have an inherent ability to contract and dilate. The state of slight contraction normally present is called capillary tone. Dilatation varies with local tissue requirements. In particular, capillaries dilate in active tissues because of the presence of tissue metabolites.

THE FLOW OF BLOOD IN VEINS

The blood in the veins of the systemic circulation is a dark bluish red because it is deoxygenated. If a vein is cut the dull red blood flows out smoothly and slowly (cf. arteries, p. 379).

The blood in veins flows slowly under a low pressure of 10 mm of mercury or less. Because the flow is so slow compared with the flow in the corresponding artery, a vein has a wider lumen than the artery. Indeed each distributing artery is usually accompanied by two veins. This ensures that, even though the blood flow in the veins is slow, in a given time as much blood can pass back along the veins as flowed rapidly along the arteries.

Maintenance of Venous Blood Flow

Because the force of the heart driving the blood along the veins is reduced to the low level of 10 mm of mercury other means of maintaining the flow are important. They are the venous valves, the muscle pump and the negative intrapleural pressure.

VENOUS VALVES: The venous valves (p. 354) allow blood to flow only towards the heart. They are particularly important in the lower limb where the flow is against the force of gravity. If the valves in the superficial veins of the lower limb become incompetent, the blood collects in the veins which become dilated and tortuous. This is the condition called **varicose veins.**

MUSCLE PUMP: In the limbs, the skeletal muscles play an important part in maintaining the blood flow in the veins. The muscles are enclosed in a firm sheath of deep fascia, for example, the fascia lata of the thigh. When the muscles contract to produce movements, their bellies swell; because they are prevented by the deep fascia from bulging outwards they tend to compress everything within the fascial sheath. The deep veins, having thin walls, are flattened and the blood is moved along; the valves ensure that the flow is only towards the heart. This whole mechanism is often called the muscle pump.

The muscle pump cannot work in this way on the superficial veins which are outside the deep fascia. It assists the flow in them in a different way. The superficial veins communicate with the deep veins by means of channels in which the valves allow blood to pass only towards the deep veins. When the muscles relax after a contraction a sucking effect is produced. This draws blood from the

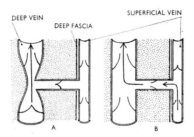

Fig. 160. The muscle pump as it acts on the veins: A, muscles contract and blood in the deep veins is driven towards the heart, valves preventing flow away from the heart; B, muscles relax and deep veins are no longer compressed; blood is sucked into them from the superficial veins.

superficial veins into the deep veins, so draining the superficial veins of blood which is then made to flow along the deep veins.

(The flow in the superficial veins is assisted also by the unusually numerous valves and the extra smooth muscle in their walls, which by its tone, prevents overdilatation.)

Soldiers standing stiffly to attention often faint because the muscle pump is being kept voluntarily out of action. Blood accumulates in the veins of the legs because there is not enough force to drive it upwards against gravity. Not enough blood reaches the heart to maintain an adequate circulation to the brain and the subject faints for lack of oxygen for the cells of the cerebral cortex.

NEGATIVE INTRATHORACIC PRESSURE: Just as the movements of respiration suck air into the lungs (p. 340), these same movements suck blood from veins outside the thorax into the heart. This suction assists particularly the upward flow of blood in the inferior vena cava.

CONTROL OF THE CARDIOVASCULAR SYSTEM

The cardiovascular system is regulated in two main ways, by nervous control and by chemical control.

NERVOUS CONTROL

The nervous control is reflex. The **reflex arcs** (p 262) concerned have their **reflex centres** in the reticular formation of the medulla of the brain. The centre which controls the heart is the **cardiac centre,** that which controls the blood vessels is the **vasomotor centre.** Together with the respiratory centre which is close to them, these centres are known as the **'vital centres'.**

The **efferent limbs of the reflex arcs** are visceromotor nerves of the autonomic nervous system. The cardiac centre and the vasomotor centre each consist of connector nerve cells belonging to both the sympathetic and the parasympathetic nervous systems.

Motor Nerves to the Heart

The heart beats automatically. The nerves to the heart serve merely to regulate the force and the rate of the beats. The parasympathetic part of the cardiac centre sends its impulses to the heart through the vagus nerve, and reduces the heart rate and the force of the contraction. This plays a part in reducing the cardiac output and in lowering the blood pressure. There is a constant discharge of these parasympathetic impulses, damping down the inherent activity of the heart.

The sympathetic part of the cardiac centre sends impulses to the sympathetic nerve cells of the lateral grey column of the thoracic part of the spinal cord and so through the sympathetic chain and cardiac nerves to the heart (p. 284). These impulses increase the heart rate and increase the force of the contraction, so playing a part in increasing the cardiac output and in raising the blood pressure.

Motor Nerves to the Blood Vessels

The nerves from the vasomotor centre to the blood vessels are almost all sympathetic. The impulses pass to the lateral horn cells, from them to the sympathetic chain and so to the blood vessels (p. 284). The majority of these fibres cause the smooth muscle in the vessel walls to contract, and are therefore known as **vasoconstrictor fibres.** The most important action of these vaso-constrictor fibres is on the walls of the arterioles. A constant stream of impulses maintains the muscle tone in their walls, and keeps the lumen partially con-stricted. This provides the peripheral resistance which is an important factor in maintaining the blood pressure (p. 382). It also ensures that the pressure of the blood entering the capillary bed is not too high (p. 354). If the vasoconstrictor nerves are stimulated more, the lumen of the arterioles is narrowed further and the blood pressure rises. Inhibition of the vasoconstrictor impulses makes the lumen wider so that the blood pressure falls.

Vasoconstriction of larger arteries is a means of reducing the blood supply to organs or regions as the need arises. Inhibition of the muscle tone in these arteries increases the blood supply to these organs and regions.

Sympathetic nerves to the coronary arteries and to the arteries in skeletal muscles are, however, unusual and are **vasodilator** (see also p. 285). This accords with the general principle that the sympathetic system alters the physiology in readiness for fright, fight or flight.

Parasympathetic nerves to blood vessels are few. They are vasodilator and are found in the salivary glands and in the erectile tissue of the genitalia.

The **afferent limbs of the reflex arcs,** that is, the pathways for the sensory impulses which act on the cardiac and vasomotor centres, come from different parts of the body.

The most important come from specialized sensory receptors, called baro-receptors and chemoreceptors. Impulses from higher centres, such as the hypothalamus and cerebral cortex, influence the vital centres. Pain impulses, especially from viscera, also have an effect.

Baroreceptors

Baroreceptors are sensitive to rises in the blood pressure. They are really stretch receptors (p. 225). The most important is the **carotid sinus,** a dilatation of the beginning of the internal carotid artery (p. 368), from which sensory impulses travel in the glossopharyngeal nerve to the cardiac and vasomotor centres in the medulla.

Stimulation of the carotid sinus by a rise in blood pressure causes reflexly, through the cardiac centre, slowing of the heart rate and a decrease in the force of the contraction. This of course tends to lower the blood pressure until the baroreceptors are no longer stimulated.

Stimulation of the carotid sinus by a rise in blood pressure also affects the vasomotor centre. It causes inhibition of the vasoconstrictor nerves, thus allowing the arterioles to dilate. This lowers the peripheral resistance and therefore causes the blood pressure to fall.

A rise in blood pressure stimulates baroreceptors like the carotid sinus and reflexly causes, through the cardiac and vasomotor centres, a decrease in the cardiac output, a decrease in the peripheral resistance and therefore a fall in blood pressure.

Chemoreceptors

Chemoreceptors are sensitive to a decreased oxygen tension in the blood. The most important is the **carotid body,** which is a collection of special cells on the wall of the internal carotid artery close to the carotid sinus. The cells are surrounded by sinusoidal capillaries and are richly supplied by filaments of the glossopharyngeal nerve which convey impulses to the cardiac and vasomotor centres.

Stimulation of the carotid body by a decreased oxygen tension causes, through the cardiac centre, an increase in the heart rate and an increase in the force of the contraction. This causes the blood pressure to rise.

Stimulation of the carotid body affects the vasomotor centre also. It causes increased vasoconstriction, which raises the peripheral resistance and causes a rise in blood pressure.

Decreased oxygen tension in the blood stimulates chemoreceptors like the carotid body and reflexly causes, through the cardiac and vasomotor centres, an increase in the cardiac output, an increase in the peripheral resistance and there-fore a rise in blood pressure.

Higher Centres

Impulses from the **hypothalamus** cause the increase in the heart rate which occurs when the body temperature rises. They also cause inhibition of the vasoconstrictor nerves, and this results in the dilation of the arterioles which occurs as part of the mechanism of losing heat from the skin.

Impulses from the **cerebral cortex** have different effects. Emotion causes a quickening of the heart rate. It may cause dilation of the arterioles, as in blushing, or vasoconstriction, as in anger. Unpleasant experiences may cause slowing of the heart and vasoconstriction as in fainting.

Pain

Painful stimuli also have different effects. Most quicken the heart rate and cause vasoconstriction.

CHEMICAL CONTROL

The heart and blood vessels respond to certain chemical substances, notably to the presence of metabolites, and to hormones such as noradrenaline and adrenaline.

Metabolites

Metabolites are the products of the metabolism of cells. When they accumulate they act on the nearby blood vessels, causing dilatation. This happens in skeletal muscle during exercise.

Noradrenaline and Adrenaline

These hormones have the same effect as stimulating the sympathetic nervous system. They cause an increase in the heart rate and in the force of the heart. They cause vasoconstriction, except in the vessels of the heart and of skeletal muscle which they dilate (see also p. 517).

Histamine is a substance found in mast cells (p. 105), and in basophil cells and platelets in the blood. The physiological function of histamine is uncertain. It can be released by minor injury and is believed to be the cause of the triple response (red line, flare and weal) to a firm stroke on the skin. It is released in urticaria (heat rash) and in allergic rhinitis (hay fever).

Histamine is also found in nettles and in bee and wasp venoms.

Regulation of the Blood Supply to Parts and Organs

The blood supply to every region and organ alters according to the needs of the moment. If the region or organ is active, its cells need a plentiful supply of oxygen, so the distributing arteries to that part dilate to allow more blood to reach it. This is brought about mainly by a reflex inhibition of the vasoconstrictor nerves to these vessels. Conversely, if an organ is resting, much less oxygen is needed and the vasoconstrictor nerves to its blood vessels are stimulated reflexly, so cutting down the blood supply.

For example, during muscular exercise, the distributing arteries to the skeletal muscles are dilated. At the same time, the arteries supplying the digestive tract are constricted, so reducing the volume of blood there, in order that more may be available for the muscles. Similarly, after a meal, the vessels of the digestive tract dilate and those to skeletal muscles contract so that the organs concerned with digestion have the necessary increased blood supply. It is not wise to indulge in muscular exercise immediately after a heavy meal, because blood is necessarily diverted to the active muscles, leaving the digestive tract inadequately supplied, and possibly causing indigestion.

THE FETAL CIRCULATION

The fetus obtains all its food and oxygen and eliminates all its waste products through the placenta (p. 75). The fetal heart, therefore, not only pumps blood to every part of the fetus but also through the extensive capillary bed in the placenta (Plate 33), and is consequently relatively large.

The fetal blood reaches the placenta through the two umbilical arteries in the umbilical cord, circulates through the capillary bed in the placenta and returns to the fetus through the single umbilical vein. It is important to realize that the blood in the umbilical vein is oxygenated and also carries food materials. From the umbilicus the umbilical vein passes in the edge of the falciform ligament (pp. 442 and 445) to the portal vein in the porta hepatis. However, the blood by passes the liver by leaving the portal vein at once in the ductus venosus, which passes upwards behind the liver to the inferior vena cava which then pours this oxygenated blood into the right atrium of the heart.

Before it enters the heart, this oxygenated blood from the umbilical vein is mixed with the deoxygenated blood travelling in the inferior vena cava from the abdomen and lower limbs. The volume of this deoxygenated blood is relatively small, however, so the stream as a whole remains well oxygenated. The foramen ovale in the interatrial septum transmits most of this blood directly to the left atrium (Plate 33). From there it passes to the left ventricle which pumps it into the aorta. The first branches of the aorta, that is, the coronary arteries and the arteries of the head, neck and upper limbs, thus have a good supply of oxygenated blood for the developing heart and brain (see also p. 116). Beyond this point the blood mixes with blood from the ductus arteriosus (see below).

From the head, neck and upper limbs a large volume of deoxygenated blood is returned, by way of the superior vena cava, to the right atrium. This passes into the right ventricle. Although there is some mixing, in the right atrium, of this deoxygenated blood with the oxygenated blood passing from the inferior vena cava through the foramen ovale to the left atrium, the orifices are so placed that the two streams remain substantially separate. The deoxygenated stream is pumped by the right ventricle into the pulmonary trunk. The pulmonary arteries are small because the lungs of the fetus are not expanded and do not function. They, therefore, receive only a little of this blood which then circulates through the lungs and is returned to the left atrium by the pulmonary veins to mix with the oxygenated blood already there.

The greater part of the deoxygenated blood from the right ventricle flows from the pulmonary trunk, into the aorta through a large communication, the **ductus arteriosus,** which joins the aorta distal to the region from which the branches to the head and upper limbs arise.

The blood in the descending aorta is therefore a mixture of the relatively well oxygenated blood left over after the head and upper limbs have been supplied, and the deoxygenated blood reaching it from the right side of the heart. The mixture as a whole is poorly oxygenated. It is distributed to the abdomen and lower limbs, but most of it is conveyed through the common and internal iliac arteries to the two **umbilical arteries,** which pass upwards on the inside of the anterior abdominal wall to the umbilicus, and from there in the umbilical cord to the placenta. The essential exchanges take place in the placenta and the blood, now oxygenated, carrying food materials and free from waste products, returns to the fetus in the umbilical vein.

The Changes at Birth

Very soon after birth, changes occur in the blood vessels which establish the post-natal pattern of the circulation. Within a few minutes the umbilical arteries contract, the cord stops pulsating and no more fetal blood reaches the placenta. The umbilical vein and ductus venosus have no further function and also contract. (When the umbilical cord is cut after delivery it is essential that the fetal end be ligatured securely, lest these large vessels bleed in spite of their contraction.) As a result much less blood enters the right atrium than before and the pressure within it is reduced.

At the same time the infant begins to breathe. The lungs expand and a much larger volume of blood begins to circulate through them. The ductus arteriosus contracts, so that all the blood from the right ventricle now goes to the lungs. This means that a much larger volume of blood than before returns to the left atrium and the pressure within it rises. The increased pressure in the left atrium, together with the decreased pressure in the right atrium, ensures that the flap of the foramen ovale is pushed to the right against the rim of the foramen which is effectively closed in this way. The atria are now completely separated from one another, and the right side of the heart has no direct communication with the left.

The fetal blood vessels which contract at birth degenerate gradually into fibrous cords. These cords persist in post-natal life as ligaments.

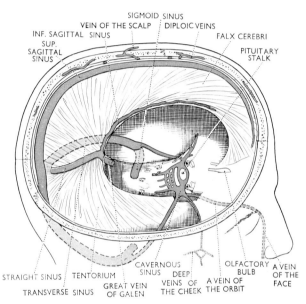

SIGMOID SINUS
VEIN OF THE SCALP   DIPLOIC VEINS
INF. SAGITTAL SINUS
SUP.   FALX CEREBRI
SAGITTAL   PITUITARY
SINUS   STALK

STRAIGHT SINUS   TENTORIUM   CAVERNOUS   OLFACTORY   A VEIN
                                SINUS   DEEP   BULB   OF THE
TRANSVERSE SINUS   GREAT VEIN   VEINS OF   A VEIN OF   FACE
                   OF GALEN   THE CHEEK THE ORBIT

Plate 29. The interior of the skull, showing the dura mater and the venous sinuses, with some of their communications with veins outside the skull.

[facing page 390

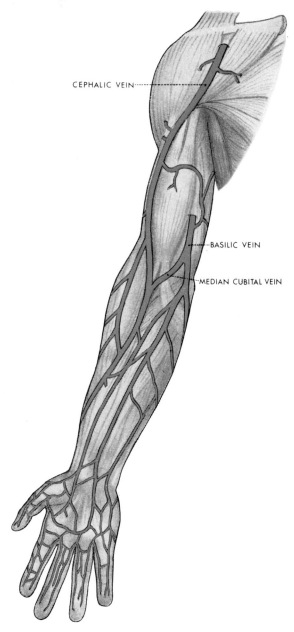

CEPHALIC VEIN

BASILIC VEIN

MEDIAN CUBITAL VEIN

Plate 30. The superficial veins of the upper limb, seen from the front.

[between pages 390/1 facing Pl. 31 & 32

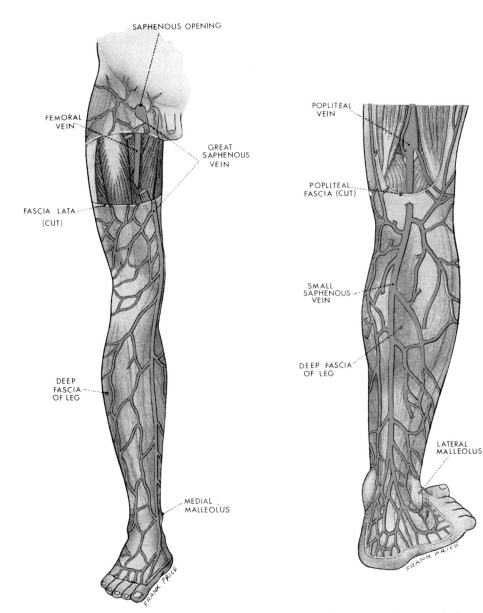

Plate 31. The veins of the lower limb seen
from in front.

Plate 32. The veins of the lower limb seen
from behind.

[between pages 390/1 facing Pl. 30

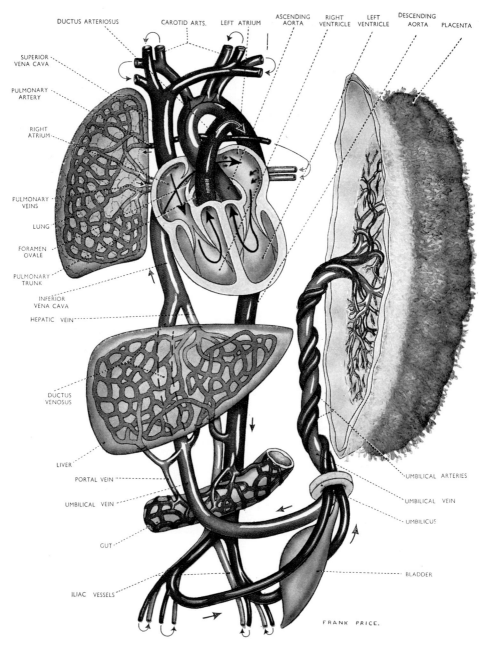

DUCTUS ARTERIOSUS   CAROTID ARTS.   LEFT ATRIUM   ASCENDING AORTA   RIGHT VENTRICLE   LEFT VENTRICLE   DESCENDING AORTA   PLACENTA

SUPERIOR VENA CAVA

PULMONARY ARTERY

RIGHT ATRIUM

PULMONARY VEINS

LUNG

FORAMEN OVALE

PULMONARY TRUNK

INFERIOR VENA CAVA

HEPATIC VEIN

DUCTUS VENOSUS

LIVER

PORTAL VEIN

UMBILICAL VEIN

GUT

ILIAC VESSELS

UMBILICAL ARTERIES

UMBILICAL VEIN

UMBILICUS

BLADDER

FRANK PRICE.

Plate 33. The fetal circulation; oxygenated blood is red; deoxygenated blood is blue; increasing degrees of deoxygenation are indicated by red/purple and purple/blue.

[facing page 391

Fetus	*Post-Natal*
Umbilical artery	Lateral umbilical ligament (p. 204)
Umbilical vein	Round ligament of the liver (p. 204)
Ductus venosus	Ligamentum venosum (p. 474)
Ductus arteriosus	Ligamentum arteriosum (p. 371)

Sometimes the ductus arteriosus remains patent in post-natal life and transmits deoxygenated blood to the systemic arteries. This is one cause of an infant's being a 'blue baby'.

The foramen ovale too may remain patent. This is one kind of 'hole in the heart'.

CHAPTER XIII

THE BLOOD AND LYMPHATIC SYSTEMS

BLOOD is an opaque reddish fluid which clots when it is outside the blood vessels. It is sticky to the touch, salty to taste and faintly alkaline in reaction.

Blood is for transport; for transport of oxygen, food materials, vitamins, hormones and antibodies to the tissues, and for transport of carbon dioxide and other waste materials, including heat, from the tissues to the organs which eliminate them from the body.

Blood also plays an important part in maintaining the acid-base equilibrium of the body, that is, in keeping the reaction of the tissue fluid close to pH 7·4.

COMPOSITION OF THE BLOOD

Blood is a tissue in which cells of two main kinds, **red blood corpuscles** (erythrocytes) and **white blood corpuscles** (leucocytes), are suspended in **plasma.** In addition, floating in the plasma, there are tiny fragments of cytoplasm called **platelets.**

PLASMA

Plasma *is the pale straw-coloured fluid obtained after removing all the cells from the blood.* It forms about half the volume of whole blood.

Plasma consists mostly of **water** (93%) in which are dissolved most of the substances carried by the blood. **Food materials** such as amino acids, glucose and lipids are dissolved in it, as well as **waste products** like carbon dioxide (see also p. 360) and urea.

Plasma contains dissolved **inorganic salts.** These are mainly the carbonates, chlorides, phosphates and sulphates of sodium, potassium and calcium. Plasma contains relatively little potassium compared with the red blood corpuscles, which contain much potassium and little sodium and calcium.

Plasma also contains **plasma proteins** which are part of the blood itself, that is, they are not being carried to the tissues for their metabolism. They are made in the liver and enter the plasma where they form a colloidal solution. The plasma proteins are **albumin, globulin,** and **fibrinogen.** (Albumins and globulins with different structures and properties can be distinguished.) Many **other proteins,** not 'plasma proteins', are dissolved in the plasma and are carried to all parts of the body. They include hormones and many enzymes.

Functions of Plasma Proteins

1. **Exertion of osmotic pressure.** Albumin, and to a lesser extent globulin, exert an osmotic pressure of about 30 mm of mercury, which draws water back into the capillaries at the venous end of the capillary bed (p. 97). This is important in regulating the blood volume and in preventing accumulation of water in the tissue spaces (œdema). The molecules of albumin and globulin in the plasma are able to exert an osmotic pressure because they are too large to pass through the capillary walls and because there is no protein in normal tissue fluid. (The molecules of the inorganic salts pass freely through the capillary walls so that their concentration in the plasma and in the tissue fluid is the same; they therefore set up no osmotic pressure.)

2. **Antibodies.** Antibodies are globulins. The globulins are important in the defence of the body against foreign proteins (p. 414) and bacteria.

3. **Coagulation of blood.** Fibrinogen is important in the coagulation of the blood. Prothrombin is a plasma globulin which also plays a part in clotting (p. 399).

4. **Buffering action.** The plasma proteins together with inorganic salts are buffers which keep the plasma pH constant.

5. **Transport of lipids.** Lipids are insoluble in water, but dissolve in plasma because they combine with the plasma proteins to form soluble compounds.

THE CELLS OF THE BLOOD (Plate 3)

> Red blood corpuscles (erythrocytes)
> White blood corpuscles (leucocytes)
> Platelets

Red Blood Corpuscles

Red blood corpuscles are orange discs about 7 micrometres (μm) (formerly microns) across. They are thicker at the edge than in the middle, that is they are biconcave. They have no nucleus. Their colour is due to the pigment hæmoglobin (p. 394) in their cytoplasm.

There are between five and six million red blood corpuscles per millilitre of normal blood.

Erythropoiesis is the production of red blood corpuscles. It takes place in the red marrow of the bones.

Hæmoglobin is a conjugated protein consisting of the protein **globin** combined with the iron-containing pigment **hæm.** It is contained entirely within the red blood corpuscles. It has the ability of combining easily with oxygen to form a loose compound, oxyhæmoglobin, and under different conditions it readily gives up the oxygen again, hæmoglobin being left. This property is due to the hæm part of the molecule. Hæmoglobin is dark bluish-red colour, whereas oxyhæmoglobin is bright red. Hæmoglobin is one of the buffers which helps to maintain the constant pH of the red blood corpuscles.

Normal blood contains 16 grams of hæmoglobin per 100 millilitres in the male and 14 grams per 100 millilitres in the female.

Life History of Red Blood Corpuscles

Red blood corpuscles are produced in the red marrow found in certain bones (p. 120). They circulate in the blood stream for about 120 days, by which time they are too old to function well. The reticulo-endothelial cells, especially those in blood-filtering lymphatic tissue, notably in the spleen (p. 411), ingest these worn out red blood corpuscles and destroy them. In health, the rate of production of red blood corpuscles in the red marrow exactly balances the rate of destruction of the worn out cells.

If the red marrow cannot produce red blood corpuscles as fast as they are normally destroyed, the number circulating falls. This is **aplastic anæmia.** If the reticulo-endothelial cells of the spleen destroy the cells more rapidly than usual, **hæmolytic anæmia** develops. This usually happens when the red blood corpuscles are abnormally fragile or strangely shaped, conditions found in some inherited diseases of the blood.

White Blood Corpuscles (leucocytes)

White blood corpuscles are transparent nucleated cells. There are several kinds, and all are a little larger than red blood corpuscles (Plate 3).

The total number of white blood corpuscles in the circulating blood is 5,000 to 10,000 per millilitre. An increase in this normal number is a **leucocytosis;** a decrease in the normal number is a **leucopenia.**

White blood corpuscles are of two main kinds, granular and agranular.

GRANULAR LEUCOCYTES: These make up about 70% of the total white cell count. They are recognized by the granules in their cytoplasm, and by their nuclei which have several lobes. According to the nature of the granules in the cytoplasm, as they are seen after the cells have been stained with a special blood stain, the granular leucocytes are classified as neutrophils, eosinophils and basophils.

Neutrophil (or polymorphonuclear) leucocytes are the most numerous, making up 60% of the total white cell count. Their cytoplasm contains very numerous fine granules which stain to a mauve colour (that is the granules are neutral—neither staining red with the acid dye eosin, nor blue with the basic (alkaline) dye methylene blue). The nucleus may have from two to five lobes; the older the cell, the more lobes has its nucleus.

Functions. Neutrophil leucocytes show **active amœboid movement.** This enables them to migrate from the capillaries into the tissues when and where they are needed. They also show **phagocytosis,** the ability to ingest particles, especially bacteria. Neutrophils are therefore an important part of the body's **defence** against acute infection.

Pus consists of tissue fluid containing harmful bacteria and very large numbers of dead neutrophils which have succumbed to the bacteria.

Eosinophil leucocytes make up about 3% of the total white cell count. Their cytoplasm contains numerous large granules which stain bright red with eosin.

An increase in their number is associated with allergic states like asthma, and with worm infestations.

Basophil leucocytes are very few in number. They form less than 1% of the total white cell count. Their cytoplasm contains large granules which stain blue with methylene blue. Basophils contain **heparin** (p. 399) and histamine (p. 388).

AGRANULAR LEUCOCYTES: The agranular leucocytes are lymphocytes and monocytes.

Lymphocytes account for about 30% of the total white cell count. They have large dense spherical nuclei and clear blue cytoplasm when they are stained with blood stains. They are of different sizes, large lymphocytes (about the same size as granular leucocytes) and small lymphocytes.

Lymphocytes play the main part in the cellular immune response. Their number is increased in typhoid fever and chronic infections.

Monocytes form about 6% of the total white cell count. They are the largest of the white blood corpuscles, and have a large kidney or horse-shoe shaped nucleus with pale blue staining cytoplasm.

They show slow **amœboid movements** and are **phagocytic.** They may be 'free' cells of the reticulo-endothelial system (p. 111).

Platelets

Platelets are tiny colourless fragments of cytoplasm without nuclei. They number 250,000 to 500,000 per millilitre of blood.

Function. Platelets are necessary for coagulation of the blood. When blood touches almost anything other than endothelium lining the blood vessels, the platelets disintegrate and from them come some of the substances essential for the formation of thromboplastin (p. 399).

Purpura is a condition in which the number of platelets is less than normal. Tiny hæmorrhages from the capillaries appear, especially in the skin and mucous membranes, looking like a purplish rash.

FORMATION AND DESTRUCTION OF BLOOD CORPUSCLES

The tissues responsible for the formation of blood cells are (*a*) the red bone marrow in which red blood corpuscles, granular leucocytes, platelets and possibly monocytes are made, and (*b*) lymphatic tissue in which lymphocytes and monocytes are made.

Blood corpuscles are destroyed by the cells of the reticulo-endothelial system (p. 111), especially in the spleen.

FORMATION OF RED BLOOD CORPUSCLES
(Erythropoiesis)

Erythropoiesis takes place in the red marrow described on p. 120. The mother cells of all the blood cells are the **hæmocytoblasts** (p. 112), (Plate 3). Within the red marrow they multiply and some form **erythroblasts** which are large cells containing nuclei and a little hæmoglobin in their cytoplasm. These develop into **normoblasts** which are smaller, contain more hæmoglobin, and have small dense degenerating nuclei. These nuclei are soon pushed out of the cells, which then assume the characteristic biconcave shape. At this stage the cells still contain in their cytoplasm a small amount of the cytoplasm characteristic of earlier stages in development. When the cells are stained in a special way it shows as a blue network, and such cells are called **reticulocytes.** Soon this immature cytoplasm disappears, and the cells are now fully formed erythrocytes, or red blood corpuscles. They enter the sinusoids of the bone marrow and are carried away in the blood stream.

In health, all red blood corpuscles found in the circulating blood are fully developed. However, if red cell production is going on faster than usual, for instance to make up the deficiency when anæmia is being successfully treated, many young, less mature cells gain entry to the blood, notably a very large number of reticulocytes.

Essential factors

For the normal development of red blood corpuscles certain substances must be present. Among them are iron, Vitamin B_{12}, Castle's intrinsic factor and erythropoietin.

Iron. This is needed for making hæmoglobin. Enough iron must be eaten, and then absorbed from the intestinal tract. Though iron is conserved by the body and stored in the liver, deficiency readily arises, for example in women as a result of the regular small loss of blood at menstruation. The result is that the red blood corpuscles are pale from lack of the pigment and unusually small, a condition called **iron-deficiency anæmia.**

Vitamin B_{12}: Extrinsic and Intrinsic Factors

Vitamin B_{12} is essential for the normal development of red blood corpuscles. If it is absent, the bone marrow produces red blood corpuscles which are larger than normal, but very few of them. This is called a **macrocytic anæmia.**

Vitamin B_{12} is also called **Castle's extrinsic factor.** It is present in many foods, especially in liver, kidney and meat in general and in yeast. It can be absorbed by the intestine, however, only in the presence of a special substance, **Castle's intrinsic factor,** which is secreted by the mucous membrane of the body of the stomach. If the stomach fails to secrete it, Vitamin B_{12} is not absorbed, and the macrocytic anæmia known as **pernicious anæmia** is the result.

Erythropoietin is a hormone, for the production of which the kidney is necessary (p. 491). It increases the production of red blood corpuscles.

FORMATION OF WHITE BLOOD CORPUSCLES
(Leucopoiesis)

The granular leucocytes are formed in the red bone marrow. The agranular leucocytes are formed in lymph nodules (p. 410).

Granular Leucocytes

Some of the blood-forming cells, hæmocytoblasts, in the red bone marrow develop through a number of stages, illustrated in Plate 3, into cells called

myelocytes which have neutrophil, cosinophil or basophil granules in their cytoplasm. From the myelocytes neutrophil, eosinophil and basophil leucocytes are formed, and make their way into the sinusoids to be carried away in the blood.

They probably circulate for about a week (neutrophils four days, eosinophils ten days, basophils fourteen days) before being phagocytosed and broken down by the cells of the reticulo-endothelial system.

Agranular Leucocytes

Agranular leucocytes develop in lymph nodules (p. 410).

Lymphocytes are derived from cells called **lymphoblasts** which are very like hæmocytoblasts and may be identical with them. These cells are found in the germinal centres of lymphatic nodules (p. 410). The lymphoblasts divide and the daughter cells, which are smaller, pass to the periphery and enter the lymphatic sinusoids and then the lymph vessels which eventually convey them to the blood via the terminal lymph vessels (p. 420).

These lymphocytes remain in the blood for less than a day before being transferred back to lymphatic tissue. They re-enter mainly into the sinusoids of lymph nodes from venules in the medulla. There is thus a continuous circulation of lymphocytes between the lymph and the blood. They probably last for a few weeks before being broken down.

Monocytes. There is much doubt about the formation and nature of monocytes.

(a) They may develop in red marrow from monoblasts which are derived from hæmocytoblasts.

(b) They may be formed in lymph nodules from lymphoblasts.

(c) They may be free cells of the reticulo-endothelial system, formed wherever reticulo-endothelial cells are found.

Leukæmia. Leukæmia is a malignant disease in which production of one of the varieties of white blood cells is uncontrolled. As well as a greatly increased number of white blood corpuscles, immature forms, usually seen only in the red marrow, are found in the circulating blood.

FORMATION OF PLATELETS

Platelets are derived from very large cells with several nuclei, called **megakaryocytes,** which are found in red marrow. They in turn are developed from hæmocytoblasts. Parts of the cytoplasm of the megakaryocytes break off and enter the blood stream, so forming the platelets.

Platelets are destroyed by the reticulo-endothelial cells.

COAGULATION OF BLOOD

Within a few minutes of leaving the blood vessels, normal blood sets into a jelly or **clot.** Soon the clot shrinks, becoming firmer and squeezing out a straw-coloured fluid called **serum.**

The **blood clot** is composed of a network of fine threads of **fibrin,** an insoluble protein which enmeshes the blood corpuscles and platelets.

Fibrin is produced from its precursor **fibrinogen,** one of the plasma proteins, by a complex process of which the main stages are as follows:

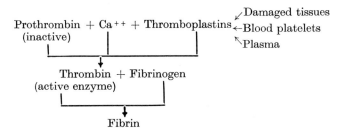

Thrombin is an active enzyme which acts on fibrinogen to form fibrin. Thrombin is formed from an inactive precursor, **prothrombin,** which is a plasma globulin made in the liver in the presence of sufficient **vitamin K** (p. 568). Prothrombin is converted to thrombin only in the presence of **calcium ions** and **thromboplastins** (thrombokinase). Thromboplastins are formed by the interaction of substances from disintegrated platelets and from plasma.

SOME SPECIAL CONSIDERATIONS

Hæmophilia is a sex-linked inherited disease (p. 59) transmitted by females who show no symptoms of it, to males who manifest it (p. 59). The blood does not clot in the normal way because of the absence of a plasma factor necessary for the formation of thromboplastin. Even minor injuries, therefore, cause serious and prolonged bleeding.

Anticoagulants are substances which prevent the blood from clotting by interfering with one of the stages in the formation of the clot. **Heparin** is an example. It is produced by the mast cells (p. 105) and is also present in the basophil leucocytes circulating in the blood. It neutralizes thrombin. Dicoumarol is an anticoagulant drug which acts by preventing the formation of prothrombin.

Blood can be prevented from clotting, after it has been withdrawn from the body, by removing the calcium ions. Potassium citrate or potassium oxalate is added to the blood so that undissociated calcium citrate or oxalate is formed.

Thrombosis

Thrombosis is the formation of a blood clot, during life, in blood flowing in blood vessels. In health it never occurs, partly because of the nature of the endothelium lining the blood vessels, and partly because of circulating anticoagulants like heparin. Thrombosis may occur:

(a) if the endothelium is damaged, for example by injury or inflammation,
(b) if the blood flow is slow, for example in varicose veins or in a patient kept in bed,
(c) if there are certain changes in the chemical composition of the blood.

All three of these factors may be present in patients after surgical operations so that thrombosis, especially in the deep veins of the legs, may then occur. For this reason, breathing exercises and early ambulation after operations are desirable.

An **embolus** is a piece of a thrombus broken off and carried along by the blood stream. If it originates in the systemic veins, it lodges in the pulmonary arteries causing a pulmonary embolism.

BLOOD SEDIMENTATION

If blood is withdrawn, prevented from clotting by the addition of an anticoagulant, and placed in a vertical tube, the blood corpuscles begin to settle to the bottom, leaving clear plasma above. The column of clear plasma is measured after one hour. In males it averages 4 mm, in females 8 mm. The blood sedimentation rate is increased in pregnancy and in many pathological states, for example in infections and after trauma.

CARRIAGE OF OXYGEN AND CARBON DIOXIDE BY THE BLOOD

One of the most important functions of the blood is to carry oxygen from the lungs to the tissues, and to carry carbon dioxide from the tissues to the lungs where it can be eliminated. The blood performs these tasks very efficiently.

The red blood corpuscles are highly specialized to this end, particularly in that they contain hæmoglobin with its unique properties. Also, the taking in and giving out of the gases by the red cells depends on diffusion; the greater the surface area the more quickly diffusion occurs; the biconcave shape of the red cells assists diffusion by presenting the maximum surface area round a given volume.

OXYGEN

The blood which leaves the lungs is nearly saturated with oxygen at a tension of 13 kilopascals (100 mm of mercury). A little of this oxygen is in simple solution in the plasma, but nearly all of it is inside the red blood corpuscles, loosely bound by chemical combination with hæmoglobin, as **oxyhæmoglobin.** The oxyhæmoglobin is bright red and gives the blood in the systemic arteries its characteristic bright colour. When the blood reaches the capillaries in the tissues, oxygen diffuses from the plasma into the tissue fluid where the oxygen tension is only 5 kilopascals (40 mm of mercury). This lowers the oxygen tension in the plasma and the oxyhæmoglobin in the red cells gives up oxygen to the plasma and this in turn passes to the tissues. The hæmoglobin which has given up its oxygen is **reduced hæmoglobin** which is a dark dull red, and gives the characteristic colour to venous blood. Oxygen is given up by the hæmoglobin until at the venous end of the capillary bed, the oxygen tension in the blood is only 5 kilopascals (40 mm of mercury), and much of the hæmoglobin is now reduced hæmoglobin. Note, however, that normal venous blood still contains considerable oxygen. If for some reason, even this oxygen is given up, the proportion of reduced hæmoglobin is greater and the blood is even darker in colour. This dark colour in the capillaries, seen through the skin, looks grey-purple and is called **cyanosis.**

The ability of oxyhæmoglobin to give up its oxygen so readily, when the oxygen tension is low, is obviously very important. The oxygen is given up even more readily if the temperature is increased, if the carbon dioxide tension is increased and if the blood becomes even a little more acid. These conditions occur in muscles during exercise.

Reduced hæmoglobin takes up oxygen just as readily in the capillaries of the lungs where the oxygen tension in the alveolar air is high, 13 kilopascals (100 mm of mercury).

CARBON DIOXIDE

Of the carbon dioxide in the blood, about two-thirds is carried in the plasma and about one-third in the red blood corpuscles.

Most of this carbon dioxide is in the form of **bicarbonate ions** carried both in the plasma and in the red cells. Some is **combined with hæmoglobin** in the red cells, and with plasma proteins in the plasma as **carbamino compounds.** A little is in **simple solution.**

In venous blood the carbon dioxide is under a tension of 6 kilopascals (46 mm of mercury); in arterial blood the carbon dioxide tension is 5 kilopascals (40 mm of mercury).

In the tissue fluid the carbon dioxide tension is high, whereas the tension in the blood capillaries is lower. Carbon dioxide diffuses into the plasma and into the red cells. Carbon dioxide dissolved in water forms carbonic acid, which in ordinary circumstances dissociates very slowly into hydrogen ion and bicarbonate ion.

$$CO_2 + H_2O \rightarrow H_2CO_3 \rightarrow H^+ + HCO_3^-$$

The red blood corpuscles contain an enzyme, **carbonic anhydrase,** which enables the dissociation to take place very rapidly. The hydrogen ion is 'mopped up' by the buffering action of hæmoglobin. The concentration of bicarbonate ions (HCO_3^-) in the red cells soon becomes greater than that in the plasma, so bicarbonate ions diffuse out of the cells into the plasma. To maintain electrical neutrality chloride ions (Cl^-) diffuse from the plasma into the red cells. This is the **chloride shift.** (Electrical neutrality in the red cells cannot be achieved by the passage outwards of hydrogen ion (H^+) or of potassium ion (K^+) in numbers to equal the bicarbonate ions (HCO_3^-) leaving, because the hydrogen ion is taken up by the hæmoglobin which buffers it, and the red cell membrane is impermeable to potassium ions.)

Carbamino Compounds

Carbon dioxide combines with the plasma proteins and with hæmoglobin to be carried in the blood as carbamino compounds. In other words, hæmoglobin combines with carbon dioxide in something like the way it combines with oxygen. Fortunately, reduced hæmoglobin combines much more readily with carbon dioxide than oxyhæmoglobin, and this adds to the efficiency of the blood in transporting the two gases.

In the alveolar capillaries, the reverse reactions occur. Carbon dioxide is given up from the blood, where its tension is 6 kilopascals (46 mm of mercury), to the alveolar air where it is 5 kilopascals (40 mm of mercury). Carbon dioxide diffuses out of the plasma into the alveoli; some therefore diffuses from the red cells to the plasma. Carbonic anhydrase catalyses the formation of carbonic acid as well as its dissociation, according to the conditions, so now we have

$$H^+ + HCO_3^- \rightarrow H_2CO_3 \rightarrow H_2O + CO_2$$

As the bicarbonate ion disappears from the red cells, more diffuses in from the plasma, is converted to carbon dioxide and is given off to the alveolar air. To maintain electrical neutrality the chloride shift occurs in the opposite direction, chloride ions passing from the cells to the plasma.

Under the conditions of lower carbon dioxide tension the carbamino compounds also give up their carbon dioxide readily.

The Reaction of the Blood

The reaction of the blood is maintained at about pH 7·4 and in health is never less than 7·3 nor more than 7·5. This is very important for homeostasis (p. 95).

There are constantly being added to the blood, carbonic acid from tissue respiration and non-volatile acids, like lactic acid from carbohydrate metabolism and hydroxybutyric acid from fat metabolism. These acids do not alter the pH because of the presence, in both plasma and red blood corpuscles, of buffering substances which mop up the hydrogen ion. The most important are bicarbonate, phosphate and plasma proteins in the plasma and hæmoglobin and phosphates in the red blood corpuscles.

It is important to realize that buffers are used up in combining with the hydrogen ions or hydroxyl ions. The acid substances named above are buffered in the blood, but since they are continuously produced, they must also be removed or the buffer substances will indeed be quite used up. The carbon dioxide is removed from the blood by the gaseous exchange in the lungs (p. 319). The nonvolatile acids are excreted by the kidney (p. 494).

ACIDOSIS AND ALKALOSIS

Sometimes in abnormal circumstances, there is a greater concentration of hydrogen ions or of hydroxyl ions in the blood than the buffers can deal with. The pH of the blood then changes towards acidity or alkalinity.

Acidosis

In acidosis the pH of the blood is less than 7·3 and at 7·0 it may be fatal.

Metabolic causes: Ingestion of ammonium chloride
                  Diabetes mellitus
                  Starvation.

In diabetes mellitus and starvation large amounts of hydroxybutyric acid are produced because fats are incompletely metabolized.

Respiratory cause: Increase in the carbon dioxide in the blood.

This occurs if there is some disturbance in the physiological mechanism of external respiration which prevents the normal loss of carbon dioxide.

Alkalosis

In alkalosis the pH of the blood is more than 7·5, and at 7·6 it may be fatal.

Metabolic causes: Ingestion of bicarbonate or of citrate.
              Vomiting, when hydrochloric acid is lost from the stomach.

Respiratory causes: Voluntary overbreathing which removes too much carbon dioxide from the blood.

BLOOD GROUPS

Agglutination *is the clumping together of the red blood corpuscles in certain abnormal circumstances.*

Hæmolysis *is the breaking up of the red blood corpuscles so that the hæmoglobin escapes into the surrounding fluid.*

When blood from two different people is mixed, either no change occurs, and the two bloods are said to be compatible; or agglutination and hæmolysis occur and the bloods are then said to be incompatible. Agglutination and hæmolysis occur when an antigen (p. 414) in the red blood corpuscles of one of the bloods is acted upon by the corresponding antibody (p. 414) which happens to be present in the plasma of the other blood. Obviously if blood transfusion is to be successful, only **compatible blood** must be given to a patient. **A mistake may result in death.**

There are four main kinds of blood, distinguished by the presence (or absence) of two **agglutinogens** (antigens) A and B in the red blood corpuscles, and two **agglutinins** (antibodies) anti-A and anti-B in the plasma. If the red blood corpuscles contain either (or both) of the agglutinogens, then the serum of that blood cannot possibly contain the corresponding agglutinins, or the blood would agglutinate spontaneously. On the other hand, if one (or both) of the agglutinogens is not present in the red blood corpuscles, the corresponding agglutinin is always present in the plasma.

The Blood Groups are named according to the agglutinogens present in the red blood corpuscles. If both are present, the Blood Group is AB, if one is present it is A or B, and if neither is present it is O.

In blood transfusion agglutination and hæmolysis of the red blood corpuscles must be avoided. If hæmolysis does occur it may have fatal results, because the free hæmoglobin damages the kidney tubules irreparably.

Blood for transfusion should be of the same group as the patient's. In addition it is always **cross-matched** with that of the patient, that is a sample of the donor's blood is mixed with a sample of the recipient's blood to make quite sure that there is no agglutination.

The effect of the donor's plasma on the recipient's red cells can usually be neglected, because the concentration of agglutinins is low and the volume of donor plasma is small compared with the recipient's. Hence it is usually possible to give Group O blood to a patient of any group.

Name of Group	Agglutinogens present in red cells	Agglutinins present in serum or plasma	Percentage of population in group
AB	AB	None	3
A	A	anti-B	42
B	B	anti-A	10
O	O	anti-A, anti-B	45

Rh Factor

Another important agglutinogen, quite distinct from the A, B, O agglutinogens, is the **Rh factor** or **rhesus factor.**

It was discovered that, if red cells from a rhesus monkey were injected into a rabbit, the rabbit developed antibodies which agglutinated not only rhesus monkey cells, but the cells of 85% of people. These people are called Rh-positive and the rest Rh-negative.

If Rh-positive cells are transfused into an Rh-negative recipient, nothing very obvious happens on the first occasion, but the Rh-positive corpuscles stimulate the production of anti-Rh agglutinins. A second transfusion of Rh-positive cells would result in their wholesale destruction by these anti-Rh agglutinins, with serious results.

Rh-factor and Pregnancy

This Rh-factor can give rise to trouble during pregnancy. If an Rh-negative mother is carrying an Rh-positive fetus (the Rh-positive factor having been inherited from the father) a few of the fetus' Rh-positive cells may gain access to the mother's circulation. (There is never in any circumstances a true mixing of maternal and fetal blood.) These cells stimulate the production of anti-Rh agglutinins in the mother. Unfortunately, the agglutinins in some cases cross the placental barrier into the fetal blood, where of course hæmolysis of the fetal red blood corpuscles occurs. In a severe case the infant dies. However, it is possible by means of transfusion immediately after birth to withdraw the infant's blood, which contains the harmful agglutinins, and replace it in stages with fresh blood, so arresting the hæmolysis. In a first pregnancy, the fetus is not usually affected.

It has been shown that the Rh positive cells from the fetus gain access to the maternal circulation at the time of delivery. If anti-Rh antibody (Rh immuno-globulin) is injected into the mother then, her cells can be prevented from producing the harmful antibodies. The risk to subsequent pregnancies is thereby almost eliminated.

Once anti-Rh agglutinins have been produced, they continue to be produced throughout life. It is important that an Rh-negative girl or woman should never be given a transfusion of Rh-positive blood. The agglutinins produced by such a transfusion might affect a future fetus.

A number of other less important blood groups have been discovered. All blood groups are inherited as alleles (p. 54) and are fixed in any individual for life.

LYMPHATIC SYSTEM

The lymphatic system comprises lymphatic tissue including the thymus and the spleen, lymphatic vessels, and the fluid, lymph, contained in the lymphatic vessels.

LYMPH

Lymph *is the fluid which is contained within the lymph vessels.* It is very like plasma, pale yellow and clear, unless it contains many fat globules following the absorption of fat from the intestines (p. 461), when it is milky. Like plasma, it is mostly water, with dissolved proteins, inorganic salts, food materials and waste products. It contains a varying number of white blood corpuscles, mostly lymphocytes.

Lymph is very like the tissue fluid which bathes all the cells, but is distinguished from it by being inside the closed system of lymphatic vessels and lymphatic capillaries. Tissue fluid enters the lymphatic capillaries by filtration and diffusion. Any protein which has leaked into the tissue fluid is also taken up.

Cellular debris, foreign particles, for example soot in the lungs, and any bacteria which may have gained entry are also taken into the lymphatic capillaries. The fluid so formed is lymph.

LYMPHATIC VESSELS

The lymphatic vessels form a second pathway for fluid returning from the tissues to the heart (veins being the first pathway). In many tissues, and especially under epithelial surfaces, there is a plexus of lymphatic capillaries, which are very like blood capillaries. These unite to form lymphatic vessels which are like very small veins in structure and have very numerous valves. Under the action of the muscle pump (p. 383) and the intra-abdominal pressure, the lymph flows along the vessels. They unite to form larger vessels which converge upon the thoracic duct. The negative intrapleural pressure associated with respiration (p. 340) assists the lymph flow upwards through the thorax in the thoracic duct to the root of the neck, where it and other regional lymph trunks (p. 421) open into the great veins (Fig. 169). In this way all the lymph is added to the blood. Before the lymph reaches the blood, however, it always passes through at least one **lymph node,** where it is filtered and any foreign particles and bacteria are removed.

LYMPHATIC TISSUE

Lymphatic tissue performs two functions:

(a) It produces certain cells, namely lymphocytes, monocytes (p. 395) and plasma cells (p. 414)

(b) It acts as a filter for (i) tissue fluid
   (ii) lymph, and
   (iii) blood.

(i) Filtration of Tissue Fluid

Lymphatic tissue for filtering tissue fluid is found under wet epithelial surfaces, especially under the epithelium lining the alimentary canal. It consists of **lymphatic nodules** (p. 409) which blend with the adjacent loose connective tissue. There is no dense connective tissue capsule round them to bar the way of the tissue fluid, which percolates through them from all sides. The nodules occur both singly, when they can be recognized microscopically, and massed together to form aggregations visible to the naked eye, for example in the appendix and in **aggregated lymphatic nodules** (Peyer's patches) in the ileum. The most striking examples of this unencapsulated lymphoid tissue are the **tonsils** (palatine tonsils), **pharyngeal tonsils** and **lingual tonsil,** which together form a ring of lymphatic tissue round the beginning of the alimentary canal.

The tissue fluid under wet epithelial surfaces is particularly liable to contamination by foreign particles and bacteria from the exterior. Its filtration by this unencapsulated lymphatic tissue obviously protects the body by preventing these undesirable elements from spreading further into the tissues.

It has been postulated that this unencapsulated 'gut associated' lymphoid tissue may play a rôle in the development of humoral immunity (p. 413) similar to that of the thymus in cell-mediated immunity.

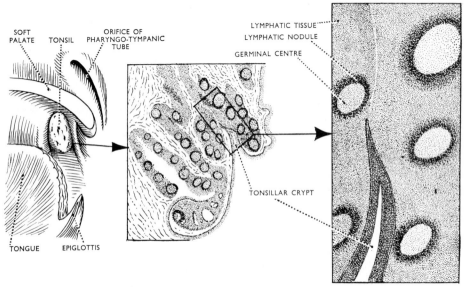

Fig. 161. The tonsil: appearance and position; microscopic structure.

(ii) Filtration of Lymph

Lymph is filtered by lymphatic tissue arranged in encapsulated masses called **lymph nodes.** (This term is preferable to the older term, lymph gland.) Lymph nodes vary in size and measure anything from a few millimetres to two centimetres across.

A lymph node (Fig. 162) is usually bean-shaped, the concave border being called the **hilum.** Here the artery enters and the vein and the efferent lymphatic vessel leave. The **capsule** is a layer of collagenous connective tissue which covers the node. From it partitions **(septa)** pass into the interior, partially

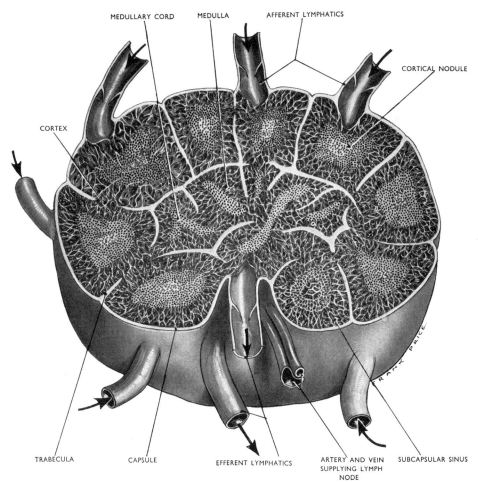

MEDULLARY CORD   MEDULLA   AFFERENT LYMPHATICS

CORTICAL NODULE

CORTEX

TRABECULA   CAPSULE   EFFERENT LYMPHATICS   ARTERY AND VEIN SUPPLYING LYMPH NODE   SUBCAPSULAR SINUS

Fig. 162. A lymph node, cut, to show the internal structure.

dividing it into compartments. In each compartment is a **lymphatic nodule** with a germinal centre. The central part of the node consists of lymphocytes arranged in **cords.** A fine reticulum supports the cells in the node. Surrounding the nodules, between them and the capsule and septa, there are wide reticuloendothelial **sinusoids.** Afferent lymphatic vessels empty their lymph into the sinusoids under the capsule. The lymph then percolates through the node into sinusoids between the cords in the central part, and eventually leaves through the efferent lymphatic vessel. While the lymph is passing through the node, cell débris, bacteria and foreign particles are taken up by the reticulo-endothelial cells, and lymphocytes and monocytes formed in the germinal centres, enter it in large numbers.

Functions of lymph nodes

Lymph nodes act as a filter for lymph. While lymph is passing through the node, cell debris, bacteria and foreign particles are taken up by the reticulo-endothelial cells.

New lymphocytes are formed in the germinal centres and lymphocytes re-enter the lymphatic system from the blood through the walls of venules in the medulla (Fig. 162). Efferent lymph therefore contains very many more lymphocytes than that entering the node. Monocytes and plasma cells (p. 414) are also formed in lymph nodes.

Lymph nodes are important in the immune response (p. 414). They produce the antibodies for the humoral response from plasma cells (p. 414) and the sensitized lymphocytes for the cell-mediated response.

(iii) Filtration of Blood

The spleen is the organ which filters blood. In addition there are, on the posterior abdominal wall, a few hæmal lymph nodes through which blood circulates instead of, or as well as, lymph.

SPLEEN

The spleen (Fig. 163) is a deep red organ, of texture similar to the liver. It is about the size of the closed fist. It is covered completely by peritoneum and lies far back in the upper left part of the abdominal cavity, close against the diaphragm which separates it from the tenth rib. Its medial end is near the midline and its anterior border does not extend further forward than the mid-axillary line. The spleen, like the liver, is therefore protected by the rib cage.

The surface of the spleen in contact with the diaphragm is convex. The surface facing the viscera has shallow concavities for the organs which lie in contact with it—the stomach, the left kidney, the splenic flexure of the colon and the tail of the pancreas, which is related to the hilum. (Figs. 163 and 192.) The **hilum** is where the splenic artery enters and the splenic vein leaves.

The spleen is covered with peritoneum. Under the peritoneum is the **capsule** made of collagenous connective tissue containing some smooth muscle fibres. (In some mammals the capsule contracts and squeezes blood out of the spleen, but this does not happen in Man.) From the capsule, partitions or **trabeculæ** extend into the spleen to give support. The cut surface of a fresh

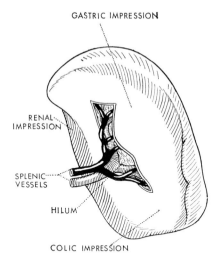

Fig. 163. The spleen seen from the front.

spleen is dark red and semi-solid, the **red pulp.** Scattered through it are tiny white nodules, the **white pulp.**

Under the microscope (Fig. 164) the white pulp is seen to be lymphatic tissue closely surrounding the arterioles, with lymphatic nodules placed at intervals. The red pulp is a delicate network of reticular fibres connected with the trabeculæ. In the mesh are found very numerous reticulo-endothelial cells (fixed macrophages) and all the kinds of cells in the circulating blood. Numerous wide **sinusoids,** with reticulo-endothelial cells forming their walls, pass through the red pulp. They are fed by the arterioles and drain into the splenic veins. Blood cells enter the red pulp either by seeping through the walls of the sinusoids or direct from arterioles with open ends (Fig. 164).

FUNCTIONS OF THE SPLEEN: As blood circulates through the spleen the reticulo-endothelial cells **ingest all the worn-out red blood corpuscles,** and destroy them. The hæmoglobin is broken down into the valuable iron-containing **hæmosiderin** and the waste pigment **bilirubin.** These are taken in the blood stream to the liver where the hæmosiderin is stored and the bilirubin is excreted in the bile (p. 480).

The white pulp provides sensitized lymphocytes for the cell-mediated immune response (p. 414) It also provides plasma cells (p. 414) and hence antibodies for the humoral immune response.

In the fetus, formation of all the different cells of the blood takes place in the spleen as well as in the liver.

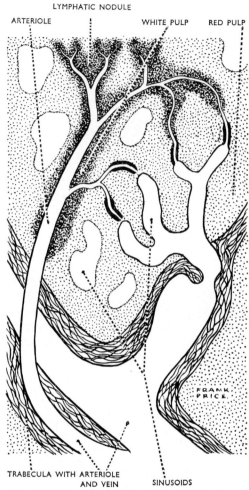

Fig. 164. Microscopic structure of the spleen.

There is no evidence that the normal spleen acts as a reservoir for blood in Man, although it does in some mammals.

THYMUS

Position and Form

The thymus is a bilobed glandular structure situated in the **mediastinum**

(p. 330). It lies behind the upper part of the sternum, separating this bone from the upper portion of the heart and pericardium, and from the great vessels.

In young children (Fig. 231) the thymus is large and occupies much of the superior mediastinal space. It attains its maximum size at puberty, after which it retrogresses slowly during adult life, until it consists only of fatty tissue covering the vessels originating from the arch of the aorta, and the related veins.

Structure

The thymus is very like other lymphatic tissue, being made up of a mass of small lymphocytes, sometimes called **thymocytes,** held together by reticulo-endothelial cells. The gland is lobulated, the cells being more densely packed at the periphery of the lobules. In the centre of the lobules are found rosettes of flattened epithelial cells called **thymic corpuscles** (Hassall's).

Function

In the newborn the thymus is necessary for the development of lymphoid tissue in other parts of the body. It is responsible for the development of the important cell-mediated immunity (p. 414) in the growing individual by supplying a special strain of 'uncommitted' lymphocytes.

A hormone is produced by the epithelial cells in the central parts of the thymus and this stimulates the production of lymphocytes both in the thymus itself and in the lymph nodes and spleen.

The lymphoblasts which form the lymphocytes in the thymus migrate to it from bone marrow. The thymic lymphocytes then populate the lymph nodes, providing cells which are immunologically competent, but uncommitted and therefore ready to become sensitized to any new potentially harmful antigen. Once sensitized, these cells multiply and form a strain of cells always ready to react to that antigen and protect that individual from it.

By adolescence the lymphoid system is fully developed and the thymus involutes.

It should be noted that plasma cells and hence the production of antibodies develop largely independently of the thymus. It has been suggested that the unencapsulated 'gut associated' lymphoid tissue (p. 408) may influence the development of humoral immunity in the way the thymus influences cell-mediated immunity.

IMMUNITY

Immunity in its modern connotation is the activity in all animals of a cell system which is concerned with preserving the integrity of the individual.

Immunity protects against all proteins and cells which are foreign to the individual, most notably against viruses and bacteria.

Different kinds of immunity are described, namely innate immunity and acquired immunity. Acquired immunity may be active or passive, and may be humoral or cell induced.

Innate immunity. Innate immunity that is, the immunity one is born with, is the first line of defence against foreign material. It is present from birth and is genetically controlled. It is non-specific, that is, it protects against a wide range of potentially harmful organisms. It varies from species to species; for example, rats are very resistant to diphtheria while guinea pigs and Man are highly susceptible to it.

Acquired Immunity. This is the second line of defence and is the result of the introduction of foreign substances into the body. The foreign substance, usually a protein, is called an **antigen.** It comes into contact with macrophages (p. 111) and lymphocytes (p. 395) and this produces an **immune response** which is specific for that particular antigen.

There are two forms of immune response. The **humoral response** results in humoral immunity, and the **cellular response** results in cell-mediated immunity.

In **humoral immunity** the antigen stimulates the production of a substance called an **antibody** which reacts with it and neutralizes it. Each antigen causes the production of a particular antibody which destroys it alone. Antibodies are plasma globulins (p. 393) and they are produced mainly by **plasma** cells. These cells, easily recognized by an eccentric nucleus with a 'cartwheel' appearance, appear in lymph nodes in response to the presence of antigens. They may develop from lymphoblasts (p. 398).

In **cell-mediated immunity** there develop in the germinal follicles of lymph nodes, lymphocytes which are sensitized to the antigen and react directly with it. These lymphocytes recognize the antigen, migrate from the blood to sites of high concentration of the antigen, and in ways not fully understood, attack it and destroy it.

Humoral immunity and cell mediated immunity usually develop together in the presence of an antigen.

Active Immunity. Humoral and cell mediated immunity together confer what is called active immunity. This gives long-standing protection because the body has learned to produce the particular antibody and particular lymphocytes needed to combat a particular organism. They are quickly produced to repel a second invasion by the same organism. This is why second attacks of diseases like measles and chickenpox are rare.

Vaccination against smallpox and immunization against diseases like diphtheria, tetanus, whooping-cough and poliomyelitis produce an active immunity in the same way. The difference is that the antigen is deliberately introduced in a form too weak to produce the disease, but active enough to induce the body to make the appropriate antibody and sensitized lymphocytes. More than one injection of the antibody is required. After the first injection, two weeks pass before antibody can be detected in the blood. Not much is present and it soon disappears unless a second dose is given. The second dose results in a remarkable increase in the amount of antibody and thus persists for many months. 'Booster' doses even at long intervals have the same result, because once the response has been produced, the 'memory' of how to do it again remains in lymphatic tissue.

Passive Immunity. If serum from the blood of someone who has had measles is injected into a subject who has not had it, a transient passive immunity to measles is produced. It lasts only as long as the injected antibody persists because the subject's cells have not learned to make the antibody.

Passive immunity is conferred at once, whereas active immunity takes time to develop.

Newborn babies have, for a few weeks, a passive immunity to some of the common infectious diseases if the mother has had them and has an active immunity. Antibodies reach the infant through the placenta and possibly also in breast milk.

Auto-immune Disease. In auto-immune diseases an immune response develops to some of the body's own constituents, and so the body destroys some of its own tissues. Acute hæmolytic anæmia is an example of one such disease.

Immunity and Cancer. Many cancer cells contain material which is foreign to the normal body tissues. This can act as an antigen. It is thought therefore that the immune response may play some part in preventing the establishment of malignant tumours.

Immunity and Transplants. Any kind of foreign tissue introduced into the body provokes an immune response. For this reason, it is not possible, in the ordinary way, to transplant skin, or any other organ from one person to another. If it is tried, a cell mediated immune response occurs in the recipient. Lymphocytes collect round the foreign tissue and attack it, so that the cells die and the tissue is cast off. Sometimes connective tissues with much intercellular substance are transplanted from one person to another, for example pieces of bone and sections of arteries. Realize that the cells in these tissues always die and that the intercellular substance persists only for a time, but for long enough to form a skeleton which surrounding recipient cells gradually invade and replace.

Blood can be transferred from one person to another, but even in this case great care must be taken to ensure that a foreign antigen is not introduced into the recipient's body (see p. 404 and p. 598).

Kidneys can be transplanted successfully in special circumstances. The tissues of donor and recipient are cross-matched (p. 405) to minimize the number of antigens as far as possible. Even then, steps must be taken to kill all the cells in the recipient's body capable of producing an immune response. This can be achieved by immunosuppressive drugs and by irradiation, but the patient must then be protected from every kind of infection.

LYMPHATIC DRAINAGE

All regions of the body except the nervous system are provided with a drainage system for lymph. This comprises lymph nodes and lymph vessels.

LYMPH NODES

Lymph nodes are found mainly in the important groups described below. In addition numerous smaller lymph nodes, often outlying members of the main groups, are found along the course of the blood vessels.

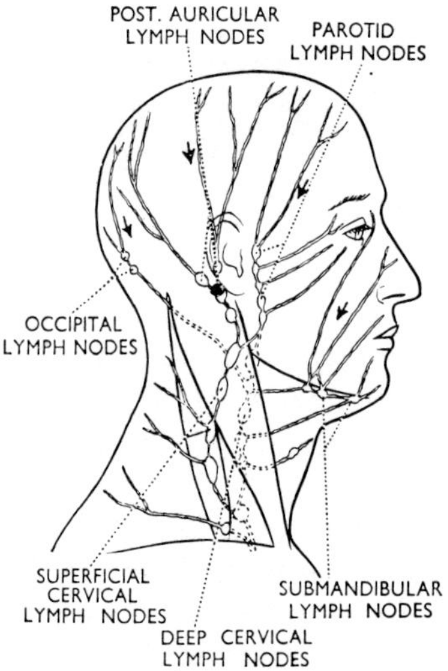

Cervical Lymph Nodes

(a) SUPERFICIAL CERVICAL LYMPH NODES

These are groups of small nodes which form a 'collar' round the junction of the head with the neck. They lie in the superficial fascia, and comprise the submental and submandibular, parotid, auricular and occipital nodes (Fig. 165). They receive lymph from the face and scalp.

(b) DEEP CERVICAL LYMPH NODES

These nodes are large and form an extensive group along the internal jugular vein, and along the subclavian vein in the root of the neck (Fig. 165). They receive lymph from the whole of the head and neck.

Fig. 165. The superficial lymph nodes and the superficial lymphatic drainage of the head and neck.

Axillary Lymph Nodes

The axillary lymph nodes are found spread out in the deep fascia in the axilla. Some sub-groups are recognized (Fig. 171). **Lateral** nodes lie close to the axillary vessels. **Pectoral** nodes lie near the chest wall. **Apical** nodes lie in the apex of the axilla, and are therefore near the nodes in the root of the neck. Some of the nodes, especially those in the lateral and pectoral groups, can be felt on deep palpation of the axilla. The axillary nodes receive lymph from the whole

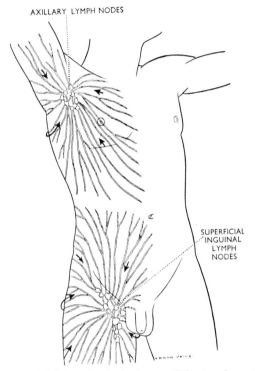

Fig. 166. The superficial lymphatic drainage of the trunk, anterior view.

of the upper limb and from the skin of the upper quarter of the body wall, including the breast (Fig. 171).

Inguinal Lymph Nodes

(a) SUPERFICIAL INGUINAL LYMPH NODES

These form a large group which lies in the superficial fascia just below the inguinal ligament (Fig. 166). The group is 'T'-shaped, the bar of the 'T' being parallel with the inguinal ligament and the stem of the 'T' lying along the proximal part of the great saphenous vein. The superficial inguinal lymph nodes receive lymph from most of the lower limb, including the buttock and from the skin of the lower quarter of the body wall, including the perineum (Fig. 84B).

(b) DEEP INGUINAL LYMPH NODES

These are a few nodes placed along the proximal part of the femoral vein. They receive lymph from the deep tissues of the lower limb.

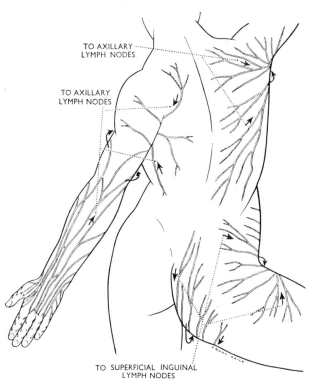

Fig. 167. The superficial lymphatic drainage of the trunk and upper limb, posterior view.

Lymph Nodes of the Thoracic Cavity

Groups of small nodes are found in relation to the blood vessels of the thoracic wall and mediastinum. They receive lymph from the deep parts of the thoracic wall and from the mediastinum.

TRACHEOBRONCHIAL LYMPH NODES

These are large nodes situated round the lower part of the trachea and round the right and left main bronchi.

BRONCHOPULMONARY LYMPH NODES

These are large and numerous nodes situated in the hilum of the lung.

The bronchopulmonary and tracheobronchial nodes receive lymph from the lungs and are often black in colour because of the soot particles trapped in them.

Lymph Nodes of the Abdominopelvic Cavity

AORTIC LYMPH NODES (Fig. 168)

An extensive group of large lymph nodes surrounds the abdominal aorta. They receive lymph from the deep parts of the abdominal wall, from the viscera and from the efferent vessels from the iliac nodes.

CŒLIAC AND SUPERIOR MESENTERIC LYMPH NODES

These are large nodes of the aortic group, arranged round the origins of the cœliac and superior mesenteric arteries, and spreading out along their main branches (Fig. 168). They receive lymph from the organs supplied by these arteries, notably from the stomach, small intestine, part of the large intestine, spleen, pancreas and liver.

INFERIOR MESENTERIC LYMPH NODES

These nodes are members of the aortic group arranged round the origin of the inferior mesenteric artery and spreading along its branches. They receive lymph from the distal part of the colon and from the rectum.

ILIAC LYMPH NODES (Fig. 169)

(a) External Iliac Lymph Nodes

These are large nodes placed along the external iliac vessels. They receive lymph mainly from the lower limb, through the efferent vessels of the superficial and deep inguinal nodes.

(b) Internal Iliac Lymph Nodes

These are placed along the internal iliac vessels and receive lymph mainly from the pelvic viscera, including the bladder, the prostate, the seminal vesicles, the uterus and the vagina.

(c) Common Iliac Lymph Nodes

This group is continuous with the other two groups of iliac nodes and is placed round the common iliac vessels. Lymph is received from the pelvic viscera and from the external and internal iliac groups of nodes.

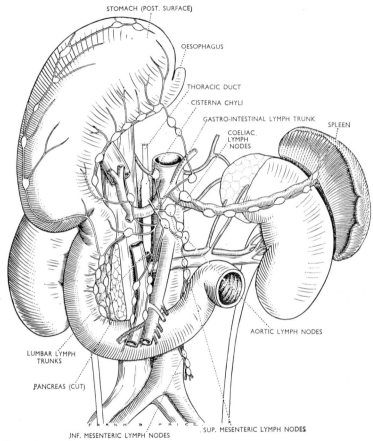

Fig. 168. Lymph nodes and lymphatic vessels associated with some of the upper abdominal viscera. The stomach has been displaced by being turned upwards.

LYMPHATIC VESSELS

Terminal Lymph Vessels

THE THORACIC DUCT (Fig. 169)

The thoracic duct is the main channel of the system of lymphatic vessels, but it is no larger than a small vein. It begins as an ovoid dilatation, the **cisterna chyli,** about 0·5 cm wide and about 7 cm long (Fig. 169). The cisterna chyli lies between the aorta and the right crus of the diaphragm opposite the first and second lumbar vertebræ. The thoracic duct emerges from its upper end and enters the mediastinum, where it ascends first on the right of the œsophagus. It crosses behind the œsophagus and ascends on its left side to the root of the neck, where it curves laterally and then downwards to open into the left brachiocephalic vein where it begins by the union of the left internal jugular vein and the left subclavian vein.

Tributaries. The cisterna chyli receives the **gastro-intestinal trunk,** two **lumbar lymph trunks** and vessels from the **posterior thoracic wall.** As the thoracic duct passes through the thorax, it receives lymph from nodes in the **mediastinum** and from the **œsophagus.** Immediately before it ends it receives the **left subclavian trunk,** the **left jugular trunk** and the **left mediastinal trunk.** These lymph trunks may open separately into the jugular or subclavian vein.

RIGHT LYMPHATIC DUCT (Fig. 169)

The right lymphatic duct is formed by the union of the **right jugular trunk,** the **right subclavian trunk** and the **right mediastinal trunk.** It opens into the beginning of the right brachiocephalic vein. Often the three lymph trunks open separately so that no true right lymphatic duct is formed.

Distribution of Lymphatic Vessels

Lymph vessels are associated with epithelial surfaces, and are most

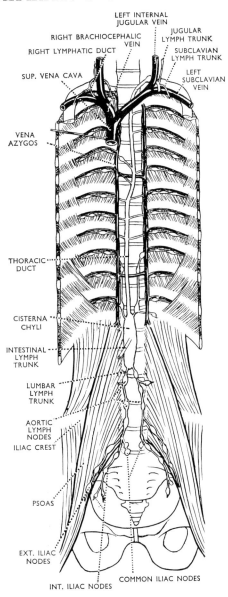

Fig. 169. The cisterna chyli and the thoracic duct on the posterior thoraco-abdominal **wall.**

numerous in the skin, in mucous membranes, in all glands and in all serous and synovial membranes.

Lymph vessels in all parts of the body can be divided into two groups: (a) **Superficial vessels** associated with the skin, and (b) **deep vessels** associated with deep tissues. In the trunk, the deep lymph vessels drain the mucous membranes and glands of the viscera, the serous membranes and the synovial membranes of the small joints. In the limbs, the deep vessels drain the synovial membranes of joints, synovial sheaths and bursæ.

LYMPH VESSELS OF THE HEAD AND NECK

The **superficial vessels** of the face and scalp drain into the 'collar' groups of nodes. The efferents from these nodes, together with the superficial vessels from the neck end in the deep cervical nodes (Fig. 165).

The **deep vessels** from the head and neck go to the deep cervical nodes; in general those from the head go to the upper members of the group, and those from the neck to the lower nodes.

The efferent vessels from the deep cervical nodes unite to form the **jugular lymph trunk** which opens into the thoracic duct on the left side and into the right lymphatic duct on the right side.

LYMPH VESSELS OF THE UPPER LIMB

The **superficial vessels** stream from the front and from the back of the limb towards the axillary lymph nodes, especially to the lateral group (Fig. 170). Note that those from the back of the shoulder sweep round the lower edge of the posterior wall of the axilla (Fig. 167).

The lymph vessels from the little finger and medial side of the hand end in the **cubital** (supratrochlear) **lymph node** which lies in the superficial fascia on the front of the arm just above the medial epicondyle (Fig. 170). From there, the lymph follows the deep stream to the lateral axillary nodes.

The superficial lymph vessels from the skin of the **upper quarter of the trunk** both front and back (below the level of the clavicle and above the level of the umbilicus) are closely associated with those of the upper limb and sweep to the axillary nodes, mainly to the pectoral group. The lymph vessels from the **breast** follow the same path to the pectoral group of axillary nodes (Fig. 171).

The **deep lymph vessels** of the upper limb follow the course of the deep blood vessels and end in the lateral axillary nodes.

The efferent vessels from the axillary nodes unite to form the **subclavian**

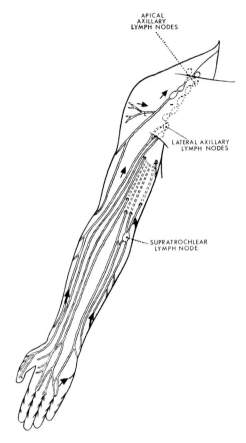

Fig. 170. The superficial lymphatic drainage of the front of the upper limb.

lymph trunk which ends in the thoracic duct on the left and in the right lymphatic duct on the right side.

LYMPHATIC VESSELS OF THE THORAX

The **superficial vessels,** including those of the breast, end in the pectoral group of axillary nodes (p. 541, Fig. 171).

The **deep vessels** follow one of two routes. Those from the posterior part of the thoracic wall and from the œsophagus join the cisterna chyli or the thoracic duct. The deep vessels from the front of the thoracic wall and from the broncho-pulmonary and tracheobronchial nodes which drain the lung, unite on each side

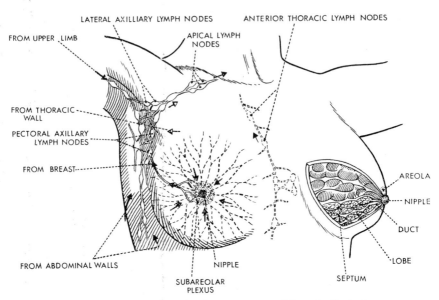

Fig. 171. The mammary gland: structure and lymphatic drainage.

to form the **mediastinal trunk** which ends in the thoracic duct on the left and in the right lymphatic duct on the right side.

LYMPH VESSELS OF THE ABDOMEN AND PELVIS

The **superficial vessels,** both from the front and from the back, drain into the **superficial inguinal lymph nodes** (Figs. 166 and 167). This includes the skin of the **perineum.** Notice that the skin of the trunk can be divided into four areas each draining to a different group of nodes, the two upper areas to the axillary nodes and the two lower areas to the superficial inguinal nodes. The lines separating these areas, that is the 'lymph sheds', are the midline, front and back, and a horizontal line at the level of the umbilicus.

The **deep vessels** of the abdomen and pelvis are the vessels which drain the viscera.

Lymph vessels from the **stomach, liver, pancreas, spleen, small intestine** and proximal part of the **large intestine** converge on the **cœliac** and **superior mesenteric lymph nodes** following the paths of the blood vessels, and being interrupted by numerous outlying lymph nodes. The lymph from the small intestine contains emulsified fat absorbed from the food, and is milky to look at. It is called **chyle.** The efferent vessels from the cœliac and superior mesenteric nodes unite to form the **gastro-intestinal trunk** which empties the chyle into the cisterna chyli.

Lymph vessels from the distal part of the **large intestine,** including the **rectum,** drain to the **inferior mesenteric nodes.**

Lymph vessels from the **kidneys, ureters, suprarenal glands** and from the **ovaries** and **testes** drain to the **aortic lymph nodes.** The long course of the lymphatic vessels of the testes and ovaries is explained by the fact that these organs originate at the level of the second lumbar vertebra and descend to the adult position.

Lymph vessels from the pelvic viscera (except the ovary) drain to the external and internal iliac lymph nodes, and efferent vessels from these go to the common iliac nodes which also receive vessels direct from the pelvis.

The **lumbar lymph trunks,** one on each side, receive the efferent vessels from all the aortic nodes, from the inferior mesenteric nodes and from the common iliac nodes, which in- cludes the lymph from the lower limbs. The lumbar lymph trunks end in the cisterna chyli.

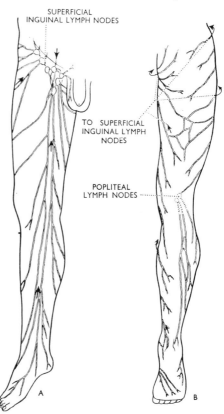

Fig. 172. The superficial lymphatic drain- age of the lower limb: A, anterior view; B, posterior view.

LYMPH VESSELS OF THE LOWER LIMB

Most of the **superficial vessels** of the lower limb stream towards the superficial inguinal nodes, especially to those forming the stem of the T-shaped group (Fig. 172). The vessels from the lateral part of the foot and back of the calf follow the small saphenous vein, and end in popliteal nodes in the popliteal fossa. The efferents of these nodes join the deep stream.

Lymph vessels from the gluteal region sweep round to the most lateral nodes of the superficial inguinal group. Lymph vessels from the **perineum,** including those from the lower part of the **vagina** and from the skin of the **anal canal,** end in the medial nodes.

The superficial inguinal nodes also receive lymph vessels from the **abdominal wall below the level of the umbilicus.**

The **deep lymph vessels** of the lower limb follow the paths of the blood vessels and end in the deep inguinal lymph nodes.

The efferent vessels from both superficial and deep inguinal nodes go to the **external iliac nodes,** from which the lymph travels along the chain of iliac nodes to reach the **lumbar lymph trunk.**

Special Considerations

LYMPH NODES AND INFECTION

In acute infections, bacteria gain access to the tissues and set up inflammation, causing pain, redness and swelling. Some of the bacteria enter the lymphatic capillaries and vessels and are carried to the nearest lymph node, where they are filtered off and trapped in the node. The node in turn may become inflamed—**lymphadenitis.** If the lymph vessels are inflamed through infection by the bacteria, they show as red streaks under the skin—**lymphangitis.**

In chronic infections, like tuberculosis, the lymph nodes of the region, through which the bacteria gained entry, are often greatly enlarged.

The lymph nodes are responsible for the immune response (p. 414). They also help to prevent bacteria from gaining access to the blood stream.

LYMPH NODES AND MALIGNANT DISEASE

When a malignant growth develops, especially in an epithelium, some of the malignant cells gain entry to the lymphatic vessels and are carried with the lymph to the nearest lymph node, where they are filtered off. In the node, they multiply and form a secondary growth or **metastasis.** In this way the growth is spread via the lymphatic system to different parts of the body.

OBSTRUCTION OF LYMPH VESSELS

This, by preventing the return of fluid and proteins which may have escaped into the tissue fluid, causes great swelling of the part (p. 97).

CHAPTER XIV

THE ALIMENTARY SYSTEM

THE alimentary system provides the means whereby the body receives the food materials it needs for body building and for energy. It is essentially a tube with an opening at one end, the mouth, where the food is taken in, and an opening at the other end, the anus, where the unwanted materials are cast out or voided. However, the contents of the alimentary canal are just as much outside the tissues of the body as materials resting on the skin would be. To be of use to the body the food must be absorbed by the cells of the mucous membrane which lines the canal. To pass through the cell membranes, the food must be dissolved in water and must be broken down, that is, digested into relatively simple compounds with small molecules, which are able to diffuse. Different parts of the alimentary canal are specialized to perform different functions to this end. In the mouth the food is broken up by the teeth into tiny pieces so that digestive enzymes can reach every part of it. Different enzymes from different parts of the canal act on the different constituents of the food. In the stomach the food is churned up with fluid and enzymes, still more fluid and digestive enzymes are added when it passes into the small intestine, until all the useful constituents are dissolved and broken down. In the small intestine too, these materials are absorbed by the mucous membrane and passed on to the blood stream. In the large intestine water is reabsorbed because the large volume poured out in the various glandular secretions is too precious to waste. This reabsorption of water continues until the contents, now consisting of waste materials only, are semisolid fæces which are expelled at intervals through the anal canal.

Outline of Development

At an early stage of development the embryo consists of an embryonic disc composed of ectoderm, mesoderm and endoderm. The cephalic and caudal ends of the disc bend round (Fig. 26), so that a space is partially enclosed in front, the **foregut,** and another behind, the **hindgut.** The part between these, which is in direct continuity with the yolk sac, is the **midgut** and the connexion is the yolk stalk. The **buccopharyngeal membrane** represents the position of the future mouth and breaks down so that the foregut opens to the exterior. Similarly the **cloacal membrane** represents

427

the site of the future anal canal, and breaks down so that the hindgut opens to the outside. The endoderm forms the epithelium lining the whole of the alimentary tract from the mouth to the end of the rectum and all the glands, including pancreas and liver, associated with it. The splanchnopleuric mesoderm in contact with it forms the smooth muscle, blood vessels and connective tissue of the gut and its derivatives. Essentially the gut is a tube which is pushed into the peritoneum from behind so that the layer of peritoneum in contact with gut becomes visceral peritoneum which in turn becomes continuous with the parietal layer by means of a mesentery (Fig. 173).

From the **cranial half** of the foregut are developed parts of the mouth, and the pharynx. The walls of the pharynx form a series of arches, the **branchial arches,** with grooves between them, rather like the gill clefts of fish, though true openings never appear. Each arch has a supporting cartilage, muscles, nerves and blood vessels. The arches form the mandible, the hyoid bone, the cartilages of the larynx, and the muscles associated with them. The most cranial of the somites move ventrally to form the tongue, which is covered, of course, by the pharyngeal endoderm.

The **caudal half** of the foregut gives rise to the œsophagus, the stomach and half of the duodenum. This part of the foregut is connected by a **dorsal mesentery** to the dorsal body wall, and by a **ventral mesentery** to the ventral body wall, in the region of the septum transversum (p. 79) which gives rise to most of the diaphragm. From most distal part of the foregut, the liver and the pancreas grow out as proliferating buds of the endoderm. The liver grows into the ventral mesentery, dividing it into the falciform ligament and the lesser omentum. Meanwhile, the stomach has enlarged and has come to lie with its right side facing dorsally and its left side facing ventrally. The interval dorsal to the stomach and lesser omentum is the beginning of the omental bursa (lesser sac). The greater omentum grows as a pouching of the dorsal mesentery of the stomach. At the same time the midgut and hindgut, which are attached to the dorsal wall only by the dorsal mesentery, have grown greatly in length and the yolk stalk has become a narrow communication with a now small yolk sac lying outside the ventral body wall. The midgut and hindgut are so long that for a time there is no room for them in the peritoneal cavity and they herniate as a long loop into the umbilical cord. When they return a twisting occurs so that the caudal half of the loop comes to lie ventral and cranial to the cranial half. The diagrams show how this affects the final position of the intestines. The mesenteries of the ascending and descending colons and of the duodenum disappear by blending with the posterior abdominal wall, but the small intestine jejunum and ileum, the transverse colon and the pelvic colon retain their mesenteries.

Each of the three parts of the gut in the abdominal cavity has its own artery from the abdominal aorta, namely for the foregut the cœliac artery, for the midgut the superior mesenteric artery and for the hindgut the inferior mesenteric artery. **From the foregut** are developed the stomach, half of the duodenum (as far as the entry of the bile duct), the liver and gall bladder and the

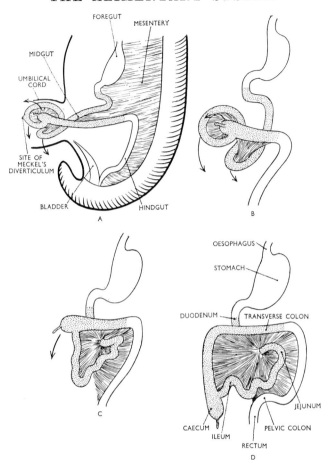

Fig. 173. The development of the intestines: A, a diagrammatic outline of the abdominal cavity seen from the side, showing the midgut herniated into the umbilical cord; B, the midgut rotating as it returns to the abdomen, seen from the side; C, the rotation continuing, seen from the front; D, the final positions of the organs seen from the front.

pancreas, all supplied by branches of the cœlic artery. **From the midgut** are developed the distal half of the duodenum, the jejunum, the ileum and the large intestine as far as the junction of the middle and distal thirds of the transverse colon, all supplied by the superior mesenteric artery. **From the hindgut** are developed the distal third of the transverse colon, the descending colon, the pelvic colon and the rectum down to the anorectal junction, all supplied by the inferior mesenteric artery. In the same way the nerves, which are distributed to the gut along these vessels, are grouped into three subdivisions, each one causing pain to be referred to a specific region of the abdominal wall, i.e. (*a*) **foregut** to the **epigastrium,** (*b*) **midgut** to the **umbilical region,** (*c*) **hindgut** to the **hypogastrium.**

LIPS

The lips surround the opening of the mouth. They contain a voluntary sphincter, which is part of the facial musculature supplied by the facial nerve. The outside is covered with skin, but the free border and the internal aspect is covered with mucous membrane, which is more transparent than skin, so that the colour of the blood in the underlying capillaries shows through. The colour of the lips can be a guide to the state of the blood, deep pink in health, blue if the blood passing through is poorly oxygenated, pale in anæmia. The lips are supplied by branches of the trigeminal nerve, and are very sensitive. Also, their blood supply is very rich so that if lacerated, they heal very well provided the edges of the wound are kept in apposition.

MOUTH

The mouth is divided into two parts, the vestibule and the buccal cavity. Both are lined throughout by stratified squamous nonkeratinized epithelium. The **vestibule** is bounded by the lips and cheeks on the one hand, and the gums and teeth on the other. It is a narrow cleft and the cheeks which form its outer wall are, like the lips, made of muscle lined with mucous membrane. The **duct of the parotid gland** opens into the vestibule opposite the crown of the second upper molar tooth. The vestibule communicates widely with the buccal cavity when the jaws are open, but if the jaws are closed, and all the teeth are present, the only passage is behind the last molar tooth. This interval can be used for inserting a feeding tube if necessary.

The **buccal cavity** is bounded by the teeth and jaws in front and at the sides, and communicates posteriorly with the oral part of the pharynx through the oropharyngeal opening. The roof is formed by the palate which separates the buccal cavity from the nasal cavity, and the floor is formed by muscles and the attachments of the tongue.

PALATE

The anterior two-thirds of the palate, the **hard palate,** is bony (Fig. 42). The posterior third, the **soft palate** (Plate 34), is composed of the insertions of a group of small palatal muscles which connect it with the base of the skull above and with the tongue and pharynx below. Movements of the soft palate (Fig. 177) are important in swallowing (p. 439) and in speech (p. 329). From the middle of the posterior free border of the soft palate, the **uvula** hangs down. At the sides this border arches downwards forming the **palatopharyngeal arch,** and completing the **oropharyngeal opening.** In front of this arch another raised arch of the mucous membrane, the **palatoglossal arch,** links the soft palate with the tongue. Together these arches are called the **fauces** and the vertical portions of the folds at the base of each arch are called the **pillars of the fauces** (Fig. 174).

TONSILS

On each side, between the pillars of the fauces, lies the tonsil, a swelling with a pitted surface (Fig. 174). It is a mass of lymphatic tissue covered by mucous membrane. It is relatively larger in children than in adults, and if it is infected it may become very large indeed (see also p. 408).

FLOOR OF THE MOUTH

The floor of the mouth is composed of a flat muscle which stretches from the inside of the body of the mandible to the hyoid bone (p. 131) forming what is sometimes called the **oral diaphragm** (Fig. 89).

TONGUE

The tongue is an organ entirely composed of striated muscle, covered with mucous membrane. In shape it is like a boot turned upside down. The toe of the boot is the tip of the tongue; the sole of the boot is the rough surface which is seen in the floor of the mouth. At the position of the heel of the boot, marked by a V-shaped groove, this surface of the tongue turns to face backwards towards the pharynx. The V-shaped groove marks the junction of the anterior two-thirds and the posterior third of the **dorsum** of the tongue (Fig. 174). The top of the boot (pointing downwards since it is inverted) represents the **root** of the tongue, which is the muscular attachment of the tongue to the hyoid bone and to the mandible behind the point of the chin. The mucous membrane which lines the mouth also covers the tongue, except for the root. On the dorsum of the tongue can be seen tiny projections of the mucous membrane, the **papillæ** of the tongue. Along the V-shaped groove is a line of larger **vallate papillæ** each surrounded by a circular groove which in turn is surrounded by mucous membrane. Taste buds (p. 310) are scattered in the mucous membrane of the dorsum of the tongue, and especially round the vallate papillæ. The faintly white appearance of the normal tongue is caused by desquamated surface cells from the stratified squamous epithelium. In disturbances of the digestive tract, these cells accumulate to give a 'furred tongue', in some cases possibly because the appetite is depressed and the usual quantities of food are not exerting the normal abrasive effect. A similar result is produced in dehydration when there is decreased salivation, and in mouth breathing in the presence of upper respiratory infections when the surface of the tongue tends to become dry. The under surface of the anterior part of the tongue is covered by thinner mucous membrane, which forms a fold, the **frenulum** attached to the floor of the mouth in the midline. On each side of the frenulum, between the tongue and the mandible, the ducts of the submandibular and sublingual salivary glands open.

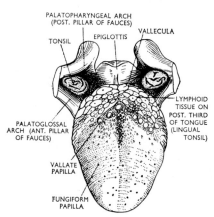

Fig. 174. The dorsum of the tongue, showing its relation to the tonsils and to the epiglottis.

The muscles of the tongue are supplied by the **hypoglossal nerve.** The mucous membrane of the anterior two-thirds is supplied with ordinary sensation by the lingual branch of the **mandibular nerve** and with taste fibres from the chorda tympani branch of the **facial.** The posterior third is supplied both with ordinary sensation and with taste by the **glossopharyngeal nerve.**

The tongue is a very mobile organ, under control of the will. It plays a part in mastication, acting with the cheeks to keep the food between the jaws. Its movements are important in speech (p. 329) and in swallowing (p. 439).

THE TEETH

The teeth are for breaking up the food. The upper teeth are carried by the maxilla and the lower teeth are carried by the mandible.

Structure

Each tooth consists of a **crown** and a **root** joined by a short **neck** (Fig. 175). The crown is the part which projects from the gums; the root fits exactly into a cavity, or **alveolus,** in the jaw. The **gum,** which is a layer of dense connective tissue attached to the periosteum of the jaw and covered with mucous membrane, forms a collar round the neck of the tooth.

The main part of both root and crown is made of **dentine,** a hard substance something like bone. Within the dentine is a cavity, the **pulp cavity,** which extends from the crown to the apex of the root, where blood vessels and a nerve enter, to branch throughout the pulp cavity. Nerves extend into the dentine which is sensitive to heat, cold, acid and sweetness. The dentine of the crown is covered by a layer of **enamel,** which is the hardest substance in the body, to withstand the wear and tear of mastication. The root is covered by a layer of **cement,** a calcified material which binds the root to the **periodontal membrane.** This is the periosteum lining the alveolus. It consists of fibres providing the means of suspending and attaching the root in the socket provided by the alveolus. The tooth can thus move or rock slightly within its socket, and this movement plays an important part in stimulating blood flow to the tooth.

Teeth are of three different shapes, according to the function they perform.

Incisors, for cutting or chiselling, have crowns with a straight sharp edge and a single root.

Canines are long and pointed, and are used by animals for grasping and tearing flesh.

Molars are for grinding and have large flattish crowns divided by grooves into rounded or pointed cusps, and two, or three, roots. The pulp cavity extends into each of the roots.

Man develops two sets of teeth—the **temporary** or 'milk' **teeth** and the **permanent teeth.** The temporary teeth are also called **deciduous teeth** because they are shed before being replaced by their permanent counterparts.

In all, there are twenty temporary teeth, five in each half of each jaw. These five are two incisors near the midline, one canine and, at the back, two molars.

There are thirty-two permanent teeth, eight in each half of each jaw, namely—two incisors, one canine, two premolars and three molars (Figs. 41 and 48). Each premolar has a single root and a crown with two cusps. The molars have from three to five cusps; those in the upper jaw have three roots, those in the lower jaw have two roots.

Nerve Supply

The teeth of the upper jaw are supplied by the maxillary division of the

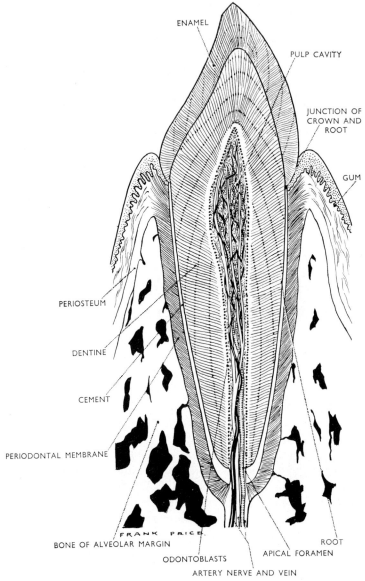

ENAMEL

PULP CAVITY

JUNCTION OF
CROWN AND
ROOT

GUM

PERIOSTEUM

DENTINE

CEMENT

PERIODONTAL MEMBRANE

FRANK PRICE.

BONE OF ALVEOLAR MARGIN

ODONTOBLASTS

ARTERY NERVE AND VEIN

APICAL FORAMEN

ROOT

Fig. 175. A section through a tooth, in position in the jaw.

trigeminal nerve; those in the lower jaw are supplied by the mandibular division. Pain from a carious tooth is usually felt in the tooth itself, but it may be referred to different parts of the face, forehead, cheek, temple, chin or external auditory meatus.

Development of Teeth

The teeth begin to develop early in fetal life. At birth the crowns of all the temporary teeth and of some of the permanent teeth are well formed, but still buried in the jaws and below the gums. During pregnancy a mother must, therefore, have a diet which supplies all the necessary calcium and phosphates and vitamins A and D to ensure proper development of the teeth as well as of the bones. If her diet is deficient in these substances, the mother's body stores will be depleted to supply the fetus. Proper dental supervision and care of pregnant women is therefore particularly important.

During the first two years the temporary teeth erupt, that is they push their way through the gums. Average ages for the eruption of the different temporary teeth are:

Lower central incisors	6–9 months
Upper incisors	8–10 months
Lower lateral incisors, first molars	15–20 months
Canines	16–20 months
Second Molars	20–24 months

During childhood the permanent teeth complete their development and, by their increasing size, encroach on the roots of the temporary teeth (Fig. 176) so that these roots dissolve, the teeth become loose and fall out. The permanent teeth erupt to take their places at the following ages:

First molar	end of 6th year
Medial incisors	end of 7th year
Lateral incisors	end of 8th year
First premolars	between 10th and 11th years
Canines	between 11th and 12th years
Second premolars	between 11th and 12th years
Second molars	between 12th and 13th years
Third molars	between 17th and 25th years

Occlusion

When the jaws are closed the teeth of the two jaws come into contact so that their biting surfaces fit together (Fig. 41). This is occlusion, and is an

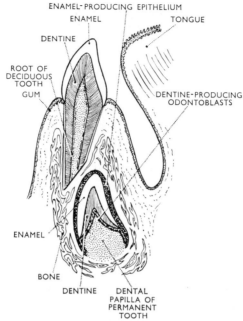

Fig. 176. A section through the lower jaw of a child, showing a deciduous tooth with its root undergoing absorption, because of the nearby developing permanent tooth.

obvious requirement for good function. In **malocclusion** *the biting surfaces do not make contact properly*, perhaps because the arches of the jaws are badly shaped or because the teeth are too crowded.

THE SALIVARY GLANDS

The salivary glands secrete the first of the digestive juices, the **saliva**. There are three pairs of salivary glands, the parotid gland, the submandibular gland, and the sublingual gland.

The **parotid gland** is the largest (Fig. 84). It is a lobulated mass of very irregular shape, packed into the interval between the posterior border of the ramus of the mandible and the external auditory meatus. The superficial surface lies under the skin, and from its anterior border the duct passes forwards across the masseter, and then through the cheek to open into the vestibule of the mouth opposite the second upper molar tooth. It is enclosed within an upward extension of the cervical fascia, which forms an inelastic investment for the gland. This is why any swelling of the gland is extremely painful.

The **submandibular gland** is an ovoid mass which lies on the inner aspect of the body of the mandible in front of the angle (Fig. 89). Its duct passes forwards above the floor of the mouth to open as a small projection or **papilla** at the side of the frenulum of the tongue.

The **sublingual gland** is almond shaped and lies on the floor of the mouth between the tongue and the mandible, close to the midline. Mucous membrane covers it and several ducts open directly into the floor of the mouth.

Saliva

Saliva is a watery secretion containing the enzyme **salivary amylase** (ptyalin), which begins the digestion of carbohydrate. It also contains mucus which acts as a lubricant. The secretion of saliva is controlled reflexly. Stimulation of the tongue by food in the mouth and the sight, smell or thought of food causes parasympathetic stimulation of the glands to secrete. If a strong tasting substance like lemon juice is placed on the tongue, a spurt of saliva can be observed from each of the orifices of the salivary ducts. Fear and excitement depress the secretion of saliva and this makes the mouth feel dry.

FUNCTIONS OF SALIVA:

1. Saliva moistens the mouth and tongue, preventing the mucous membrane from drying and cracking.
2. It moistens the food so that it can be moulded into a bolus for swallowing, and it lubricates the bolus.
3. By means of the enzyme salivary amylase, it begins the digestion of carbohydrate. The saliva is mixed with the food before swallowing, and the digestion goes on inside the bolus after swallowing until the hydrochloric acid in the stomach inhibits the enzyme. The carbohydrate is hydrolized by salivary amylase to **dextrin** and **maltose.**
4. The taste buds are stimulated only by dissolved substances. Saliva acts as a solvent to facilitate tasting.
5. Saliva is a cleaning agent, to wash away débris. If salivation is suppressed, as it is in fevers, the mouth becomes dirty.
6. If the body is growing short of water, salivation is depressed and the awareness of the need for water is felt as a drying of the mouth.
7. A few chemicals, iodides for example, are excreted in the saliva.

THE PHARYNX

The pharynx is a wide muscular tube, most of it behind the nose and mouth (Plate 34). It conducts air from the nose to the larynx and food from the mouth to the œsophagus. It stretches from the base of the skull above, to the level of the cricoid cartilage in the neck below, where it is continuous with the œsophagus. It lies immediately in front of the first six cervical vertebral bodies. The posterior and side walls are continuous but the anterior wall is deficient. The upper part of the anterior wall, above the level of the palate, communicates with the nose, and this part of the pharynx is the **nasopharynx.** Below the soft palate and above the larynx, the anterior wall communicates with the mouth through the **oropharyngeal isthmus;** this part of the pharynx is the **oropharynx.** The **laryngeal part** of the pharynx lies behind the larynx. Surgeons refer to this part as the **postcricoid space.**

The walls of the pharynx are composed of thin curved sheets of striated muscle called the **superior, middle** and **inferior constrictors** of the pharynx (Plate 34). They are arranged to overlap, one inside the other from above down, much as flower pots might be when stacked. The upper margin of the superior constrictor is connected with the base of the skull. The anterior edges of the muscles are connected to the pterygoid processes of the sphenoid, to the mandible, to the hyoid bone, to the thyroid cartilage and to the cricoid cartilage. The lowest part of the inferior constrictor blends with the beginning of the œsophagus.

The muscles of the pharynx are supplied by a branch of the vagus nerve.

The **nasopharynx** is described with the respiratory system on p. 323.

The **oropharynx** communicates in front with the mouth through the oropharyngeal isthmus (see above). Below this opening the back of the tongue is connected with the front of the epiglottis by a midline fold of mucous membrane. On each side of this is a hollow, the **vallecula** (Fig. 174). The tongue is very mobile and its posterior surface readily makes contact with the back wall of the oropharynx, for example in swallowing. Consider too an **unconscious patient** lying on his back (Fig. 177, c). The tone in all muscles including those of the tongue is lost, and the tongue, being flaccid, flops backwards against the pharyngeal wall, thus blocking the airway. It is essential to prevent this; the patient's head is turned to one side so that the tongue falls sideways rather than backwards; the tongue is held forwards by lifting the mandible forwards at its angle because the muscles, which in normal circumstances pull the tongue forward, are attached to the front part of the mandible. If the patient lies prone the tongue will fall forward automatically.

The **laryngeal part** of the pharynx is narrower than the other parts. The laryngeal aditus is in the midline in the anterior wall, with the epiglottis projecting upwards above it. On each side of the aditus, where the pharynx partly surrounds the larynx, there is an elongated hollow, the **piriform fossa** (Plate 34).

Sometimes parts of the food, especially fish-bones, stick when they are being swallowed and cause great discomfort. Common sites for this are the tonsillar crypts, the vallecula and the piriform fossa.

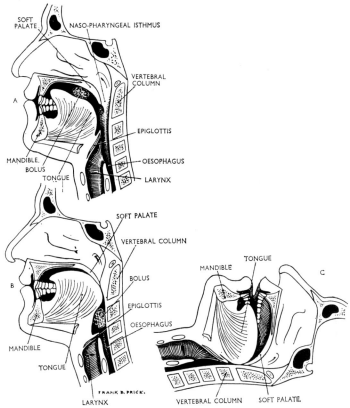

Fig. 177. A, the first stage in swallowing; B, the second stage in swallowing; C, the relaxed tongue of a recumbent, unconscious patient blocking the airway.

SWALLOWING

The oropharynx is a channel both for air on its way to the larynx and for food on its way to the œsophagus. Swallowing is the process of temporary interruption of breathing with closing of the air passages, while food is propelled from the mouth to the œsophagus and stomach. Swallowing occurs in three stages with no pause between stages.

First, the food is passed from the mouth into the oropharynx (Fig. 177, A).

This stage is voluntary. The food is moulded by the tongue into an ovoid mass, or **bolus,** which rests on the dorsum of the tongue. The tongue is then pressed against the palate from before backwards and this drives the bolus through the oropharyngeal isthmus.

Secondly, the food passes from the oropharynx to the œsophagus. This stage is involuntary and is controlled reflexly as a result of the presence of food in the oropharynx. The bolus is driven downwards to the œsophagus by contraction of the constrictors of the pharynx. Meanwhile, however, the naso-pharynx has been shut off by the raising of the soft palate until it makes close contact with the pharyngeal wall (Fig. 177, B). The laryngeal aditus is also pro-tected; the whole larynx is drawn upwards and at the same time a little for-wards under the posterior part of the tongue; the laryngeal muscles round the aditus contract, reducing the opening; the epiglottis tilts backwards to form a shelter over the aditus. The oropharyngeal isthmus is narrowed at the same time to prevent any return of food to the mouth.

Thirdly, the food passes down the œsophagus involuntarily by peristalsis. Fluids may pass down very rapidly without the aid of peristaltic contractions.

THE PERITONEAL CAVITY

The **peritoneum** is the serous membrane which lines the abdominal cavity and covers the viscera. Like all **serous membranes,** it has a smooth shiny surface composed of a layer of simple squamous epithelium supported by a thin layer of areolar tissue. The peritoneum forms the walls of a closed sac, with the epithelial surface facing into the cavity, which is called the peritoneal cavity. We can imagine this sac placed inside the abdominal cavity, lining its walls.

Next we must consider the relationship of the viscera to the peritoneum. An organ like the kidney, which lies in direct contact with the posterior abdo-minal wall, has peritoneum covering only its anterior surface. It is said to be **retroperitoneal.** The small intestine, on the other hand, might be considered to have pushed forwards from the posterior abdominal wall, carrying the peritoneum in front of it until, surrounded by peritoneum, it is suspended by a two-layered fold from the posterior abdominal wall (Fig. 178). Such a fold is a **mesentery.** The peritoneum covering the intestine or any other viscus is called **visceral peritoneum;** that lining the walls of the abdominal cavity is **parietal peritoneum;** visceral peritoneum and parietal peritoneum are merely different parts of the same serous membrane. Many organs, some of them large, like the stomach and the liver, are invested with visceral peritoneum in a similar way, so much so that their serous surfaces are everywhere in contact with those of adjacent organs or with the parietal peritoneum (Fig. 180). The peritoneal cavity is, therefore, only a potential space in health. If fluid collects in it or if

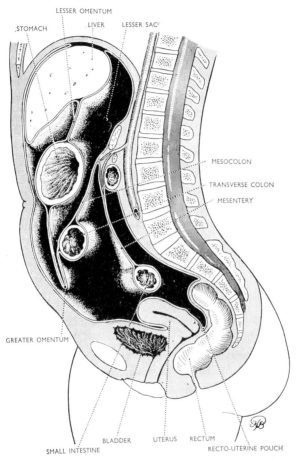

Fig. 178. A midline sagittal section of the abdominopelvic cavity to show the arrangement of the peritoneum in the female. The lesser sac is now called the omental bursa.

air enters it, as it does when the abdominal wall is opened at operation, it becomes a true space. The smooth surface of the peritoneum allows the viscera to move easily in relation to each other and to the abdominal walls. Friction is reduced still further by a thin layer of fluid between the contiguous surfaces.

A fold in the peritoneum is a **peritoneal ligament,** for example the falciform ligament (Fig. 194) and the broad ligament of the uterus (Fig. 214). Such peritoneal ligaments (unlike the collagen ligaments associated with joints) have no tensile strength, are easily stretched and play no part in supporting the viscera. All mesenteries and some peritoneal ligaments convey blood vessels, lymph vessels and nerves from the abdominal wall to the viscera.

With the growth and development of the viscera, the basically simple arrangement of the peritoneum becomes more complex. In early development the whole gut from the œsophagus to the rectum has a **dorsal mesentery.** Some parts of it remain as the **mesentery** (that is, the mesentery of the jejunum and ileum), the **transverse mesocolon** (the mesentery of the transverse colon) and the **pelvic mesocolon** (the mesentery of the pelvic colon). The mesenteries of the duodenum and of the ascending and descending colons disappear by blending into the parietal peritoneum. The dorsal mesentery of the stomach is attached to the border which becomes the greater curvature. The cephalic part of the dorsal mesentery is divided lengthways into two parts by the spleen which develops in the middle of it. The dorsal part which connects the posterior abdominal wall, and the left kidney lying on it, with the spleen is the **lieno-renal ligament;** the ventral part between the spleen and the stomach is the **gastrosplenic ligament.** The caudal part of the dorsal mesentery of the stomach forms a large pouch, with the concavity facing to the right. The pouch is flattened and its walls largely fuse, to form the apron-like **greater omentum** (Fig. 178). The transverse mesocolon later fuses with the greater omentum.

The stomach and the more cranial part of the duodenum have also a **ventral mesentery** connecting their ventral border (which, in the case of the stomach, becomes the lesser curvature) with the anterior abdominal wall. It has a free border caudally. The liver grows into the ventral mesentery, dividing it into the **falciform ligament** (Fig. 194) which connects the anterior abdominal wall with the anterior surface of the liver, and the **lesser omentum** (Fig. 178) which connects the liver (at the porta hepatis and the fissure for the ligamentum venosum, p. 474) with the lesser curvature of the stomach.

The stomach meanwhile has come to lie so that its right surface faces backwards and its left surface forwards. A recess, the **omental bursa** (lesser sac) of the peritoneum, is found between the stomach and the posterior abdominal wall. (The general peritoneal cavity is sometimes called the greater sac.) The posterior wall of the omental bursa consists of peritoneum covering part of the posterior abdominal wall, including the beginning of the abdominal aorta with the cœliac artery, the crura of the diaphragm, the right suprarenal gland, the upper part of the left kidney and the body of the pancreas. The anterior wall of the

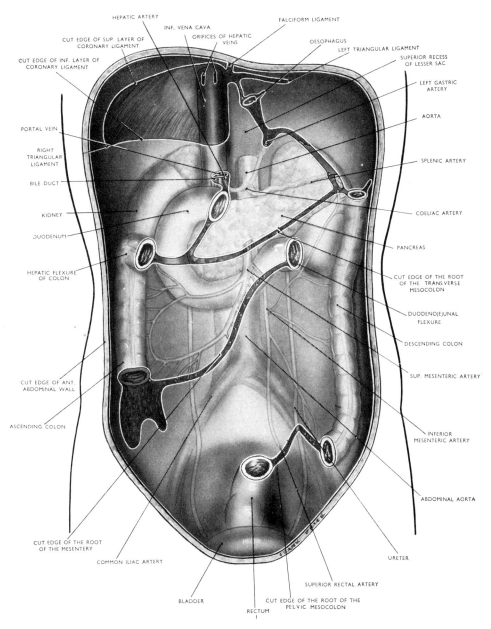

HEPATIC ARTERY

INF. VENA CAVA

CUT EDGE OF SUP. LAYER OF
CORONARY LIGAMENT

ORIFICES OF HEPATIC
VEINS

FALCIFORM LIGAMENT

OESOPHAGUS

LEFT TRIANGULAR LIGAMENT

CUT EDGE OF INF. LAYER OF
CORONARY LIGAMENT

SUPERIOR RECESS
OF LESSER SAC

LEFT GASTRIC
ARTERY

PORTAL VEIN

AORTA

RIGHT
TRIANGULAR
LIGAMENT

SPLENIC ARTERY

BILE DUCT

KIDNEY

COELIAC ARTERY

DUODENUM

PANCREAS

HEPATIC FLEXURE
OF COLON

CUT EDGE OF THE ROOT
OF THE TRANSVERSE
MESOCOLON

DUODENOJEJUNAL
FLEXURE

DESCENDING COLON

CUT EDGE OF ANT.
ABDOMINAL WALL

SUP. MESENTERIC ARTERY

ASCENDING COLON

INFERIOR
MESENTERIC ARTERY

ABDOMINAL AORTA

CUT EDGE OF THE ROOT
OF THE MESENTERY

COMMON ILIAC ARTERY

URETER

SUPERIOR RECTAL ARTERY

BLADDER

CUT EDGE OF THE ROOT OF THE
PELVIC MESOCOLON

RECTUM

Fig. 179. The peritoneum on the posterior abdominal wall, showing its reflections and the
retroperitoneal viscera.

omental bursa is composed of peritoneum covering from above downwards, the caudate lobe of the liver, the lesser omentum and the stomach. The cavity of the omental bursa continues downwards into the greater omentum until the walls of the pouch, from which it is formed, fuse. To the left, the omental bursa is limited by the lienorenal and gastrosplenic ligaments. To the right, the cavity of the omental bursa retains its continuity with the general peritoneal cavity through a small foramen—the **epiploic foramen** or aditus to the

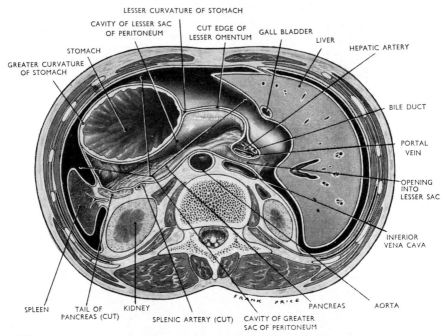

Fig. 180. A horizontal section through the trunk at the level of the upper part of the first lumbar vertebra, to show the viscera and the arrangement of the peritoneum, especially the omental bursa (lesser sac) and its aditus. The section is viewed from above. Compare it with Fig. 196 which is seen from below.

omental bursa (Fig. 180), large enough to admit one or two fingers. The boundaries of the epiploic foramen are, in front, the free border of the lesser omentum which contains the hepatic artery, the bile duct and the portal vein; behind, peritoneum covering the inferior vena cava; above, peritoneum covering the liver (the caudate process) and, below, peritoneum covering the first part of the duodenum.

Peritoneum of the Liver

The liver is almost wholly covered by peritoneum. The lesser omentum, attached to the porta hepatis and to the fissure for the ligamentum venosum, connects the liver with the lesser curvature of the stomach; the falciform ligament connects the anterior surface with the anterior abdominal wall. As the

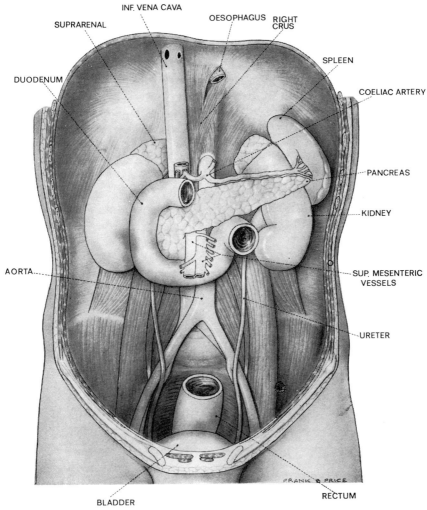

Fig. 181. The posterior abdominal wall with some of the retroperitoneal viscera. The spleen is also shown, although it is covered in peritoneum, except at the hilum.

falciform ligament is traced upwards to the upper surface of the liver, its two layers separate. The left layer extends to the left and then back on itself to form a small fold, the **left triangular ligament** which connects the upper surface of the left lobe with the diaphragm. On the right the corresponding layers form the **coronary ligaments** which are widely separated (Fig. 194, A); the surface of the liver between them is not covered by peritoneum and is called the **bare area.**

Subphrenic Spaces

The upper surface of the liver is in contact with the diaphragm, part of the general peritoneal cavity being of course between them. This part of the peritoneal cavity is, however, partially divided up by the falciform and coronary ligaments where they connect the liver with the diaphragm. Between the liver and the diaphragm, therefore, we find a number of spaces more or less separated from each other by the ligaments. These are the **subphrenic spaces.** They are important because infection is often localized in one or other of them, forming a subphrenic abscess. On the **right side** the coronary ligaments divide the space into an **anterior** and a **posterior space;** on the **left side,** the lesser omentum separates an **anterior subphrenic space** from the **omental bursa** (lesser sac) (see Fig. 194).

Peritoneum of the Pelvis

The peritoneum of the lesser pelvis is continuous with that of the abdominal cavity. The lesser pelvis is shaped like a pudding basin, and contains the pelvic viscera.

In the male, the bladder lies in front and the rectum behind. If it is now imagined that the peritoneum is pushed in as a sheet from above to line the cavity which already contains the viscera, the arrangement of the peritoneum is readily visualized. It clothes the side walls of the pelvis, the upper surface of the bladder and the front and sides of the upper half of the rectum (Fig. 203). The deep hollow, where the peritoneum passes from the rectum to the bladder, is the **rectovesical pouch.**

In the female, the uterus and vagina are placed between the bladder and rectum. From the upper lateral angles of the uterus the uterine tubes stretch laterally, nearly to the side walls. If the peritoneum were pushed in from above as before, it would be draped over the uterus and uterine tubes, clothing them front and back and forming a partition across the cavity. The fold of peritoneum so formed on each side of the uterus, and containing the uterine tube in its upper free border, is the **broad ligament.** The shallow hollow between the uterus and the bladder is the **uterovesical pouch.** A very deep recess is formed where the peritoneum is reflected from the back, not of the uterus, but of the vagina (Fig. 201) to the front of the rectum. This is the **recto-uterine pouch** (pouch of Douglas). It is the lowest part of the peritoneal cavity and in it any fluid formed in the peritoneal cavity in response to disease is likely to collect. In addition, only the thickness of the wall of the vagina separates the peritoneum here from the outside world.

STRUCTURE OF THE ALIMENTARY CANAL

The mouth and pharynx are highly specialized parts of the alimentary canal. The other parts have the same basic structure, being tubular in shape with walls made of four layers. From within outwards these are:

1. mucous membrane,
2. submucous coat,
3. muscle coat, and
4. serous coat.

1. Mucous Membrane

The mucous membrane is the innermost coat. Its surface layer, the **epithelium,** comes into contact with the food materials, and is of the stratified squamous kind where the food is rough and being merely conducted along the tube, but columnar where digestion and absorption take place. A **brush border** is present at sites where absorption takes place. The brush border, made up of tiny projections called **microvilli,** greatly increases the free surface area of the cell. A layer of connective tissue, the **lamina propria,** supports the epithelium and contains blood vessels, lymph vessels and nerves to supply the epithelium. Diffuse lymphatic tissue (p. 407) is found throughout the lamina propria and in some places lymph nodules occur as well. It also contains many simple glands which dip in from the epithelium on the surface. These glands are of different kinds to produce different secretions in different parts of the alimentary canal. Most of the glands derived from the epithelium lie in the mucous membrane in this way. A few lie in the submucous layer, for example, in the duodenum and in the œsophagus. Some large glands, like the pancreas and the liver, lie beyond the gut wall and have ducts leading back through the wall to the lumen. The outside layer of the mucous membrane is a thin layer of smooth muscle, the **muscularis mucosae,** which produces localized movement of the mucous membrane.

2. Submucous Coat

This layer is of loose connective tissue which binds the mucous membrane to the muscle layer. It contains many elastic fibres and forms the core of any folds in the mucous membrane. It contains plexuses of blood vessels to supply the mucous membrane and the **submucous plexus** (Meissner's) of nerve fibres—both sympathetic and parasympathetic—for glands, smooth muscle and blood vessels.

3. Muscle Coat

The muscle coat is of smooth muscle arranged in two layers. In the **inner circular layer** the fibres are arranged circularly round the wall; in the **outer longitudinal layer** the muscle fibres are arranged along the length of the organ. Between the layers is the **myenteric plexus** (of Auerbach) of sympathetic and parasympathetic nerve fibres.

Functions of the Muscle Coat

(a) The **tonus** of the muscle coat is important in regulating the size of the lumen to allow proper functioning of the organ.

(b) **Rhythmic contraction.** Even without nervous stimulation, smooth muscle undergoes spontaneous rhythmic contractions. Contracting in this way the muscle coat keeps the contents of the alimentary canal thoroughly mixed.

PERISTALSIS: *Peristalsis is the process by which the contents are propelled along the alimentary canal.* A wave of relaxation followed by a wave of contraction passes along the gut wall. The contraction squeezes the contents into the ready dilated region in front. Normally, peristalsis passes from the mouth towards the anus. Peristalsis is of two types; a slow wave over a short length of the gut moves the contents onwards a few inches; a **peristaltic rush,** sometimes called mass peristalsis, is a rapid movement which may involve the whole intestine. **Antiperistalsis,** that is movement in the opposite direction, may occur, but it is unimportant. In addition, there are simple contractions, or **segmentation movements,** and **pendular movements** in which the contents are passed to and fro over short segments of gut, thus enabling thorough mixing of the contents. Peristalsis depends on co-ordination of the contraction of the smooth muscle fibres by the autonomic nervous system. Parasympathetic impulses increase the movements, sympathetic impulses diminish them.

SPHINCTERS: In certain places the muscle fibres of the circular coat are increased in number to form a thickened ring of muscle round the canal, called a **sphincter.** When its fibres contract the lumen is occluded and the intestinal contents cannot pass. The sphincters are under control of the autonomic nervous system, sympathetic impulses causing them to contract, parasympathetic to relax.

4 Serous Coat

The visceral layer of the peritoneum (p. 440) forms a complete covering for some parts of the alimentary canal and a partial coat for others. The peritoneum allows the viscera to move easily in relation one to the other.

THE ŒSOPHAGUS

The œsophagus is a flattened tube about 25 cm long, which begins in the neck as the continuation of the pharynx at the level of the cricoid cartilage, and passes through the root of the neck, through the thorax and into the abdominal cavity, to the stomach. It lies near the midline in front of the bodies of the vertebræ. It is behind the trachea, as far as its bifurcation, then behind the pericardium which separates it from the left atrium of the heart. It swings to the left of the midline just before it pierces the muscular part of the diaphragm opposite the tip of the eighth left costal cartilage, and ends almost at once in the stomach, at the cardiac orifice. The cardiac orifice is about forty centimetres from the incisor teeth.

Structure

The œsophagus has the coats characteristic of the alimentary canal, except that it has no serous coat apart from the short intra-abdominal part. The mucous membrane has a stratified squamous epithelium, which is kept moist by the secretion from mucous glands in the submucosa. The peristaltic action of its muscle coat, which consists of striated muscle in the upper part, propels food into the stomach during swallowing.

THE STOMACH

The stomach is the widest part of the alimentary canal. It is J-shaped (Figs. 159 and 182). The œsophagus enters it on its right border near its upper end at the **cardiac orifice,** and the lower end is continuous with the duodenum at the **pyloric canal.** The rounded upper part, above the level of the cardiac orifice, is the **fundus,** the vertical part is the **body** and the part leading to the pyloric canal is the **pyloric antrum.** The right border, short and concave, is the **lesser curvature,** the left border, much longer and convex, is the **greater curvature.**

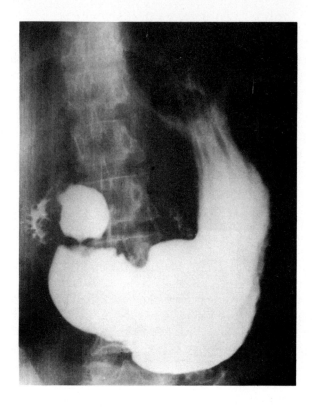

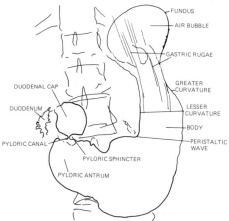

FUNDUS
AIR BUBBLE
GASTRIC RUGAE
GREATER CURVATURE
LESSER CURVATURE
BODY
PERISTALTIC WAVE
DUODENAL CAP
DUODENUM
PYLORIC CANAL
PYLORIC SPHINCTER
PYLORIC ANTRUM

Fig. 182. A radiograph of the stomach after a barium meal. The barium sulphate shows the outline of the **interior** of the organ.

The stomach lies in the upper left quadrant of the abdominal cavity. The fundus is under the left dome of the diaphragm. Behind the stomach is the omental bursa of peritoneum; in front is the anterior abdominal wall. The lesser

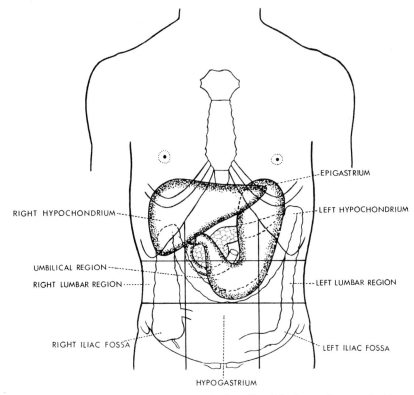

Fig. 183. The regions of the anterior abdominal wall, with the surface projections of the main abdominal viscera.

curvature is connected to the liver by the lesser omentum; the peritoneum stretching from the greater curvature forms the gastrosplenic ligament to the left, and the greater omentum inferiorly. The surface marking of the stomach is shown in Fig. 183.

Structure

The stomach has four coats, the mucous membrane, the submucous coat, the muscle coat and the serous coat (Fig. 184).

The mucous membrane is raised into irregular longitudinal ridges, the **gastric rugæ** (Fig. 184). Microscopically it is seen that the epithelium is tall and columnar. There are very numerous simple tubular glands which secrete the **gastric juice.** The glands in the fundus and body of the stomach contain three kinds of cells; **chief cells** secreting fluid containing **enzymes; parietal cells** secreting **hydrochloric acid;** and **mucous neck cells** secreting **mucus**

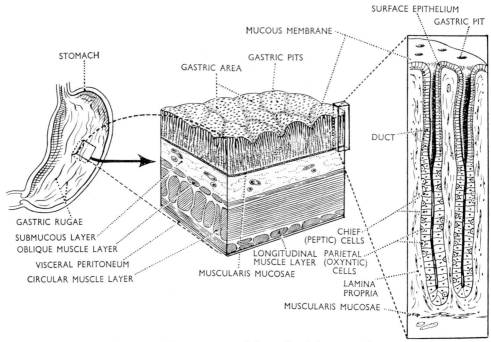

Fig. 184. The structure of the wall of the stomach.

to protect the surface epithelium from digestion. The glands in the pyloric antrum secrete only mucus.

The muscle coat, besides the two characteristic inner circular and outer longitudinal layers, has an extra oblique layer internally. At the cardiac orifice the inner circular fibres form a weak sphincter, the so-called **cardiac sphincter.** Round the pyloric canal the circular fibres are greatly thickened to form the **pyloric sphincter** (Figs. 159 and 182).

Gastric Digestion

Food reaching the stomach is semi-solid. In the stomach it is mixed with the gastric juice to form a thick fluid—**chyme.** The pyloric sphincter remains closed and repeated waves of peristalsis passing over the stomach churn the contents. From time to time, the pyloric sphincter relaxes to allow some of the chyme to pass into the duodenum. After a meal, the stomach takes two to five hours to empty.

SECRETION OF GASTRIC JUICE: A small amount of gastric juice is secreted continuously. The flow of juice needed for digestion is started by reflex stimulation of the vagus nerve by the pleasurable taste, sight, smell or anticipation of food. Distaste for food inhibits this flow. If meals are pleasant, therefore, digestion is improved. Next, certain foods, especially meat extracts, in contact with the mucous membrane of the pyloric antrum cause it to produce a hormone **gastrin** which acts on the fundus and body of the stomach to cause secretion of more gastric juice. Hence the value of appetizers, like meat soups, at the beginning of a meal. Thirdly, the presence of food in the duodenum causes the secretion there of a hormone which stimulates gastric secretion.

FUNCTIONS OF GASTRIC JUICE:

1. Protein Digestion

The chief cells secrete **pepsinogen,** the precursor of **pepsin** which is formed from it in the lumen of the stomach in the presence of the **hydrochloric acid** secreted by the parietal cells. Pepsin acts best at the low pH produced by the hydrochloric acid. It begins the digestion of proteins, hydrolysing them to **proteoses** and **peptones** (p. 42).

2. Clotting of Milk

In young animals **rennin** is secreted in the stomach. This causes clotting of milk, in preparation for protein digestion. It is not present in human infants but pepsin plays the same rôle.

3. Hæmopoiesis

One of the normal constituents of gastric juice is **Castle's intrinsic factor.** It is essential for the absorption from the intestine of vitamin B_{12} which is necessary for the proper development of red blood corpuscles. If the intrinsic factor is not secreted in the gastric juice, pernicious anæmia develops.

4. Antiseptic Action

The hydrochloric acid in the gastric juice kills bacteria ingested with the food.

The gastric juice has no direct action on fats, but it digests the connective tissue surrounding fat and sets it free, ready to be acted upon by the pancreatic juice.

In the stomach the action of **salivary amylase** (p. 437) on carbohydrates continues until the acidity of the gastric juice inhibits the enzyme.

ABSORPTION: Very little absorption occurs in the stomach. Water and alcohol are absorbed to some extent in the pyloric antrum.

Vomiting

In vomiting, the contents of the stomach are evacuated through the mouth. It is a reflex act, the afferent impulses coming from many different parts of the body, for example, from the stomach itself, from other viscera, from fauces and pharynx, or from the vestibular apparatus (p. 309), to the vomiting centre in the medulla. Efferent impulses pass in the vagus to the stomach, in the phrenic nerve to the diaphragm and in the spinal nerves to the abdominal muscles.

A deep breath is taken, and the nasopharynx and larynx are closed (cf. swallowing, p. 439). The abdominal muscles and diaphragm contract, raising the intra-abdominal pressure and compressing the stomach. The pyloric end of the stomach contracts, the cardiac sphincter relaxes and the contents are expelled with the aid of antiperistalsis of stomach and œsophagus.

Vomiting is accompanied by nausea and excessive salivation, by retching, which is spasmodic contraction of the diaphragm, and by sweating, pallor and feeble pulse.

Fractional Test Meal. A stomach tube is passed in the fasting patient and the fasting stomach contents are drawn off. Then a flow of gastric juice is stimulated by giving the patient a test meal, such as a standard quantity of tea and toast or thin gruel, or by an injection of histamine or of insulin. A small volume (15 ml) of stomach contents is withdrawn at 15-minute intervals until the stomach is empty. The samples of stomach contents are examined for the presence and amounts of normal constituents such as hydrochloric acid and pepsin, and for abnormal constituents, such as blood. The response to the test meal gives an indication of the function of the stomach.

THE INTESTINE

The intestine has two parts, the small intestine which is about 2·5 cm in diameter, and the large intestine which in parts is more than twice as wide, hence its name. The small intestine, though narrower than the large intestine, is longer.

SMALL INTESTINE

The small intestine has three main functions: to complete the digestion of food, to absorb the digested materials and to move the chyme through it from one end to the other. The small intestine is about one and a half metres long. The measurement after death is some six metres, but it is likely that the extra length is due to relaxation of the smooth muscle which is normally in a state of tone. The first twenty-five centimetres of the small intestine is the duodenum. Of the rest, the proximal two-fifths is the jejunum and the distal three-fifths, the ileum.

Duodenum

The duodenum is a tube, shaped like the letter C, continuous with the stomach at the pyloric sphincter. It lies behind the peritoneum, close against the bodies of the first, second and third lumbar vertebræ, and surrounds the head of the pancreas. The bile duct, passing down from the liver, lies behind the upper part of the duodenum and opens into the lumen at the middle of the concave border, in common with the pancreatic duct (Fig. 192). In the interior of the duodenum, the orifice of the confluent bile and pancreatic ducts (**ampulla of Vater**) is marked by a small conical projection of the mucous membrane, the **duodenal papilla.**

Jejunum and Ileum

At the distal end of the duodenum, the intestine bends sharply forwards at the **duodenojejunal flexure** (Fig. 192) to become the jejunum. The jejunum and ileum are suspended from the posterior abdominal wall by the **mesentery** which is attached obliquely across it from the left side of the second lumbar vertebra to the right iliac fossa. This attachment is called the **root of the mesentery** (Fig. 179). The mesentery is some twelve centimetres wide at its broadest and its free border contains the jejunum and ileum. This border is much longer than the root, so that the mesentery looks like a frill. Nerves, blood vessels and lymphatics reach the intestine through the mesentery. The jejunum and ileum are similar to look at, and lie coiled behind the greater omentum which hangs down in front of them. The jejunum lies mainly in the upper left quadrant of the abdominal cavity and the ileum in the lower right quadrant. The ileum enters the large intestine just above the cæcum in the right iliac fossa (Fig. 188). The opening is guarded by the **ileocæcal valve** formed of folds of the mucous membrane. The valve prevents regurgitation of the contents of the cæcum into the ileum, but its resistance may be overcome, for example by an enema.

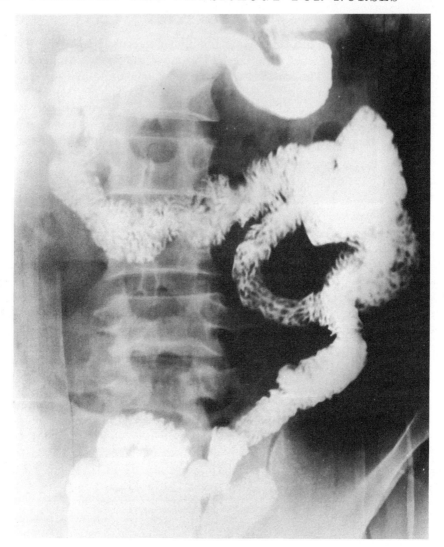

Structure of the Small Intestine

The small intestine has the characteristic four coats, namely mucous membrane, submucous coat, muscle coat and serous coat (Fig. 187).

The **mucous membrane** is thrown up into **circular folds** (Fig. 187). This increases the area of the epithelium in contact with the chyme, and by

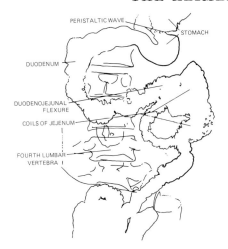

PERISTALTIC WAVE

STOMACH

DUODENUM

DUODENOJEJUNAL
FLEXURE

COILS OF JEJENUM

FOURTH LUMBAR
VERTEBRA

Fig. 185. A radiograph, taken after a barium meal, showing the small intestine.

increasing the number of cells engaged in absorption, increases the rate of absorption. The surface of the mucous membrane is not smooth but looks like velvet. Each of the hairs of the pile is a **villus.** The villi greatly enlarge the area of the epithelium available for absorbing.

Microscopic examination (Fig. 187) shows that the villi are finger like processes projecting from the surface. They are covered by the surface epithelium which is composed of tall columnar cells. Among these are scattered **goblet cells** each of which contains a large drop of colourless mucus. The mucus secreted by them acts as a lubricant. Each villus has a core of loose connective tissue and, in the centre of this, is a wide lymph capillary with a blind end—a **lacteal,** into which some of the absorbed fat passes (p. 461). To each villus comes a tiny **arteriole** which feeds the **capillary plexus** lying close to the epithelium. Food materials absorbed from the lumen by the columnar cells are passed on to the blood in these capillaries. The plexus is drained by a **venule** of the **portal system** which conveys the blood to the liver (Plate 24). In the connective tissue are some smooth muscle fibres which produce shortening and lengthening movements of the villus. These movements, by intermittently compressing the lacteal and venule, help to promote the flow of chyle and portal blood.

Between the bases of the villi, the epithelium dips into the lamina propria forming simple tubular glands, the **intestinal crypts** (crypts of Lieberkuhn). The cells lining the crypts secrete the **intestinal juice (succus entericus)** which is alkaline and contains inorganic ions, mucin and many enzymes (p. 460) which complete the breaking down of fats, carbohydrates and proteins to simple molecules which can be absorbed (p. 460).

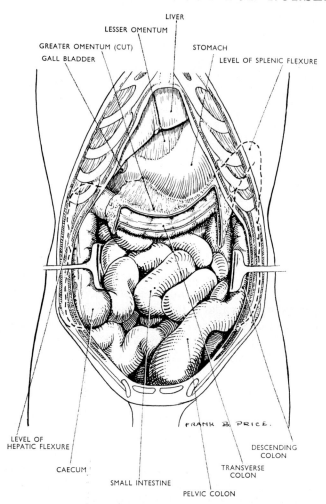

Fig. 186. The arrangement of the abdominal organs as seen after removing the anterior abdominal wall. Most of the greater omentum has been cut away.

Diffuse lymphatic tissue and small lymph nodules occur throughout the lamina propria. In the ileum there are in addition, especially in children, many large lymph nodules known as **aggregated lymphatic nodules** (Peyer's patches).

The muscularis mucosæ, by its contractions, produces local movements of

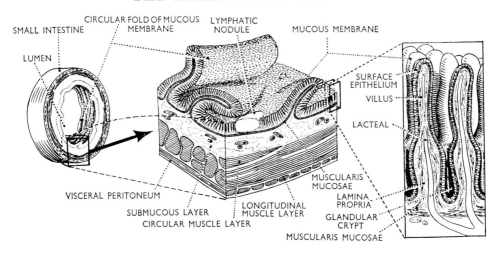

Fig. 187. The structure of the wall of the small intestine.

the mucous membrane. This aids absorption by bringing fresh chyme continuously into contact with the villi.

The **submucous coat** binds the mucous membrane to the muscle coat and forms the core for each of the circular folds of the mucous membrane. In the duodenum this coat contains the **duodenal glands** (Brunner's glands), which secrete an alkaline mucus to protect the mucous membrane from the acidity of the chyme from the stomach.

The **muscle coat** has inner circular and outer longitudinal layers of smooth muscle, whose tone maintains the intestine in a functional state. Frequent rapid **peristalic waves** (Fig. 185) in the muscle move the chyme along a few inches at a time. **Segmentation** is a characteristic movement of the small intestine. A length is divided into a number of small segments by localized constrictions where the circular muscle has contracted. The segments bulge, then a constriction appears in the middle of each bulging segment and the original constrictions disappear. This is repeated several times a minute. Segmentation causes no forward movement of the chyme, but it mixes it with the intestinal juices, aiding digestion; it also brings the chyme into contact with the villi, aiding absorption. **Pendular** movements have a similar function.

The **serous coat.** Except for the duodenum which has peritoneum only on its anterior surface, the small intestine is surrounded by peritoneum which is reflected from it as the mesentery.

Functions of the Small Intestine

The small intestine has three main functions, to complete the digestion of food, to absorb the digested food and to move the chyme along from one end to the other.

The chyme is moved along by peristalsis of the muscle coat.

DIGESTION: In the small intestine the chyme is mixed with the intestinal juice, with the pancreatic juice and with bile (p. 479). Segmentation and pendular movements ensure thorough mixing. The intestinal juice is alkaline and contains inorganic ions, mucin and many enzymes, namely enterokinase, lipase, amylase, sucrase, lactase, maltase, erepsin and alkaline phosphatase. Intestinal juice is secreted reflexly after ingestion of food. Secretin (p. 471) also stimulates the flow.

Since the intestinal juice, the pancreatic juice and the bile are all alkaline, the acid chyme from the stomach is neutralized. The enzymes in the intestinal and pancreatic juice are most active in an alkaline mixture.

Carbohydrates. Some digestion of carbohydrates to dextrin and maltose has already taken place under the influence of salivary amylase (p. 437). In the small intestine **amylase** from the pancreatic juice and intestinal juice hydrolyses all the **starch** and **dextrin** to **maltose.** Then the **disaccharides,** maltose, lactose and sucrose, are hydrolysed by the appropriate enzymes in the intestinal juice to the **monosaccharides,** glucose, galactose and fructose. *Only monosaccharides can be absorbed.*

Fats. Bile is essential for the digestion of fats. The **bile salts** lower the surface tension and allow the fat, which is liquid at body temperature, but insoluble in water, to form an emulsion, that is, a suspension of very fine droplets. The **lipase** from the pancreatic juice (and some from the intestinal juice) is then able to act on these droplets. In addition, the bile salts increase the digesting activity of lipase. Lipase hydrolyses **neutral fats** to **glycerol** and **fatty acids.**

Proteins. The pepsin and hydrochloric acid in the stomach have already hydrolysed the proteins to **proteoses** and **peptones.** In the duodenum, **enterokinase** from the intestinal juice acts on the **trypsinogen** of the pancreatic juice to form **trypsin,** an enzyme which breaks down the **proteoses** and **peptones** to **polypeptides. Erepsin** in the intestinal juice completes the process by hydrolysing the **polypeptides** to **amino acids.**

ABSORPTION: Almost all the absorption of digested food takes place in the small intestine. The area of epithelium to do this is greatly increased by the presence of the villi and of the circular folds. **Water,** up to 10 litres a day, and the relatively **simple products of digestion** pass into the columnar cells of the epithelium and are transferred to the blood in the capillary plexus underneath. They are then taken in the veins of the portal system to the liver.

The process of absorption into the columnar epithelial cells is complex. To some extent monosaccharides and amino acids pass into the cells according to the laws of diffusion and osmosis. However, some substances, like glucose, are absorbed much more quickly than this, and it is clear that the protoplasm of the cells plays an active part in the absorption both of monosaccharides and of amino acids.

Absorption of fat. Bile is essential for the absorption of fat. In its presence neutral fat forms a very fine emulsion in the chyme. Some of the very fine particles of neutral fat are taken directly into the epithelial cells. The rest of the fat is hydrolysed to fatty acids and glycerol. The bile salts by their hydrotropic action render the fatty acids soluble, so that they can be absorbed into the cells. There they may combine again with glycerol to form particles of neutral fat. The neutral fat is passed from the epithelial cells to the lacteal in the villus, where it gives the lymph a milky appearance. Such lymph is called **chyle.** It is carried by the lymph vessels to the cisterna chyli and via the thoracic duct, to be emptied into the blood stream at the root of the neck. About two thirds of the fat enters the lymphatic vessels in this way.

Some of the fatty acids in the epithelial cells form other compounds, such as phospholipids, and then pass to the blood capillaries to be carried to the liver. About one third of the absorbed fat follows this path.

THE LARGE INTESTINE

The large intestine has the general shape of an inverted U. Its constituent parts are the cæcum, the appendix, the colon, which has ascending, transverse, descending and pelvic parts, and the rectum (Figs. 188 and 189).

Cæcum

The cæcum lies in the right iliac fossa. It is a bag whose lumen is continuous above with that of the ascending colon. The ileum enters on the left side of the junction of the cæcum and ascending colon. The ileocæcal orifice is guarded by the ileocæcal valve (p. 455). About two centimetres below the ileocæcal orifice the root of the appendix (p. 465) is attached to the cæcum. The cæcum is clothed with peritoneum and the peritoneal pocket, between its posterior wall and the iliac fossa, is the **retrocæcal recess.**

Ascending Colon

The ascending colon passes upwards on the right side of the abdominal cavity until it reaches the right lobe of the liver, where it bends sharply at the **hepatic flexure** to become the transverse colon. The ascending colon has no

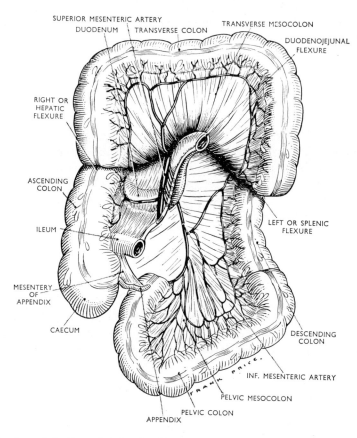

Fig. 188. The large intestine, showing its different parts and its blood supply. The transverse colon, which hangs down, has been displaced upwards, and the small intestine has been removed. Compare this with Fig. 190).

mesentery but is covered by peritoneum. Along its right side, there is a groove lined by the parietal peritoneum between it and the abdominal wall, the **right paracolic gutter.** Followed upwards this leads to the right posterior subphrenic space (p. 446).

Transverse Colon

The transverse colon stretches across the abdominal cavity from the hepatic flexure on the right to the spleen on the left side, where it bends sharply downwards at the **splenic flexure** to form the descending colon. As it crosses, it loops downwards in front of the small intestine. It is suspended from the posterior abdominal wall by the transverse mesocolon which is fused to the posterior surface of the greater omentum (Figs. 188 and 179).

Descending Colon

This passes down the left side of the posterior abdominal wall to the brim of the lesser pelvis, where it becomes the pelvic colon. It has no mesentery. It is narrower than the rest of the colon and its firm wall may often be palpated in the left iliac fossa.

Pelvic Colon

The pelvic colon, suspended by the pelvic mesocolon from the brim and posterior wall of the lesser pelvis, lies coiled in the pelvis.

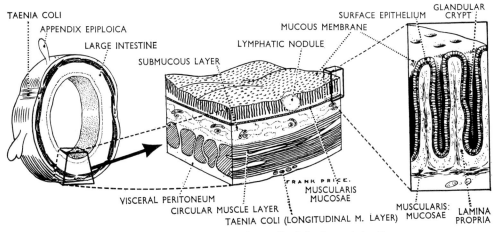

Fig. 189. The structure of the wall of the large intestine.

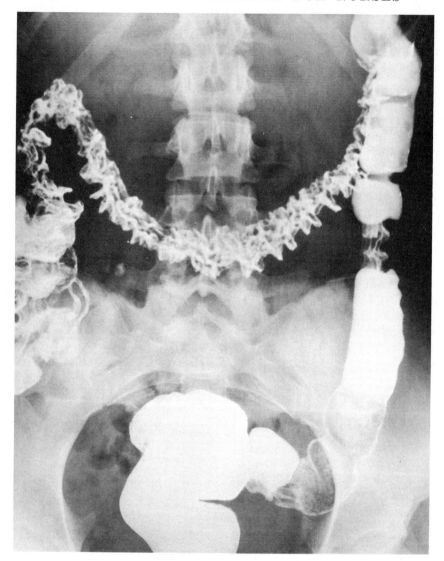

Rectum

The rectum begins at the middle of the sacrum and follows its curve down-wards to the tip of the coccyx, where it bends backwards at a right angle, the **anorectal junction,** to become continuous with the **anal canal.** The rectum

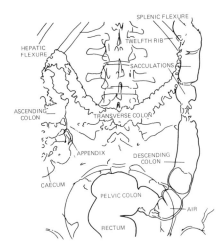

Fig. 190. A radiograph of the abdomen taken after a barium enema. There is some air in the colon, and some of the barium has been evacuated.

also bends from side to side as it descends (Fig. 190) and its mucous membrane is raised into three semicircular horizontal folds, the **rectal valves** (Fig. 203).

Structure of the Large Intestine

The large intestine can be distinguished at once from the small intestine by its external appearance (Fig. 188). It is wider; attached to the surface are numerous small processes, the **appendices epiploicæ,** which are of lobulated fat covered with peritoneum; the walls are **sacculated** (Fig. 190) because the longitudinal muscle coat is incomplete. The longitudinal muscle fibres form three narrow bands, the **tæniæ coli,** which run the length of the cæcum and colon. Between them the circular muscle bulges outwards to form the sacculations.

The mucous membrane has columnar epithelium with very many goblet cells to secrete mucus for lubricating the contents which are becoming more solid. **Intestinal crypts** are present, but there are no villi (Fig. 189).

Appendix

The appendix is a narrow blind tube attached to the medial aspect of the cæcum about two centimetres, below the ileocæcal valve. It varies in length from two to twenty-two centimetres, but is usually about ten centimetres long. It has a covering of peritoneum and is attached by a mesentery, the **meso-appendix,** to the lower end of the ileum. Blood vessels from the superior mesenteric vessels and nerves reach it through the mesentery. Although the root of the appendix is fixed by its attachment to the cæcum in the iliac fossa, the tip is free and may lie almost anywhere on the periphery of a circle of which the root is the centre. Thus the tip of the appendix may point towards the spleen, lying in front of or behind the end of the ileum, it may lie in the retrocæcal recess (p. 462), it may point towards the inguinal ligament or dangle over the brim of the lesser pelvis.

STRUCTURE: The appendix has the characteristic four coats. The mucous

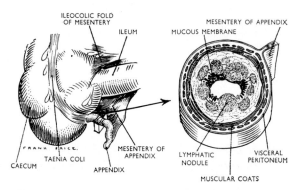

Fig. 191. The cæcum and the appendix; the structure of the appendix.

membrane is similar to that of the colon with columnar epithelium, goblet cells, intestinal crypts (a few) and no villi, but the lamina propria is greatly thickened by lymphatic tissue, the nodules surrounding and bulging into the lumen.(Fig. 191). The muscle coat has inner circular and outer longitudinal layers. The longitudinal fibres form a complete coat and can be traced into the tæniæ coli. Indeed, to find the appendix any one of the tæniæ can be traced downwards to its root, where all three tæniæ meet.

THE ANATOMY OF APPENDICITIS: Appendicitis is inflammation of the appendix. It starts very often because the narrow lumen has been blocked by something sticking in it or because the lymphatic nodules have become inflamed and swollen. Bacteria multiply in the stagnant lumen distal to the block, tissue fluid is poured out and the appendix is distended. Distension of a hollow viscus gives rise to pain. In this case the pain is not felt in the appendix, but is referred to the skin which is innervated by the same segment of the spinal cord as the appendix, namely the skin round the umbilicus (midgut pain—see p. 430). As the inflammation progresses, it spreads through the wall of the appendix and, after a few hours, the structures surrounding the appendix are irritated,

Usually the parietal peritoneum is involved and its sensory nerves, that is the nerves of the body wall, are stimulated, so that the pain is now felt in the right iliac fossa. Thus the pain of appendicitis moves from the umbilical region, in the early stages, to the right iliac fossa later. If the appendix irritates the ileum or organs in the lesser pelvis, as it may according to its variable position, the symptoms resemble those of disease of these organs.

The Anal Canal

The anal canal is about three centimetres long and is directed downwards and backwards, at right angles to the direction of the rectum (Fig. 203). The lower half is lined with skin which is very sensitive and is supplied by a branch of the **pudendal nerve.** (This is in contrast with the rectum which is lined by mucous membrane supplied by visceral sensory nerves.) The muscle coat is modified. In the upper part, the circular smooth muscle fibres of the gut wall are increased to form the **internal sphincter** which is of course under control of the autonomic nervous system. The lower part of the muscular wall is striated muscle which forms the **external sphincter** (Plate 8). This is supplied by a branch of the pudendal nerve, and is, like most other striated muscle, under voluntary control. The upper part of the external sphincter blends with the puborectalis fibres of levator ani (p. 209).

The walls of the lower anal canal are supplied by branches of the pudendal artery and drained by the corresponding veins. The lymph vessels pass to the superficial inguinal nodes (Fig. 97), while those from the upper portion pass to the abdominal lymph nodes (Fig. 168).

Tributaries of the portal vein, which drains the rectum and upper anal canal, and tributaries of the pudendal vein (a systemic vein) communicate in the walls of the anal canal. A rise of pressure in the portal system may cause, in these communicating veins, varicosities known as **hæmorrhoids** or **piles.**

Movements of the Large Intestine

Slow peristalsis occurs in the proximal colon, and three or four times a day a peristaltic rush drives the contents on to be stored in the distal colon. The gastrocolic reflex produces a strong peristaltic rush (see defæcation, below).

Functions of the Large Intestine

The main function of the large intestine is to **absorb water** from the fluid chyme which enters it from the small intestine. By the time the contents reach the descending colon, they are of the consistency of fæces. Besides water, glucose and salt can be absorbed, as in rectal feeding. The descending and pelvic parts of the colon store the fæces until they are discharged at defæcation.

Bacteria flourish in the large intestine, breaking down further the contents of the chyme. Some perform an important function in synthesizing **vitamin K** (p. 568) and **vitamin B** (p. 565).

Fæces are the waste materials from the alimentary tract. They contain:

Water (up to 70%).

Bacteria (mostly dead).

Mucin, leucocytes and desquamated epithelial cells all derived from the mucous membrane.

Undigested and unabsorbed food residues, notably cellulose and the products of bacterial putrefaction.

Substances excreted in the bile like cholesterol, and bile pigments which give the fæces their characteristic brown colour.

Substances excreted by the intestinal mucosa like iron and calcium.

DEFÆCATION: This is the expulsion of fæces through the anal canal. It occurs once a day as a rule, but there is a wide range of normal variation from twice a day to once every two or three days. The act is partly involuntary and partly voluntary.

The rectum is usually empty. The taking of a particular meal (often breakfast, but this is a matter of habit) reflexly stimulates a strong peristaltic rush. This is the **gastrocolic reflex.** The resulting filling and stretching of the rectum by the contents of the pelvic colon gives the call to defæcate. Defæcation is resisted, until the moment is opportune, by contraction of the external sphincter which is under voluntary control. Meanwhile, the tone of the rectal wall is adjusted to its contents, and the sensation passes off until another peristaltic wave stretches it further. At the right moment, the external sphincter is voluntarily allowed to relax. Parasympathetic impulses relax the smooth muscle of the internal sphincter and stimulate peristalsis, so that the fæces are evacuated from the descending and pelvic parts of the colon. This is aided greatly by contractions of the diaphragm and of the muscles of the abdominal wall which raise the intra-abdominal pressure. This effort begins reflexly, but can be voluntarily controlled.

RECTAL EXAMINATION: A well-lubricated finger gently pressed through the external sphincter into the rectum feels the shape and position of several structures. In the male the coccyx and sacrum can be felt behind, and in front the prostate, with the seminal vesicles and trigone of the bladder above it.

In the female the sacrum and coccyx are felt behind and in front the cervix of the uterus and its external os can be examined. During labour the extent of dilatation of the cervix can be gauged per rectum.

THE BLOOD SUPPLY OF THE ALIMENTARY TRACT

Arteries

Three branches of the abdominal aorta supply nearly the whole of the alimentary tract. The cœliac artery supplies the structures derived from the foregut, namely the stomach, part of the duodenum, the liver and the pancreas. (The œsophagus receives branches from the descending thoracic aorta.) The superior mesenteric artery supplies the midgut, namely the rest of the duodenum, the jejunum, ileum, appendix, cæcum, ascending colon and proximal two-thirds of the transverse colon. The inferior mesenteric artery supplies the hindgut, namely the distal third of the transverse colon, the descending colon, the pelvic colon and the rectum (see also p. 372).

Veins

The alimentary canal is drained by the **portal system** of veins (p. 377, (Plate 27).

Lymphatic Drainage

The mucous membrane of the alimentary canal is richly supplied with lymphatic capillaries and with lymphatic tissue, both diffuse and in nodules, to filter lymph. The lymph vessels which collect the lymph follow back along the path of the arteries, through groups of lymph nodes, to reach the main groups of lymph nodes round the origins of the cœliac, superior mesenteric and inferior mesenteric arteries. From these nodes vessels pass to the **cisterna chyli** (Fig. 169) which is the dilated lower end of the largest lymph vessel in the body, the **thoracic duct** (p. 420). The lymph from the small intestine contains droplets of fat absorbed from the lumen, and is, therefore, milky to look at. It is called **chyle** and is carried with the rest of the lymph via the cisterna chyli and the thoracic duct to the root of the neck (Fig. 169) where it is poured into the junction of the left internal jugular and left subclavian veins.

THE PANCREAS

The pancreas is a large elongated gland which lies across the posterior abdominal wall (Fig. 192) behind the peritoneum of the posterior wall of the omental bursa. The largest part, which is circular, is the **head,** which lies in the concavity of the duodenal loop. A narrow portion, the **neck,** joins it to the long **body** which stretches across to the left, across the left kidney, to end in the conical **tail** which touches the spleen at its hilum.

The pancreas has both endocrine and exocrine cells. The endocrine cells secrete **insulin,** which is essential for the proper metabolism of carbohydrates,

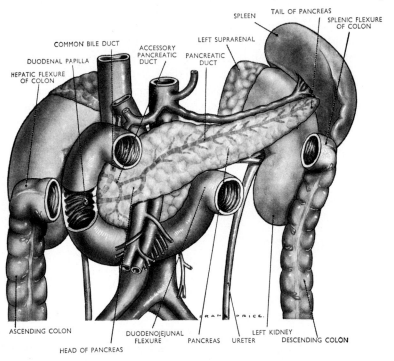

Fig. 192. The organs related to the upper part of the posterior abdominal wall.

and **glucagon** (p. 471); the exocrine cells secrete **pancreatic juice** which contains enzymes for the digestion of proteins, carbohydrates and fats in the small intestine.

The pancreatic juice is secreted into the tributaries of the pancreatic duct which runs along the length of the pancreas and opens, in common with the bile duct, into the middle of the duodenum at the duodenal papilla (Fig. 192).

The pancreas is supplied by branches of the hepatic and splenic arteries from the cœliac artery, and the blood, containing of course the insulin and glucagon from the endocrine cells, is drained by the portal system to the liver.

Structure

The pancreas is whitish and lobulated. Under the microscope (Fig. 193) can be seen groups of exocrine cells and the ducts which drain their secretion, the **pancreatic juice**. Scattered among them are spherical masses of smaller cells arranged in cords, the **pancreatic islets** (of Langerhans). These are the endocrine cells which secrete insulin and glucagon.

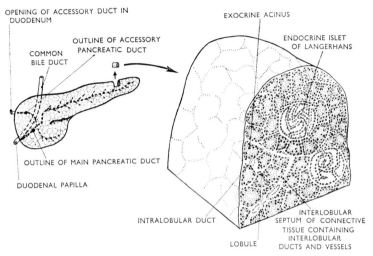

OPENING OF ACCESSORY DUCT IN DUODENUM

OUTLINE OF ACCESSORY PANCREATIC DUCT

COMMON BILE DUCT

EXOCRINE ACINUS

ENDOCRINE ISLET OF LANGERHANS

OUTLINE OF MAIN PANCREATIC DUCT

DUODENAL PAPILLA

INTRALOBULAR DUCT

LOBULE

INTERLOBULAR SEPTUM OF CONNECTIVE TISSUE CONTAINING INTERLOBULAR DUCTS AND VESSELS

Fig. 193. The structure of the pancreas.

Pancreatic Juice

Pancreatic juice is secreted both reflexly through the vagus in response to the taste, thought or sight of food, and when the hormones **secretin** and **pancreoxymin** act on the cells. These hormones are produced by the mucosa of the duodenum in response to the presence of acid chyme containing partly digested protein from the stomach.

FUNCTIONS: Pancreatic juice is alkaline and contains inorganic ions, mucin and the enzymes trypsinogen, amylase, maltase and lipase. It is essential for adequate digestion in the small intestine.

1. With the bile, it **neutralizes** the acid secreted by the stomach.
2. **Proteins.** The trypsinogen is converted to trypsin by enterokinase from the intestinal juice. Trypsin continues the digestion of proteins, hydrolysing proteoses and peptones to polypeptides.

3. **Carbohydrates.** Amylase hydrolyses starch and dextrin to maltose. Maltose then splits into two molecules of glucose.

4. **Fats.** In the presence of bile, lipase hydrolyses neutral fats to glycerol and fatty acids.

Insulin

Insulin, the endocrine secretion produced by the **pancreatic islets** (of Langerhans), is described on p. 557. It regulates carbohydrate metabolism, mainly by lowering the blood sugar.

Glucagon, another hormone secreted by the pancreatic islets, raises the blood sugar.

THE LIVER

The liver is a large glandular organ which lies in the upper right quadrant of the abdominal cavity, close under the right dome of the diaphragm and protected by the ribs. Its cells act like those of an exocrine gland in secreting bile into the hepatic ducts; they also act like those of an endocrine gland in manufacturing new materials and secreting them into the blood stream.

The liver is soft and flabby and is reddish brown in colour. In shape (Fig. 194), it is like a wedge with the thin edge to the left. The upper surface is rounded and is smoothly continuous with the anterior surface and with the right surface, so that these surfaces fit against the domed lower surface of the diaphragm. The inferior surface, or visceral surface, faces the other abdominal viscera and is continuous with the posterior surface. As well as facing downwards, the visceral surface faces to the left. The right part of the liver is, therefore, more massive than the left which ends in the thin part of the wedge. The liver has a thin anterior or lower border where the superior and anterior surfaces meet the inferior one.

Surface Anatomy

The surface marking of the upper surface of the liver corresponds with that of the diaphragm (p. 188) extending to the left as far as the midclavicular line (Fig. 183). The surface marking of the lower border is a finger's breadth below the costal margin of the right side, round to the tip of the ninth right costal cartilage; it crosses the epigastrium to the tip of the eighth left costal cartilage and joins the superior surface marking in the midclavicular line.

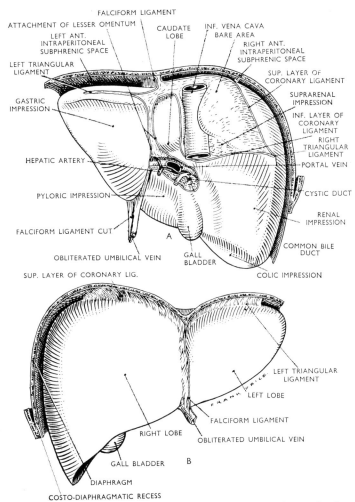

FALCIFORM LIGAMENT
ATTACHMENT OF LESSER OMENTUM
LEFT ANT.
INTRAPERITONEAL
SUBPHRENIC SPACE
CAUDATE LOBE
INF. VENA CAVA
BARE AREA
RIGHT ANT.
INTRAPERITONEAL
SUBPHRENIC SPACE
LEFT TRIANGULAR LIGAMENT
SUP. LAYER OF CORONARY LIGAMENT
GASTRIC IMPRESSION
SUPRARENAL IMPRESSION
INF. LAYER OF CORONARY LIGAMENT
RIGHT TRIANGULAR LIGAMENT
HEPATIC ARTERY
PORTAL VEIN
PYLORIC IMPRESSION
CYSTIC DUCT
RENAL IMPRESSION
FALCIFORM LIGAMENT CUT
A
OBLITERATED UMBILICAL VEIN
GALL BLADDER
COMMON BILE DUCT
COLIC IMPRESSION

SUP. LAYER OF CORONARY LIG.
LEFT TRIANGULAR LIGAMENT
FRANK BALCE
LEFT LOBE
FALCIFORM LIGAMENT
OBLITERATED UMBILICAL VEIN
RIGHT LOBE
GALL BLADDER
B
DIAPHRAGM
COSTO-DIAPHRAGMATIC RECESS

Fig. 194. A, the liver seen from behind, showing the posterior and visceral surfaces; B, the liver seen from the front.

Form and Relations

The liver is entirely clothed with peritoneum, except for the bare area on its posterior surface between the layers of the right coronary ligament (p. 446, Fig. 194, A). The bare area is in direct contact with the lower posterior part of the right dome of the diaphragm. The peritoneum is reflected from the liver

(Fig. 194) to form the falciform ligament, the right coronary ligaments, the left triangular ligament and the lesser omentum (p. 442). Under the peritoneum, the whole liver is covered by a thin layer of connective tissue, the **liver capsule,** from which prolongations extend inwards throughout the liver to provide a support for the liver cells and paths for its blood vessels and ducts.

The falciform ligament divides the anterior aspect of the liver into a large right lobe and a small left lobe. These lobes can be distinguished on the inferior visceral surface too, separated by the fissure for the round ligament of the liver and the fissure for the ligamentum venosum (Fig. 194, B).

Near the middle of the visceral surface is an oblong area about three centimetres long, the **porta hepatis,** where the hepatic artery and portal vein enter the liver and the hepatic ducts leave. From the left end of the porta hepatis a deep groove, the **fissure for the round ligament,** runs forwards to the lower margin of the liver where the free edge of the falciform ligament begins. The **round ligament,** which is the remnant of the umbilical vein of the fetus, passes from the umbilicus in the free edge of the falciform ligament and then, in this fissure, to the portal vein in the porta hepatis. From the left end of the porta hepatis a second deep groove, the **fissure for the ligamentum venosum,** passes backwards and over the posterior surface of the liver. It contains a fibrous cord, the **ligamentum venosum,** which is the remains of the fetal ductus venosus, the channel which carries the blood of the umbilical vein from the portal vein to the inferior vena cava. The lesser omentum is attached to the margins of the porta hepatis and to the fissure for the ligamentum venosum.

Between the right end of the porta hepatis and the lower margin of the liver is a shallow groove in which the pear-shaped **gall bladder** lies (Fig. 194). The **cystic duct,** the 'stem' of the pear, ends in the **common hepatic duct** at the porta hepatis, where this confluence of the ducts forms the **common bile duct**.

Behind the right end of the porta hepatis, but separated from it by a narrow bridge of liver tissue, the **caudate process,** is a deep groove in which lies the inferior vena cava.

The **quadrate lobe** of the liver is the rectangular area bounded by the porta hepatis, the gall bladder, part of the lower margin and the fissure for the round ligament. The **caudate lobe,** the area between the fissure for the ligamentum venosum and the inferior vena cava, is connected with the right lobe by the **caudate process** (Fig. 231, A).

The visceral surface of the right lobe of the liver is in contact with the right kidney behind and with the hepatic flexure of the colon in front. The visceral surface of the left lobe is in contact with the fundus of the stomach.

The front of the quadrate lobe is in contact with the pylorus and the beginning of the duodenum. The caudate lobe forms the anterior wall of the upper part of the omental bursa which separates it from the right crus of the diaphragm.

Blood Supply

Blood comes to the liver through two different vessels, the **hepatic artery** and the **portal vein,** which enter it at the porta hepatis. Blood is drained away by the **hepatic veins,** one from the right lobe and one from the left, which empty into the inferior vena cava where it lies in the groove in the liver just before it pierces the diaphragm (Fig. 179).

To the porta hepatis come the hepatic artery, bringing oxygenated blood, and the portal vein, bringing blood depleted of some of its oxygen (which has been used up by the cells of the walls of the gut) but rich in food materials absorbed from the gut and insulin from the pancreas. The blood of the portal vein contains the material on which the liver cells must work; the blood of the hepatic artery and portal vein contains the oxygen the cells need for burning food materials to give them energy to do the work. The branches of the hepatic artery and portal vein are carried in the connective tissue to every part of the liver and pour their blood into wide capillaries, called **sinusoids,** between the liver cells. The two kinds of blood mix in the sinusoids. From the sinusoids the blood drains into a completely new set of veins which drain into two large **hepatic veins,** one from each lobe; these empty into the inferior vena cava.

Structure

The liver is composed of large many-sided cells arranged in lobules which are just big enough to give the liver surface a granular appearance to the naked eye. In microscope sections (Fig. 195) the liver lobules are seen to be roughly six-sided and partly separated by thin walls of connective tissue. At certain points on the periphery of adjacent lobules the connective tissue encloses a branch of the hepatic artery, a branch of the portal vein, and a tributary of the hepatic duct. These are **portal areas.** In such a section, the liver cells seem to be arranged in columns radiating from the centre of each lobule. Each column consists of two rows of liver cells and is separated from the neighbouring columns by spaces which are the **liver sinusoids.** The sinusoids are lined by the endothelium which lines all blood vessels, but at intervals are placed large phagocytic cells of the reticulo-endothelial system called **stellate cells** (of Kupffer) (p. 111). The sinusoids drain into the vein in the middle of the lobule, the **intralobular vein,** which is a tributary of a **hepatic vein.** Mixed blood from branches of the hepatic artery and portal vein, therefore, circulates past the cells of a lobule by entering the sinusoids at the periphery, flowing slowly towards the centre and then being carried away by the intralobular vein to the hepatic vein and the inferior vena cava.

It was said that each of the columns of liver cells in a lobule was composed of two rows of cells. Between these two rows runs a very fine **bile canaliculus** from near the centre of the lobule to the periphery. Into it the adjacent liver cells secrete bile. The bile canaliculi unite and pour the bile into the tributaries

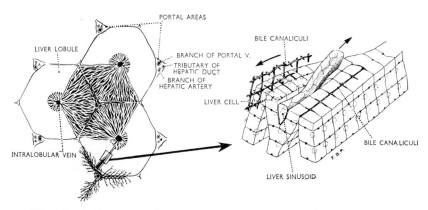

Fig. 195. A diagrammatic representation of the structure of the liver.

of the **hepatic ducts** which are seen in the portal areas. These hepatic ducts follow the path of the hepatic artery and portal vein back to the porta hepatis (see also p. 478).

Each liver cell is placed extremely well to carry out its work. One surface, facing a sinusoid, is bathed by mixed blood which contains oxygen (from the hepatic artery) and food materials and insulin (from the portal vein). From it the cell takes in all it needs, and into it discharges some of the substances it has made or stored (for example glucose, urea, ketones, iron). The opposite surface of the cell faces a bile canaliculus, and into it the liver cell secretes the exocrine secretion, bile.

This description has taken into account only a single flat section of the liver. In three dimensions the liver cells form not columns but interconnected plates (Fig. 195). The principles of the relationship of the cells to the sinusoids and bile canaliculi are, however, the same.

From the point of view of blood supply and drainage, the left lobe of the liver includes the quadrate and caudate lobes.

Functions of the Liver

The functions of the liver are very numerous. It is the principal organ of metabolism and has a part to play in many different bodily processes.

1. Metabolism

The liver plays an important part in the metabolism of **carbohydrates, fats** and **proteins** (see below).

2. Storage

The liver stores glycogen, fat, iron and vitamins A, D and B (especially B_{12}).

3. Bile Secretion (p. 478)

4. Synthesis

The liver synthetizes the plasma proteins, fibrinogen, albumin, globulin and prothrombin.

5. Detoxication

The liver enables the body to get rid of unwanted and possibly harmful substances such as certain drugs, in two ways: the substance may be combined with another to form a compound which is excreted in the urine, or it may be destroyed in the liver.

6. Excretion

The liver eliminates some substance from the body in the bile, for example bile pigments and cholesterol.

7. Heat Production

Because of the biochemical activity of the liver cells, considerable heat is produced in the liver.

8. Blood Formation

In fetuses two to four months old, the liver is one of the main sites for the formation of red blood corpuscles. In post-natal life the liver does not manufacture red cells under normal circumstances (also see p. 589).

METABOLISM:

(*a*) **Carbohydrate.** Glucose brought to the liver from the intestine is converted to glycogen (**glycogenesis**) and stored there. As need arises the glucose is reformed from glycogen (**glycogenolysis**) and released into the blood stream.

Galactose and fructose are converted to glucose.

Glucose is synthetized (**gluconeogenesis**) from glycerol and amino acids.

(*b*) **Fat.** Neutral fat to be used by the body is first brought to the liver either from the stored body fat or from the intestine. It is broken down in the liver cells into glycerol and fatty acids. The glycerol is converted to glucose and the fatty acids are oxidized either to carbon dioxide and water with the release of much energy, or only to ketones, like acetone, which are then taken in the blood to be oxidized in other tissues of the body.

Saturated fatty acids undergo **desaturation** in the liver as a stage in being broken down. This is effected by removing hydrogen from the molecule, and may be a necessary preliminary to oxidation.

Phospholipids are formed from neutral fat in the liver by the addition of phosphorus and nitrogen. Fats in this form are easily carried in the plasma and are readily hydrolysed by enzymes.

(*c*) **Protein.** Amino acids, which are not used as such, are deaminated in the liver, that is the amino group (NH_2) is removed. The rest of the amino acid molecule is converted into glucose, fat, ketone bodies or other amino acids.

The amino groups form ammonia which is highly toxic and must be removed. This is done by liver cells which convert it to harmless **urea,** which is then excreted by the kidneys. Urea is formed only in the liver.

The liver synthetizes many proteins, among them the plasma proteins, albumin, globulin, fibrinogen and prothrombin.

BILIARY TRACT

The biliary tract is the series of ducts which conveys the bile from the liver cells, which secrete it, to the lumen of the duodenum. Within the liver **the bile canaliculi** join the tributaries of the hepatic ducts, which then join to form larger and larger ducts; these finally unite to form the **right hepatic duct,** from the right lobe of the liver, and the **left hepatic duct** from the left lobe. These emerge from the liver into the porta hepatis, where they unite to form the **common hepatic duct.**

Gall bladder

The gall bladder is a thin walled, pear-shaped sac which lies in contact with the visceral surface of the liver (Fig. 194). The broad rounded end of the sac, the **fundus,** projects from under the lower edge of the liver. It is opposite the tip of the ninth right costal cartilage. From the narrow end of the gall bladder, the **cystic duct** emerges into the porta hepatis.

Between the layers of the lesser omentum, close to the porta hepatis, the common hepatic duct and the cystic duct unite to form the **common bile duct.** The common bile duct passes downwards, first in the free border of the lesser omentum, then behind the first part of the duodenum and through the head of the pancreas, to enter the duodenum at the **duodenal papilla** (p. 455). Just before it opens into the duodenum it is joined by the pancreatic duct to form the **hepatopancreatic ampulla** (of Vater). The end of this channel in the duodenal papilla is surrounded by a **sphincter** (of Oddi) which can close it. There is also a sphincter round the bile duct immediately above the site of its junction with the pancreatic duct.

FUNCTIONS OF THE GALL BLADDER: The gall bladder **stores bile,** which is secreted continuously by the liver, until it is needed for digestion. It also **concentrates the bile** by absorbing water through its mucous membrane. The gall bladder contracts and empties the concentrated bile into the duodenum in response to the eating of fat. When the fat enters the duodenum, its mucosa secretes a hormone, **cholecystokinin,** which is carried by the blood to the gall bladder and makes it contract.

Bile

Bile is a yellowish green fluid. It is alkaline and contains, dissolved in water, bile salts, bile pigments, fatty acids, cholesterol and inorganic salts.

FUNCTIONS OF BILE: The **bile salts** are essential for the digestion and absorption of fats in the small intestine.

Emulsifying action. By lowering the surface tension, the bile salts allow neutral fat to form an emulsion of particles so fine that some are absorbed directly into the epithelial cells. The emulsified fat also presents a large surface for enzyme action.

Hydrotropic action. The bile salts combine with insoluble fatty acids in such a way that they dissolve in water. This helps in their absorption. In the same way, they are important in facilitating the absorption of the fat soluble vitamins A, D, E and K.

Activation of lipase. Bile makes pancreatic lipase more active.

Excretory function. Certain waste products of liver metabolism are excreted in the bile, notably bile pigments and cholesterol. Some drugs too are excreted in the bile.

BILIARY OBSTRUCTION: Sometimes some of the dissolved substances in the bile, particularly cholesterol and calcium, are precipitated in the gall bladder to form gall stones. If one of these passes into the common bile duct and sticks, it may block the duct completely, causing biliary obstruction. This has serious effects.

1. The digestion and absorption of fat is upset because no bile reaches the duodenum. The stools lose their brown colour, which is due to the bile pigments, and become clay coloured.

2. Substances usually excreted in the bile are reabsorbed into the blood-stream, notably the bile pigments. These pigments, circulating in the blood, stain all the tissues a yellowish green colour; this is obstructive jaundice, which shows first in the whites of the eyes and then in the skin. The bile pigments and bile salts are also excreted in the urine, making it brown in colour and frothy when shaken.

3. If the obstruction is not relieved, the back pressure of the bile on the liver cells interferes with their essential metabolic functions.

Radiology of the Alimentary System

On ordinary 'straight' radiographs, only the parts of the alimentary tract which contain air can be made out. Thus the lumen of the mouth and pharynx and the outline of the tongue and palate can be seen. The fundus of the stomach usually contains an air bubble which shows as a translucent area under the left dome of the diaphragm (Fig. 142). The coils of the small and large intestines contain a variable quantity of gas which may outline the lumen of localized parts.

The whole alimentary tract may be examined radiologically by introducing into the lumen a radio-opaque substance. On a radiograph, or on a fluorescent screen, the shape of the lumen of the organs can then be seen (Fig. 182). Barium sulphate is used because it is suitably radio-opaque, and, being insoluble, cannot be absorbed by the gut.

Barium swallow. A rather thick suspension of barium sulphate is swallowed mouthful by mouthful. The three phases of swallowing (p. 439) can be observed on a fluorescent screen and also the outline of the œsophagus.

Barium meal. A larger volume of thinner suspension of barium sulphate is drunk (Figs. 182 and 185). The shape of the inside of the stomach can then be seen, and the peristaltic waves can be watched. Irregularities of the mucous membrane caused by ulcers or by growths may be observed. The pyloric canal shows up intermittently as a very narrow channel when the pyloric sphincter relaxes. Barium sulphate in the first part of the duodenum casts a characteristic uniform conical shadow, known as the 'duodenal cap'. Radiographs may be taken at intervals after the barium meal, to follow its course along the alimentary canal. This is known as a 'follow through', and it shows the size, movements and tone of the small and large intestines (Fig. 185).

Barium enema (Fig. 189). A suspension of barium sulphate is given as an enema. The outline of the lumen of the whole of the large intestine can then be seen. The appendix is sometimes visible, depending on its position.

Gall bladder—Cholecystogram. The gall bladder can be seen on a radiograph if the subject has been given, either intravenously or by mouth, a radio-opaque substance which the liver excretes in the bile. If the subject then eats a fatty meal, the gall bladder contracts, emptying the radio-opaque bile, and is then either no longer visible or a smaller shadow is observed, because of the contracted state of the gall bladder's wall.

CHAPTER XV

THE URINARY SYSTEM

The urinary system consists of (1) two excretory organs, the right and left **kidneys** which filter the blood circulating through them and produce **urine.** (2) Two collecting ducts, called **ureters,** which convey the urine from the kidneys to (3) the **bladder,** which is the organ in which the urine is stored till it is voided by the act of **micturition,** when the urine is passed to the exterior by way of (4) the **urethra.**

Development

The development of the urinary system is linked with that of the caudal or lower portion of the alimentary tract, and with that of the genital system. At a very early stage of development, the parts which will become the bladder and the urethra form with the rectum a common cavity, called the **cloaca.** This cavity is later divided by a partition, called the **urorectal septum**, which separates the future bladder and urethra (**urogenital sinus**) in front from the rectum behind (Fig. 210). Incomplete development of this septum leads to abnormal communications or fistulæ between the urogenital system and the lower bowel.

The part of the cloaca which later becomes the urogenital sinus is joined by a duct, the **mesonephric duct,** which grows down from the **mesonephros** near which the gonad develops (see Chapter XVII). Proximal to the junction of this duct with the cloaca a new duct, **the ureteric bud,** grows out (Fig. 210) towards the developing kidney, the **metanephros.** When the ureteric bud has reached the metanephros, the ureteric bud divides repeatedly to give rise to the ureter, pelvis, calyces and collecting tubules within the kidney. The dividing ureteric bud also causes the metanephros to form **nephric vesicles** which become the glomerular capsules, proximal convoluted tubules, loops of the nephrous (of Henle) and distal convoluted tubules. Nephric vesicles may fail to develop properly and may fail to link up with the collecting ducts formed from the ureteric bud. Such vesicles may either degenerate or secrete urine to form cysts. Marked degrees of this condition give rise to congenital polycystic kidney.

The renal corpuscles develop by the invagination of loops of capillaries (glomeruli) into the dilated blind ends of metanephric tubules (Fig. 200).

The further development of the urethra will be considered in Chapter XVII.

THE KIDNEYS

Form

There are two kidneys. Each is a brownish red organ, 10–11 cm long, 6 cm wide and about 3 cm thick. It has the characteristic bean shape, its lateral border being convex, and its medial border concave in the middle and convex at each end. The concavity is the **hilum,** through which the renal artery enters the kidney and the renal vein and the ureter leave.

Position

The kidneys lie on the posterior abdominal wall behind the peritoneal cavity (Figs. 181 and 199). The hilum of each is opposite the first lumbar vertebra, but the right kidney is about 2 cm lower than the left. This lower position of the right kidney is associated with the presence, on the right side, of the liver which takes up much of the space in the upper right part of the abdominal cavity.

Palpation

The lower pole of each kidney can often be felt during abdominal examination of the living subject, since, placed as it is on the forward-projecting vertebral bodies of the lumbar curvature, it is not far from the abdominal wall. The right kidney, being lower, is more easily felt than the left. Both kidneys are more easily palpated in women than in men, because women have a more marked lumbar curvature and a less muscular abdominal wall. The kidney can be felt to move with the diaphragm during breathing.

Relations

The kidney is invested by fascia, the **perirenal fascia,** within which it is held firmly by the **perirenal fat.** In emaciated individuals, depletion of this fat store may lead to a kidney's becoming abnormally mobile (floating kidney).

The superior and posterior relations of the two kidneys are similar, in that each upper pole is capped by a suprarenal gland (Plate 27 and Figs. 181 and 206) and each posterior surface is related above to the diaphragm, behind which is the pleural cavity (especially on the left side) and below to the muscles forming the posterior abdominal wall. These are, from medial to lateral, the psoas muscle, the quadratus lumborum and the transversus abdominis (Fig. 181). The anterior relations of the two kidneys differ. The **right kidney** has in front of it the liver above, the hepatic flexure of the colon below, and the duodenum medially. The **left kidney** has in front of it the stomach and spleen, below which is the pancreas and lower still is the jejunum; the most lateral part of the anterior

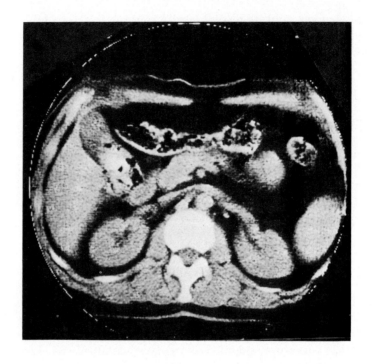

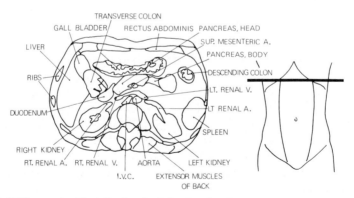

TRANSVERSE COLON
GALL BLADDER
RECTUS ABDOMINIS PANCREAS, HEAD
LIVER
SUP. MESENTERIC A.
PANCREAS, BODY
RIBS
DESCENDING COLON
LT. RENAL V.
DUODENUM
LT RENAL A.
SPLEEN
RIGHT KIDNEY
RT. RENAL A. RT. RENAL V.   AORTA   LEFT KIDNEY
I.V.C.   EXTENSOR MUSCLES
              OF BACK

Fig. 196. A CAT scan (p. 7) at the level of the first lumbar vertebra, showing the relations of the viscera at this level.

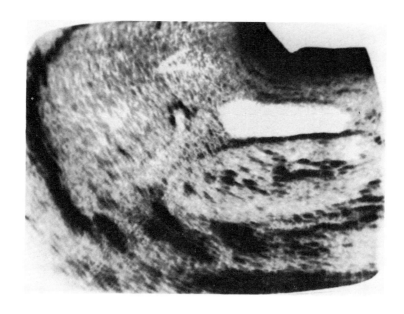

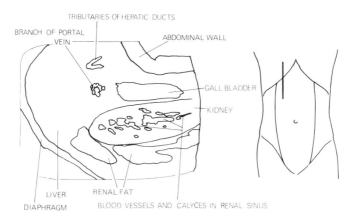

TRIBUTARIES OF HEPATIC DUCTS

BRANCH OF PORTAL
VEIN

ABDOMINAL WALL

GALL BLADDER

KIDNEY

LIVER

RENAL FAT

DIAPHRAGM

BLOOD VESSELS AND CALYCES IN RENAL SINUS

Fig. 197. A longitudinal ultrasound scan (p. 8) of the upper abdomen, to the right of the midline.

surface is related to the descending colon. The CAT scan and the ultrasound scan illustrated in Figures 196 and 197 show how these relations can now be demonstrated in the living subject. Because of its relations, the kidney is approached at operation more easily from behind, so that the usual incision is an oblique loin incision, parallel to the last rib and to the nerves of the abdominal wall.

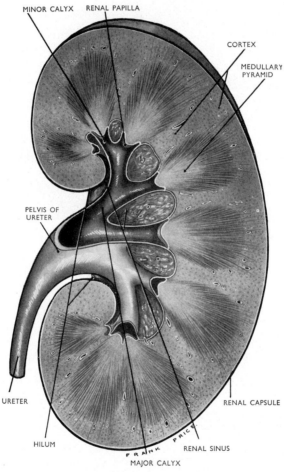

Fig. 198. Section through the kidney to show the relationships of the cortex, medulla, papillæ, sinus and hilum. The pelvis of the ureter has been cut open to show the relationships of the minor calyces to the renal papillæ.

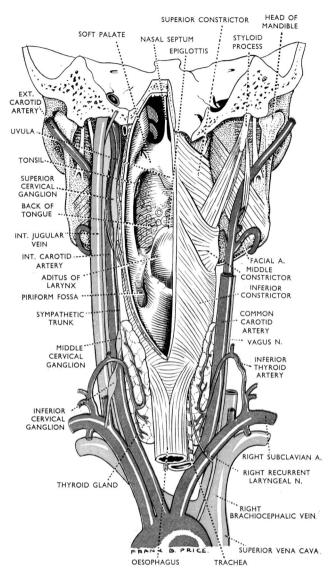

SUPERIOR CONSTRICTOR
HEAD OF MANDIBLE
SOFT PALATE
NASAL SEPTUM
STYLOID PROCESS
EPIGLOTTIS
EXT. CAROTID ARTERY
UVULA
TONSIL
SUPERIOR CERVICAL GANGLION
BACK OF TONGUE
INT. JUGULAR VEIN
INT. CAROTID ARTERY
ADITUS OF LARYNX
PIRIFORM FOSSA
SYMPATHETIC TRUNK
MIDDLE CERVICAL GANGLION
INFERIOR CERVICAL GANGLION
THYROID GLAND
FACIAL A.
MIDDLE CONSTRICTOR
INFERIOR CONSTRICTOR
COMMON CAROTID ARTERY
VAGUS N.
INFERIOR THYROID ARTERY
RIGHT SUBCLAVIAN A.
RIGHT RECURRENT LARYNGEAL N.
RIGHT BRACHIOCEPHALIC VEIN
FRANK B. PRICE.
OESOPHAGUS
TRACHEA
SUPERIOR VENA CAVA

Plate 34. The pharynx seen from behind, with the great vessels. The left half of the posterior pharyngeal wall has been removed, to reveal the interior and the communications with the nose, the mouth and the larynx The arrow indicates the opening of the pharyngotympanic tube.

[facing page 486

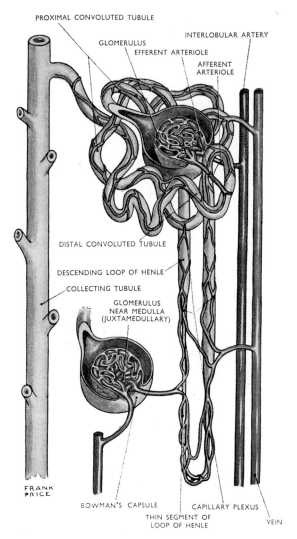

PROXIMAL CONVOLUTED TUBULE

GLOMERULUS

EFFERENT ARTERIOLE

INTERLOBULAR ARTERY

AFFERENT ARTERIOLE

DISTAL CONVOLUTED TUBULE

DESCENDING LOOP OF HENLE

COLLECTING TUBULE

GLOMERULUS NEAR MEDULLA (JUXTAMEDULLARY)

FRANK PRICE

BOWMAN'S CAPSULE

THIN SEGMENT OF LOOP OF HENLE

CAPILLARY PLEXUS

VEIN

Plate 35. Diagram to show the different parts of the nephron and their relations to blood vessels in the substance of the kidney. Note that a loop of a nephron, descending into the medulla, is surrounded by capillaries derived from the efferent arterioles of glomeruli situated near the medulla. Bowman's capsule is now called the glomerular capsule and Henle's loop is called the loop of the nephron.

[between pages 486/7 facing Pl. 36

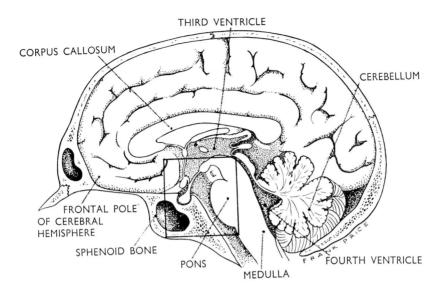

THIRD VENTRICLE

CORPUS CALLOSUM

CEREBELLUM

FRONTAL POLE
OF CEREBRAL
HEMISPHERE

SPHENOID BONE

PONS

MEDULLA

FOURTH VENTRICLE

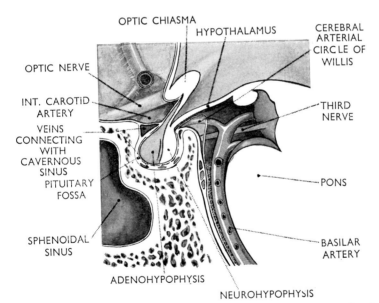

OPTIC CHIASMA

HYPOTHALAMUS

CEREBRAL
ARTERIAL
CIRCLE OF
WILLIS

OPTIC NERVE

INT. CAROTID
ARTERY

THIRD
NERVE

VEINS
CONNECTING
WITH
CAVERNOUS
SINUS
PITUITARY
FOSSA

PONS

SPHENOIDAL
SINUS

BASILAR
ARTERY

ADENOHYPOPHYSIS

NEUROHYPOPHYSIS

Plate 36. Diagrams to show the position and relations of the pituitary gland (hypophysis cerebri).

[between pages 486/7 facing Pl. 35

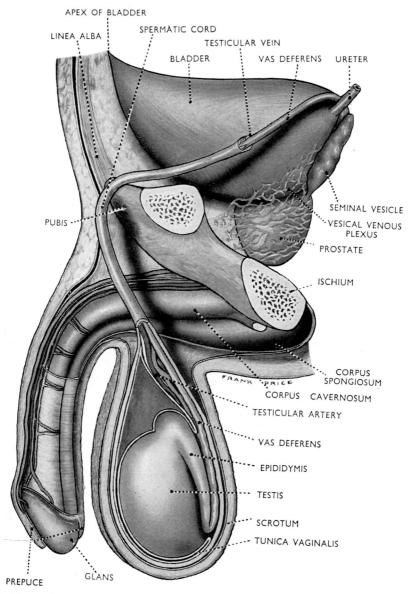

APEX OF BLADDER
LINEA ALBA
SPERMATIC CORD
TESTICULAR VEIN
BLADDER
VAS DEFERENS
URETER

PUBIS

SEMINAL VESICLE
VESICAL VENOUS PLEXUS
PROSTATE

ISCHIUM

FRANK PRICE

CORPUS SPONGIOSUM
CORPUS CAVERNOSUM
TESTICULAR ARTERY
VAS DEFERENS
EPIDIDYMIS
TESTIS
SCROTUM
TUNICA VAGINALIS

PREPUCE
GLANS

Plate 37. The male genital organs and bladder, seen from the left side. The coverings of the testis have been cut away to show the relationships of the testis, epididymis and distal end of the spermatic cord.

[facing page 487

STRUCTURE OF THE KIDNEYS

The kidney is surrounded by a thin capsule of connective tissue.

If the kidney is cut in half, longitudinally in the coronal plane, much of its structure can be seen (Fig. 198). The **hilum** leads into a hollow in the kidney substance, known as the **sinus** of the kidney. The cut surface of the kidney itself presents two zones, an outer **cortex** and an inner **medulla,** of different colour and texture. The cortex, often paler, is granular to the naked eye (p. 490). The medulla consists of between twelve and twenty medullary **pyramids,** which are often darker in colour and are striated from base to apex. The base of each pyramid is towards the cortex and the apex, called a **renal papilla,** projects into the sinus of the kidney. The pyramids are separated by columns of cortical substance, the **renal columns.** From the bases of the pyramids, **medullary rays** of medullary tissue extend into the cortex.

The sinus of the kidney contains the funnel-shaped upper end of the ureter, called its **pelvis.** The pelvis divides into two or three parts, the **major calyces,** and each of these divides into several **minor calyces.** Each minor calyx has a cup-shaped end which fits over a renal papilla. The pelvis of the ureter and its subdivisions are well illustrated in the intravenous pyelogram shown in Fig. 199.

The renal artery and vein also pass through the sinus of the kidney (p. 373).

The human kidney is complex, but the rabbit kidney is easier to understand. It has only one medullary pyramid, surrounded, except at its apex, by a layer of cortex, into which medullary rays extend. The pelvis of the ureter fits over the apex of the pyramid. The human kidney is made up of between twelve and twenty parts, or lobes, each of which is like the whole kidney of the rabbit. These lobes are placed side by side, so that each pyramid is separated from its neighbours by a column of cortex. To cap each pyramid separately, the pelvis of the ureter is divided into calyces.

The Nephron

The nephron is the functional unit of kidney tissue. It is too small to be seen with the naked eye, but is easily demonstrated with a microscope. Each kidney contains about one million nephrons, closely packed and intertwined.

STRUCTURE OF THE NEPHRON: A nephron is a tubule about 3 cm long. One end is closed and the other opens into a collecting duct. The closed end, formed of a single layer of flat cells, is dilated to form the **glomerular capsule** (Bowman's capsule) which is invaginated by a knot of capillary loops, called a **glomerulus** (Fig. 200 and Plate 35). The spherical structure so formed is a **renal corpuscle** (Malpighian corpuscle). The function of the renal corpuscle is **filtration.**

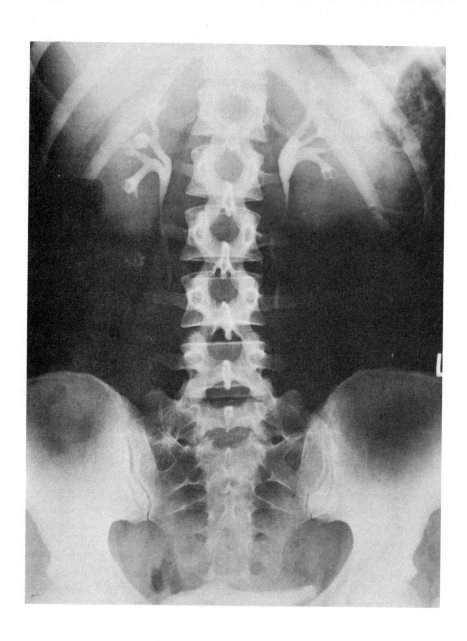

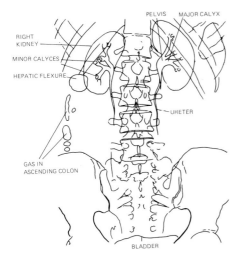

Fig. 199. An intravenous pyelogram (IVP).

The rest of the tubule is coiled and looped (see Plate 35). The section next to the renal corpuscle has a wall of cubical cells and lies coiled close to the corpuscle. It is called the **proximal convoluted tubule.** This leads into the thin walled **loop of the nephron** (of Henle) which extends, with straight sides, into a medullary pyramid and back again. The tubule then forms near its own glomerulus a second coil, the **distal convoluted tubule,** which ends by joining a collecting duct. The proximal and distal convoluted tubules and the loop of

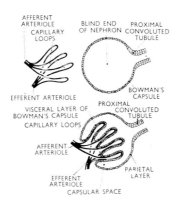

Fig. 200. Diagrams to show how capillary loops between the afferent and the efferent arterioles are invaginated into the blind end of the nephron.

the nephron **concentrate** the urine by **selective reabsorption,** and also add substances to it by **secretion** (p. 492).

Each **collecting duct** receives many tubules and passes straight through a pyramid to open into a minor calyx at the papilla.

The spherical glomeruli and the coiled proximal and distal convoluted tubules lie in the cortex, the cut surface of which has therefore a granular appearance. The straight limbs of the loops of the nephron and the straight collecting ducts are in the medullary rays and medullary pyramids which therefore look striated.

Each medullary ray has clustered round it the renal corpuscles and convoluted tubules of the nephrons whose loops and collecting ducts it contains. This constitutes a **lobule** of the kidney.

Blood Supply of the Kidney

Each kidney is supplied by a short wide **renal artery** direct from the abdominal aorta. In the sinus of the kidney it divides into several branches **(interlobar arteries)** which enter the renal columns and then form arcades **(arcuate arteries)** across the bases of the pyramids. From these arcuate arteries, branches pass into the medulla and also, between the lobules (as **interlobular arteries**) into the cortex. From the interlobular arteries an **afferent arteriole** goes to each glomerulus. The blood passes through the **capillary loops** of the glomerulus and is carried away by an **efferent arteriole** which leads to a **capillary network** round the rest of the nephron. From this plexus the blood is drained away by **venules** which eventually join up to form the **renal vein.**

Blood flows through the kidneys not only to nourish them, but so that they can alter its composition, by removing unwanted substances according to the needs of the body (p. 491). The total volume of blood in the body flows through the kidneys once every five minutes. This explains why the renal vessels are so large.

An adequate blood supply to the kidney is essential. If for any reason it is less than usual, the kidney secretes a hormone-like enzyme called **renin** (see p. 492), which raises the blood pressure and so helps to ensure that more blood reaches it. Unfortunately, if the nephrons receive insufficient blood because of disease in the kidney, they secrete renin in an ineffective attempt to improve the function. Serious hypertension results, but this can be relieved by removing the offending kidney, if the other kidney is healthy.

FUNCTIONS OF THE KIDNEYS

The principal functions of the kidneys are excretion and the maintenance of homeostasis.

Excretion

Excretion is the elimination of unwanted substances from the body. The kidneys excrete by producing a watery fluid, called **urine** (p. 494), which has dissolved in it the nitrogen-containing waste products of protein metabolism (e.g. urea, uric acid and creatinine), excess salts and other unwanted substances.

(Other organs of excretion are the lungs which excrete carbon dioxide and water; the sweat glands which excrete water and small amounts of salt and urea; and the alimentary tract which excretes water and some drugs through its mucous membrane, as well as cholesterol, bile pigments and some drugs by means of the bile.)

Maintenance of Homeostasis

By **excreting unwanted substances** and **conserving others** the kidneys maintain the composition of the plasma. This in turn maintains the composition of the tissue fluid, so that it is always a suitable environment for the body cells. In other words the kidneys play an essential part in the maintenance of homeostasis (pp. 95 and 97). To this end the kidneys perform the following functions:

(*a*) They help to regulate the **water content** of the body by varying the volume of urine produced (p. 493).

(*b*) They vary the **kinds and the amounts of electrolytes** excreted in the urine (p. 493) and may excrete glucose if the blood concentration is too high (p. 493)

(*c*) They maintain the **acid-base balance** (p. 494) of the plasma and of the tissue fluid.

Detoxication

The kidney renders some toxic substances, for example certain drugs, harmless by altering their chemical form and then excretes them.

Hormone Production

The kidney is responsible for the production of two hormones, **angiotensin** and **erythropoietin**.

A decrease in blood flow to the kidney causes the kidney to liberate an enzyme called **renin** which is responsible for the appearance of a hormone called angiotensin. Angiotensin acts upon the suprarenal cortex and stimulates the release of **aldosterone** (see p. 515). The secretion of aldosterone leads to sodium retention by the kidney and when sodium is retained so is water. This in turn leads to an increase in the circulating blood volume and necessitates an increased cardiac output. The blood pressure rises because of this increased cardiac output combined with the increased peripheral resistance to circulating blood caused by constriction of the peripheral blood vessels.

The kidney is necessary for the production of an erythropoietic substance which is able to raise the number of red blood corpuscles in normal individuals. The rôle of the kidney in blood formation is of practical importance because chronic renal failure is accompanied by an anæmia which cannot be attributed simply to a deficiency in excretion by the kidney. Conversely, in the presence of a renal carcinoma, a malignant tumour of the kidney, there may be too many red corpuscles in the circulating blood.

In Infants

The kidneys of new-born infants are relatively inefficient, and cannot deal effectively with more than minor variations in normal physiology. The careful management of water and electrolyte balance in the treatment of infants who are ill is therefore essential.

Function of the Nephron

The nephron is the functional unit of kidney tissue and the functions of the kidney as a whole are carried out by its different parts.

The **nephron produces urine in two stages:** (1) filtration under pressure, (2) selective reabsorption.

FILTRATION UNDER PRESSURE: This takes place **in the renal corpuscle.** The blood pressure in the capillary loops of the glomerulus is high, because the afferent arteriole is larger than the efferent arteriole. This pressure forces water and all the other constituents of plasma, except the large protein molecules, through the capillary walls and through the overlying flat epithelium of the glomerular capsule (Fig. 200 and Plate 35) into its lumen. This fluid in the glomerular capsule is called **glomerular filtrate** and has the composition of plasma without any protein. The two kidneys produce about 170 litres of glomerular filtrate in 24 hours.

SELECTIVE REABSORPTION: This takes place **in the tubule.** As the glomerular filtrate passes through the tubule, its composition is altered until urine is found in the collecting ducts. Substances useful to the body, such as water, glucose, amino acids, sodium and chloride ions, are re-absorbed by the cells of the tubule and passed back into the blood in the capillary network round them. Some substances are reabsorbed completely and others only partially. Most of this reabsorption takes place in the proximal convolutions of the tubules which roughly separate the substances which must be conserved from those which are to be rejected in the urine. Waste materials, like urea, uric acid or creatinine, and unwanted electrolytes pass on. The loops of the nephron, the distal convolutions and the collecting ducts are concerned mainly with the fine regulation of water, electrolyte and hydrogen ion balance.

SECRETION: Although **the tubules** function mainly by selective reabsorption, they also actively secrete certain substances into the urine, for example hydrogen ions, potassium ions, creatinine and some toxins and drugs.

DETAILS OF TUBULAR FUNCTION: **Water.** Whereas about 170 litres of glomerular filtrate are formed in 24 hours, the volume of urine produced is only about 1·5 litres. Most of this water is reabsorbed by the proximal convoluted tubules, an important function since the body could not afford to lose such a large quantity of water. The urine must contain a certain minimum amount of water to keep in solution the substances dissolved in the glomerular filtrate. Any water in excess of this minimum is reabsorbed by the tubules, unless the body already has enough water. The exact amount reabsorbed, and therefore the volume of urine formed, is controlled by the **antidiuretic hormone** of the posterior lobe of the pituitary, which acts on the distal convoluted tubules and collecting ducts. If the body needs to conserve water (for example after much sweating) the antidiuretic hormone causes these cells to reabsorb water, and a smaller volume of concentrated urine is left in the tubules and collecting ducts. On the other hand, if there is an excess of fluid (for example after many cups of tea) the antidiuretic hormone is no longer secreted, the cells of the distal convoluted tubules and collecting ducts do not reabsorb water and a greater volume of dilute urine results. In this way, the kidney regulates the water content of the body. The **mineralo-cortico-steroid hormones** of the suprarenal also influence the kidney tubules. They cause the retention of sodium ions and of water, and increased urinary loss of potassium.

Threshold substances. These are substances which are present in the glomerular filtrate and are wholly or partly reabsorbed by the tubules. They include water, glucose and electrolytes. Substances like creatinine, which are not reabsorbed, are non-threshold substances.

Glucose, when it is present in normal amounts in the plasma, passes into the glomerular filtrate and is **all reabsorbed** by the tubules, so that none appears in the urine. If there is an excess of glucose in the plasma, as for example in diabetes mellitus, the extra glucose is not reabsorbed and appears in the urine (**glycosuria**). The urine then also contains more water to keep the glucose dissolved; in other words the volume is increased. To provide this extra water the patient has to drink more than is usual.

Acid-base balance. The pH of the blood and of the tissue fluid is kept constant within narrow limits. Acid substances are constantly being produced during metabolism. Alkaline substances are ingested in the food. These are buffered, it is true, but as the buffering substances are used up the need to eliminate the acids and free the buffers for further action becomes urgent. The kidneys play an important part in eliminating acids, and indeed fresh normal urine is acid, the pH being between 5 and 7. In acidosis the kidney excretes a more acid urine and in alkalosis the urine becomes alkaline.

The cells of the kidney tubules vary the reaction of the urine by the nature of the ions excreted in the urine. Also they produce ammonium, which can combine with ions such as chloride for excretion and so conserve sodium for the body.

Concentration gradients. The processes by which concentrated urine is produced are complex and are dependent on the fact that the loops of the nephron and the collecting ducts lie close together in the medulla. These structural and functional features result in the establishing of concentration gradients for sodium and urea. The gradient of osmotic pressure, or osmolarity, increases from the cortex, through the medulla, to the tips of the renal papillæ. This fact is also important when considering the excretion of toxic substances, which may damage the renal **papillæ** because of increased concentration in this region.

THE URINE

Urine is an excretion, and not a secretion, because it is of no further use to the body.

Urine is a **yellow** fluid, varying in shade from a pale straw colour, when it is dilute, to a deep amber when it is concentrated. The **specific gravity** is about 1·020 (normal range 1·012 to 1·025) and its **reaction** is acid. A normal adult passes about 1·5 litres (50 oz) in 24 hours. Fresh urine has a faintly aromatic smell.

The volume and composition of the urine varies widely in health, depending on the amount and kind of food eaten, the amount of fluid taken and the amount of fluid lost by other means, for example by sweating. Certain normal constituents are always present.

Normal Constituents

Water.

Waste products of protein metabolism (p. 554), i.e. urea (2%), uric acid and creatinine.

Salts: sodium chloride (1%), sulphates and phosphates.

Urinary pigments.

WATER: This forms 96% of urine. A minimum volume of water is essential to keep the other constituents in solution.

UREA: This is the most abundant dissolved substance, forming 2% of urine. By means of it, most of the waste nitrogen from protein metabolism is eliminated.

If urine is allowed to stand, bacteria multiply in it and break down the urea to form ammonium carbonate. This makes the urine, usually acid when fresh, alkaline and makes it **smell of ammonia.** The same chemical reaction occurs in a baby's wet napkin. Unless the napkin is changed, the ammonia burns the skin and produces nappy rash.

SALTS: Sodium chloride is the most abundant, forming 1%. The presence and concentration of other salts determines the reaction of the urine.

URINARY PIGMENTS: The origin of the colouring matter is unknown. Traces of pigments derived from bile pigments are present.

If concentrated urine is allowed to cool, some of the dissolved substances, for example uric acid and certain salts, precipitate (form solid particles). This makes the urine look cloudy.

Abnormal Constituents

Abnormal constituents in the urine are **indicative of disease** of the kidney or of other parts of the urinary tract.

Blood in the urine (**Hæmaturia**), if present in considerable amounts, colours it pink or red.

Pus in the urine (**Pyuria**) makes it cloudy and, if the urine stands, the pus forms a whitish yellow, sometimes 'ropy' precipitate.

Casts are tiny cylinders of material shed from the lining of the kidney tubules in some diseases. They can be identified if the urine is examined under a microscope.

With a microscope too, red blood cells and pus cells can be recognized, even when their numbers are too small to alter the naked eye appearance of the urine.

Protein. Plasma proteins, especially albumin because it has the smallest molecule, may pass into the glomerular filtrate if the renal corpuscle is damaged. This protein passes on into the urine. Albumin in the urine is called **albuminuria.**

TEST FOR PROTEIN: The urine is boiled. Any protein present forms a white cloud, which does not dissolve and disappear when the urine is acidified by adding acetic acid.

Glucose. Sometimes not all the glucose in the glomerular filtrate is re-absorbed, and some passes on to appear in the urine. This is known as **gly-cosuria.** It happens when the blood sugar is high in diabetes mellitus and the glomerular filtrate therefore also contains an excess of glucose, which is not all reabsorbed; or it may happen when the kidney has an abnormally low threshold for sugar, and sugar, as it were, 'spills over' into the urine.

TEST FOR GLUCOSE: Glucose is identified in urine by adding 8 drops of urine to 5 ml of Benedict's reagent, and then boiling the mixture for 2 minutes. Glucose produces a red, a yellow or a green precipitate according to the amount present.

The 'clinitest' for glucose is a proprietary adaptation of Benedict's test. It is important to realize that a positive result may be due to substances other than glucose in the urine, for example aspirin or lactose (p. 39).

Factors Influencing the Production of Urine

DIURNAL OR CIRCADIAN RHYTHM: Urine production decreases during sleep at night and is at its greatest during the first few hours after waking (see also p. 562).

INCREASE IN VOLUME (POLYURIA) OCCURS:

if the fluid intake is increased;

if the renal blood flow is increased;

if the skin is cold; this causes constriction of the blood vessels to the skin and reflex dilatation of the vessels in the internal organs with a resulting rise in pressure in the glomerular capillaries of the kidney;

if there are nervous influences such as excitement or fear.

in disease, for example diabetes insipidus, diabetes mellitus and chronic nephritis, because of changes in the concentration of osmotically active substances in the renal tubules. These changes impede the reabsorption of water.

DECREASE IN VOLUME (OLIGURIA) OCCURS:

if the fluid intake is reduced;

if the fluid loss is increased, for example by sweating, diarrhœa, or vomiting;

if the renal blood flow is reduced, for example in the low blood pressure of shock;

in disease, for example in acute nephritis and in fevers.

ANURIA is the term used to describe the complete failure of urine production.

Investigation of Renal Function

1. VOLUME AND SPECIFIC GRAVITY OF THE URINE: Under ordinary conditions, an adult passes 1·5 litres of urine of specific gravity 1·020 in 24 hours. If the water intake is restricted, healthy kidneys concentrate the urine very much, and a small volume of urine of high specific gravity (1·030) is formed. After the ingestion of much fluid, the kidneys excrete a large volume of dilute urine of low specific gravity (1·005). Diseased kidneys cannot alter the volume and specific gravity of the urine in this way.

2. ABNORMAL CONSTITUENTS IN THE URINE: The presence of protein or of casts indicates some abnormality of renal function.

3. BLOOD UREA: If the kidney is excreting waste products including urea satisfactorily, the amount of urea in the blood is kept to a normal low level (20 to 40 mg. per 100 ml.). If kidney function is upset, waste products accumulate in the blood and the amount of urea rises. The blood urea is estimated in hospital laboratories. The measurement of the **rate** at which urea is cleared from the body—**the urea clearance test**—gives even more precise information about the state of functioning of the kidneys.

4. THE EXCRETION OF X-RAY OPAQUE SUBSTANCES (intravenous pyelogram): The excretion of a substance, such as uroselectan, should take place within minutes of its injection into a vein, and show an outline of the renal pelvis and calyces on radiographs (Fig. 199). This shadow is delayed or poor when kidney function is impaired.

Some Disorders of Kidney Function

NEPHRITIS: The various kinds of the disease, known as nephritis, throw an interesting light on the normal functions of the constituent parts of a nephron.

In **acute, type 1 nephritis,** the glomeruli are inflamed so that there is impairment of glomerular filtration with diminished output. The urine is also bloodstained and contains albumen. More fluid than normal is retained in the plasma, which leads to œdema or water-logging of the tissues.

In **type 2** nephritis, both glomeruli and tubules are affected by the inflammation. The output of urine may be normal or slightly reduced, but, because the nephron has an increased permeability to protein, there is a marked albuminuria. The loss of protein from the plasma reduces its osmotic pressure and leads to gross œdema (see p. 97).

In **chronic nephritis,** there is degeneration of the nephron. This leads to increased urinary output, because the tubules can no longer concentrate the glomerular filtrate. Thus the urine is dilute and has a low specific gravity. There is also loss of protein in the urine, which eventually leads to œdema, and the kidney function continues progressively to fail. The nitrogenous waste products in the blood accumulate and give rise to the condition of **uræmia.**

THE 'CRUSH SYNDROME': It has been found that people who have had part of the body crushed, say a limb, often suffer afterwards from failure of urinary excretion. This is accounted for by the fact that these injuries cause reflex spasm of the arteries in the cortex of the kidney, which thus suffers from an insufficient supply of blood, and little or none of it goes to glomeruli. Whatever blood does circulate through the kidney in these circumstances passes through the vessels in the medulla, which is devoid of glomeruli, and so little or no urine is produced.

THE URETERS

The ureters convey the urine from the kidneys, where it is formed, to the bladder where it is stored.

The ureter begins at the medial border of the kidney by the joining of the calyces to form the funnel-shaped upper end of the ureter, called the **pelvis of the ureter** (Fig. 198). This leads into the ureter itself which is a narrow muscular tube, 25 cm long. The ureter passes downwards over the posterior abdominal wall and into the lesser pelvis, where it enters the bladder through its posterior wall.

On the posterior abdominal wall the ureter lies on the psoas muscle, behind the parietal peritoneum. It crosses the iliac vessels at the brim of the lesser pelvis and curves forwards and medially. Just before it reaches the bladder it lies, in the female, close to the cervix of the uterus and the upper end of the vagina, and in the male the vas deferens passes above it. It enters the bladder by passing obliquely through the muscle of its posterior wall. This, together with a tiny flap of bladder mucosa over the opening, prevents regurgitation of urine from the bladder into the ureter.

Structure

The ureter has three coats: (1) an outer fibrous coat; (2) a smooth muscle coat; (3) a lining of mucous membrane which has waterproof transitional epithelium (p. 103).

Function

The ureter aids the flow of urine by peristaltic contraction of its smooth muscle. The contractions become excessive and very painful if the ureter contains a stone—a condition known as **renal** or **ureteric colic.**

URINARY BLADDER

The bladder is a hollow organ which collects the urine from the ureters, stores it, and, at a convenient moment, voids it. The average capacity of a healthy adult male bladder is about 300 ml. If it is distended, its capacity may be very much more.

Form

The bladder, when empty, is the shape of a pyramid. The **apex** points forwards and the **base** faces backwards. The surfaces are the base, a superior surface and two inferolateral surfaces. The ureters enter through the upper lateral angles of the base and the urethra emerges at the inferior angle of the base, this region being known as the **neck** of the bladder. The apex of the bladder is connected to the umbilicus by a cord of connective tissue, the **median umbilical ligament.** When the bladder is full it is larger and much more rounded in shape.

Interior of the Bladder

The interior of the bladder can be seen in the living subject by means of an instrument called a **cystoscope.** The lining of mucous membrane is loosely attached and is thrown into folds when the organ is empty. The internal surface of the base differs from the rest and is called the **trigone.** The mucous membrane here is firmly attached and is always smooth. It is a darker colour because of its rich blood supply and it is more richly supplied by nerves than the rest of the bladder. The orifices of the ureters can be seen at its upper lateral angles and the urethra leaves at its inferior angle.

The trigone is developed from the mesonephric (genital) ducts and pain from it, having a genital character, is referred to the perineum. The rest of the bladder

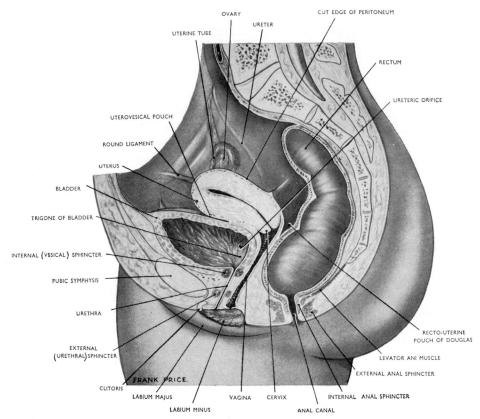

Fig. 201. A median sagittal section through the female pelvis, seen from the left side.

is developed from the cloaca, like the hindgut, and pain from it, like pain from the hindgut, is referred to the lower abdominal wall.

Microscopic Structure

The wall of the bladder is made up of four layers, namely:

1. An outer layer of **peritoneum** on its upper surface only.
2. A **muscle coat** of smooth muscle, called the **detrusor muscle.** Near the neck of the bladder, the muscle fibres surround the beginning of the urethra to form the **sphincter vesicæ.**
3. A **submucous coat** of loose connective tissue.

4. A lining of **mucous membrane,** the epithelium of which is transitional
   (p. 103).

Nerve Supply

The bladder is supplied both by sympathetic and by parasympathetic
nerves. Stimulation of the parasympathetic nerves empties the bladder by
causing the detrusor muscle to contract and the sphincter vesicæ to relax.

Stimulation of the sympathetic nerves prevents emptying by causing the
sphincter vesicæ to contract and the detrusor to relax (see also pp. 282 and 285).

Position and Relations

The bladder lies in the anterior part of the lesser pelvis, but when it is full,
and especially when it is overdistended, it bulges upwards into the abdominal
cavity. In infants and young children, in whom the pelvis is very small, the
bladder lies in the abdominal cavity.

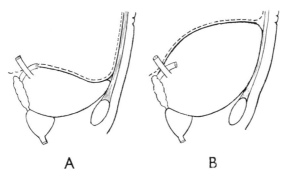

Fig. 202. Schemes to show the relations of the bladder to peritoneum (represented by an
interrupted line), to the pubic symphysis and to the part of the abdominal wall below the
navel. A, when the bladder is empty; B, when the bladder is full.

Only the superior surface is covered by peritoneum. As the bladder fills it
bulges upwards between the peritoneum and the posterior surface of the
anterior abdominal wall. When it is overdistended the apex may reach the
umbilicus. When it is distended in this way, an opening can therefore be made
into it through the abdominal wall without opening the peritoneum (Fig. 202).

The two inferolateral surfaces are related to the pubic bones, separated
from them by an interval, the **retropubic space** (Fig. 203), which contains
loose connective tissue and the floor of which is formed by the ligaments connecting the bladder to the pubis (see below).

The other relations differ in the two sexes.

In the male (Fig. 203), the base is related to the ends of the vasa deferentia and to the seminal vesicles. Behind these is the rectum. The neck of the male bladder is closely applied to the upper surface of the prostate gland (p. 531).

In the female the base is close against the anterior wall of the vagina, and behind the vagina is the rectum (Figs. 201 and 216). The body of the uterus bends forwards above the superior surface of the female bladder, separated from it by the uterovesical pouch of the peritoneum.

Ligaments of the Bladder

The neck of the bladder is connected to the pubic bone by a series of ligaments, which in the female are termed **pubovesical ligaments,** but in the male they are called **puboprostatic** as they are also connected to the base of the prostate gland. The **apex of the bladder** (where the superior and inferolateral surfaces meet) is connected to the umbilicus by the **median umbilical ligament,** which is the obliterated urachus or allantoic remnant (see p. 71 and Fig. 210). Obliteration may not be complete and give rise to cysts or a diverticulum extending from the bladder.

THE URETHRA

The urethra is a narrow canal which leads from the bladder to the exterior. It differs in the two sexes.

The Female Urethra

The female urethra is short (about 4 cm in length) and straight. It transmits urine only. It runs downwards and forwards behind the symphysis pubis, very close to the anterior wall of the vagina, and opens in the vulva, behind the clitoris and in front of the vaginal orifice (Fig. 219).

The Male Urethra

The male urethra is long (about 20 cm in length) and bent like the letter 'S' (Fig. 203). It transmits both semen and urine, but not simultaneously. It has three parts, namely:

1. The **prostatic part** (3 cm long) which passes through the prostate gland.
2. The **membranous part** (1 cm long) which is surrounded by the external sphincter (see below) and then pierces the perineal membrane.

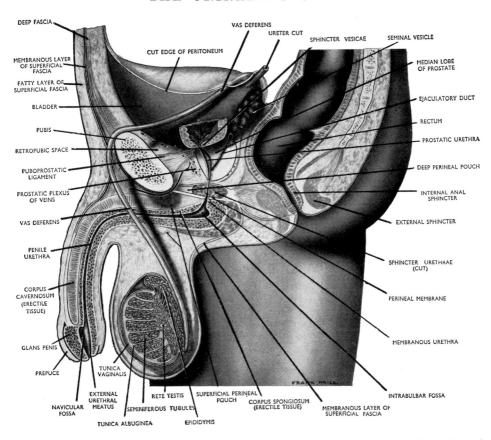

Fig. 203. Sagittal section through the male pelvis, seen from the left side. The region of the bladder neck has been cut open to show the relations of the inside of the bladder to the sectioned urethra and prostate. The left testis has also been sectioned to show its internal structure.

3. The **spongy part** which enters the substance of the corpus spongiosum of the penis (p. 532) and traverses its length to open at the external urethral orifice on the tip of the glans. The external orifice is the narrowest part of this long 'S'-shaped tube, so that any catheter or sound which can be introduced at all, should pass into the bladder without difficulty if the urethra is normal.

Sphincters of the Bladder and of the Urethra

In each sex, two sphincters control the escape of urine from the bladder, the sphincter vesicæ (or internal sphincter) and the sphincter urethræ (or external sphincter) (Figs. 201 and 203).

THE SPHINCTER VESICÆ: The sphincter of the bladder is composed of part of the smooth muscle wall of the bladder. The **smooth muscle** fibres are arranged circularly round the beginning of the urethra at the neck of the bladder. The sphincter vesicæ is supplied by **sympathetic nerves** and is not under voluntary control.

THE SPHINCTER URETHRÆ: The sphincter of the urethra is composed of **striated muscle** which surrounds the urethra just before it pierces the perineal membrane. It is attached, at each side, to the inferior ramus of the pubis. It is supplied by a branch of the **pudendal nerve** (p. 279), and is under voluntary control.

MICTURITION

Micturition is the process of **passing urine.** It is essentially a reflex act which has been brought under voluntary control.

The bladder fills slowly as urine reaches it through the ureters. Under control of the sympathetic nerves, the sphincter vesicæ remains closed and the detrusor muscle of the bladder wall relaxes a little to accommodate the increasing volume of urine. When the volume reaches about 300 ml, the walls do not relax so readily and the pressure then rises. The increased pressure stimulates stretch receptors in the bladder wall. In infants, before voluntary control is established (p. 585), this forms the afferent limb of a simple reflex arc (p. 262). The impulses are carried to the spinal cord, and relayed to the parasympathetic nerve cells in the sacral region of the spinal cord. Their axons, the pelvic splanchnic nerves, then carry the impulses to the detrusor muscle, causing it to contract to push the urine out. At the same time, the sphincter vesicæ and the sphincter urethræ reflexly relax, so that the urine is evacuated.

However, once voluntary control of micturition is established, the reflex can be suppressed, for a time at least. The first afferent impulses, as the bladder becomes full, are interpreted by the brain as the desire to micturate. Until time and place are suitable, inhibitory impulses are sent from the cortex to the para-sympathetic cells preventing contraction of the detrusor muscle. At the same time the sphincter urethræ is contracted voluntarily.

At the right moment this control is removed and reflex emptying of the bladder occurs as before. It can be assisted voluntarily by increasing the intra-abdominal pressure through simultaneous contraction of the diaphragm and anterior abdominal wall.

Disorders of Micturition

Inability to micturate is called **retention of urine.**

Loss of control of micturition is called **incontinence of urine.**

Damage to the brain or spinal cord, which interferes with the corticospinal tracts, results in incontinence. At first there is retention of urine due to spinal shock, but later the bladder is emptied reflexly at intervals, as in an infant.

The Prostate and Micturition

Enlargement of the prostate prevents normal micturition by narrowing the prostatic part of the urethra. Very often, enlargement of the middle lobe of the prostate blocks the upper end of the urethra. Retention of urine is the result. Sometimes there is **retention with overflow,** a kind of incontinence in which the bladder is grossly distended and a little urine dribbles away continuously.

EXAMINATION OF THE URINARY TRACT IN LIVING SUBJECTS

Abdominal Examination

The kidneys can often be palpated (p. 483). A distended bladder produces a swelling in the midline above the symphisis pubes.

Examination of the Urine

The urine is examined for normal and abnormal constituents (p. 495).

Cystoscopy

An instrument called a cystoscope is passed into the bladder. The interior of the bladder, including the ureteric orifices, can then be inspected. Ureteric catheters can be passed up along each ureter, so that a sample of urine can be taken separately from each kidney.

Radiological Examination

The outline of the kidneys can be seen on an ordinary 'straight' radiograph of the abdominal cavity (Fig. 98).

Excretion Pyelogram

A nontoxic radio-opaque substance which the kidney excretes in the urine is injected intravenously. The outline of the kidney, the calyces and pelvis of the ureter, the ureter and the bladder can then be seen on a radiograph (see also p. 487 and Fig. 199).

Retrograde Pyelogram

During cystoscopy (see above) with ureteric catheters in position, a radio-opaque fluid is introduced into the ureter. A radiograph then shows the outline of the calyces and pelvis of the ureter, ureter and bladder.

CHAPTER XVI

THE ENDOCRINE SYSTEM
(DUCTLESS GLANDS)

A N **endocrine gland** *is a gland which delivers its secretion directly into the blood stream.* In the course of development from an epithelial surface, the gland has lost the connexion or duct linking it to such a surface, either on the outside or the inside of the body—thus, an endocrine gland is said to be **ductless.** As the secretions of the gland cannot be poured out along a duct, they pass directly into the blood-stream and are known as **internal secretions** or **hormones.** In the blood-stream, hormones are distributed to relatively remote sites throughout the body, so that organs and tissues far from the gland may be stimulated by its secretion. An organ which responds to such a hormone is known as a **target organ.** An endocrine gland is so designed that its constituent cells are very closely related to blood capillaries and a rich blood supply is characteristic of endocrine glands (Fig. 33).

This system includes not only such glands of internal secretion as the hypophysis (pituitary), the thyroid, parathyroid and suprarenal glands, but the ovary and testis which are described in the next chapter, the pancreatic islets (p. 471) and possibly the thymus (described on p. 412).

Classification of Endocrine Glands, and their Development

As was described in Chapter V endocrine glands develop as cellular cords growing from an epithelial surface into the underlying connective tissue, 'pushing' it and its blood vessels before them, so that these come to lie in intimate contact with the cords of glandular cells (Fig. 33).

The connexion with the surface is lost, and if the endocrine cells do not need to store secretions to any appreciable extent, they maintain their basic relationship to one another by forming **anastomosing cords of cells** (Fig. 33). If on the other hand they store their secretions before liberating them into the blood-stream, they secrete into a communal central storage cavity, forming a **follicle** (Fig. 33), and from this the secretion is extracted and liberated into the blood-stream as required. The parathyroid and suprarenal provide examples of the first type and the thyroid an example of the second type of ductless gland.

It is also possible to classify endocrines according to the germ layer of the embryo from which they are derived; from **ectoderm**—the hypophysis and suprarenal medulla; from **mesoderm**—the gonads and suprarenal cortex; from **endoderm**—the thyroid, parathyroid and pancreatic islets.

The third method of classification is according to the chemical nature of the endocrine secretions, but as it has not yet been possible to identify chemically the active principle of some endocrine secretions, notably those of the hypophysis, all that can be stated is that:

Phenolic derivatives are secreted by the thyroid and the suprarenal medulla.

Proteins are secreted by the hypophysis (anterior and posterior lobes), the islets of the pancreas and the parathyroid glands.

Steroids are secreted by the suprarenal cortex, the ovary and the testis.

Clinical Importance of Endocrines

Although all the endocrine secretions (hormones) circulate through all the tissues of the body, most of the hormones are selective in their action and only affect certain organs or tissues. A number of diseases are due either to **over functioning (hyperfunction)** or **under functioning (hypofunction)**. Thus hyperfunction of the thyroid may be termed hyperthyroidism and hypofunctioning of the pituitary may be termed hypopituitarism.

Endocrine glands interact on one another, so that the secretion of one gland may stimulate or depress the activity of another. Thus, the hypophysis produces a hormone that stimulates the thyroid to produce its hormone; in turn, the thyroid secretion induces the hypophysis to produce less thyroid stimulating hormone. This is known as the **'negative feed-back'**.

THE THYROID GLAND

Development

The thyroid develops as an outgrowth from the floor of the mouth in the region of the developing tongue. The **foramen cæcum** of the tongue, at the junction of its anterior two-thirds with its posterior one-third, indicates the site of origin of this endocrine gland. The thyroid normally grows down into the neck to its position in front of the trachea, its path being indicated by a fibrous cord, called the **thyroglossal duct,** which extends from the tongue to the isthmus of the thyroid. This duct may contain remnants of thyroid tissue which sometimes give rise to cysts. Rarely the thyroid fails to migrate to the neck and remains situated in the substance of the tongue.

Form and Relations

The thyroid consists of two lobes situated one on each side of the trachea and joined across the front of the trachea by a narrow connecting band termed the isthmus. This lies opposite the 2nd, 3rd and 4th rings of the trachea (Fig. 204).

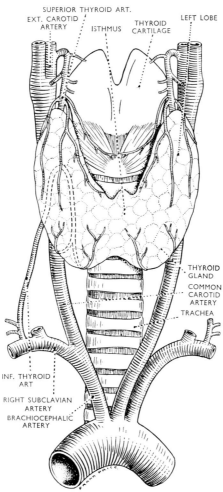

Fig. 204. The thyroid gland and trachea, with related arteries, seen from in front.

It is connected by a fascial sheath to the larynx above it, so that it moves with the latter on swallowing. It is covered in front by the infrahyoid muscles (p. 188 and Fig. 89), the platysma and skin; laterally and posteriorly it is related to the cartoid sheath containing the common carotid artery, internal jugular vein and vagus nerve; posteriorly and medially it is related to the œsophagus and the recurrent laryngeal nerve where this ascends to the larynx in the groove between the trachea and the œsophagus. The parathyroid glands are situated on the posterior surface of the lobes of the gland.

Blood Supply

It is richly supplied with blood by the superior thyroid arteries descending to the upper poles of the lobes from the external carotid arteries, and by the inferior thyroid arteries ascending to the lower poles from the subclavian arteries (Figs. 204 and 205).

Structure

The secreting cells are cubical in shape and arranged to form hollow vesicles called follicles, which are filled with a homogenous viscous colloid in which the hormone **thyroxine** is stored. Between the follicles there are small clumps, of parafollicular cells which secrete a second hormone, **calcitonin**. The height of the cells varies with activity of the gland; in general, the more active the gland is, the taller are the cells. Closely applied to the outside of the follicles are numerous capillaries.

Physiology

Thyroxine is the principal hormone secreted by the thyroid gland, and its action is to increase the metabolic rate of the organs and tissues of the whole body. In this way it also promotes growth and development in the young.

Some 60% of thyroxine consists of iodine, an element which is essential to the gland to enable it to synthetize its hormone. No other organ in the body stores iodine, and adequate amounts of it must be ingested in the diet.

The **basal metabolic rate** (B.M.R.) of the body (discussed on p. 550) is estimated in clinical practice to assess the function of the thyroid. The B.M.R. is increased in hyperthyroidism and reduced in hypothyroidism.

Calcitonin, secreted by the parafollicular cells, lowers the blood calcium level, and with parathormone (p. 513) helps to control calcium metabolism.

A normal thyroid gland cannot be felt; only when it is enlarged is it palpable.

ENLARGEMENT OF THE THYROID

1. PHYSIOLOGICAL: The thyroid gland may become slightly enlarged in response to the physiological needs of the body. This occurs when the metabolic rate of the body is increased, for example, at puberty and during adolescence, and in women during pregnancy and lactation.

2. GOITRE: Enlargement of the thyroid other than the physiological variety is termed a *goitre*, and may be simple or toxic (see below).

Simple goitre, which is prevalent in certain countries and districts, usually remote from the sea, is due to a deficient intake of iodine and is cured by the administration of iodine. In this deficiency disease the gland, though enlarged, does not produce more hormone than is produced by a normal gland; indeed it usually produces less.

HYPOFUNCTION OF THE THYROID: Hypothyroidism is manifested differently in children as compared with adults. **Cretinism** affects children and is due to a congenital absence or defect of the gland. Growth is stunted, the features are coarse, frequently the child has a protruding tongue and an enlarged abdomen; the mentality of the child is low and retarded.

It is very important to treat these children with thyroid hormone at the earliest opportunity, as then they may develop into normal adults if treatment is kept up. The longer treatment is deferred the less chance there is for the child to develop and mature normally.

Myxœdema is the condition caused by thyroid deficiency in adults. It affects women more frequently than men, and may occur spontaneously or as a result of surgical removal of too much of the gland. It is characterized by a puffy, bloated appearance, associated with coarsening of the features and skin which is doughy and dry. There is loss of hair from the scalp and eyebrows and usually a tendency to obesity. The subject usually 'feels the cold' and there is loss of appetite and often constipation. In fact, the metabolic rate of the whole body is depressed, with consequent slowing of mental as well as of physical activity.

All the symptoms of the condition can be relieved by the regular administration of thyroid hormone, which is effective when taken by mouth.

HYPERFUNCTION OF THE THYROID GLAND: This is usually associated with its moderate enlargement. An excessive amount of thyroxine is poured into the blood and the metabolism of the body is speeded up. The patient dislikes heat, usually loses weight, has an increased pulse rate, suffers from nervous excitability and fine tremor of the hands, and in some cases has protrusion of the eyeballs. These 'toxic' signs and symptoms are responsible for the condition being known as **toxic goitre** or **thyrotoxicosis.** Other names are exophthalmic goitre and Graves' disease.

The disease may be treated either by the administration of drugs, such as thiouracil or neomercazole, which inhibit the production of thyroxine, or by the surgical removal of part of the gland—partial thyroidectomy. When this operation is performed, the posterior portion of each lobe is left *in situ* to ensure that the parathyroid glands are not removed and that the recurrent laryngeal nerves are not damaged with consequent impairment of the voice.

THE PARATHYROID GLANDS

Development

The parathyroid glands develop as cellular outgrowths from the endoderm lining lateral pouches in the walls of the embryonic pharynx. These cellular outgrowths migrate down to the neck and come to lie behind the thyroid gland. The lower parathyroids develop in conjunction with the thymus gland, which has a comparable origin from the pharynx and, in the course of its development, descends into the mediastinum of the thorax.

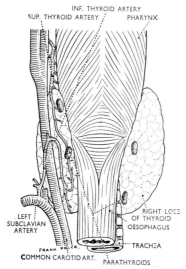

Fig. 205. The pharynx, œsophagus, trachea, thyroid gland and related arteries seen from behind. Note the variable position of the parathyroid glands.

Form and Position

Usually the parathyroid glands consist of four pea-like bodies found closely related to the posterior aspect of the thyroid gland, and they are in fact frequently embedded within its capsule of fibrous tissue. They derive their rich blood supply from the superior and inferior thyroid arteries (Fig. 205).

Structure

This is typical of the structure of an endocrine gland and consists of irregularly disposed **columns of cells,** between which there is a rich plexus of capillaries. After puberty, there are two types of cells in the cellular columns (**chief cells** and **oxyphil cells**), but as far as is known there is only one type of parathyroid secretion. After middle age some adipose tissue accumulates in the substance of the gland.

Physiology

The parathyroid secretion, **parathormone**, exerts two main actions. Firstly, it regulates the balance between the calcium in bones and that in extracellular tissue fluid, thus affecting the amount of calcium in the blood. Secondly, it controls the excretion of phosphates in the urine, probably by reducing tubular reabsorption of phosphorus by the kidney tubule (see p. 493).

Derangement of Parathyroid Function

HYPOFUNCTION: This may be caused as an unusual complication of operations on the thyroid, either by accidental removal of parathyroids, or by interference with their blood supply. The level of calcium in the blood drops (**hypocalcæmia**) with consequent increase in the excitability of nerves. This results in a condition known as **tetany** in which the patient is the subject of violent, generalized, painful muscular spasms.

HYPERFUNCTION: This is usually due to a tumour of parathyroid tissue which secretes an excess of parathormone. This leads to an abnormal rate of calcium withdrawal from bones which consequently become decalcified, softened, deformed, painful and often develop cysts—a condition known as **osteitis fibrosa cystica**. The level of calcium in the blood is raised, and the excess is excreted in the urine and some in the fæces. The greatly increased concentration of calcium in the urine may lead to the formation of stones, or **calculi,** in the urinary tract. The raised calcium level in the blood has the effect of reducing the excitability of nerves and these patients often suffer from lassitude and weakness.

The condition is cured by removal of the tumour.

THE SUPRARENAL GLANDS

Development

These glands have a composite origin. The outer part **(cortex)** is derived from the epithelial lining of the cœlomic cavity (see p. 84) of the embryo in the vicinity of the developing gonads (see p. 523). The inner portion **(medulla)** has a completely different origin, being developed from neural crest cells (p. 82) which have migrated from the developing neural tube and have become enclosed within the developing cortex. The cortex of the fetal suprarenals is very bulky and has different histological characters from the cortex seen in the postnatal gland. The bulkiness accounts for the relatively huge size of the gland in a new-born infant. The large size of the suprarenal cortex in the fetal gland is related to the fact that the cortex possibly secretes hormones, that counteract the maternal hormones which gain access to the fetal circulation, and it probably plays a role in the sexual differentiation of the fetus.

Position

As their name suggests, the glands are situated above the kidneys, one being related to the upper pole of each kidney (Plate 27 and Fig. 206).

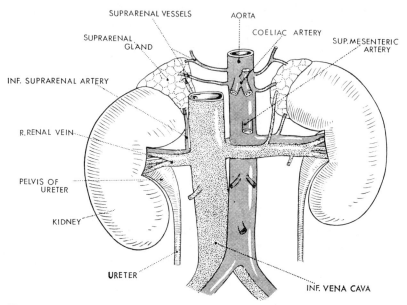

Fig. 206. A diagram to show the suprarenal glands and their blood supply.

Blood Supply

They derive their blood supply from the renal artery, the phrenic artery and directly from the aorta. These arteries enter the cortex of the glands and give rise to capillaries which permeate the cortex, and thence the medulla, where venules are formed which form a single suprarenal vein. The suprarenal vein drains into the renal vein on the left side and directly into the inferior vena cava in the case of the right gland. The suprarenal glands share with the thyroid the distinction of being the most vascular organs in the body.

THE SUPRARENAL CORTEX

Structure

The cortex has typical structure of an endocrine gland consisting of cords of cells in intimate contact with capillaries; these run from the surface towards the central medulla (Fig. 207). Three zones are discernible within the cortex: below the capsule, the cells form more or less spherical collections (**zona glomerulosa**); in the middle, they form parallel columns (**zona fasciculata**) and deeper still, where the cortex abuts on the medulla, the columns run in all directions (**zona reticularis**).

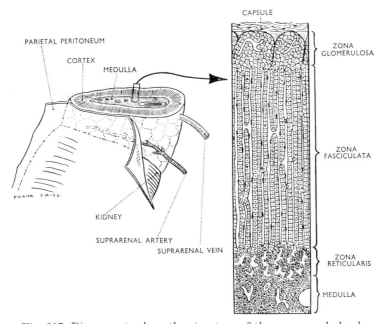

Fig. 207. Diagrams to show the structure of the suprarenal gland.

Secretions of the Suprarenal Cortex and their Physiological Actions

The cortex of the suprarenal secretes three different kinds of hormone, known as **corticosteroids.**

1. The first group, known as **mineralocorticoids,** regulate the sodium and potassium balance in the body. The most potent is known as **aldosterone.**
2. The second group consists of substances known as **glucocorticoids,** the principal one being called **hydrocortisone.** The effects of this group are complex and not well understood. For instance, hydrocortisone tends also to cause sodium retention and potassium excretion; it stimulates conversion of protein to carbohydrate and so has a diabetogenic effect (see p. 557); it brings about a reduction in the size of lymphatic tissues, and

also inhibits the proliferation of fibroblasts and so affects healing processes (see p. 595); it has an inhibitory effect on allergic phenomena; it also affects the quality of intercellular substances, hence its use in the treatment of rheumatic diseases.

3. The third group are **sex hormones.** In some way, not well understood, the suprarenal cortex can, and in certain circumstances does, supplement the production of sex hormones by the gonads. Some tumours that arise in cortex produce substances which have a male sex hormone activity. They masculinize women.

HYPOFUNCTION: This occurs classically when the cortex is destroyed by some pathological process such as tuberculosis. The condition is known as **Addison's disease** and is characterized by bronzing of the skin and a lowered blood sugar level. Sodium and chlorides are excreted in excess, but potassium is retained. Without treatment death follows.

HYPERFUNCTION: This is a condition in which there is an excessive production of aldosterone, due to a tumour of the cortex. This results in an excessive loss of potassium in the urine with consequent depletion of potassium in the plasma. This condition is known as **primary aldosteronism.**

Another cause of increased production of cortical hormones may be a tumour or hyperplasia of suprarenal cortex associated with **Cushing's syndrome.** This condition usually afflicts women and, not only is normal hormone production increased, but substances resembling male sex hormones are also produced. Masculinization, including growth of hair on the face and chest, is accompanied by obesity, hyperglycæmia and glycosuria (from excess production of glucocorticoids).

ABNORMAL FUNCTION: This may cause the **adrenogenital syndrome,** in which a tumour or hyperplasia of the cortex produces abnormal substances resembling sex hormones, particularly male ones. In young children of either sex, precocious puberty results with increased muscular development (**infant 'Hercules'**). In adult women the condition is known as **adrenal virilism** because these women develop a masculine build and appearance, which includes a masculine distribution of hair.

THE SUPRARENAL MEDULLA

Structure

The medulla consists of loosely arranged cords of cells between which are large sinusoidal capillaries and venules. The cells contain granules which stain brown with chromic acid and its salts. They are, therefore, known as **chrom-affin cells.**

Secretion of the Suprarenal Medulla

The suprarenal medulla secretes noradrenaline and adrenaline. The name adrenaline comes from the fact that in some animals the gland is alongside the kidney rather than above it as in Man, and so is called the adrenal gland.

ACTIONS OF NORADRENALINE AND ADRENALINE: The chemical structure of these two hormones is similar but the effects they produce are somewhat different. However, together, in general they mobilize the resources of the body to enable it to cope with emergencies—the **'fight or flight'** response to fear.

Thus the heart-rate is increased; the blood supply to the organs vital for coping with the emergency is increased by vasodilation, e.g. to muscles of limbs; the blood supply to parts of the body not so required, e.g. to skin and gut, is cut down by vasoconstriction (adrenaline can thus be used to stop bleeding from the latter regions). Peristalsis of the alimentary tract is inhibited, but the muscle in sphincters contracts. The pupil dilates to allow more light into the eye and to widen the angle of vision. The smooth muscle of the bronchial tree is relaxed to allow more air to reach the alveoli of the lungs, hence the use of adrenaline to relieve bronchospasm. Sweating is stimulated and this makes the skin of an animal slippery and more difficult to hold. Adrenaline increases the level of glucose in the blood by mobilizing glucose from the liver. This explains the **emotional glycosuria,** which affects certain individuals at times of stress.

HYPERFUNCTION OF THE SUPRARENAL MEDULLA: This may occur when a rare tumour of the medulla—a **phæochromocytoma**—develops. It causes excessive secretion of both adrenaline and noradrenaline, resulting either in persistently raised blood pressure, or hypertension occurring in paroxysms associated with increased heart rate, vasoconstriction and dilated pupils.

THE HYPOPHYSIS OR PITUITARY GLAND

Development

The hypophysis is developed as two separate rudiments. One, responsible for the anterior lobe, grows up from the roof of the embryo's mouth. This upgrowth meets a down-growth from the forebrain vesicle, which gives rise to the posterior lobe and stalk of the pituitary. This stalk connects the gland to the hypothalamus (p. 252) and this connexion is not lost in the course of development, but the anterior lobe does lose

its connexion with the roof of the mouth. Small remnants of cells along its development track may give rise to a tumour of anterior lobe pituitary cells, known as a
craniopharyngioma.

Form and Position

The gland, which is about the size and shape of a large somewhat flattened
pea, is situated in the hypophyseal fossa of the sphenoid bone in the middle
cranial fossa (Plate 36). The hypophyseal stalk connects the gland to the
hypothalamus in the floor of the third ventricle. This stalk passes through a
diaphragm of dura mater which separates the upper surface of the gland from
the under surface of the brain. The sides of the gland are flanked by the cavernous venous sinuses (p. 376). The optic chiasma (p. 264) is situated just anterior
to the hypophyseal stalk and may be damaged by tumours of the hypophysis.
These tumours may also change the saddle-shaped fossa (**sella turcica**) of the
sphenoid bone in which the gland is accommodated.

THE ADENOHYPOPHYSIS (ANTERIOR LOBE)

Structure and Functions

The anterior lobe accounts for about 70% of the bulk of the gland. It has the
typical structure of an endocrine gland, made up of cords of cells permeated by
numerous capillaries. There are three types of cells: some take up little stain
and are called **chromophobe cells:** others take up stain—**chromophil cells,**
which may be either acidic—**acidophil cells,** or basic—**basophil cells.**

There is evidence to suggest that chromophobes can change into chromophils
by accumulating granules and that chromophils can revert to chromophobes.

Chromophil cells produce a number of hormones:

1. The **growth hormone** stimulates skeletal growth, and growth in the
   proportions of the various parts of the body.
2. The **lactogenic hormone** stimulates and maintains milk secretion,
   but only after the breasts have been primed by the action of ovarian and
   chorionic hormones during pregnancy (see p. 540). It may also have a
   maintaining effect on the corpus luteum.
3. **Trophic hormones,** by which the hypophysis influences and controls
   the other endocrine glands. The stimulation of other endocrine glands by the
   hypophyseal trophic hormones is associated with a 'feed back' mechanism,
   so that increasing concentration in the blood of the hormone produced by
   the other gland results in the diminished production of trophic hormone
   by the hypophysis (see Fig. 221). By virtue of these trophic secretions the

hypophysis earns itself the nickname of 'Leader of the endocrine orchestra'. At least three types of these hormones are produced:

(a) **Adrenocorticotrophic hormone** (A.C.T.H.) stimulates the adrenal cortex to secrete corticosteroid hormones.

(b) **Thyrotrophic hormone (T.H.)** stimulates the thyroid to produce thyroxine.

(c) **Gonadotrophic hormones,** of which there may only be one in the male, but of which there are definitely two in the female, namely a **follicle-stimulating hormone (F.S.H.)** and a **luteinizing hormone (L.H.).** Both of these play an important rôle in the regulation of the sexual cycle in women (p. 541). Gonadotrophins stimulate the production of sex hormones and gametes by the gonads, be they testes or ovaries. F.S.H., which stimulates the production of gametes, stimulates the development of ovarian follicles in females and its equivalent in the male stimulates sperm production. L.H. stimulates the development of corpora lutea in females; in males there may be an equivalent of L.H. known as **interstitial cell stimulating hormone (I.C.S.H.).**

The acidophil cells produce growth and lactogenic hormones, whereas the basophil cells produce the trophic hormones.

HYPERPITUITARISM: This is a condition resulting from over secretion of the growth hormone. If it occurs before the epiphyses of bones have fused **gigantism** is produced, but if it occurs in an adult, enlargement is confined to the extremities, notably the face, hands and feet, giving rise to a condition known as **acromegaly.**

HYPOPITUITARISM: In childhood, this deficiency leads to **dwarfism,** but though such individuals sometimes look older than they are, they are well proportioned and intelligent.

DYSTROPHIA ADIPOSOGENITALIS (FRÖHLICH'S SYNDROME): A condition, exemplified by the 'fat boy' of the Pickwick Papers, has been attributed to pituitary deficiency, but it is more likely that it is, at least in part, attributable to a lesion in the hypothalamus. Cases of this condition are somnolent, have a voracious appetite, are obese and have poorly developed genitalia.

THE NEUROHYPOPHYSIS (POSTERIOR LOBE)

Its developmental relationship to the hypothalamus has already been described. Structurally it presents the appearance of nervous tissue, and it is linked to the hypothalamus (p. 252) by means of nerve fibre tracts, which enable the two regions to be closely linked functionally.

Secretions and functions

Two hormones are produced by the neurohypophysis.

1. The **antidiuretic hormone (A.D.H.,** vasopressin, pitressin) controls loss of water from the body by regulating the amount of water reabsorbed by the kidney tubules (p. 493).
2. The **oxytocic hormone** (Pitocin) induces uterine muscle to contract during labour and so helps to expel the contents of the uterus. After

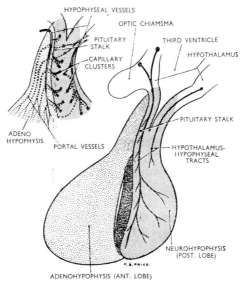

Fig. 208. Schemes to show the hypophyseal portal system of vessels and the nervous connexions of the neurohypophysis.

delivery it helps the uterus to contract down and to stop uterine bleeding from the site from which the placenta has separated. It also causes the ejection of milk from the breast.

DIABETES INSIPIDUS: This is a condition which results from malfunction of the neurohypophysial–hypothalamic complex, and diminished secretion of anti-diuretic hormone. Very large quantities of dilute urine, which contains no abnormal constituents, are voided.

Blood Supply to the Hypophysis

The adenohypophysis is linked to the neurohypophyseal stalk by a **portal system** of vessels (i.e. vessels which are formed by the coming together of capillaries in the neural stalk and which break up again into capillaries when they reach the adenohypophysis) (Fig. 208). This enables the hypothalamic region of the brain, which is linked to the neurohypophysis by fibre tracts, to control the adenohypophysis by means of hormonal secretions liberated in the neurohypophyseal stalk. There do not appear to be any nerve fibre connexions between the nervous system and the adenohypophysis.

THE PINEAL BODY

The pineal body is a small gland attached to the roof of the third ventricle of the brain and related to the roof plate of the midbrain (p. 238 and Fig. 107). The functions of the pineal body are poorly understood, but evidence is mounting that it plays a part in regulating gonadal development. From early adulthood, calcareous deposits in the gland render it progressively more radio-opaque and it provides a useful landmark for radiologists.

The other endocrine glands such as the gonads (pp. 527 and 533), the pancreatic islets (p. 471) and the thymus (p. 412) are described elsewhere.

CHAPTER XVII

THE REPRODUCTIVE OR GENITAL SYSTEM

THE human species ensures its continued survival by means of sexual reproduction.

THE ADVANTAGES OF SEX

The human body is made up of an immense number of cells which have a limited span of life. Indeed the whole organism has a limited span and, if human beings or animals are to survive, they must produce young, who will go on living when the parents die. This reproductive pattern needs to be carried on from generation to generation.

When the whole body is considered it becomes evident that, although all the cells of the whole organism are derived from a single cell—the fertilized egg or zygote (see p. 49)—most of the daughter cells have become specialized to form the differently functioning tissues of the body such as muscle, bone, heart, gut, nerves, etc. These cells are specialized and most can reproduce themselves to maintain the tissue to which they belong, but they no longer retain the capacity to reproduce a complete individual, as the first cell or zygote could. Individuals, however, develop special organs, called **gonads,** which maintain a stock of cells which retain the faculty of reproducing a complete individual, if and when it unites with a comparable cell from an individual of the opposite sex in the process of fertilization (see p. 49). The primitive reproductive cells from the gonads are called **germ cells** and they mature through a series of special changes to form **gametes** (see p. 51).

If an individual produced offspring from his own cells alone, the offspring would have the same genetic make-up as the parent, and this would mean that both parent and offspring would flourish or perish in comparable environments. In sexual reproduction, the process of **genetic inheritance** (see p. 54) ensures that the offspring receive characteristics from both father and mother, and in various combinations. This makes for variety in the species, tends to prevent one characteristic from being predominant, and produces individuals who are sufficiently different for some of them to thrive in altered environments. This process also tends to even out defects which would otherwise lead to extinction. Sexual reproduction makes the race adaptable.

THE ADVANTAGES OF INTRA-UTERINE DEVELOPMENT

As well as benefiting from the advantages of sexual reproduction, the human race derives great advantages from the fact that human embryos and fetuses develop in a specially adapted incubating chamber, called a womb or uterus. By this means, the growing individual is kept in a relatively constant environment; is protected from physical injury and relatively protected from outside noxious influences, such as bacteria, by the placental barrier (see p. 73). However, drugs and certain organisms, such as viruses and spirochætes, can and do pass this barrier and consequently damage the embryo.

CONSTITUENT PARTS OF THE GENITAL SYSTEM IN THE TWO SEXES

In both sexes, the genital system is made up of a primary sex organ, the **gonad** which produces gametes, together with a number of **glands** which produce secretions to carry and nourish the gametes, and a system of tubes, the **genital ducts,** to convey the gametes to the outside of the body. Together, all these parts of the genital system make up the **internal genitalia.**

The parts of the genital system, called the **external genitalia,** permit the act of copulation, by which sperms are deposited inside the female genital duct system.

DEVELOPMENT OF GONADS AND GENITAL DUCT SYSTEM

Developmentally, a gonad consists of **primitive germ cells,** which migrate from the yolk sac (p. 69) to the epithelium lining the abdominal part of the cœlomic cavity (p. 84) near the region from which the primitive excretory organ called the **mesonephros** develops. The germ cells develop into sperms in testes, and into ova or eggs in ovaries (Fig. 209). The cœlomic epithelium, carrying with it the germ cells, grows into the underlying mesenchyme and forms supporting tissue for the germ cells. Thus in males, this epithelium forms the supporting **sustentacular** (of Sertoli) **cells** in the seminiferous tubules which produce sperms, and in females, it forms the cells lining the **ovarian follicles.** The **mesenchymal cells,** into which the cœlomic

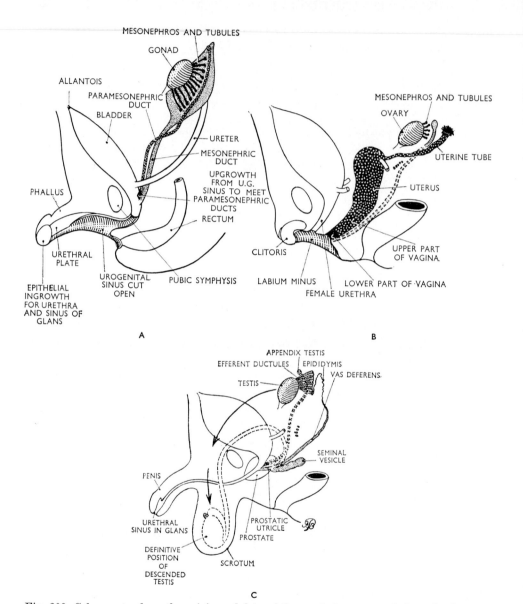

Fig. 209. Schemes to show the origin and fate of the genital organs and ducts in the two sexes. A, disposition of the gonad and genital ducts in the undifferentiated state which is common to male and female fetuses; B, fate of the organs and ducts in the female; C, fate of the organs and ducts in the male.

epithelium grew, give rise not only to connective tissue stroma, but to **endocrine gland cells—interstitial cells** in the testis and **thecal cells** in the ovary.

The tubules of the mesonephros drain into a duct, the **mesonephric duct** (Fig. 209). This duct becomes the **vas deferens** in males, but disappears in females. Consequently a new duct is required to convey the female gametes. This is the **paramesonephric duct** which develops alongside the mesonephric duct. Although this paramesonephric duct develops at first in male embryos too, it soon disappears in them except at its caudal end where it contributes to a structure in the prostate—the utriculus masculinus. In females, the caudal parts of these tubes fuse to give rise to the **vagina** and **uterus**, and the cranial parts remain separate to form the **uterine tubes.**

Determination of Sex

Enough has so far been said to make it clear that, although the sex of an embryo is determined at fertilization (p. 58), only the nuclei of cells (sex chromatin) can give a clue as to the sex of the embryo, till the gonads begin to diverge in development, when the embryo is 6 to 8 weeks old. Even then, the genital ducts and external genitalia look identical and do not differ till the fetus is about 3 months old. Up to this age, all fetuses have a protruding phallus (Fig. 210) which makes them all look male, even if they are female. This may account for the fact that aborted fetuses of this age are almost invariably reported as being male.

Further Developments of the Urogenital Tract

The genital ducts described above open into a wide channel at the tail end of the embryo, called the **cloaca** (Fig. 210). This channel is continuous with the **allantois** (see p. 71 and Fig. 26) cranially and with the hindgut caudally. A partition—the **urorectal septum**—grows down, dividing the channel into a primitive bladder and urethra in front and a rectum behind (Fig. 210). A duct—the **ureteric bud**—grows out from the back of the mesonephric duct. This grows up to the developing kidney and develops into the ureter, calyces and collecting ducts of the kidney. The mesonephric duct's caudal part is then absorbed into the posterior wall of the primitive bladder to form the trigone, and the ureteric bud and remainder of the mesonephric duct twist around one another so that the ureter opens in the bladder and the vas into the urethra (Figs. 209, 210 and Plate 37).

The mesonephric ducts (future vas) and paramesonephric ducts (future vagina and uterus) open into the primitive urethra, or **urogenital sinus**, at the same level (Fig. 210). As the vaginal orifice needs to be in the perineum, the lower part of the urogenital sinus opens out in females and the part of the urogenital sinus above the point of entry of the true genital ducts forms the whole of the female urethra. In males, however, the genital ducts open into the middle of the prostatic urethra, and the lower part of the urogenital sinus is devoted to the formation of the lower prostatic and membranous urethra (Figs. 203 and 209).

The first indications of the future external genital organs are in the form of three hillocks. The most anteriorly placed hillock lies in the midline and is known as the **phallic tubercle.** The two posterior ones are situated one on each side of the midline and are called **genital swellings.**

As the phallic tubercle elongates to form a **phallus** (Fig. 210), the urogenital sinus is drawn out along the under surface of the phallus as a shallow **urethral groove.** This groove is then deepened by the breakdown of a solid **urethral plate,** which lies just above the urethral groove (Figs. 209 and 210). The margins of this groove are called **urethral folds** and, in a male fetus, they grow together by folding over the urethral groove. They meet in the midline along the under surface of the phallus to form the penile urethra in the fully developed penis. This fusion brings together the

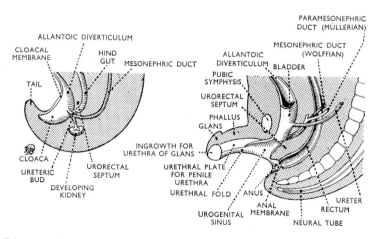

Fig. 210. Diagrams illustrating the early development of the urogenital tract in either sex.

genital swellings, which previously lay on each side of the open urogenital sinus, and so form a single fused scrotum. The line of fusion is indicated by the **perineal raphe.**

Such fusion does not occur in female fetuses. Thus it will be seen that the essential difference in the development of the external genitalia of the two sexes is that, in the female, the lower urogenital sinus remains not only open, but expands to allow the vaginal orifice to reach the surface at the perineum, this being associated with a retrogression of the phallus to form a small clitoris (Fig. 209); the urethra stops short at the base of the clitoris with the unfused urethral folds forming the labia minora. Also, the genital swellings remain separate and form the two labia majora. In the male, the lower urogenital sinus is closed in and carried forward along the enlarged phallus, so that a urethra is produced which opens at the tip of the penis.

After the scrotum has been formed the testes migrate from their position on the posterior abdominal wall down to the brim of the pelvis, then forwards to the inguinal region where they pass through the inguinal canals (p. 202) to reach the scrotum. They draw down a **processus vaginalis** of peritoneum with them, which forms the tunica vaginalis testis and then loses its connexion with the peritoneal cavity. If it does not, it affords a channel along which abdominal viscera can reach the scrotum, thus giving rise to a **hernia** or **rupture**. In contrast, the ovary descends only as far as the pelvic inlet, and so women are not liable to this kind of inguinal hernia.

THE MALE GENITAL SYSTEM

THE SCROTUM

The scrotum is a pouch of dark skin situated below the root of the penis and the pubic symphysis (Plate 37). It contains the testis and its coverings, the epididymis and the lower end of the spermatic cord.

The size of the pouch varies in size and shape from time to time, due mainly to the presence in the subcutaneous layer of smooth muscle fibres constituting the **dartos muscle.** When this muscle relaxes, the scrotum elongates and the wrinkles in the scrotal skin are smoothed out. On the other hand, when the muscle contracts, as a result of cold or exercise, the scrotum becomes smaller and its skin becomes puckered into numerous wrinkles.

The scrotum is divided into two by a midline septum, and the division is indicated on the surface by a ridge called the **raphe** (p. 526). This raphe is continued forwards along the under surface of the penis, and backwards, to the anus.

In the scrotum, the testis and its tunica vaginalis are covered by layers of fascia which are continuous with the oblique abdominal muscles. The layer continuous with the internal oblique muscle (p. 201), consists of the cremasteric fascia and cremaster muscle (see below).

THE TESTIS

The testis is the gonad of the male and it is a laterally compressed ovoid organ about 4 cm long. There are two testes, one on each side, and normally they are situated in the scrotum in the perineum (Plate 37) where they hang obliquely with the upper pole forwards. In the scrotum, they are kept at a temperature that is slightly lower than the intra-abdominal temperature. This is an important consideration, for this 'cooling' is necessary for the testis to produce normal fertile sperms. If the testis does not descend properly in the course of its development, it does not produce spermatozoa satisfactorily, and the administration of gonadotrophic hormones (p. 519), which encourage descent, or an operation may be necessary to place the testis in the scrotum to encourage it to function properly.

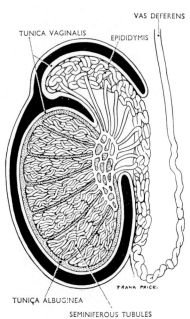

Fig. 211. A diagram of the testis to show the arrangement of its tubules and ducts, and their relation to the epididymis.

As the testis lies in the scrotum, it is surrounded by a serous sac, consisting of a parietal and a visceral layer of peritoneum, which is called the **tunica vaginalis** (Fig. 211 and Plate 37) and is derived from the processus vaginalis (p. 527). Normally it contains only a thin film of fluid, but under abnormal circumstances, such as inflammation of the testis (**orchitis**), fluid may accumulate in the tunica vaginalis. Such a pathological effusion of fluid is a **hydrocœle**.

Structure and Function of the Testis

The male gonad is surrounded by the visceral layer of the tunica vaginalis inside which there is a very tough white capsule, the **tunica albuginea.** From this, partitions extend inwards to separate the numerous coiled **seminiferous tubules,** in which sperms are produced by the process of spermatogenesis (see below). Scattered between the seminiferous tubules are endocrine cells called **interstitial cells.**

Spermatogenesis is the process by which the male germ cells, or **spermatogonia,** become transformed into sperms or **spermatozoa.** In the course of this transformation, spermatogonia containing 46 chromosomes give rise to **spermatocytes** containing only 23 chromosomes (see p. 53 and Fig. 12). These then give rise to **spermatids** which, by a series of complicated changes, lose most of their cytoplasm and acquire a tail to become spermatozoa (Fig. 212).

It should be noted that the sperms in the testis are incapable of fertilizing an ovum till they have **matured** by relatively slow passage along the male efferent ducts to be described later. In addition they need to be inside the female genital tract for a number of hours before they are capable of fertilizing an ovum. This phenomenon is known as **capacitation.** It is thought that the

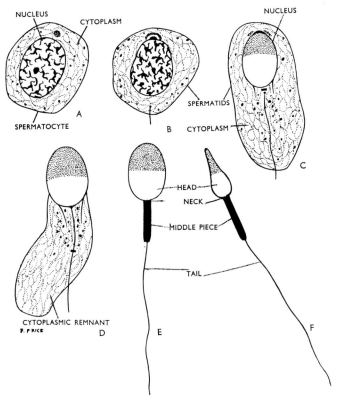

Fig. 212. Stages in the conversion of a spermatocyte (A) into a sperm (E, from above; F, sideview).

survival period of human sperms within the female tract is not more than 24–48 hours.

The Endocrine Function of the Testis

The interstitial cells secrete the male sex hormone **testosterone.** They probably function in fetal life to ensure the proper differentiation of the genital tract, but in post-natal life they become fully active at the age of puberty. The testosterone as well as stimulating the further development of the genital organs, is also responsible for what are known as the **secondary sex characteristics** of the male. These are such things as the growth of hair on the face and chest; the male distribution of hair on the pubis (hence the term puberty) and lower abdomen; the 'breaking' of the voice and general heavier development of skeletal structures.

THE EPIDIDYMIS AND VAS DEFERENS

The sperms are conveyed to the female genital tract in a fluid called **seminal fluid,** which with the sperms constitutes **semen.** Part of it is produced in the seminiferous tubules, but secretions from the epididymis and vas deferens, and further along the tract from the seminal vesicles and prostate, are added to it.

The seminiferous tubules empty their contents by way of small **efferent ducts** into a highly coiled tube which leads to the vas deferens. This coiled tube is known as the **epididymis** and it covers the poles and back of the testis (Plate 37 and Fig. 211).

The **vas deferens** leads off from the lower pole or tail of the epididymis and ascends in the spermatic cord (Plate 37) to reach the inguinal canal (p. 202) which it then traverses. It crosses the brim of the pelvis and runs medially towards the back of the bladder. Here it hooks over the ureter and then descends towards the back of the prostate, where it is joined by the seminal vesicle (Fig. 213).

The vas is a very muscular tube with a narrow lumen and thick wall which renders it cord-like on palpation. Its muscle wall is capable of strong expulsive contractions in the course of ejaculation.

The **spermatic cord** contains, as well as the vas, blood vessels to and from the testis, lymphatic vessels from the testis ascending to the para-aortic lymph nodes, and a leash of muscle (**cremaster**) which regulates the level at which the testis hangs. This muscle may actually retract the testis to the inguinal canal in young boys, this being both a protective reflex and a response to cold.

THE SEMINAL VESICLES

Each seminal vesicle is a wide tube which lies coiled behind the prostate and bladder (Plate 37 and Fig. 213) and in front of the rectum. Each contributes its secretions to semen by way of a short narrow duct that joins the vas deferens to form the **ejaculatory duct.** This then enters the substance of the prostate (Fig. 203). A normal seminal vesicle is not easily felt on rectal examination, but, because its lymphatic drainage is linked to that of the vas and epididymis, infective disease of these often spreads to a seminal vesicle, and then it is tender to palpation.

THE PROSTATE GLAND

Form and Position

The gland is about the size and shape of a large sweet chestnut and surrounds the urethra as it leaves the neck of the bladder (Figs. 203 and 213, and Plate 37). It is related anteriorly to the lower part of the pubic symphysis and posteriorly

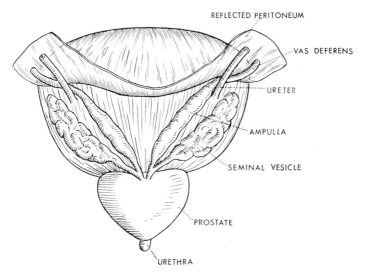

Fig. 213. The bladder, prostate and seminal vesicles seen from behind.

to the seminal vesicles and rectum. It is readily palpable on rectal examination. It is enclosed by a condensation of connective tissue, which forms a capsule for the gland, and is surrounded by a rich plexus of veins which receive veins from the penis. In prostatectomy, the gland containing the prostatic urethra is shelled out of its capsule, which henceforth acts as a substitute for this part of the urethra.

Function

The prostate develops as a group of diverticula from the prostatic urethra into which the glands consequently discharge their secretions, one of the components of seminal fluid. An infection of the urethra (urethritis) may thus spread to the prostate (prostatitis), as for example in gonorrhoea, and such an infection is usually difficult to eradicate.

Structure

The prostate consists of glandular tissue embedded in a fibromuscular stroma. The ejaculatory ducts traverse the substance of the gland from its postero-superior aspect, obliquely downwards, towards the middle of the posterior wall of the prostatic urethra, where the latter is raised to form a **urethral crest.** At this level, they open on either side of a blind glandular diverticulum—the **prostatic utricle.**

The course of the ejaculatory ducts through the substance of the gland demarcates a **median lobe** which is related to the trigone of the bladder (Fig. 203). This is the part of the gland most subject to the condition known as **simple** or **senile enlargement.** This, as explained on p. 505, may interfere with micturition and its control.

THE PENIS

The penis is a cylindrical organ, slightly expanded at its tip to form the **glans** (Plate 37). The **root** of the penis is situated under the pubic symphysis in the superficial perineal pouch (Fig. 203). The **penile urethra** traverses the whole length of the penis. The substance of the penis is made up of **cavernous tissue** (i.e. a sponge-work of collagenous partitions) into which blood vessels can pump blood to make it turgid; this type of tissue is therefore also known as erectile tissue. This erectile tissue forms three bodies, two **corpora cavernosa,** and the **corpus spongiosum** below and between them. The penile urethra passes along the length of the corpus spongiosum and is therefore also called the **spongy urethra.**

THE MALE URETHRA

The urethra in the male (Fig. 203) is about 20 cm (8 in) long and is made up of a **prostatic part** which passes through the prostate, a **membranous part** which passes through the deep perineal pouch surrounded by the external sphincter (p. 502), and a **penile** or **spongy part.** Where the spongy urethra joins the membranous part it is expanded and called the **bulb.** The bulb lies almost at right angles to the membranous part and it is important to note that the bulb projects backwards from its junction with the membranous part (see Fig. 203). The **bulbo-urethral glands,** which are situated one on each side in the deep perineal pouch, open into the urethra in this region.

A number of blind diverticula extend from the roof of the penile urethra and there is a particularly large one in the glans (the **lacuna magna**). These diverticula are important because when a curved catheter (coudé or bicoudé) is passed, the curved tip must be directed downwards so as not to catch in such a diverticulum. Also, it is necessary to pull the penis forwards to obliterate the posterior projection of the urethral bulb and so prevent the tip of the catheter from becoming lodged in it.

Extravasation of Urine

If an individual falls astride on a hard object, his urethra may be crushed between this object and the lower margin of the pubic symphysis, with consequent rupture of the urethra. If urine is passed from the bladder, it will leak out through the rupture into the perineum from which it may spread forwards in front of the pubis, to reach the anterior abdominal wall, where it will spread between the superficial fascia and the deep fascia.

THE FEMALE GENITAL SYSTEM
THE OVARY

The two ovaries are ovoid organs situated, one on each side, in relation to the wall of the pelvis in the angle made by the external iliac artery and the ureter (Fig. 201). The ovaries are attached to the posterior superior surface of a fold of peritoneum, called the broad ligament, in whose free margin is situated the uterine or Fallopian tube (Fig. 214). Blood vessels, lymphatics and nerves reach the ovary by means of the broad ligament.

Structure

The ovary is a solid organ consisting of a **connective tissue stroma,** covered on the outside by cubical **germinal epithelium. Ovarian** or **Graafian follicles** are embedded in the stroma (Fig. 215). **An ovarian follicle** consists essentially of a female **germ cell,** which forms the ovum or egg, and a layer of cells surrounding the germ cell, which constitutes the **membrana granulosa.** Outside the membrana granulosa the stromal cells condense to form the **theca.**

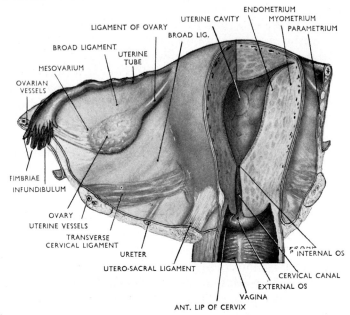

Fig. 214. The uterus, upper part of the vagina and broad ligament seen from behind. The right half of the posterior wall of the uterus has been removed to show the appearance of the cervical canal and of the endometrium.

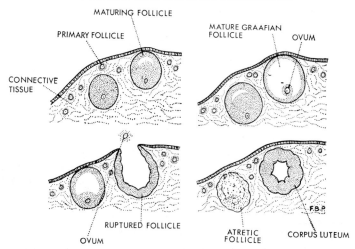

Fig. 215. A schematic representation of the development of the ovarian follicle, its growth, maturation and rupture, with the subsequent formation of the corpus luteum.

THE UTERINE (FALLOPIAN) TUBES

These two muscular tubular structures extend, one on each side, from the uterine cavity (Fig. 214). They are about 10 cm long and are contained in the free margin of the broad ligaments. The lateral extremity of each tube is funnel-shaped and called the **infundibulum.** Its opening is surrounded by finger-like processes, **fimbriæ,** which are related to the corresponding ovary. The part of the tube medial to the infundibulum is called the **ampulla** and it is continuous with the medial third of the tube or **isthmus.**

Structure and Function

Being contained in the free margin of the broad ligament, the uterine tubes are almost completely surrounded by peritoneum. Within the peritoneal coat, there is a smooth muscle coat which is lined on the inside by a highly folded mucous membrane.

When an ovum is shed by the ovary at **ovulation,** it is engulfed by the lateral end of the tube (infundibulum) and **fertilization** will take place in the outer portion of the ampulla if sperms capable of penetrating the ovum are present. The inside or lumen of the tube is lined by a highly folded mucous membrane, the epithelium of which is ciliated columnar and contains goblet cells. The mucous membrane produces a fluid secretion which provides **nutriment** for the ovum and tubal **motility** ensures that it reaches the uterine cavity. The narrowest part of the uterine tube is where it traverses the uterine wall to reach the uterine cavity. This is, therefore, the part of it most liable to become blocked as a result of scarring after inflammation. This blockage may be complete or partial. If both tubes are completely blocked the woman will be sterile, because sperms cannot reach the ovum to fertilize it. Such a blockage can be discovered by injecting a non-irritating radio-opaque substance into the uterus and observing it radiologically, to see whether any of it passes out into the peritoneal cavity through the uterine tubes. This is known as a **salpingogram.** Another method is to determine whether gases can be blown through the tubes via the uterine cavity, this investigation being known as **tubal insufflation.** If blockage of the tube is only partial, sperms may be able to pass the obstruction and reach an ovum to fertilize it in the lateral part of the tube. The resulting zygote may, however, be too bulky to pass the obstruction on its way down to the uterine cavity. The blastocyst being unable to reach the endometrium, implants (see p. 67) in the lining of the uterine tube. The tube accommodates the developing embryo until it can expand no further to contain the growing conceptus, and consequently ruptures. Implantation and continued gestation in an abnormal site is known as an **ectopic pregnancy.**

THE UTERUS

This organ has external measurements of about 8 cm in length, 5 cm in width and is about 3 cm thick. In pregnancy it grows to more than four times this size. In the non-pregnant woman it is situated within the lesser pelvis.

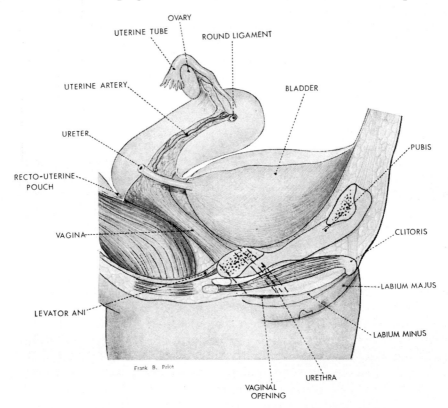

Fig. 216. The pelvic viscera of the female seen from the right.

Constituent Parts

It consists of two parts:

(*a*) The **body** to which the uterine tubes are attached and which is about 5 cm long; and (*b*) the **cervix,** the lower half of which projects into the vagina. The cervix is about 2·5 cm long.

The part of the body which projects above the uterine tubes is known as the **fundus.**

Form and Relations

The uterus lies at right angles to the vagina (Figs. 201 and 216) with the fundus projecting forwards just above the pelvic brim, thus it is said to be **anteverted** (Fig. 217, A); in addition the uterine body is curved forwards on the cervix so that it is described as being **anteflexed** (Fig. 217, B). In this normal position the cervix projects backwards into the vagina. Sometimes the uterus is tilted in the opposite direction, so that the cervix is directed downwards and forwards and the fundus is directed towards the sacrum. This is described, as **retroversion** of the uterus. This has the effect of pulling the broad ligaments, the uterine tubes and the ovaries backwards towards the recto-uterine pouch.

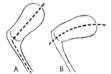

Fig. 217. Diagrams to show that the uterus is A, anteverted
in relation to the vagina, and B, anteflexed.

The front and back of the uterine body are covered by the visceral peritoneum which is continued on to the posterior aspect of the cervix and on to the posterior aspect of the upper part of the vagina, where it forms the anterior wall of the **recto-uterine pouch** (of Douglas) (see Fig. 201 and p. 447).

The anterior and posterior layers of this visceral peritoneum are continued laterally as the two layers of the **broad ligaments** which connect the sides of the uterus to the lateral pelvic wall (Fig. 214). Enclosed within its layers lie the uterine tubes at the free margin and the **round ligament,** which is a fibro-muscular cord, running laterally from the uterus, near the attachment of the uterine tube, to reach the inguinal canal and through it the labium majus. Because of its position and direction, shortening of the round ligament by an operation may help to keep the uterus anteverted.

Round the uterus there is condensed connective tissue which blends with that round the bladder and with the connective tissue within and below the broad ligament. It is called the **parametrium** and contains lymph vessels and nerves. The uterine artery runs through it to reach the cervix (Fig. 214) from the internal iliac artery, and the ureter passes forwards through it to reach the bladder. These are important relations because carcinoma of the cervix spreads readily into the parametrium and may obstruct the ureter.

Structure

Like the uterine tube, the uterus has three coats, namely peritoneum, muscle and mucous membrane. The muscular coat is very thick and the mucous membrane is called **endometrium** and undergoes cyclical changes to be described later (p. 541).

The cavity of the uterus (Fig. 214) is very narrow from front to back but wide from side to side, so as to have an inverted triangular shape with its base related to the fundus and the apex related to the cervix. The lumen of the cervix is a canal constricted at each end. The upper constriction, the **internal os,** communicates with the uterine cavity and the lower, the **external os,** with the vagina. The lining of the lower part of the cervix is different from that of the uterus and the boundary between the two is known as the **histological os.** It is situated in the cervical canal between the external os and the internal os. The part of the cervix between the histological os and the internal os is known as the **lower segment** of the uterus (Fig. 218) because in pregnancy it is incorporated into the uterine body. Its behaviour, especially during labour, is described on p. 546.

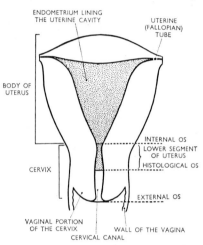

Fig. 218. Diagram to show the various parts of the uterus.

The Supports of the Uterus

These are of two kinds: (1) muscular, (2) ligamentous.

The **muscular support** is the **levator ani** muscle, that is, the **pelvic diaphragm** (p. 207). This muscle is inserted into the **perineal body,** situated between the vagina and the anal canal. The perineal body, in turn, is held in position by the **transverse perineal muscles** (Plate 8). (It is, therefore, very important to repair these muscles if they have been torn during labour.)

The **ligamentous supports** of the uterus form three pairs of slings attaching the cervix to the walls of the pelvis. In front are the **pubocervical** ligaments, which skirt round the neck of the bladder to connect the cervix to the pubis. The **transverse cervical** ligaments extend laterally from the cervix, while the posterior pair, the **uterosacral ligaments,** skirt round the rectum to connect the cervix to the sacrum. These ligaments are fused with the peritoneum above them (Fig. 214).

Other structures, such as the round ligaments, may play a minor part in supporting the uterus.

THE VAGINA AND VULVA

The **vagina** is a fibromuscular tube lined by stratified squamous epithelium. The cells of the epithelium are laden with glycogen, which provides food for certain beneficial bacteria that produce lactic acid by fermentation. The lactic acid, by preventing the growth of harmful organisms, promotes the health of the vagina.

The vagina is inclined upwards and backwards and its posterior wall 10 cm is much longer than the anterior 5 cm. The cervix protrudes backwards into the upper part of the vagina through the anterior wall. The part of the vagina above and behind the cervix is the **posterior fornix,** which is separated from the rectum by a pouch of peritoneum. This is the **rectovaginal** or **recto-uterine pouch** (of Douglas) (Fig. 201). Lower down posteriorly the vagina is separated from the rectum by connective tissue only, and from the anal canal by a fibromuscular condensation called the **perineal body** (central tendon of the perineum). Anteriorly the vagina is related from above downwards to the uterus, the bladder and the urethra.

The **vulva** is the collective term used to describe the external genitalia of the female (Fig. 209). It consists of two folds of skin on each side, the outer pair

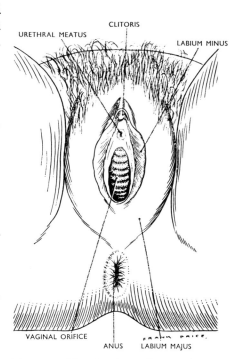

Fig. 219. The female perineum showing the relationships of the vulva.

being called **labia majora** and the inner ones **labia minora.** They can be traced forwards on each side of the urethral orifice to a small projection called the **clitoris.** Deep to the posterior end of each labium majus is a **greater vestibular gland** (of Bartholin), whose duct opens deep to the labium minus between it and the posterior margin of the vaginal orifice. In a virgin the vaginal orifice is partially occluded by a fold of mucous membrane termed the **hymen.**

Vaginal Examination

Two fingers introduced into the vagina can palpate, not only the vagina itself, but also the cervix, the uterus and the ovaries. The vagina and cervix can also be inspected with the aid of a speculum.

THE BREASTS OR MAMMARY GLANDS

These are modified sweat glands, which develop as 15 to 20 cellular buds extending into the underlying dermis of the pectoral region. In males, they remain rudimentary, but they are accessory parts of the reproductive system of females, being adapted to secrete milk to feed infants.

Because of its developmental history, each breast consists of 15 or 20 **segments** or **lobes,** each opening by a separate duct on to a projection, which is called a **nipple.** This nipple surmounts the hemispherical projection of the adult female breast. The skin of the nipple and of the circular area surrounding its base (**areola**) is thin and very sensitive. It becomes heavily pigmented in pregnancy. The substance of the nipple contains smooth muscle which enables it to protrude more and so be grasped easily by a baby's mouth in suckling; because of this the nipple is said to be erectile.

Structure and Function

The breasts are under the control of sex hormones. Up to puberty, they consist of only a rudimentary duct system. At puberty, under the influence of œstrogenic hormones (p. 542), the duct system becomes more complex, but the growth of the breast, visible at this time, is mainly due to accumulation of fat within its fibrous stroma. It is only when a woman becomes pregnant, that secretory units develop from the ends of the ducts. The secretory units are surrounded by contractile cells, **myo-epithelial cells,** which express the milk or eject it when a woman is breast-feeding a baby. Although secretion of milk is stimulated by the lactogenic hormone of the adenohypophysis (p. 518) the ejection of milk is caused by the oxytocic hormone (p. 520) of the neuro-hypophysis which is released by a nervous reflex initiated by suckling or even psychological anticipation of suckling. This is probably why emotional stress may disturb lactation.

The breast is one of the commoner sites for the occurrence of cancerous growths. These spread along lympatics mainly to the axilla and thence to the base of the neck (see p. 417 and Fig. 171).

MILK: This is an opaque white liquid which contains all the necessary food materials for a growing infant. Thus it contains proteins such as **lactalbumin** and **caesin,** carbohydrates in the form of **lactose;** fat in the form of **fat globules** which rise to the surface when left to stand—this is the cream of the milk; **inorganic substances** particularly calcium and phosphorus, but little iron, and the **vitamins** A, B, C and D, although their concentration in milk depends on the mother's diet.

In comparison with cow's milk, human milk contains more carbohydrate but less inorganic substances and protein. In addition, the proportions of proteins are different, there being more lactalbumin than casein in human milk but more casein than lactalbumin in cow's milk. Therefore, to make cow's milk as like human milk as possible for a young infant, it should be diluted with water (1 part water to 2 to 3 parts milk) and sugar should be added, 1 teaspoonful to 100 ml ($\frac{1}{4}$ pint).

THE ENDOCRINE FUNCTION OF THE OVARY AND THE MENSTRUAL CYCLE

In the **newborn** female infant the genital organs are rudimentary. The uterine body is very small, the greater part of the uterus consisting of cervix. The ovary contains thousands of **primary ovarian follicles** in which each germ cell is surrounded by a membrana granulosa composed of a single layer of cells.

At the time of **puberty,** under stimulation of gonadotrophic hormones of the hypophysis (p. 519), the ovary begins its cyclical activity which results in cyclical changes in the uterus known as the **menstrual cycle.** This cycle is evidenced by the **menses,** or periods, and their onset is known as the **menarche.** This cyclical activity continues until the 'change of life' or **menopause** (see p. 605), when it stops.

The menstrual cycle is the result of synchronized activity in the hypophysis, ovary and uterus, and a normal cycle lasts **28 days.** In the ovary, a number of primary follicles become active under the stimulation of **follicle stimulating hormone** (p. 519). The cells of the **membrana granulosa** multiply and produce **liquor folliculi** which accumulates in the centre of the follicle, so that it becomes a hollow, fluid-filled little bag. The ovum, with some of the granulosa cells surrounding it, projects into the fluid filled cavity (Fig. 215). The cells of the theca (p. 533) round the follicle, and also possibly the granulosa cells, produce the **œstrogenic sex hormones,** which cause the female sex organs and secondary sex characteristics (p. 10) to develop, and also induce the endometrium of the uterus and its tubular glands to proliferate (Figs. 220 and 221).

Every month, a whole group of follicles begins to ripen in this fashion, but only one completes the process and enlarges enough to project on the surface of

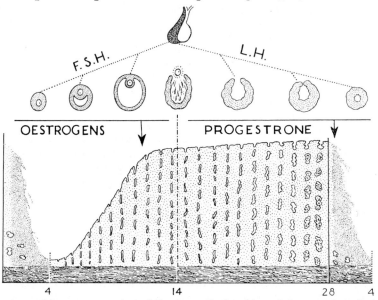

Fig. 220. A graphic representation of the interrelationships of the anterior pituitary, the ovarian follicle, the corpus luteum and the endometrium during the menstrual cycle.

the ovary. At **ovulation** this follicle bursts, and the ovum, surrounded by a few granulosa cells—the **corona radiata cells,** is liberated into the peritoneal cavity. Those follicles which have failed to complete the process then degenerate but the cells of the theca become **interstitial cells** and continue to produce œstrogen. The liberated ovum is taken into the uterine tube, and the granulosa and thecal cells of the follicle that has discharged the ovum are reorganized and enlarge to form a **corpus luteum** which secretes the hormone **progesterone.** This happens under the influence of the other hypophyseal gonadotrophin, **luteinizing hormone** (p. 519).

Progesterone, in contradistinction to œstrogen which is produced continuously during the reproductive years, is secreted only after ovulation. Its function is to stimulate the endometrium to enter its secretory phase, in which its glands become distended with secretion and the stroma becomes œdematous. It prepares endometrium to receive the implanting blastocyst about a week after ovulation, if the ovum has been fertilized. The corpus luteum then continues to play a rôle in maintaining the pregnancy for the first three months, after which

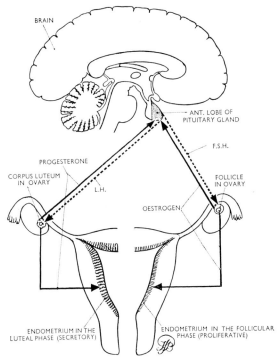

Fig. 221. Scheme to show the hormonal interrelationships between the anterior lobe of the pituitary gland and the ovary; the consequent changes in the uterus are also shown.

the placenta takes over the role of the corpus luteum by secreting progesterone itself. If pregnancy does not follow ovulation, the corpus luteum retrogresses after a few days, the endometrium degenerates and breaks down for lack of progesterone, and menstruation ensues. During pregnancy, progesterone and œstrogens together cause the mammary glands to proliferate in readiness for lactation.

CHORIONIC GONADOTROPHINS: The reason the corpus luteum continues to produce progesterone during pregnancy is that the trophoblast of the embryonic chorion (p. 71) produces gonadotrophin similar to L.H., and this maintains the corpus luteum. This gonadotrophin is excreted in the urine of a pregnant woman and this is of great clinical importance, because the urine can be used to carry out **biological tests of pregnancy.** The urine of a pregnant woman, when injected into female mice or rabbits, produces characteristic changes in their ovaries, or, when injected into toads and frogs, causes them to lay eggs if they are females, or to liberate sperms if they are males. More recently, reliable tests based on immunity reactions have been introduced.

Menstruation

This is the external sign that the preceding ovulation has not been followed by pregnancy. It consists of a shedding of the superficial two-thirds of the endometrium, the loss of 60 to 80 ml of blood. This is the menstrual flow which, normally, lasts about four days. It is followed by a renewed building up of the endometrium under the influence of œstrogenic hormone.

Menstruation usually starts 14 days after an ovulation that has failed to result in pregnancy.

When a pregnancy is established, both ovulation and menstruation are suppressed for the whole length of pregnancy, and also for a number of months during lactation.

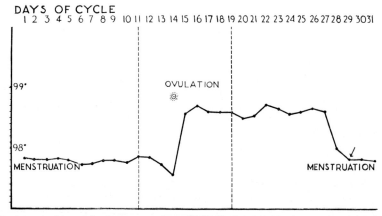

Fig. 222. A typical basal body temperature chart during an ovarian cycle which is followed by menstruation. (On this chart the body temperature is recorded in degrees Fahrenheit. 98°F = 36·6°C; 99°F = 37·2°C.)

The Timing of Ovulation and Relation to Fertility

As has been stated, ovulation takes place 14 days before the onset of the next menstruation but, as it may be important to determine the time of ovulation, further indications of its occurrence will be considered. The importance of determining precisely the time of ovulation derives from the fact that the ovum can be fertilized only within 24, or at most 48 hours, of ovulation.

One of the simplest means of determining that ovulation has taken place is by recording the basal body temperature of a woman (in the mouth or, better, in the rectum) each morning before rising (see Fig. 222). The temperature may drop slightly just before ovulation, but as soon as ovulation has taken place, there is a distinct rise of about 0·5°C, and this rise is maintained till a day or so before the onset of the next menstruation. Also the secretions of a healthy cervix are characteristic at the time of ovulation, being then crystal clear.

SOME ASPECTS OF PREGNANCY AND PARTURITION

A number of the changes that occur in the body of a pregnant woman have already been described, namely, that ovulation and menstruation cease, the post-ovulatory rise in basal body temperature is maintained (Fig. 223), the breasts develop secretory units, and the nipples and areolæ become pigmented.

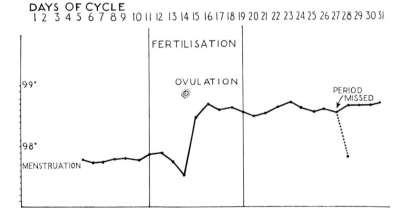

TEMPERATURE CHART

Fig. 223. A typical basal body temperature chart during an ovarian cycle which results in pregnancy. (On this chart the body temperature is recorded in degrees Fahrenheit. 98°F = 36·6°C; 99°F = 37·2°C.)

Gonadotrophins produced by the trophoblast are excreted in the urine. The cervix of the uterus acquires a softer texture and as the pregnancy proceeds, especially beyond the third month, the lower segment (p. 538) stretches and becomes incorporated into the uterine body as it changes its shape from a sphere to a more pear-shaped structure. As peritoneum does not extend on to the front of the cervix (see Fig. 201) it means that as the lower segment of the uterus stretches (see below) it becomes possible to approach the baby by an extraperitoneal incision, a procedure known as a lower segment cæsarian section. The change in the shape of the uterus is associated with the uterus rising out of the pelvis into the abdominal cavity with consequent stretching of the urethra. The nerves controlling micturition tend to be irritated by this stretching and displacement, so that pregnant women often experience some difficulty in controlling micturition or are subject to increased frequency of micturition.

A hormone, **relaxin,** is produced in the latter half of pregnancy which relaxes ligaments, and this has a particularly important effect on the pubic symphysis and sacro-iliac joints, so that the pelvis forms a less rigid canal for the passage of the baby through it during **parturition** (the process of birth).

Labour

During labour there are three phases called **stages.** During the **first stage,** the contractions of the uterine muscle, or labour 'pains', result in dilatation of the cervix, in stretching of the lower segment (see p. 538), and in organization of the rest of the uterine body into a propulsive component. The amnion and chorion rupture towards the end of this stage and this results in 'breaking of the waters', so that amniotic fluid escapes through the vulva.

During **the second stage,** the baby is expelled from the uterus by 'bearing-down' contractions of the abdominal musculature, which accompany strong contractions and progressive shortening of the uterine muscular fibres. During this second stage it is important that the head of the fetus be kept flexed, so that the smallest diameter of the elongated fetal head passes through the pelvic cavity and through the vaginal orifice. It is also important that the bony pelvis of the mother have a characteristic female shape (p. 12 and Fig. 59) so that it causes no obstruction to the passage of the fetal head. The important features are that there should be a sufficiently large rounded pelvic inlet, that the sacrum and ischial spines be directed backwards, that the ischial tuberosities be sufficiently distant from one another and that the subpubic angle be wide enough to be able to accommodate the baby's head.

During **the third stage,** the placenta is expelled from the uterus.

During parturition the endometrial lining of the uterus is lost with the fetal membranes (see p. 71 and Fig. 24) and the uterus is left with a raw bleeding inner surface which is liable to infection (puerperal sepsis) till its epithelial lining has been reconstituted. The bleeding stops as a result of uterine muscle contraction under the influence of the posterior pituitary hormone **oxytocin** (p. 520).

After delivery the uterus, whose muscle fibres have grown considerably, involutes and the ligamentous supports of the uterus, which have been relaxed and stretched, contract down to their original dimensions and relations. It is, therefore, important that the uterus should be in its normal position at this stage, so that it can become 'set' again in its correct relations. The muscles of the pelvic diaphragm and perineum also need to be repaired, if at all damaged, and subsequently 'toned up' by exercises.

Failure to take these precautions, especially after repeated births, may lead to the uterus and other pelvic viscera being inadequately supported, so that they prolapse (i.e. descend towards the perineum).

Suckling appears to have a reflex effect which encourages the uterus to involute.

SEXUAL DIFFERENTIATION AND INTERSEX CONDITIONS

It has already been described how sex is determined in the embryo (p. 58) and how the genital organs develop (p. 525). As embryos of both sexes develop the same basic genital duct systems before they become adapted to the needs of the particular sex of the embryo or fetus, it is not surprising that occasionally individuals develop organs that are intermediate in character between those typical of either male or female. These are intersex conditions. Even in normal individuals the external genitalia of the two sexes can be seen to correspond, though they look completely different. Thus the clitoris corresponds to the penis of the male, the labia minora to the penile urethra, the labia majora to the scrotum and the greater vestibular glands to the bulbo-urethral glands of the male.

The basic difference between the external genitalia of a man and those of a woman is thus seen to be that a woman's urethral groove does not close, its margins becoming labia minora, whereas in the male, the margins fuse to form a penile urethra. At the same time, the scrotal swellings fuse to form a single scrotum. The midline fusion of the external genitalia of the male is not possible in the female because of the migration of the vaginal orifice into the perineum. If a male fetus is feminized by some adverse influence, the bilateral external genital rudiments fail to fuse in varying degrees; contrariwise, masculinization of a female fetus leads to enlargement of the clitoris. There is plenty of evidence that the administration of masculinizing hormones to pregnant women tends to masculinize female fetuses.

SECTION III

CHAPTER XVIII

METABOLISM—NUTRITION—DIET

METABOLISM

Metabolism *is the total of the chemical changes which occur in a living cell, in a group of cells or in the body as a whole.* The chemical changes are of two kinds, namely catabolic and anabolic. **Catabolism** is the *breaking down* of substances taken into the cell to produce energy and waste products. **Anabolism** is the *building up* of new substances, including new protoplasm, within the cell; for this the energy released by catabolism is essential.

ROLE OF ENZYMES IN METABOLISM

Enzymes (see p. 27) are of prime importance in the processes of metabolism—probably all enzymes are proteins and many have been isolated in pure form and crystallized. More and more of the proteins in cells are found to have enzymic activity and it is evident that cells contain vast numbers of enzymes. The other remarkable fact is that an enzyme is extraordinarily specific and is usually concerned with the build up, or break down, of a particular substance. Reactions, which when effected in a test-tube require drastic procedures such as the application of great heat and of strong chemicals, are brought about in cells at body temperature through the action of enzymes.

It seems that protoplasm is made up largely of enzymes which bring about, step by step, the sum of reactions which we call metabolism. As protoplasm grows or is replenished, enzymes must be synthetized. This is done by devoting part of the anabolic (building up) activity to this synthesis, energy for it being derived by the enzyme-governed catabolism (break-down) of food substances which are brought to the cell by means of the blood stream.

Thus in general terms, metabolism can be said to comprise all those chemical and physical processes by which protoplasm is made and maintained, and it provides the means by which **energy** is made available to the organism.

ENERGY (also see p. 28)

Energy is derived from the breakdown of the bond or link between Carbon (C) and Hydrogen (H), which uses up oxygen (O_2) to form water (H_2O) and Carbon dioxide (CO_2) with the liberation of heat. C—H bonds are found most commonly in carbohydrate foodstuffs, which thus provide the main source of energy for the body.

Energy takes many forms, and each form can be changed into any of the others. All forms of energy, including heat are measured in joules (see p. 28).

Energy Values of Foodstuffs

The amount of heat energy which is liberated by a foodstuff when it is broken down into its simplest compounds, is its energy value. This can be determined by breaking down the foodstuff outside the body, that is, by burning it and measuring the amount of heat given off. Thus:

1 gram of fat gives 38 kilojoules (9 Calories).
1 gram of carbohydrate gives 17 kilojoules (4 Calories).
1 gram of protein gives 17 kilojoules (4 Calories).

In the course of metabolism in the body, of course, the foodstuffs are broken down inside the cells by the gentler action of the enzymes. Only some of the energy stored in the foodstuffs is released as heat; much of it appears as muscular work, and some is used for building up new complex compounds.

The energy which does appear as heat is useful in so far as it keeps the body warm, i.e. at the right temperature for the cells to perform their work best. However, since the chemical reactions of metabolism always produce heat, it follows that when cells are especially active, for example the muscle fibres during exercise, much more heat is produced than is necessary. This heat must be got rid of (p. 318) and it represents wasted energy.

The Basal Metabolic Rate

Basal metabolism is the amount of chemical activity in the cells which enables the body to maintain its basic vital functions such as the beating of the heart, breathing, forming urine and keeping the body warm, when the subject is completely relaxed mentally and physically, i.e. **at rest.** The **basal metabolic rate (B.M.R.)** is expressed as the numbers of kilojoules (or Calories) given out per square metre of body surface per hour, when the body is at rest, in an equable temperature about 12 hours after food. In normal adult males, the B.M.R. is 170 kilojoules (40 Calories) per square metre per hour. It is slightly lower in females and higher in children. After the age of 40, the B.M.R. decreases slightly. The daily basal metabolic output for an average man is of the order of 7200 kilojoules (1728 Calories) per day: that is, even completely at rest he uses up that amount of energy every day.

Many conditions affect the basal metabolic rate; some of them raising it and others lowering it.

It will be remembered that it was stated above that the Basal Metabolic Rate referred to the body at rest. That is because any **muscular activity** raises the metabolic rate of the body.

FACTORS RAISING THE B.M.R.:

Age. The B.M.R. is at its highest at the age of 2, when it has a value of 210 kilojoules (50 Calories) compared with 170 kilojoules (40 Calories) for an adult male.

Sex. The B.M.R. of Males is about 7% higher than that of females.

Hormones. Increased secretion of certain hormones raises the B.M.R. The most important of these is **thyroxine,** the secretion of the thyroid gland. An increase in the secretions of the anterior pituitary gland and of sex hormones also raises the B.M.R. Related to this are the variations in the B.M.R. occurring during the **ovarian cycle** in women and the increased B.M.R. in **pregnancy.**

Low external temperature. The B.M.R. is also raised in response to lowering of the external temperature surrounding the body.

The ingestion of foodstuffs. The intake of food raises the B.M.R. and this effect is known as the **specific dynamic action** of foodstuffs. The mechanism producing this phenomenon is not known, but it takes place only if the liver is present. It is demonstrated by the fact that when 420 kilojoules (100 Calories) worth of protein are fed to a fasting individual, 546 kilojoules (130 Calories) are given out by that individual. The equivalent figures for carbohydrate and fat are 441 (105) and 437 (104). Thus protein has by far the highest specific dynamic action and so induces the body to 'burn up' more calories. This is an important factor when planning diets, and has a bearing on the well known fact that proteins are 'less fattening' than fats and carbohydrates.

The administration of certain drugs and chemical substances increase the B.M.R., notable examples being adrenaline and caffeine.

Fever raises the B.M.R. to the extent of about 14% per 1°C rise in body temperature and certain **diseases,** not necessarily characterized by fever, e.g. lymphatic leukæmia, also raise the B.M.R.

FACTORS LOWERING THE B.M.R.:

Age. Premature babies have a low B.M.R. and there is a small progressive decrease after the age of 40.

Sleep reduces the metabolic rate of the body.

Starvation and **undernutrition** progressively lower the metabolic rate.

Hormones. Reduction in the secretions from the thyroid, adrenal and pituitary glands have the same effect.

METABOLISM OF PROTEINS

Protein, being an important constituent of protoplasm, is concerned in the growth and repair of tissues and in the formation of specific substances such as enzymes, but it is also involved in the provision of energy.

Protein is therefore one of the most important nutrients. As was described on p. 42, the protein molecule is made up of long chains of amino acids joined by peptide linkages. Protein is required in the diet to provide the amino acids with which new tissue protein can be built up in the body. According to the type of protein eaten, the proportions of the various amino acids reaching the tissues vary, and the nutritional value of a particular protein varies greatly according to the nature of its constituent amino acids and to their relative proportions.

The element **nitrogen** is an important constituent of all proteins and the mammalian organism is dependent on organic nitrogen, i.e. nitrogen bound in organic compounds, for all its nitrogenous requirements. This organic nitrogen is obtained from the **amino acids** which constitute the proteins ingested in the diet or the proteins contained in the tissues of the body. Thus in **starvation,** when no proteins are ingested or are ingested in only inadequate quantities, the amount of nitrogen excreted by the body is reduced to a minimum. It cannot be stopped completely, so that there is a wasting of the tissues of the body. Not all tissues waste equally in these circumstances, and heart and brain, for instance waste much less than say liver.

Nitrogen Equilibrium or Balance

On any given diet, there are three possible resulting states for an individual:

1. The intake of nitrogen in the diet may be just sufficient to counterbalance the amount of nitrogen lost by the body by excretion. The individual is then in a state of **nitrogen equilibrium.**
2. The intake of nitrogen may be insufficient to counterbalance the nitrogen lost by the body. This state is referred to as a **negative nitrogen balance.**
3. The intake of nitrogen may exceed the loss of nitrogen by the body, in which case the individual is storing nitrogenous compounds. This state is referred to as a **positive nitrogen balance.**

The ingestion of a quantity of protein, which supplies that amount of nitrogen just equal to the minimum amount of nitrogen excreted by the body, is not sufficient to allow the body to establish a nitrogen balance. The amount of nitrogen ingested usually needs to be at least twice as much as the amount excreted. This is because the nutritional value of different proteins is variable and not all their contained nitrogen is necessarily absorbed; also proteins may be used by the body to provide energy. Therefore, if the diet contains sufficient carbohydrate and fat for the provision of energy, less protein is required to attain nitrogen equilibrium. This effect of carbohydrate and fat is known as their **protein-sparing action.**

Nitrogen is excreted as urea, ammonium salts, creatinine, creatine and uric acid in the urine. In addition, some is lost in the sweat, hair, desquamating cells from the body surfaces and in the fæces.

A negative nitrogen balance, or tendency for the body to become depleted of nitrogen, occurs in fasting and starvation, lack of insulin, excess of adrenal cortical secretions and of thyroid secretion and as a result of wounds, infections, burns and fractures. A less obvious cause of a negative nitrogenous balance is the intake of proteins of low **biological value** (p. 42). This value of proteins varies according to the digestibility, absorbability and amino acid make up of the protein. In general, proteins obtained from animal tissues have a higher value than those obtained from vegetable material, but the proteins of potatoes have quite a good value. In general, mixed proteins have a higher value than single proteins. It is important to remember that nitrogen equilibrium can be attained relatively rapidly in man by the intravenous administration of human plasma.

Essential Amino Acids

Proteins are made up of amino acids, many of which can be synthetized by the human body out of the materials ordinarily available to the cells and at a speed commensurate with the demands of ordinary growth. This is not true of all amino acids and some have to be ingested simultaneously in a balanced mixture—these are known as essential amino acids (see also p. 42).

Fate of Proteins in the Body

Proteins are broken down to **amino acids** in the stomach and small intestine. The amino acids are then absorbed selectively by the intestinal mucosa whence they pass into the blood stream and so on to the liver.

The amino acids are then utilized in the body in the formation of new **tissue protein, enzymes** and those **hormones** which are of a protein nature. They are utilized by the liver and by the reticulo-endothelial system to synthetize **plasma proteins.** They are also used in the synthesis of specific substances such as histamine.

Some amino acids can, with the aid of enzymes, transfer their NH_2 or amino group to other substances by a process known as **transamination,** while non-essential amino acids can lose their amino group (NH_2) by **deamination** and later be reaminated to meet the requirements of the body. Deamination is an oxidative process which takes place in the liver and which yields **urea.** The non nitrogen-containing residues of amino acids can be used by the body to reform amino acids by reamination, or they can be converted to **glucose** or **glycogen,** or they can be transformed by way of esters to **carbon dioxide** and **water.**

SOME ASPECTS OF THE METABOLISM OF SPECIAL PROTEIN DERIVATIVES: Three different amino acids are used to synthetize **creatine** which is found in muscle as a phosphate in **phosphagen.** Creatine is found normally in the urine of young children and intermittently in adult females. It is found constantly in the urine of pregnant and lactating women and in individuals suffering from wasting diseases of muscles.

The anhydride of creatine—**creatinine** is a normal constituent of urine and its concentration is constant for any individual.

Glutamic acid and **glutamine** are important constituents of brain tissue. Apart from brain tissue itself, the kidneys play an important part in their metabolism. Glutamine, which penetrates all membranes more readily than glutamic acid, is synthetized from the latter and **ammonia** (NH_4). Glutamine is hydrolysed back to glutamic acid and ammonia. The concentration of ammonia is high in the kidney where it is utilized to conserve the body's sodium.

Purines and **pyrimidines** are both found in the **nucleic acids** of nucleoproteins present in nuclei and cytoplasm. The breakdown of purines in the body yields **uric acid.** This endogenous uric acid production is increased in severe or unwonted muscular exercise, fever and leukæmia. Uric acid is excreted in the urine, but accounts, under normal circumstances, for only about 2% of the total nitrogen in the urine.

Unlike purines, dietary pyrimidines are not incorporated into the nucleic acids of the body, but they are readily synthetized in the liver. The breakdown of pyrimidines in the body yields **urea** and **carbon dioxide.**

METABOLISM OF CARBOHYDRATES

At the outset it should be realized that carbohydrates supply at least 70% of the fuel for the body.

Functions of Carbohydrates

1. **Source of energy.** Carbohydrates supply energy especially for muscular work, and glucose is the sole source of energy for the brain, the retina and embryonic tissues.
2. **Source of heat.**
3. **Formation of integral part of special complex compounds.** Many complex substances found in the body are formed partly of carbohydrate. Examples are nucleoprotein of nuclei and cytoplasm, cerebrosides of nervous tissue, mucoproteins (e.g. some hormones), mucopolysaccharides of intercellular substance, the vitamin riboflavine, etc.
4. **Protection of tissue protein.** Nitrogen equilibrium can be maintained on much smaller amounts of protein if the diet contains a sufficiency of carbohydrate.
5. **Formation of fat.** When excess carbohydrate is ingested, it is converted to fat for storage.
6. **Prevention of ketosis** (see section on insulin p. 557).

As has been explained, in the chapter on Biochemistry, there are three main types of carbohydrates.

1. **Monosaccharides,** which are the simplest sugars and made up of single basic carbohydrate molecules or sugar units, e.g. glucose, fructose, galactose.
2. **Disaccharides,** which consist of two sugar units linked together, e.g. sucrose (ordinary sugar), lactose, maltose.
3. **Polysac .rides,** which consist of three or more sugar units linked together, e.g. starch, glycogen, cellulose.

Sources of Carbohydrate in the Body

1. INTAKE IN THE DIET: Polysaccharides, such as starches and glycogen, and disaccharides are converted by the digestive juices into monosaccharides which are practically completely absorbed by the small intestine. Fructose and galactose may be partly converted to glucose by the intestinal mucosa, but the process is completed in the liver. Normal absorption of carbohydrate does not take place in thyroid or adrenocortical deficiency, nor in deficiency of certain representatives of the Vitamin B complex.

2. GLUCONEOGENESIS: The glycogen in the liver can be built up from non-carbohydrate precursors such as amino acids and possibly fats. These precursors are first converted into glucose and then converted into glycogen, in which form carbohydrate is stored in the liver. A large part of the protein ingested in the

diet is used for the synthesis of liver glycogen. When the body needs glucose, the liver glycogen is converted back to glucose and is carried away by the blood.

Blood Sugar

For practical purposes, **glucose** is the only form in which carbohydrate is transported in the body. It is equally distributed between the water of the plasma and that contained in the red blood corpuscles, and the fasting level is usually **somewhat less than 100 mgm per 100 ml.**

'Glucose Tolerance.' To determine this, the blood glucose concentration is determined before, and every 15 minutes after, the ingestion of 1 gm of glucose per kgm of body weight. In a normal individual, the maximum level is reached in 30 minutes and the value returns to the 'resting' level in about 2 hours. The maximum value varies with the diet the subject has been taking previously, but it **should not exceed 160 mgm per 100 ml** of blood—a value which is known as the normal **renal threshold.** If the renal threshold is exceeded, sugar is excreted in the urine. This is known as **glycosuria.**

In some individuals the renal threshold is abnormally low and glycosuria readily occurs.

In certain diseases, e.g. diabetes mellitus, acromegaly, hypercortico-adrenalism, the glucose tolerance of the individual is altered so that the resting or fasting blood sugar level is higher, the maximum is higher and the return to the initial value is delayed.

When the blood sugar level falls **below 40 mgm per 100 ml of blood,** **hypoglycæmic** symptoms appear (see section on insulin p. 557).

THE CONTROL OF THE BLOOD SUGAR LEVEL is effected by a balance of three sets of factors:

1. Normal **liver** function and normal glycogen storage.
2. The pancreatic endocrine secretion **insulin** which **lowers** the level of the blood sugar.
3. The secretions of the suprarenal cortex termed **11-oxysteroids, glucagon** from pancreatic islet tissue (p. 470), and the **glycotrophic hormone** of the anterior lobe of the pituitary, all of which **raise** the level of the blood sugar.

FATE OF THE GLUCOSE IN THE BLOOD: Firstly, glucose diffuses into **tissue fluid** and so reaches the cells of the body; secondly, glucose may be converted to **glycogen** (which is the form in which carbohydrate is stored) in liver and muscle. Thirdly, glucose is oxidized in the cells to **carbon dioxide** and **water** with the liberation of **energy.** Surplus carbohydrates are converted to

fat. When the level of sugar in the blood exceeds the renal threshold, sugar is excreted in the urine.

Insulin

Insulin is essential for normal carbohydrate metabolism. It is secreted continuously by the **pancreatic islets** (p. 470), and the amount is regulated by the concentration of glucose in the blood reaching the pancreas—more glucose in the blood, more insulin is secreted.

ACTIONS OF INSULIN: Insulin *lowers the concentration of glucose in the blood and tissue fluid* in a number of different ways:

1. Insulin promotes the oxidation of glucose in the tissues.
2. Glucose is converted to glycogen in the liver and in the muscles under the influence of insulin.
3. Insulin promotes the conversion of carbohydrate to fat.
4. Insulin prevents the formation of glucose from amino acids in the liver.

DIABETES MELLITUS: In this disease, the pancreas does not produce enough insulin to keep the blood sugar down to its normal value. The blood sugar exceeds the renal threshold and glucose appears in the urine. In the treatment of diabetes, insulin must be administered by injection because, when given by mouth, it is destroyed by the digestive juices.

Ketosis

During the metabolism of fats (see p. 560) fatty acids are oxidized. Their level of oxidation is reduced when carbohydrate metabolism is depressed in **diabetes mellitus,** or in **starvation,** with the resulting accumulation in the tissues and blood of aceto-acetic acid, acetone and hydroxybutyric acid. These compounds are known as **ketone bodies** and their accumulation in the blood and appearance in the urine is referred to as **ketosis.** Ketosis in diabetes mellitus is associated with severe metabolic disturbances which lead to deepening coma and, eventually, death.

Ketone bodies are produced mainly in the liver and their disposal by oxidation occurs principally in the kidneys and muscles.

In the tissues, fatty acids and carbohydrates compete for the available oxygen and normally carbohydrate is oxidized preferentially. In starvation when carbohydrates are in short supply, or in diabetes when they cannot be properly utilized, fatty acid oxidation may lead to the production of such a quantity of ketone bodies, that their production far outstrips the body's ability to dispose of them.

The production of ketone bodies, **ketogenesis,** is checked by the administration of carbohydrate, provided that it can be utilized properly because enough insulin is present in the blood and tissues. Carbohydrates are thus said to be **antiketogenic.** The glycerol portion of the fat molecule (see p. 560) is also antiketogenic, as are the products of deamination of amino acids which are metabolized by way of carbohydrate derivatives.

It is probable that these antiketogenic substances are metabolized in preference to fat, cutting down fatty acid oxidation and so causing decreased ketone body production.

Glycogen in Liver and Muscle

The distribution of carbohydrate in a well-fed human body is such that, out of a total of about 270 grams, about 150 grams are in the form of glycogen in muscle, about 100 grams are in the form of glycogen in the liver and about 20 grams are in the form of glucose in extracellular fluid.

Muscle glycogen is not depleted by fasting but is diminished by convulsions severe exercise or adrenaline. Insulin has the effect of increasing it.

Liver glycogen is almost absent after 24 hours of fasting. It is diminished by severe exercise, anoxia, increased secretion of adrenaline, glucagon or thyroid hormone, a diet poor in carbohydrate, a low renal threshold for glucose. Liver glycogen is, however, increased by a rich carbohydrate diet, insulin, the 11-oxysteroids of the suprarenal cortex and the hyperglycæmic factor of the anterior lobe of the pituitary gland.

GLYCOGEN METABOLISM: The formation and breakdown of glycogen in the body takes place through a fairly complex series of intermediate steps, constituting a cycle in which glucose, lactic acid and pyruvic acid are involved. Oxidation of pyruvic acid plays an important rôle in energy production, and liberated lactic acid may enter the blood stream and be resynthetized to glycogen in the liver.

Glucose may thus have a cycle in the body which has been summarized simply as follows:

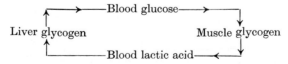

The muscles are also able to **synthetize** glycogen from lactic acid, but only slowly.

METABOLISM OF LIPIDS OR FAT

As was explained in the chapter on biochemistry, lipids are classified as:

1. Simple lipids or true fats (neutral fats) which are esters of fatty acids and alcohols.
2. The compound lipids such as phospholipid.
3. Sterols.

The Functions of Fat may be Summarized as Follows:

1. Some, e.g. phospholipids, constitute an essential part of cell structure.
2. Fats provide a store of potential chemical energy.
3. The subcutaneous fat of the superficial fascia provides an insulating layer which prevents heat loss.
4. This same subcutaneous layer provides, with other pads of fat, a 'shock absorbing' or 'padding' layer which protects other tissues against mechanical trauma.
5. Fat acts as a vehicle for the transport of certain important chemical substances, such as the fat soluble vitamins A, D, E and K.

Source of Body Fat

Fat is ingested as such in food, but can also be synthetized from the carbohydrate and from the protein of the diet.

Neutral Fats and Adipose Tissue

Adipose tissue is made up of cells which contain globules, mainly of **neutral fats,** and in an individual who is in a state of energy balance (see p. 561) an equilibrium exists between the fat metabolized and that deposited in adipose tissue.

Obesity represents an excess of energy intake over output or expenditure, as the result of eating more energy producing food than is used up. There is evidence that early food habits, rather than genetic factors, influence human 'fatness'. There is also evidence that the dorsal parts of the hypothalamus prevent excessive eating and obesity, while the ventrally situated parts and the hypophysis prevent loss of appetite and **cachexia** or pathological 'thinness'.

The amount of fat varies more than any other constituent of the human body, being minimal in the fetus. It constitutes a reserve or depot of fuel for the body, about half of it being present as subcutaneous fat. The rest is found round the kidneys as perirenal fat, and in the mesenteries and omenta of the peritoneum. A small amount is present in intermuscular connective tissue.

Phospholipids

Phospholipids form an integral part of the constituents of the cells of the body, being present in the organelles known as mitochondria and in cell membranes. They also act as a transport form for lipids in blood, and play an important rôle in the formation of adipose tissue and in the oxidation of fats in the body.

Active phospholipid synthesis occurs in liver, kidney, small intestine and nervous tissue.

FATE OF FAT IN THE BODY:

Absorption. Fat is absorbed in the jejunum, either in the form of particulate neutral fat, as bile-salt–fatty acid complexes, as phospholipids, or as cholesterol esters. Normally at least 70% of absorbed fat passes as neutral fat into the lacteals of intestinal villi and thence to the thoracic duct. This neutral fat makes the lymph milky in appearance and such lymph is known as **Chyle.** As little as 10% of absorbed fat may pass into the portal circulation as fatty acids and phospholipids.

Bile is essential for the absorption of fat. During digestion, fat is hydrolysed and broken down to fatty acids. If bile is absent, insoluble calcium salts of the fatty acids produced by digestion appear in the fæces.

Blood fats. Fat is transported in the blood, either as neutral fat, as phospholipid, as free cholesterol, or as cholesterol bound to other substances. **Lipæmia,** or raised blood fat, occurs in starvation, pregnancy, diabetes mellitus, hypothyroidism and in certain kidney diseases.

Utilization of fats.—The ultimate products of the oxidation of fat are CO_2 and **water** with liberation of **energy.** To reach this stage, however, a number of intermediate steps have to be taken. Hydrolysis of the fat yields **fatty acids** and **glycerol,** the latter being utilized in the same way as carbohydrate and being thus antiketogenic. The early stages in the utilization of fatty acids are not clear, but it is usually accepted that neutral fat is converted into **phospholipid,** which mixes readily with plasma and forms a ready means of transport of insoluble fats. Phospholipid is also more easily **hydrolysed.** Phospholipids may be formed in the tissue cells or in the liver. In the **liver** the phospholipids undergo a process of **desaturation** (see p. 478).

The **unsaturated fatty acids** obtained from the breakdown of fats are **oxidized** with the resultant liberation of energy and production of **ketone bodies.** The oxidation takes place mainly in the liver, but there is evidence that the process can also take place in skeletal muscle, heart, kidney, lung, brain and spleen. It is thought to take place exclusively in the **mitochondria of intact**

cells. In other words, damaged or diseased cells cannot dispose of fatty acids by oxidizing them.

Traces of ketone bodies are normally present in the urine. If the metabolism of carbohydrates is greatly reduced, as may happen in starvation or in diabetes mellitus, ketone bodies, intermediary products of fat metabolism, are produced in large amounts to give rise to the condition known as **ketosis** (see also p. 557). Large amounts of ketone bodies are then excreted in the urine—**ketonuria.**

It is important to realize that an adequate intake of protein containing the amino acid **methionine** is essential for the biosynthesis of **choline** (p. 567), which in turn permits the synthesis of the phospholipid **lecithin.** These are known as **lipotropic factors** and help to prevent fatty infiltration of the liver.

Sterols

CHOLESTEROL: **Cholesterol** is present in the cells of all vertebrates and is easily synthetized in the body.

In Man, about 20% of the cholesterol taken in the diet is absorbed in the presence of bile-salts. Not all sterols ingested in the diet are absorbed, but the related substance vitamin D is.

In the body, cholesterol may undergo conversion to adrenal cortical hormones, bile-salt and progesterone. It is excreted in the bile and also by the mucosa of the small intestine.

ADRENAL CORTICAL HORMONES: The suprarenal gland cortex can synthetize **hydrocorticosterone** and **corticosterone** from cholesterol in the presence of the adrenocorticotrophic hormone of the hypophysis. The suprarenal can also synthetize these hormones without first forming cholesterol.

ANDROGENS: **Testosterone** is formed in the testes in the presence of hypophyseal gonadotrophic hormone. Testosterone is oxidized and the resulting products are excreted in the bile and the urine.

ŒSTROGENS: **Œstrogens** are synthetized by the ovary in the presence of hypophyseal gonadotrophic hormone. The liver is the main site of their conversion to glucuronides or sulphates which are excreted in the urine.

PROGESTERONE: **Progesterone** may be synthetized in the body from cholesterol. Excretion in the urine takes place after it has been converted by the liver to glucuronide, or sulphate of hydroxyallopregnane, or pregnanediol.

METABOLIC BALANCE

In this context, balance refers to the state of **equilibrium** which results when the intake of food substances and water exactly matches the requirements of the body for its basic needs, for its energy output, and for its losses by secretion and excretion.

If the intake exceeds these requirements, a state of **positive balance** is achieved. The body then either excretes the excess of the particular substance or stores it, either as such or in the form of a storage material, for example as glycogen or as fat.

If the intake is insufficient, a state of **negative balance** results and, if the body cannot synthetize the particular substance, stores are depleted and eventually deficiency ensues.

CIRCADIAN OR DIURNAL RHYTHMS

Day and night follow one another in a fairly precise 24-hour cycle, even though the proportion of light and darkness varies with the seasons. Work, meals, sleep and leisure are all geared to this cycle, so it is not at all surprising that many physiological processes vary in intensity during this 24-hour period. Thus each of these physiological processes has a rhythm around the 24-hour day period—this is a circadian rhythm. (*Circadian:* from the latin *circa*, around or round about, and *diem*, the day.)

It is fairly well known that in health the body temperature is usually lower on waking than at bedtime, and that this rhythm persists even when the temperature is raised in fever. This is an indication of the rhythm in the total metabolic activity of the body and this rhythmicity affects many other functions. It is important to be aware of this rhythmicity in biological activity, because it makes a substantial contribution to the variations observed in a number of biological measurements. Thus the content of a particular substance in the blood may be quite normal for one time in the day, but may be of pathological significance at another.

The alternations of light and darkness, and the consequent habitually rhythmic activities of working, eating and sleeping, can be subjected to an abrupt shift of phase by round the world air travel into a different time zone. It is now common knowledge that some physiological rhythms take days or even weeks to adapt fully after such a flight.

Mention has already been made of the rhythmic variations in the daily temperature cycle and in the section on the kidney (p. 496) attention was drawn to the fact that urine production is reduced during the night. Circadian variations are also known to affect the functions of the suprarenal cortex and medulla. It is generally supposed that the suprarenal rhythm is responsible for many of the other circadian variations, including the rhythm of the eosinophil count, which normally falls to a low level after waking. This corresponds to a time of high corticosteroid production. Sleep–wakefulness rhythms also seem to reflect variations in corticosteroid production.

Circadian periodicity also appears to affect the pulse rate, pulse pressure, blood pressure, cardiac output and most hæmatological values.

THE DIET

The body needs a balanced diet that will supply it with its requirements. It needs to be **balanced** in the sense that the constituents must be present in the correct proportions. Thus the diet should supply the body with enough **water** and sufficient **protein, carbohydrate** and **fat** to satisfy the requirements of **basal metabolism, tissue building** and **repair** by the formation of protoplasm and enzymes, the requirements of the **specific dynamic action** of the food, the provision of **glandular secretions** both endocrine and exocrine and the replacement of **secretory** and **excretory losses.**

It must supply various regulators of bodily function such as **vitamins** and **salts.**

For a diet to be considered satisfactory, it must therefore fulfil certain conditions:

It must have sufficient **energy value** to maintain body weight, body temperature and enable the body to function efficiently, both physically and mentally. On the other hand, the energy value should not exceed these requirements and so lead to obesity.

It should contain a balanced mixture of protein, carbohydrate and fat and the protein should be of adequate biological value (see p. 42 and p. 529) and maintain the nitrogenous equilibrium of the body. As well as containing an adequate supply of vitamins, it must contain a balanced mixture of inorganic salts, particularly providing sodium, potassium, magnesium, calcium, iron, copper, cobalt, zinc, phosphate, chloride, iodine, bromine. The diet must be palatable and satisfying. Lastly, but most important, it must contain sufficient water.

CONSIDERATION OF CERTAIN ESSENTIAL FACTORS IN THE DIET

Protein. The diet must contain the proteins that will supply the **essential amino acids** that the body cannot synthetize (p. 42). The biological value of the protein in the diet must be adequate, but there is a difference of opinion about the amount of protein that should be ingested. In general, the League of Nations Standard for adults can be taken as a useful guide. According to this, not less than **1 gram per kilogram** of body-weight should be taken each day and it is desirable that part of the protein be of animal origin.

Carbohydrates. Carbohydrates are cheap and usually form the largest part of any diet. It is always necessary to take in sufficient carbohydrate to avoid excessive gluconeogenesis from body protein (p. 555), and to ensure the efficient oxidation of fat (p. 557).

Fat can be formed from carbohydrate in Man, but a certain amount of fat in the diet appears to be essential, if only to supply fat soluble vitamins. Fat is more slowly absorbed than carbohydrates and, weight for weight, it has twice the energy value of carbohydrate. It is difficult to say how much fat an individual should take in, but, as a rough guide, the same quantity as the protein in the diet seems to be about right.

Fats constitute the second largest source of energy in most diets. About half the fat is eaten as table fat and the other half in 'hidden fat' present in cakes, puddings, sauces etc. Foods rich in fat are expensive and there is a close association between average national income and fat intake. There are some so-called **'essential fatty acids'** which animal tissues cannot synthetize and which should be supplied in the diet. These are **unsaturated fatty acids** (p. 40). Diets rich in these unsaturated fatty acids lower the concentration of cholesterol and other lipids in the plasma and this may have a protective action against the development of arterial disease (atherosclerosis).

The diet contains many lipids, but the most important as a source of energy are the **true fats or triglycerides** (p. 39). A high proportion of saturated fatty acids in the molecule of a true fat makes it solid at room temperature.

All animal and dairy fats, except marine fats, contain a high proportion of saturated fatty acids. The true fats present in plants and in marine oils contain relatively more unsaturated fatty acids and are liquid at room temperature. The artificial hardening of these oils by hydrogenation, i.e. saturation of the unsaturated fatty acids, is the basis of margarine manufacture.

Energy Requirements

As has been stated above, the basal metabolic rate of an adult male is 170, i.e. he gives out 170 kilojoules (40 Calories) per square metre of body surface per hour. This, of course, applies to a body at complete rest. All activity increases the metabolic rate and hence the energy requirements to meet the body's metabolism. Some examples of additional kilojoules (Calories) expended per hour by the average body, are as follows: sitting 126 (30, standing 170 (40), brisk walking 630 (150), dancing (waltz) 840 (200), running 2100 (500), swimming 2310 (550), writing 126 (30), sweeping floors 420 (100), doing carpentry 630 (150), working as a blacksmith 1260 (300).

From this it is obvious that the energy requirements will vary enormously from one individual to another, and that occupational and spare-time activities need to be considered in addition to the age, size and build of the individual, when estimating individual requirements. Generally speaking, men leading a moderately active life require to take in about 12 600–14 700 kilojoules (3000–3500 Calories) a day, women 8400–10 500 (2000–2500). However, women need to increase their intake by 1050–2100 kilojoules (250–500 Calories) in pregnancy and by 4200 kilojoules (1000 Calories) during lactation.

Infants require about 420 kilojoules (100 Calories) per kilogram of body weight; children between 1 and 3 require 5460 kilojoules (1300 Calories) a day; at 10, the requirement has risen to 10 500 kilojoules (2500 Calories) and youths of 16–19 require 15 120 kilojoules (3600 Calories) per day.

The Vitamins

Vitamins have been described as *accessory food substances which are essential to health* although they are found in only *small quantities in a well-balanced diet.*

Vitamin A

SOURCE: The precursor of vitamin A, **β-carotene,** is present in carrots, spinach and green leafy vegetables, but only about a fifth of the ingested carotene is absorbed, bile-salts being required for its absorption. The β-carotene is converted to vitamin A in the liver. Vitamin A occurs as such in some animal fats, milk, eggs, butter, cheese, cod and halibut liver oils.

FUNCTIONS: It is necessary for normal growth, is a constituent of visual purple (p. 298) and is necessary for the maintenance of normal epithelia.

Lack of this vitamin, therefore, causes disturbances of growth, especially of the vertebral column, with attendant degenerative changes especially in afferent (or sensory) nerves. Its lack causes night blindness through lack of visual purple, and susceptibility to infections because the epithelia of the skin and of the mucous membranes of the respiratory and alimentary tracts are not in good condition. A rarer, but well known, sequel of absence of this vitamin in the diet is **xerophthalmia,** which consists of the loss of lacrimal secretion, keratinization of the cornea and blindness.

The Vitamin B Complex

This consists of a group of factors, the known ones being **aneurin** (vitamin

B_1), **riboflavine** (vitamin B_2), **nicotinamide** (P-P factor); **pyridoxine** (vitamin B_6), **pantothenic acid, folic acid, biotin** and **choline**. Other factors probably remain to be isolated. **Vitamin B_{12}** was isolated only in 1948.

These substances are water soluble and are found in the germ and the husk of cereals, in yeasts, in animal tissues and in bacteria. Some of them are important as parts of the enzyme system of cells.

Aneurin (Thiamine, Vitamin B_1)

FUNCTIONS: Aneurin plays a part in the metabolism of pyruvic acid (part of carbohydrate metabolism). Lack of this vitamin causes loss of appetite and fatigue. There is a bradycardia (slow pulse rate) at rest and marked tachycardia (rapid pulse rate) on exertion; there is decreased motility of the gastro-intestinal tract, muscular weakness, paræsthesia of legs and loss of tendon reflexes. There is a reduction of the basal metabolic rate, macrocytic hyperchromic anæmia and hypoproteinæmia. Extreme effects of deficiency of this vitamin are seen in **beri-beri,** which is in fact a multiple deficiency of the vitamin B complex, minerals, protein and fats affecting people who live almost exclusively on polished rice, that is rice from which the husk and germ have been removed. The condition affects the cardiovascular and nervous systems and may be associated with marked œdema or dropsy.

Riboflavin (Vitamin B_2)

SOURCE: The best sources are meat, milk, carrots, yeast and wholemeal flour.

FUNCTIONS: Riboflavin plays a part in the enzyme system of cells, and deficiency of the vitamin is manifested in extreme cases by muco-cutaneous lesions of the mouth region and vascularization of the cornea.

Nicotinamide (P-P Factor)

SOURCE: The best sources are yeasts, cereals (not maize), liver and meat.

FUNCTIONS: It forms part of the enzyme system of cells and extreme deficiency of the vitamin, associated with protein deficiency, gives rise to **pellagra** (hence the synonym P-P or pellagra-preventing factor) characterized by stomatitis, glossitis, diarrhœa, dermatitis and dementia.

Pyridoxine (Vitamin B_6)

SOURCE: The best sources are meat and yeasts.

FUNCTIONS: It forms part of the enzyme system of cells, and deficiency may lead to microcytic hypochromic anæmia and demyelinization of peripheral nerves.

Pantothenic Acid

SOURCE: The best sources are liver extract, meat, yeast, eggs and royal jelly.

FUNCTIONS: It forms part of the enzyme system of cells. It is concerned particularly with the acetylation of choline and with the biosynthesis and oxidation of fatty acids (p. 560).

Folic Acid

SOURCE: The best sources are concentrated liver extract and meat.

FUNCTIONS: Deficiency is associated with failure to grow and with anæmia of the macrocytic type.

The chemically related **folinic acid,** found in yeast and liver, is thought to be the intermediary in the transfer of a carbon (formyl) radical (p. 25) in metabolic reactions.

Biotin

SOURCE: The best sources are meat and yeasts.

FUNCTIONS: It plays a part in the metabolism of pyruvic acid and thus in carbohydrate metabolism (p. 558). Deficiency causes loss of weight, skin changes and muscle pain.

Vitamin B_{12}

SOURCE: The best source is concentrated liver extract.

FUNCTIONS: It is essential for animal life and plays a part in normal erythropoiesis. It requires intrinsic gastric factor (p. 453) for adequate absorption.

Choline

SOURCE: It is a constituent of lecithin, and is widely distributed in the human body and in animal tissues.

FUNCTIONS: It is an integral part of the myelin sheath of nerves and its ingestion by mouth prevents the abnormal deposition of fat in the liver, which would otherwise result from the ingestion of a high fat diet.

Vitamin C (Ascorbic Acid, Cevitamic Acid)

SOURCE: Vitamin C is found in the juice of citrus fruits, tomatoes, black currants, in the leaves of green vegetables. Some is found in potatoes.

PROPERTIES: It is water-soluble and is rapidly destroyed by heat, especially by boiling in the presence of oxygen (with no lid on the saucepan) and in an alkaline medium (e.g. by adding bicarbonate in cooking). It is also destroyed by drying and storage.

FUNCTIONS: It is necessary for the maintenance of the normal state of intercellular cement substance, and lack of this vitamin leads to **scurvy.** Lack of vitamin C leads to the failure by cells, such as fibroblasts, osteoblasts and odontoblasts, to lay down their fibrous proteins, i.e. collagen, ossein and dentine. It is obviously important in wound healing.

Vitamin D

Vitamin D is made up of at least two closely related sterols, vitamin D_2 or calciferol, derived from the irradiation of ergosterol with ultra-violet light, and vitamin D_3 which occurs naturally.

SOURCES: It is present in halibut liver oil (most concentrated source), cod liver oil, egg yolk, milk, butter and cream (in summer for the last three). British margarine has vitamin D added to it. It is absent from vegetable oils.

PROPERTIES: It is fat soluble and may be synthetized in the body by the action of the ultra-violet rays of sunlight on the ergosterol in the skin.

FUNCTIONS: It is primarily concerned with favouring the absorption of calcium. As a consequence of increased calcium absorption, phosphate absorption is increased. Vitamin D may also have a direct action on bone cells, thus accelerating bone formation. Insufficient vitamin D in the food of infants prevents the normal development of the growing bones and results in **rickets**. Very large amounts are poisonous.

Vitamin E (α-tocopherol)

SOURCE: It is present in wheat germ oil.

FUNCTIONS: It is an intracellular anti-oxidant, and deficiency may lead to defective fat absorption and creatinuria. There is evidence that it plays a rôle in ensuring fertility in the male, and in the maintenance of pregnancy with normal development of the fetus.

Vitamin K

SOURCE: It is present in small amounts in cabbage, spinach and in still smaller amounts in animal tissues. Biosynthesis of this vitamin is said to occur in the gut in the presence of the normal bacterial flora.

FUNCTIONS: It is fat soluble and is absorbed from the small intestine only in the presence of bile-salts. It is necessary for maintaining a normal level of prothrombin in the plasma and hence for the normal coagulation of blood.

REQUIREMENTS FOR INORGANIC CONSTITUENTS IN THE DIET

Mineral, Salt and Water Metabolism

Most minerals and water are so plentifully distributed in nature that any diet contains them in sufficient amount.

Exceptions to this statement are calcium, iron and iodine. In certain circumstances the intake of ordinary salt (sodium chloride) and of water must also be supplemented.

INORGANIC CONSTITUENTS are needed by the body to maintain the osmotic pressure of the body fluids and, in addition, to perform specific functions.

Calcium

Calcium is necessary for the formation of bone and teeth, for the regulation of excitability at neuromuscular junctions, for cardiac muscular contraction and for blood coagulation.

SOURCE: Sources of the element are milk, cheese, nuts, pulses and cereals.

METABOLISM: **Absorption** depends on a number of factors, such as the presence of sufficient vitamin D, the pH of the contents of the small intestine, the ratio of calcium and phosphorus in the diet, and the **phytic acid** content of the diet. This acid, which is present in cereals, tends to reduce calcium absorption, but the body soon adapts itself to an increased amount of phytic acid in the diet. It should be noted that decreased absorption of fats produces a decreased absorption of calcium. Probably not more than 30% of ingested calcium is absorbed.

The parathyroid gland secretion, **parathormone,** raises the level of calcium in the blood; calcitonin from the thyroid lowers it. Calcium is **secreted** in the intestinal juices and only a proportion of it is reabsorbed by the gut. Calcium is also **excreted** in the urine.

The **daily requirement** is about 1 gram a day with a 50% increase in pregnancy and lactation.

Phosphorus

Phosphorus is necessary for the **organic phosphorus compounds** forming an integral part of cellular structures, as a reserve store of **phosphoric acid** for the organism, as **glycerophosphates** in bone formation, as **hexose phosphates** in carbohydrate metabolism, and as **phosphatides** for fat transport and metabolism. It is also necessary as **inorganic phosphate** in acid-base equilibrium, in the absorption of glucose and to provide the inorganic part of bone.

SOURCE: Sources of phosphorus are milk, meat, eggs, pulses and cereals.

METABOLISM: Its **absorption** depends on the calcium-phosphorus ratio of the diet and the pH of the intestinal contents.

Excretion is by way of urine as inorganic phosphates.

Adults require to take in about 1 gram of the element per day.

Iron

Iron is required for the formation of hæmoglobin, to form part of the chromatin in nuclei and to form such cellular constituents as cytochrome and myoglobin.

SOURCE: Sources are provided by lean meat (especially beef), peas, beans, spinach, kale, whole egg, whole wheat.

METABOLISM: The amount of iron **absorbed** from the diet appears to depend on the level of iron in the body reserves and the ferrous variety is better absorbed than the ferric.

Excretion is mainly in the bile, but minute amounts are lost in the urine.

Adults require 10–15 mgm of iron daily. Women need more to compensate for the iron lost in menstruation and they need even more during pregnancy, when the fetus depletes the maternal stores.

Iodine

Iodine is required for the formation of thyroid hormone.

SOURCE: Sources of iodine are fish and shellfish, vegetables grown and milk obtained in non-goitrous areas. At the sea-shore it is possible to inhale minute amounts of iodine in the air.

METABOLISM: It is rapidly absorbed from the small intestine as iodine and the body requires an average daily intake of 0·1 mgm.

Other Elements Performing Specific Functions:

Sodium is essential for the normal functioning of all cells.

Potassium is also necessary for normal cell function. It also promotes muscular relaxation.

Copper is needed in traces for the maturation of normoblasts in hæmopoietic tissue.

Magnesium activates some phosphates.

Salt and Water

Sodium chloride, or ordinary table salt, is required to provide both sodium and chloride ions in tissue fluid and in cells. They are usually ingested in sufficient quantity in the diet, but it must be remembered that salt is being lost, not only in the urine if the body has an adequate level of these ions, but it is lost in sweat and various other glandular secretions. Salt loss is thus increased very considerably in profuse sweating, in vomiting and in diarrhœa, and the body may become rapidly depleted of salt in these conditions.

In the tropics, salt intake may have to be increased considerably by taking salt tablets or by drinking dilute salt solutions. The same is true for individuals whose occupation make them sweat a lot, e.g. stokers.

The body is constantly losing water, not only in urine (average 1·5 litres per day), but also in the fæces, in expired air, and as invisible or insensible perspiration from the skin, so that the body loses about 3 litres per day. Vomiting, diarrhœa, diuresis and increased sweating all increase the loss of water, and therefore much more needs to be taken in. The small intestine can absorb up to 10 litres of water per day.

The body's water balance is controlled by **osmoreceptors** in the hypothalamus. These are stimulated by raised osmotic pressure of the blood and cause the hypothalamic neurohypophyseal system to secrete antidiuretic hormone (p. 520), which acts on the renal tubules and so causes increased retention of water by the kidney.

STARVATION

Starvation may be complete or partial. Complete deprivation of both water and foodstuffs leads to death fairly rapidly. The survival time depends on such variables as the condition of the person, climate, work, etc. In a hot climate, the individual may survive up to three days, but in a temperate zone this period may be extended to between 6 and 14 days.

CHAPTER XIX

GROWTH AND GROWTH CHANGES

Growth normally consists of a change, usually an increase in the size, and a change in the shape and proportions of the body as a whole, or of the cells and organs constituting it.

The tendency to grow in size is a fundamental characteristic of a living organism. The process of growth involves an increase of three kinds, namely the addition of material to existing cells, an increase in the number of cells in the individual and an increase in the intercellular material.

Although simple organisms continue to grow indefinitely so long as the required nutrients are provided, a human life is characterized by a period of growth, followed by decline and cessation of growth, followed in turn by ageing, senescence and eventual death.

The different parts of the body grow at varying rates and these rates change as the individual ages (see Fig. 224). Some organs grow at a steady rate throughout development, but others grow at greatly varying rates. Some tissues develop early, presumably because of the need for early function. For example, the tissues of the lymphatic system develop greatly, soon after birth, as a defence mechanism against potential infections. On the other hand, the gonads develop late, presumably because the individual is not ready to reproduce till relatively late in his life span.

Another point that is noteworthy is that growth is not necessarily a continuous process, and in many tissues periods of activity are followed by periods of quiescence. Thus, we talk of **'growth cycles'**.

A special feature of the development of Man is that, after a long period of steady but relatively slow growth, the rate is suddenly increased at about the time of puberty before falling to zero at maturity.

Individuals vary greatly in their rates of growth and development, but they tend to pass through the same stages in roughly the same order. A variety of features can be used to assess the stage and degree of development attained by a given individual. Thus we speak of a **dental age,** because the milk and the permanent teeth erupt in a given regular sequence; we talk of a **skeletal age,** because the ossification of the bones proceeds in a regular, ordered sequence. We may refer to the **morphological age,** as determined from measurements of size, height and proportions of the parts of the body. The stage of **sexual development** may also be used as an index.

The pattern of growth in Man is unique. Childhood is greatly prolonged compared with the period of growth and development in other species. This makes possible the development of the brain to a remarkable degree which is Man's main biological characteristic. The long childhood determines much of Man's way of life, because during this long time children must be cared for and protected until they can fend for themselves.

THE PRENATAL PATTERN OF GROWTH AND DEVELOPMENT OF FUNCTION

In Chapter IV it was described how it takes 266 days for a fetus to develop from a single cell, a fraction of a millimetre in diameter, to a baby of over two hundred million cells and weighing about 3·2 kgm (7 lb) at birth.

When fertilization has been successfully accomplished, the newly conceived, one-celled individual proceeds to develop by the repeated successive division of the fertilized egg, and of the cells resulting from division of the egg.

Thus, there is at first growth by a process of **multiplication** of cells. Then as development proceeds, growth by multiplication of cells is accompanied by the progressive setting apart and specialization of groups of cells to form the various organs and tissues of the body. This diversification and specialization is known as **differentiation.**

Growth and differentiation go on till a complete adult individual is produced, but, for the sake of convenience, life, which is really a continuous process, is divided up into somewhat artificial periods called pre-natal life, infancy, childhood, adolescence, adulthood, etc. In fact, life is a continuous process, which starts for any given individual at conception and evolves progressively until death supervenes.

The **first four weeks** after conception are devoted to conveying the new individual to the womb, **implantation** there (see p. 67) and conversion of the circular embryonic disc (see p. 78) into a more cylindrical embryo. This has a definite **embryonic axis,** i.e. a front, a back, a head end and a tail end, a right and a left side.

The embryo is growing fast at this stage and is dependent on oxygen and food supplies from the mother's blood-stream conveyed to it by way of the developing placenta (see p. 71). Therefore the blood vessels in the placenta, blood vessels linking the placenta to the embryo through the umbilical cord, blood vessels in the embryo, **blood** to fill those **vessels** and a pump, or **heart,** to push this blood round all those blood vessels, need to be and are very rapidly developed. In fact, within less than four weeks after conception, the embryo has a rudimentary blood vascular system and a rudimentary heart which is already beating. It will be appreciated that this is less than two weeks after the mother has missed her first period and she is only beginning to suspect that she may be pregnant.

The **second month** of embryonic life is devoted to converting a tiny embryo of less than 5 mm in length and which does not yet look much like a baby to a **fetus** (see p. 50) which at the end of this second month is just over 30 mm long and has a form that makes it clearly recognizable, even to a lay person, as a small human baby. Its **head** and **face** are well formed. The limbs are well differentiated into **arms** and **legs,** with elbows and knees, wrists and ankles, hands and feet with fingers and toes.

It is at about this time that the fetus begins its **earliest movements,** but these are too weak at this stage to be felt by the mother. The **brain,** which is already well developed, appears to be sending out impulses to different parts of the body. The **heart** is now beating sturdily and is well developed. The **liver** produces blood cells and the rudimentary **kidneys** are thought to begin their excretory function. Also, the **internal reproductive organs** of male and female fetuses begin to differentiate differently according to their sex. The developing parts of the fetus are very soft and almost of the consistency of jelly at this stage. The **skeleton** is therefore laid down early to reinforce and support the tissue of the developing baby. At first, the skeleton consists of cartilage, but from the end of the second month of life in the uterus it becomes progressively converted to bone.

During the **third month,** the process of differentiation nears completion in most organs and systems, and it is now that the **external differences** between developing male and female fetuses are established. Other **finishing touches** are the appearance of nails, eyelids which close the eyes, and the fact that the ears come to lie at their proper level on the sides of the head. And so, three months after conception, the fetus measures about 60 mm from the crown of the head to its rump and, apart from certain details, most of the organs are developed and more or less in position.

The **remaining two-thirds of pregnancy** are devoted principally to increasing the bulk of the baby and to perfecting the various organs so that it will become progressively better able to live independently of its mother.

After about **four months** of pregnancy, the **fetal movements** become strong enough for the mother to become aware of them. This is known as 'quickening' and it used to be thought that it was at this time that life was instilled into the baby.

The baby learns to **swallow** and **suck** while in the uterus and probably also performs **breathing movements,** but, as the fetus is contained in a protective bag of amniotic fluid, when it inhales it draws fluid into its lungs. The fetus does not drown, because its lungs are not required for breathing, all the oxygen it requires reaching it via the placenta.

Late in the **seventh month,** the baby is said to become **viable** because, although it still weighs less than 1 kg ($2\frac{1}{2}$ lb) its organs and in particular its lungs would be sufficiently developed to enable the baby to survive were it born at this stage.

Such a **premature baby** would however be at a considerable disadvantage compared to a baby born at the proper time. Its digestive tract does not function very efficiently yet, so that there may be feeding difficulties; it may still be difficult for it to breathe (p. 321) and it may be necessary to administer oxygen to it; it has not had time to accumulate an insulating layer of fat under its skin and its temperature regulating mechanism is particularly inefficient, so that it needs to be kept in an incubator to keep it at an even temperature. The baby is also particularly subject to infection as it has not yet received sufficient protective substances, such as antibodies, which are thought to be conveyed to it particularly during the last three months of pregnancy.

During pregnancy, maternal hormones reach the fetus through the placenta. That such hormones can and do affect the fetus is evidenced by the stimulation of the breasts of infants of both sexes to produce 'witch's milk', by the relatively large size of the cervix of the uterus and by changes in the vaginal epithelium of female fetuses, and by histological changes in the prostate of male fetuses.

THE POSTNATAL PATTERN OF GROWTH

After birth, the growth rate shows four phases.
1. Rapid growth in infancy.
2. Slower growth 2–12 years.
3. Increased rate at puberty.
4. Slowing down to completion from adolescence to adulthood.

This pattern refers principally to stature, as, after an individual has reached adulthood, his girth and weight may still increase as the result of deposition of fat.

Different tissues grow at different rates and during different periods.

Nervous tissue reaches almost full development during the **first decade.**

Lymphoid tissue, which grows rapidly during early childhood, reaches maximum development at puberty and then regresses.

Reproductive organs are dormant till puberty, development being very slow during infancy and childhood. Maximum growth occurs during adolescence and regression takes place at the end of the reproductive period of life.

The production of new tissue is dependent on an adequate food supply and it is interesting to note that, in this country, as social conditions and medical care have improved, not only has the expectation of life been almost doubled in little over 100 years, but the relative duration of childhood and adolescence has decreased. Individuals are maturing sooner and their average stature is increasing.

THE CONTROL OF GROWTH AND MATURATION

The whole course of growth after the early pre-natal stages is probably regulated by some time mechanism within the brain. The execution of the brain's control is through the hypothalmus, which exerts hormonal influences on the anterior pituitary gland, which in turn affects the other endocrine glands.

There is a need to emphasize that in Man, the mechanism for controlling maturation ensures that maturity is achieved only after a relatively long interval, and it may be assumed that such a delay is biologically advantageous for the species.

A child's rate and degree of development almost certainly depends mainly on genetic factors, but the processes may be influenced and, in particular, limited by nutritional influences. Temperature and other climatic factors seem to have little influence. For instance there is a high correlation for the age at the menarche (p. 541) between mothers and daughters, between sisters and especially between identical twins. There is plenty of evidence of the effect of malnutrition in slowing growth and development. If, after a short period of malnutrition, conditions improve, growth accelerates and the child catches up and returns to the developmental rate and pattern from which the malnutrition had forced it to depart. The adolescent changes then take place when the child reaches the appropriate size.

It is of interest that the growth of boys is more easily inhibited than that of girls, but they catch up in growth faster.

It seems therefore that growth and maturation are controlled by factors which may be classified as genetic (inherited), socio-economic (diet, etc.), endocrine and disease.

GENETIC FACTORS

No one has yet discovered how many genes determine body height, but it is clear that they are numerous, and intermarriage can rapidly eliminate genetic differences of this kind.

Genetic factors presumably control growth processes, at least in part, by affecting the metabolism of dividing cells. They are also presumably responsible for the variations in the hormones which affect growth, and for variations in the ability of tissues to respond to hormones.

SOCIO-ECONOMIC FACTORS

Professional, semi-professional and skilled men, who enjoy better diet and housing, are taller and heavier than unskilled workers. The quantity and quality of the food, consumed during and after the period of growth, have a profound effect on the rate of growth, on the height and on the weight of the body. The accelerated maturation, that is taking place in rich countries, can be attributed in large part to improved nutrition. Per unit of body-weight, an infant requires twice as many kilojoules (Calories) as an adult man doing moderately active work.

ENDOCRINE FACTORS

The most important hormones for growth are the pituitary growth hormone, the thyroid hormone and the sex hormones.

The **pituitary growth hormone,** or **somatotrophin,** controls the general increase of body tissue through the stimulation of protein synthesis from amino acids. It is able to induce growth on diets that otherwise would permit no growth. Excess of the hormone before puberty acts on the bones before the epiphyses of long bones have fused and leads to **gigantism.** Excess of the hormone acting after puberty leads to distortion of the skeleton, associated with overgrowth of the hands, feet and mandible, a condition known as **acromegaly.**

Thyroid hormone influences the metabolism of all tissues, and there is little doubt that it is necessary for normal differentiation and growth. Insufficiency of this hormone in infancy and childhood leads to a condition, known as **cretinism,** in which physical and mental development are impeded and distorted. The mental defects are due to altered vascularity of the cerebral cortex and to impeded development of the axons and dendrites of cortical neurones.

Gonadal or **sex hormones** have a considerable effect on the growth of the body. **Androgens,** the male hormones, stimulate tissue synthesis in general, and stimulate the development of the male secondary sexual characteristics.

Œstrogens, which are female hormones, probably hasten epiphyseal union and so restrict growth; they also stimulate the development of female secondary sexual characteristics.

The adrenocortical hormone, **cortisone**, also depresses growth, and tends to be an antagonist to the pituitary growth hormone.

DISEASE

A serious illness may delay growth and maturation. Part of the cause may be that large amounts of corticosteroids are secreted under the stress of an illness and these hormones inhibit growth.

NERVOUS FACTORS

There is reason to believe that there may be a control centre for growth in the brain, possibly in the hypothalamus. This part of the brain is certainly closely associated with the pituitary gland, and it is postulated that the 'growth centre' is responsible for keeping a child along its genetically determined growth pattern. If, for some reason such as illness, a child strays from its genetically determined growth curve, recovery from the adverse influence is associated with a period of increased growth to make good the deficiency. Once the child is 'back on schedule', the accelerated growth stops.

The peripheral nervous system also influences the growth of tissues and it is affected markedly by interruption of the nerve supplying the said tissues. It is now accepted that the nervous system exerts 'trophic' influences (pertaining to nutrition) on other tissues, and it seems probable that this is effected by the passage of chemicals from the nerve terminals to the cells in the tissue concerned.

OTHER FACTORS

There is much evidence that children mature more rapidly now than they did formerly. Diet is not the whole story, since this increased rate is not confined to any particular socio-economic group, although children in the 'top' group are taller than those of unskilled labourers at adolescence. The factors involved in this differential growth rate are not fully understood. There is also evidence that growth in height is faster in the Spring than in Autumn, while growth in weight is faster in the Autumn than in Spring. Exercise can increase both the size and weight of the muscles, and can reduce the storage of fat.

Finally, emotion is a factor in growth, and worried or apprehensive children under emotional strain do not grow as fast as those who have no anxieties.

THE HUMAN BODY AS A GROWING ENTITY

Growth may well be described as a change, normally an increase, in the size and shape of the body, or in that of the cells and organs constituting it. This change may be effected by an increase in the **number of cells (hyperplasia)**, by an increase in the **size of the cells (hypertrophy)**, or by an increase in the amount of intercellular substance of tissues.

It is necessary to state that growth usually results in an increase in size, because in certain circumstances, e.g. early development, the number of cells may increase, but the total size of the organism may diminish because the cells, though more numerous, are much smaller. It must be emphasized that the first three months of intra-uterine life are devoted mainly to the differentiation of tissues and organs, and that the remaining six months of pregnancy are mainly devoted to an increase in the size of the baby and to maturation of its tissues so that it will be viable.

The convention is that for the first two months the developing individual is called an **embryo.** From the beginning of its third month of existence, when its external appearance, especially its face, is recognizable as that of a human being, it is called a **fetus.** At this time it measures about 30 mm from the crown of its head to its rump (known as its **crown-rump** (C.R.) length). This measurement is the best guide to the **age of an embryo,** although the relative proportions of the different parts of the body are constantly changing.

At 32 days after conception, an embryo measures 5 mm. After this, its C.R. length increases by 1 mm a day up to 55 mm, when the rate of growth becomes $1\frac{1}{2}$ mm a day. Thus, if the C.R. length of an embryo is 20 mm, its age must be $20 - 5$ (5 mm at 32 days) $= 15 + 32 = 47$ days.

The **length of gestation** is on an average 266 days from fertilization, that is about 10 lunar months, or 9 calendar months, counting from the first day of the last menstruation. The duration of pregnancy is variable, however, and the longer the pregnancy, the larger and heavier the baby will be at birth. Other factors which affect birth size and weight are parity (number, if any, of previous pregnancies) and multiple births, i.e. the first-born child is usually smaller than its subsequently born brothers or sisters, and twins are smaller than babies produced by single pregnancies. The **average birth weight** is 3·2 kg (7½ lb) and the **average total length** is 50 cm (20 inches).

Prematurity is more frequent than delayed parturition, and is more common among the babies of young mothers. Premature babies are characteristically under weight, even if they are of normal length.

Normal babies usually lose about 5% of their birth weight during the first few days of life. This is mainly because the fluid intake during this period, when lactation is being established, is small. It usually takes a week or ten days for the birth weight to be regained, but premature babies take longer to regain their initial weight, partly because they lose relatively more weight than full-term babies.

During post-natal growth, the weight of the body increases 20 times, the surface area 7 times and the height 3·5 times. Thus, the surface area per unit of body weight is drastically reduced as the individual grows. The relatively huge surface area of babies and children must be remembered when questions of metabolism and heat regulation in children are under consideration. **Babies and children lose heat very much more readily than adults.**

At birth, the relative size of the head is enormous compared with that of an adult. Also, the upper limb is longer and more fully developed than the lower limb. These changes are no doubt related to the fetal circulation which ensures a rich blood supply to the head, neck and upper limbs. The head accounts for about a quarter of the stature of the baby at birth, but for no more than an eighth of that of an adult. The lower limb accounts for only a third of the baby's length at birth, but for a half of that of an adult. Reference to Fig. 224 will show that, whereas the navel is well below the midpoint of the body of a baby, it is well above it in an adult. In contrast to the head and lower limbs, the trunk and arms maintain approximately the same relative size throughout the period of post-natal growth. As a result of these various factors, the centre of gravity shifts from the level of the lower thorax in a newborn to the top of the pelvis in an adult.

General body growth is subject to a **cyclical rhythm.** Each year, until the child reaches puberty, there is evidence that growth is accelerated in the spring and early summer and depressed in winter.

Postnatal growth is at its height **during infancy** and the rate of growth is never again reached in subsequent 'spurts' of growth. The baby doubles its weight in the first 3–4 months of life and trebles it by the end of the first year.

During and **after puberty,** there is a sustained period of growth, called the **adolescent growth spurt.** This is usually between the ages of 11 and 14 years in girls and between 13 and 16 years in boys, so that girls of 11 to 13 tend to be

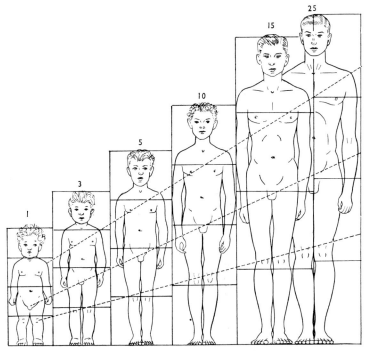

Fig. 224. Scheme to show the changing proportions of the body at different ages.

taller than boys of a same age. After this spurt, the rate of growth gradually decreases till it stops at about 18 in girls, because of the effect of œstrogens, but not until 20 in boys. Increases in weight continue past these ages, as does 'broadening out' of the shoulders, because the clavicles do not stop growing till the age of 25.

It would be wrong to convey the impression that **puberty** and **adolescence** refer to precise periods in the life of the individual. In the narrow sense, puberty refers to the appearance of hair on the pubis, but in practice is used to refer to the whole process of maturation of the reproductive organs. This usually lasts from 2 to 4 years. It is heralded both in boys and in girls by a burst of growth, which in girls stops when the ovaries become functional. In boys, however, the growth phase continues into the period called adolescence (a term derived from the latin verb, *to grow—olescere*). The pubertal and adolescent phases are associated in boys with development of the reproductive organs, with breaking of the voice as a result of the growth of the larynx, with growing of facial hair and the development of the masculine type of body build. In girls, these phases are associated with the development of the breasts as well as of the reproductive organs, and with deposition of subcutaneous fat to conform to the contours of the mature woman.

The general increase in weight, as a result of growth from the infant at birth to the adult, is about twenty fold, but the increase in the musculature amounts to thirty times. The skeleton accounts for about a fifth of the body-weight throughout the growth period, but muscle, which accounts for only a quarter of the body-weight in the newborn, accounts for nearly half of the weight of an adult. The relative weight of the viscera is reduced from 10% at birth to about 5% in the adult.

In **middle age,** the stature begins to decrease because of changes in the intervertebral discs and probably also in the joints of the limbs.

SOME SPECIAL REGIONS

The growth patterns of certain regions are sufficiently different to merit special consideration.

THE HEAD AND NECK REGION

At birth, the most striking features are the **large size of the head** in relation to that of the body and the relatively **large size of the cranium** compared with the face. This is due to the fact that the brain, eyes and ears have grown rapidly before birth, but the mouth and jaws are still very small. A baby has a very **short neck,** and cervical structures such as the trachea and œsophagus are short and little developed. The epiglottis and the larynx are consequently placed relatively high, close to the back of the tongue, so that the epiglottis can be seen through the mouth.

At birth, the **circumference of the head** is approximately 33 cm (13 inches). This measurement is approximately 45 cm (18 inches) at 1 year, 50 cm (20 inches) at 2 years, 53 cm (21 inches) at 6 years and 58 cm (23 inches) in an adult. Caps and hats are the one article of clothing that children wear out or lose rather than outgrow. There are two unossified portions in the cranial vault at birth known as **fontanelles** (Fig. 226). The anterior fontanelle, which is about 2·5 cm (1 inch) across at birth, normally closes during the second year of life. The posterior fontanelle is smaller and is closed by 3 months.

Growth during the first few years of life affects the **face** more than the **cranium.** Their respective size ratio at birth is 1 : 8; this becomes 1 : 4 at about 5 years and 1 : 2 in the adult. In infancy, the skull lacks the bony part of the

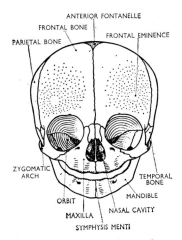

Fig. 225. The skull of a newborn infant seen from in front.

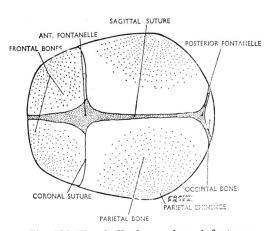

Fig. 226. The skull of a newborn infant seen from above.

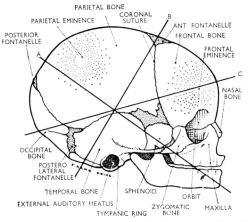

Fig. 227. The skull of a newborn infant seen from the right side. The solid lines indicate diameters, the measurements of which are important in the practice of midwifery. A, occipitomental; B, suboccipitobregmatic; C, occipitofrontal. B is the smallest diameter of the fetal head, and therefore, the one which will pass most easily through the mother's birth canal. This is why it is important to keep the baby's head well flexed on the neck during birth.

external auditory meatus and the mastoid process. Consequently, the ear drum and facial nerve are very close to the surface and more liable to damage; e.g. the application of forceps to the baby's head to facilitate delivery may result in a facial nerve palsy in the baby. The **mastoid process** starts to grow towards the

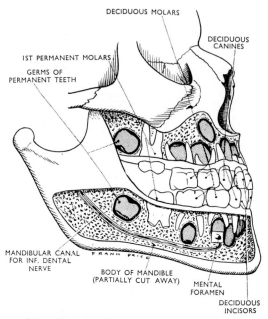

DECIDUOUS MOLARS

DECIDUOUS CANINES

1ST PERMANENT MOLARS

GERMS OF PERMANENT TEETH

MANDIBULAR CANAL FOR INF. DENTAL NERVE

BODY OF MANDIBLE (PARTIALLY CUT AWAY)

MENTAL FORAMEN

DECIDUOUS INCISORS

Fig. 228. The skeleton of the face of a child. Portions of the bones have been removed to show the developing permanent teeth in relation to the roots of the deciduous teeth.

end of the first year, but does not reach an appreciable size until the child is five; there is another burst of growth at puberty.

Of the **paranasal air sinuses,** only the maxillary and sphenoidal are present at birth. The others develop in infancy and, by 5, a child has reasonably developed sinuses. They undergo a period of considerable growth at about the time of puberty. This and the establishment of the permanent dentition account for the 'lengthening' of the face that occurs at this time. The **mandible** of the newborn is small and consists of two halves joined by fibrous tissue at the **symphysis menti.** This is replaced by bone at the end of the first year. The body of the mandible joins the very short ramus at an obtuse angle at birth. During growth, the mandible increases in breadth, in height and especially in anteroposterior length with reduction of the angle from 140° at birth to 120° at maturity.

Growth of the **upper jaw** is mainly in its posterior part, and is associated with the expansion of the maxillary sinus. The growth of the upper jaw is closely correlated with that of the mandible. If the two jaws do not grow in unison, their inequality leads to **malocclusion,** which is the failure of the upper and lower teeth to close together properly. Unequal growth of the jaws also results in irregularities in the timing of eruption and in misplacement of the teeth.

The order and times of **eruption of the teeth** of the deciduous milk and permanent dentitions are given on p. 435.

There is no great difference in the times at which deciduous teeth erupt in male and female babies. There is considerable variation in the order in which the permanent teeth erupt, but all permanent teeth, except for the first upper molar, erupt later in boys than in girls. Also, on average, the teeth of the upper jaw erupt after those of the lower jaw.

As has been stated, the **larynx** is placed very high in the neck of the newborn child, the cricoid cartilage lying opposite the interval between the 3rd and 4th cervical vertebræ (cf. opposite 6th cervical vertebra in the adult). In the course of development, their faster rate of growth makes the larynx and trachea appear to descend in relation to the cervical vertebræ.

THE CENTRAL NERVOUS SYSTEM

The **brain** doubles its weight in the course of the first year of life, by the end of the third year it weighs three times as much as at birth and by the sixth year it has almost reached its adult size. It should be realized that this increase in size is not associated with an increase in the number of neurones, as these almost certainly do not divide after birth. All the main lobes and fissures of the cerebral hemisphere are well developed at birth, but **myelinization** of the fibre tracts, which is to some extent related to the development of function, is far from complete. At birth, the main ascending sensory tracts are myelinated, but myelinization of the corticospinal tracts is not completed until the infant is 2 years old, by which time it should have acquired proper motor control. It is of interest, that the optic nerves undergo myelinization at about the time of birth.

At birth, the **spinal cord** is about 15 cm (6 inches) long and reaches down to the level of the third lumbar vertebra (see Fig. 229). As a result of postnatal growth, it trebles its length to 45 cm (18 inches), but as the vertebral column grows faster still, the spinal cord reaches down only to the upper border of the second lumbar vertebra in the adult.

ORGANS OF SPECIAL SENSE

The eye and the inner ear are well developed at birth, tending, as they do, to follow the pattern of brain growth. At birth the ear drum, middle and internal

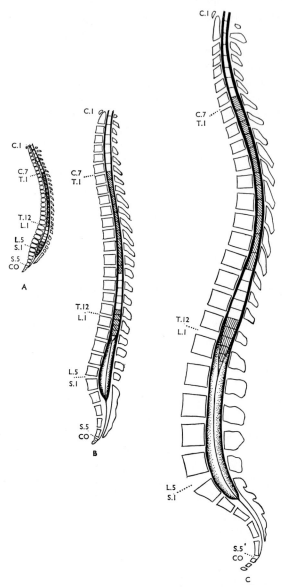

Fig. 229. Schemes to show the levels of the segments of the spinal cord in relation to the vertebræ. A, in a fetus; B, at birth; C, in an adult. The front is to the left of the illustration in each case.

ears are fully formed and almost of adult size although the bony part of the external ear is absent. Consequently, the ear drum, or **tympanic membrane,** is very near the surface and liable to be damaged by any object inserted into the auditory meatus.

THE VERTEBRAL COLUMN

The spine increases in length by about $3\frac{1}{2}$ times between birth and adulthood and continues to grow until after most of the other bones of the body have stopped growing. The lumbar and sacral vertebræ grow most and the cervical vertebræ least.

At birth, two curvatures of the vertebral column are present, the **thoracic curve** and the **sacral curve;** they are both concave forwards. They are the **primary curves** (see Fig. 229, A) and they are associated with the characteristic 'curled up' attitude of the fetus within the uterus. When the baby holds its head up at 3–4 months, the **cervical curve,** which is convex forwards, appears in the cervical part of the spinal column. The **lumbar curve,** also convex forwards, appears when the child starts to walk at 12–18 months. These **secondary curves** only become permanent considerably later in childhood.

THE CHEST, HEART AND LUNGS

The chest, heart and lungs all present interesting growth patterns.

The **chest** looks small compared with the abdomen in a newborn baby. It is barrel-shaped and the ribs are almost horizontal. The shoulder girdles are set high with consequent great obliquity of the clavicles. The manubrium of the sternum lies high opposite the first thoracic vertebra (cf. 2nd or 3rd in an adult).

With the assumption of the erect posture the chest becomes progressively flattened antero-posteriorly, because transverse growth exceeds antero-posterior growth. This has the effect of moving the centre of gravity backwards. Associated with this, the vertebral column comes to lie more anteriorly within the thoracic cage (see Fig. 230) and this brings it into line with the centre of gravity for efficient weight bearing.

As these changes in the chest take place, anterior ends of the ribs descend so that they come to lie more obliquely. At the same time, the shoulders descend and the clavicles come to lie horizontally in women, and almost so in men.

The **thymus** occupies a large part of the superior mediastinum and is relatively largest at birth. It continues to grow rapidly during early childhood, attaining its maximum size at or shortly before puberty. It is said to become

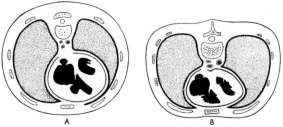

Fig. 230. Drawings of transverse sections through the chest to show the general shape of the thoracic cavity and the relative size of the heart. A, in a young child; B, in an adult.

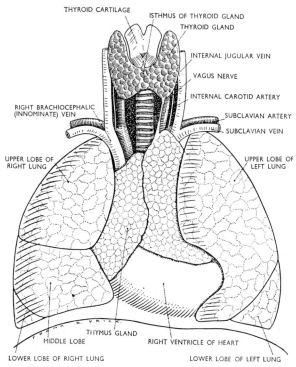

THYROID CARTILAGE

ISTHMUS OF THYROID GLAND

THYROID GLAND

INTERNAL JUGULAR VEIN

VAGUS NERVE

INTERNAL CAROTID ARTERY

RIGHT BRACHIOCEPHALIC
(INNOMINATE) VEIN

SUBCLAVIAN ARTERY

SUBCLAVIAN VEIN

UPPER LOBE OF
RIGHT LUNG

UPPER LOBE OF
LEFT LUNG

THYMUS GLAND

MIDDLE LOBE

RIGHT VENTRICLE OF HEART

LOWER LOBE OF RIGHT LUNG

LOWER LOBE OF LEFT LUNG

Fig. 231. The thoracic contents with the thyroid gland, trachea and great vessels of an infant.

larger in males than in females. After puberty, it retrogresses (involutes), so that the proportion of the superior mediastinum occupied by it diminishes progressively and the thymic tissue (see p. 413) is replaced to a large extent by fatty tissue.

The **heart** multiplies its birth weight only twelve times (cf. $\times 25$ for other tissues), i.e. it is relatively larger in the newborn (p. 389) and in young children. In a newborn baby, the right ventricle is nearly as large and muscular as the left, but in adult life, its weight is only half and the thickness of its wall only a third of that of the left. In young infants, the cardiac shadow seen on radiographs is relatively much larger than in adults, and may extend over more than half of the transverse diameter of the thoracic shadow. On palpation, the apex beat is found to lie in the 4th or even in the 3rd intercostal space, i.e. at least one space higher than in an adult. This relatively large size of the fetal heart reflects the size of its task. It pumps the blood not only round the fetal body but through the umbilical cord and round the placenta as well.

In contrast, the **lungs** follow the general body rate of increase during growth, namely an increase of 20–25 times the birth weight.

ABDOMINAL ORGANS

The alimentary tract conforms to the general pattern of body growth. It is important to realize, however, that at birth the **stomach** has a capacity of only about 30 ml (1 fluid oz). This has increased to 85 to 115 ml (3 or 4 oz) within two weeks and by three months the stomach has a capacity of about 200 ml (7 oz). The **cæcum** is relatively small in infants, but the **appendix** is well developed at birth and communicates with the cæcum through a wide funnel-shaped opening which is very unlikely to become obstructed.

The **liver** is the largest abdominal organ at birth and accounts for 5% of the body weight. This proportion is reduced to $2\frac{1}{2}\%$ in the adult. The large size of the liver at birth is an indication of its importance during fetal life, when it is a blood-forming organ. This **erythropoietic function** ends at birth and, during subsequent growth, the left lobe of the liver becomes relatively smaller, possibly because of the enlargement of the stomach. During the entire period of growth, the **kidneys** increase their weight twelve times. At birth the kidneys are lobulated, but these lobulations disappear in early childhood and the kidneys assume their adult form at puberty. The cortex of the kidney is much thinner at birth than it is in later life, and the epithelium of Bowman's capsule of the glomeruli is cubical in contrast to the pavement epithelium found after the first year. This may account for the relatively poor renal filtration during the first year of postnatal life.

The **suprarenal** is relatively enormous at birth and declines in weight in the first few months of life. An adult suprarenal is not much larger than that found in a newborn baby. The large size of the gland at birth is associated with the development, during fetal life, of a special type of cortex, whose secretions may play a rôle in sexual differentiation and in counteracting the influence of the mother's female hormones, which reach the fetus through the placenta.

THE PELVIS AND ITS CONTENTS

The bony pelvis already shows sex differences in fetal life, but the definite remodelling of the female pelvis to become more capacious takes place at puberty. At birth, the pelvic capacity of infants of both sexes is relatively small,

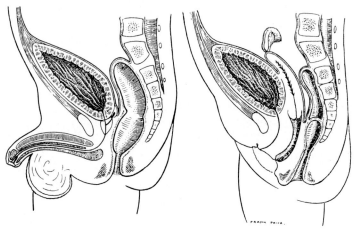

Fig. 232. Diagrams of median sagittal sections through the pelvis and lower abdomen of male and female infants, to show the position of the 'pelvic' organs.

so that organs such as the bladder are predominantly abdominal organs (see Fig. 232). As the pelvis enlarges in childhood, the sigmoid colon, the bladder and other structures between them 'descend' and come to lie in the positions they occupy in an adult. This is associated with the disappearance of the 'pot-belly' characteristic of children under six, and with the development of a waist.

THE LIMBS

The limbs have already been mentioned in the general consideration of the pattern of growth, but it should be emphasized that, although the lower limb is slightly shorter than the upper limb at birth, it grows faster and in adult life it is considerably longer than the upper.

Centres of Ossification

The long bones of the limbs have each a **primary** or **diaphyseal centre of ossification** which gives rise to the shaft of the bone. In addition, each bone has two **secondary** or **epiphyseal centres of ossification,** one at each end. Primary centres almost invariably appear before birth, whereas secondary centres usually appear after birth (Figs. 233 and 234). A notable exception is the centre for the **lower end of the femur,** which appears just before birth, and its presence may be used as a **criterion of maturity** in a newborn baby.

It will be appreciated that, while the bone is growing, there persists a disc of cartilage between the bony shaft and the bony epiphysis; this is known as the **growth** or **epiphyseal cartilage.** This appears, on a radiograph, as a dark line crossing the bone between the light shaft and the light epiphysis (Fig. 234). When the bone stops growing, the cartilage disappears as the bony shaft and bony epiphysis fuse with one another (Fig. 57). The plane of fusion is marked by a thin layer of dense bone easily seen on radiographs and called the **epiphyseal line** (Figs. 78 and 79).

Centres of ossification appear and fuse earlier in girls than in boys. It should also be appreciated that illnesses can retard the development of long bones, in which case, there remain permanent marks on the shaft called **Harris's lines.** They are in the form of transverse bands in the part of the bone which was closest to the epiphyseal cartilage at the time of the illness. Within these limits the sequence and time relations of the appearance and fusion of the centres of ossification, as revealed by X-rays, can be correlated with the age of normal subjects and can be used as an **index of maturity** in the case of individuals.

General Conclusions

The rate of growth of the body as a whole and its proportions are obviously of great interest to anyone looking after children. If a child is too short, too tall, or indeed if an adult is too heavy or too light in relation to his stature, it may immediately throw light on the nature of a disorder affecting the person. When consulting the tables, that are available for establishing the correct relation between weight and stature, it is important to be sure that the table is applicable to the population group under consideration, e.g. tables compiled from data obtained from American children are not applicable to British children of corresponding ages.

It is generally recognized that the developmental stage of a child is reflected far better by the X-ray appearances of its bones than by measurements of its height and weight.

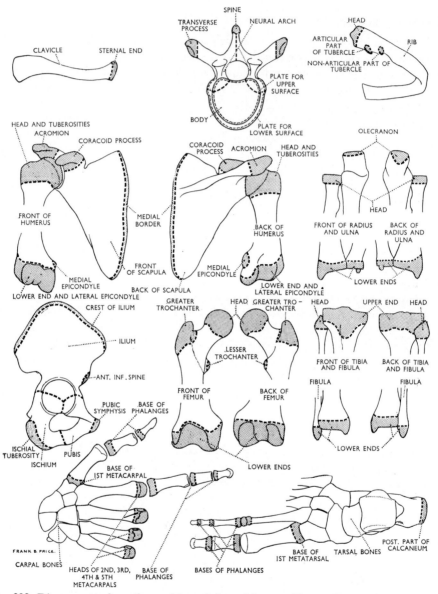

Fig. 233. Diagrams to show the position of the epiphyses of bones. Parts of bones ossified from epiphyses are stippled. Interrupted lines indicate lines of fusion, either between an epiphysis and the part of the bone ossified from the primary centre of ossification, or between parts ossified from different primary centres of ossification.

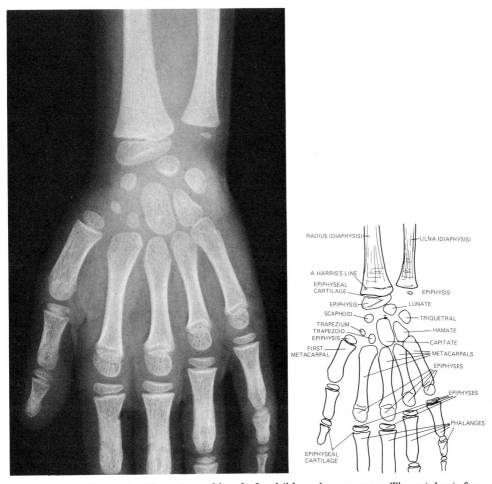

Fig. 234. A radiograph of the wrist and hand of a child aged seven years. The epiphysis for the head of the ulna has recently appeared. The carpal bones ossify from primary centres which appear after birth, between the ages of one and seven years.

Adults vary considerably in size and shape because, not only do they vary in their degree of development, but because they tend to accumulate fat after middle age, especially in 'affluent' societies. Nevertheless, there is a reasonable correlation between weight and stature, and, in general, the girth measurement correlates fairly well with weight.

CHAPTER XX

REPAIR, REGENERATION, AGEING

BECAUSE various events result sooner or later in the loss and destruction of some constituent parts of an organism, survival depends on an adequate system of replacement. Hence growth, repair and regeneration are interrelated processes which operate at a variety of levels. There is a continuous replacement of substances by turnover within cells; there is a continuous replacement of cells within the body.

Continuous replacement of materials in the body is absolutely essential for self-maintenance, and in a complex organism, such as a human being, the processes of replacement and growth must be regulated so as to preserve an integrated system of tissues and organs, differentiated for particular functions (see p. 90). In this sense, differentiation is the inverse of growth, growth usually preceding differentiation or specialization of tissues. As a tissue differentiates and specializes, it tends to lose its ability to grow and, when cells such as those of a cancer lose their normal growth control mechanisms, they tend to revert to a less differentiated and less specialized state.

The study of the mechanisms that control normal growth and repair is therefore very relevant to the problem of cancer. Also, the study of the processes, by which the body and its cells lose their ability to grow and to replace their constituents is closely related to understanding the changes, that occur in ageing and degeneration, leading eventually to death. It is of some significance that most cancers arise in individuals and organs that are past their biological prime. Thus, the problem of ageing is also related to that of cancer, in the sense that carcinogenesis (the production of cancer) might be associated with disordered ageing of cells.

Maintenance, repair, replacement and regeneration are similar processes, linked through the methods by which they operate in the body. They are all processes by which the individual life is enabled to continue despite wear and tear.

In most tissues there is a continuous turnover of constituent materials and, in some, the cells are regularly replaced. These maintenance operations, in a sense, anticipate damage and are particularly evident in vulnerable areas, such as the skin or the lining of the gut. Other parts of the body may suffer damage only by accident, i.e. occasionally or not at all. In these, there is genetic information for healing, repair and replacement, but these are only brought into effect when called for as a result of accidental damage.

In a sense, the powers of repair and replacement are a second line of defence to be brought into play, when the ordinary anticipatory mechanisms to avoid damage have failed. Thus, normal development provides the body with bones that are strong enough to meet most of the stresses and strains that are likely to fall upon them. When subjected to greater stresses than anticipated, a bone breaks and mechanisms of repair and regeneration are available to enable it to heal and mend.

Maintenance and repair are geared to deal with minor, recurrent and temporary damage. Replacement and regeneration constitute major acts of differentiation and resemble processes that are observed in the course of development (see p. 573).

Before considering any details of the processes of repair and regeneration in wounded tissues of the body, a few general principles should be emphasized.

The first has already been mentioned and is that, as a cell assumes specialized functions, it tends to lose its capacity for reproducing itself. For example, the primitive unspecialized mesenchymal cell (see Plate 3 and p. 104), which is the stem or parent cell of connective tissues, is capable of reproducing itself very readily but, as the daughter cells mature and differentiate into specialized connective tissue cells, they become less able to divide. One kind of cell, that has become so specialized as to be incapable of dividing, is the neurone in the central nervous system. It is thus fairly obvious that a tissue consisting of specialized cells, like nervous tissue, is far less likely to repair itself and regenerate, than a tissue containing many primitive undifferentiated cells, such as loose areolar tissue. A tissue usually regenerates by the multiplication of its less specialized constituent cells, e.g. in a gland, the duct cells are less specialized than the secreting cells to which they have given rise and, if the secreting cells are damaged, more secreting cells are produced by the duct cells.

WOUND HEALING

If the surface of the body is breached, the edges of the wound usually separate and bleeding takes place into the resulting gap. The blood then clots in the gap, and the clot is **organized** by the growth into the clot of **fibroblasts** (primitive connective tissue cells derived from mesenchyme) and blood **capillaries**. This forms **granulation tissue**. The fibroblasts then lay down fibres of collagen and **scar tissue** is formed. If the breached surface is covered by an epithelium, the cells from its cut edges produce new epithelial cells that grow over the granulation tissue and scar, and thus epithelial continuity is re-established.

There are many theories about what constitutes the stimulus for healing, but it is unfortunately true that at present we do not know what initiates or controls repair mechanisms. It is possible that the stimulus consists of a 'wound hormone' liberated by damaged cells. On the other hand, the tissue may have a system that enables it to 'sense' a structural defect or a functional lack.

Experimental studies have demonstrated that, in some tissues, cells are prevented from dividing by the inhibitory action of metabolites produced by the cells themselves. Such substances are known as **chalones,** and represent a local chemical control system maintaining the balance between cell division and differentiation. This mechanism is of great importance in the repair of injuries.

Some specific instances of repair and regeneration will now be considered as .they are of direct relevance to clinical medicine.

THE SKIN

In the healing of skin wounds and burns, a very important consideration is the extent to which the **epidermis** of the skin is damaged. If the skin is blistered, it means that plasma and tissue fluid have accumulated between the dermis and epidermis. In thick skin, however, the accumulation may be between the superficial and basal layers of the epidermis. Part or the whole of the epidermis superficial to the collection of fluid will be shed, but, providing the epithelium of the hair follicles or sweat glands persists, a new layer of epidermis will regenerate from these surviving structures. If the damage to the skin extends deeper than the hair follicles and sweat glands, regeneration of epidermis can be effected only by ingrowth from surviving epithelium at the margins of the wound or burn. In regenerated epithelium of this kind, sweat glands may be present, but hair will not, as these grow in regenerated skin only if the deep part of the original follicles has survived. In general, however, the external root sheaths of hair follicles play a much more energetic part in re-epithelializing denuded areas than do the sweat glands.

Enough has been said to indicate that the epithelium of skin, i.e. the epidermis, shows a marked ability to regenerate and repair itself. The **dermis,** because it is made up of connective tissue, also has a high capacity for regeneration. If the epidermis is scraped off, shaved off or burnt off, the dermal **papillary ridge pattern** (basis of finger prints) is accurately reproduced.

On the other hand, if the dermis is destroyed or severely damaged, new papillary ridges are formed, but they do not correspond to the original pattern.

Skin Grafting

In conditions where the epidermis regenerates from the margin of a wound or burn which is extensive, the slowness of the process means that considerable time will elapse before healing is complete. It may, in fact, take months or even years, during which time the dermis is exposed to infection, with consequent inflammation, to mention but one hazard, and huge scars are likely to result. Nowadays, to obviate this, large defects of skin resulting from injury or burning are made good much more quickly by skin grafting.

There are two main types of skin graft. In the one—a **free graft**—the portion of skin to be grafted is completely disconnected from its original blood supply before being transferred; in the second—a **pedicle graft**—the transplanted skin is never severed completely from its blood supply. Usually, free grafts are thin—so-called split skin grafts—and consist of epidermis with only a thin shaving of dermis. They are thin enough for the constituent cells to be kept alive by means of the tissue fluid produced by the capillaries of the host site, until capillaries from this host site have grown into the transplanted tissue.

By means of a pedicle graft, the full thickness of the skin can be moved to the site of injury by detaching it only partially from the donor site, so that blood vessels can still feed it from one end.The other end is attached to the new site and allowed to establish a new blood supply. Once this new attachment has been effectively vascularized, the persisting connexion to the donor site can be severed. Relatively large pieces of skin can be transplanted from one part of the body to another in this way, and several steps may be necessary before the graft is established at the desired site. For instance, the graft may be taken from the thigh to the face. To do this, the graft may have to be fixed by one end to the arm, allowed to be vascularized from the arm, disconnected from the thigh, connected to the face and allowed to be vascularized from the face before being disconnected from the arm.

It has been emphasized that, if a graft is to 'take', capillaries must grow into it from the host site. This takes place if skin is transplanted from one part of an individual to another site in the same individual (**autograft**). This does not take place, however, if skin from one individual is transplanted to another (**homograft**). Homografts are rejected because of the immune response (p. 414) An immune response does, however, not usually take place between **identical (monovular) twins,** who have the same genetic make-up. The immune response can be prevented by such means as irradiation of the reticulo-endothelial system of the body or the administration of immunosuppressive drugs. The grafting of tissues and organs successfully, e.g. a kidney, from one individual to another is now a well established procedure.

Corneal Grafts

So far, the only exceptions to the rejection of all homografts, without the suppression of the immune response, are homografts in identical twins and **homografts of cornea**. The latter phenomenon is explained by the fact that corneal tissue is avascular and normally survives by diffusion from tissue fluid bathing it. It should, however, be noted that the corneal cells of the donor survive for only a limited time and are gradually replaced by cells of the recipient or host (also see p. 291).

BONE REPAIR

Usually a fracture involves the breaking of a single bone into two parts which are known as the fragments. Not only is the bone damaged, but the periosteum is torn. The blood vessels crossing the line of fracture are also torn, with the result that bleeding occurs at the site of fracture. This blood and the blood in the ends of the torn vessels clots. Consequently, the ends of the fragments near the fracture line are deprived of a blood supply and die (see Fig. 235, A, B and C).

The fracture is repaired by the growth of new tissue, termed **callus,** which is called **external callus**, if it is outside the ends of the fragments, and **internal callus,** if it is between the two ends of the bony fragments, and in and between the two marrow cavities.

Callus is formed by three types of cell:

1. Osteogenic cells from the cellular layer of the periosteum.
2. Osteogenic cells derived from the endosteum, i.e. 'periosteum' on the internal surface of the bone.
3. Mesenchymal cells from the marrow cavity.

These cells multiply and, with new capillaries budding from nearby blood vessels, replace the blood clot. The periosteal cells, by multiplying, raise the fibrous layer of periosteum (Fig. 235, B and C) and lay down a periosteal cuff, or collar, of bone that bridges the gap at the fracture line. The other osteogenic cells, which have invaded the clot with the capillaries, lay down a spongy network of bony trabeculæ uniting the two fragments and replacing the devitalized ends of the fragments (Fig. 235, D). Once union has been established

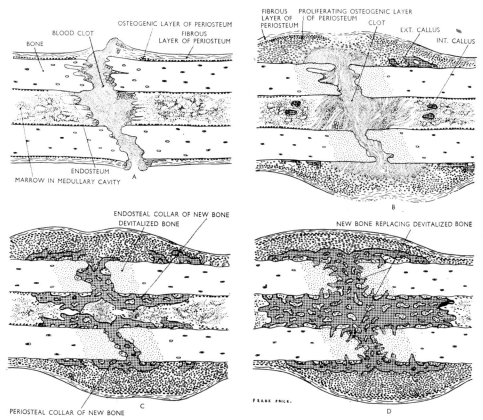

Fig. 235. Diagrams showing stages in the healing of a fractured bone.

satisfactorily, the bone is remodelled so as to have an outer cortex of compact bone and a central marrow cavity. Providing the two fragments were well aligned before healing began, the original shape of the bone is re-established and, after a period of months, the site of the fracture may no longer be identifiable by a thickening of the bone.

If the repair process is understood, it will be seen why it is important for the two fragments of a broken bone to be brought back into alignment, if they have been displaced. It will also be understood how, when periosteum, or some other tissue, becomes interposed between the fragments in the course of injury, the interposed tissue forms a barrier to the repairing osteogenic cells and capillaries trying to bridge the gap, and union may be prevented.

Bone Grafting

When the fragments of a broken bone fail to unite, a transplant of healthy bone from another part of the body can be used to facilitate union, or indeed may be used to repair a defect caused by accident or disease. It used to be thought that such a transplant of bone continued to live, but now it is generally accepted that most of the osteocytes die and that, sooner or later, the dead transplanted bone is replaced by new bone growing into it. The transplanted fragment thus serves as a kind of scaffolding round which new bone can be built.

REGENERATION AND REPAIR IN THE NERVOUS SYSTEM

As has been mentioned several times, specialization of cells is associated with a loss of regenerative capacity. The cells of the nervous system—**neurones** —have lost the power of regeneration more or less completely and probably never divide after birth in Man. The only kind of repair possible, for practical purposes, is replacement of nerve cells by the connective tissue elements of the nervous system, i.e. **neuroglia,** with consequent loss of neural function. Provided the neurone is not damaged permanently, section of its processes, or nerve fibres, may be followed by regeneration, if the fibre is surrounded by a **neurilemmal sheath** (see p. 224 and Fig. 236). Fibres **within the central nervous system,** i.e. in the brain and spinal cord, are not surrounded by such a sheath and **therefore do not regenerate. Outside the central nervous system,** i.e. in peripheral nerves, fibres **can regenerate,** for every fibre acquires a neurilemmal sheath as soon as it leaves the central nervous system.

In this connexion, it is interesting to note that the optic nerve is really an outgrowth of the brain and not a true cranial nerve (see Fig. 124 and p. 288). Consequently, it is incapable of regeneration—damage to this so-called 'cranial nerve' is permanent, when it occurs.

The Process of Nerve Regeneration (Fig. 236)

If a peripheral nerve is cut, or crushed severely enough, not only do the portions of the nerve fibres distal to the injury degenerate, but the degeneration also spreads 'back' up the nerve to the first **node of Ranvier** (see p. 224) above the level of the injury. The degeneration affects not only the nerve fibre, but also the **myelin sheath. The neurilemmal cells** are mobilized to bridge the gap, and

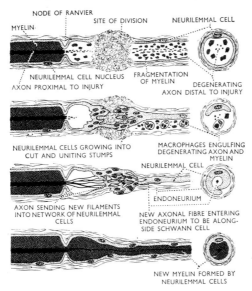

NODE OF RANVIER
MYELIN
SITE OF DIVISION
NEURILEMMAL CELL
NEURILEMMAL CELL NUCLEUS
AXON PROXIMAL TO INJURY
FRAGMENTATION OF MYELIN
DEGENERATING AXON DISTAL TO INJURY

NEURILEMMAL CELLS GROWING INTO CUT AND UNITING STUMPS
MACROPHAGES ENGULFING DEGENERATING AXON AND MYELIN

NEURILEMMAL CELL
AXON SENDING NEW FILAMENTS INTO NETWORK OF NEURILEMMAL CELLS
ENDONEURIUM
NEW AXONAL FIBRE ENTERING ENDONEURIUM TO BE ALONGSIDE SCHWANN CELL

NEW MYELIN FORMED BY NEURILEMMAL CELLS

Fig. 236. Diagrams showing stages in the regeneration of a sectioned peripheral nerve fibre.

macrophages from the **endoneurium** 'mop up' the débris of broken up nerve fibres and myelin.

The mesh formed by the proliferating neurilemmal sheath cells in the gap provide a means for the nerve fibres to grow across it. Beyond the bridged gap, the regenerating fibres grow down the persisting tunnels in the endoneurium, where they come in contact with further neurilemmal cells. These cells eventually enclose the fibre and produce myelin around it.

Nerve Grafting

For a nerve to regenerate, it is essential for the distal degenerating part of the nerve to be close to the proximal end, so that the neurilemmal cells can grow across the gap and establish a network down which the regenerating fibres can grow.

If a whole segment of a nerve has been destroyed, a length of nerve may be grafted to re-establish the physical continuity of the nerve. The neurilemmal cells of the graft appear to survive and provide a mesh for the regenerating fibres to grow down, but the resulting network is obviously much longer and more complex than when the cut ends of nerves are sutured. The results of grafting are therefore not nearly as satisfactory.

REPAIR AND REGENERATION OF MUSCLE

Effects of Paralysis and Ischæmia

As well as being damaged directly by injury, muscle, especially skeletal striated muscle, can be affected by interference with its **nerve supply (paralysis)** or with its **blood supply (ischæmia).**

Interruption of the peripheral nerve supplying a skeletal muscle can lead, not only to **paralysis** of the said muscle, but to **wasting (atrophy)** of its muscle fibres. Such a muscle is flabby (**flaccid**). The atrophy of the muscle fibres is associated with a relative increase in the proportion of connective tissue within the muscle. Interruption of the blood supply to a skeletal muscle may lead to death of the muscle fibres. Neutrophils and macrophages remove the débris of the degenerating fibres, and this is followed by replacement by fibroblasts and capillaries. The fibrous tissue, which is laid down by the fibroblasts, tends to contract and thus, **ischæmic contractures** deform the limb to which the degenerate muscle belongs.

Regeneration and Repair of Striated Muscle

It is generally believed that striated muscle fibres do not undergo proliferation by cell division after fetal life, growth taking place by enlargement of the individual fibres. Just like nerve cells, striated muscle fibres are highly specialized; hence their relative inability to divide and regenerate.

If, however, a muscle fibre is only partially destroyed, it can regenerate. An important factor in successful regeneration of a muscle fibre is the preservation of the endomysial connective tissue tube, which enclosed the original fibre, as this tube provides a pathway for the guidance of the growing fibre. It is a fact that fibrosis and obliteration of the endomysial tubes usually takes place before the regenerating fibre grows very far. This accounts for the fact that little or no striated muscle regeneration takes place in Man.

Regeneration and Repair of Tendons

As tendons are often severed by accident, it is fortunate that, if properly treated, they heal very well. After the tendon is cut, fibroblasts from the inner tendon sheath grow into the gap with capillaries and lay down new collagenous fibres, which cement together the free ends of cut fibres. As more and more collagen is laid down, the blood supply is cut down and soon the 'scar' is as avascular as the rest of the tendon.

Regeneration and Repair of Smooth muscle

Smooth muscle is much less specialized than striated muscle, and smooth muscle cells can increase both in size and number in post-natal life, either in response to a physiological need (uterus in pregnancy) and in repair processes after damage, or as part of a pathological process (in walls of arteries in raised blood pressure). The increase in number of smooth muscle fibres can occur as the result of their mitotic division or by the differentiation of residual mesenchymal cells to form new muscle cells (see Plate 3).

REGENERATION OF GLANDS

As stated earlier, **exocrine glands** are capable of regenerating secretory units by proliferation and differentiation of cells from the less specialized ducts.

Although the cells of the **liver** do not usually exhibit mitosis, they fail to conform to the pattern just mentioned for glands. When the liver has been extensively damaged, the actual glandular cells of the liver divide by mitosis in an attempt to make good the damage.

Endocrine glands, which by definition do not possess ducts, regenerate, in those cases where it is possible, by mitotic proliferation of the surviving cells. In the **suprarenal cortex** this is effected by the cells of the zona glomerulosa, just underneath the capsule of the gland (see Fig. 207).

The **islets of the pancreas** present a fascinating problem of regeneration. There is little evidence that the β cells, which are deficient in a diabetic, regenerate in these individuals. There is evidence, however, that complete islets can regenerate and, when they do, it is from the ducts of the exocrine portion of the gland that they grow, subsequently losing their connexion with these ducts. In fact, the cells of the islets reappear by the same process as that by which they originally developed.

AGEING

The changes of old age affect all parts of the body and it is not always easy to see the biological connexion between the facts that old people have wrinkled skin, behave peculiarly, are short of breath on exertion, are no longer able to reproduce and are increasingly prone to die. Yet, behind all these features of old age probably lie, in varying proportions, three categories of fundamental biological change

1. Changes in the mitotic activity of cells and in the quality of the daughter cells.
2. Loss or damage of post-mitotic cells with changes in the intracellular information store.
3. Changes in the molecules of intercellular substances.

Perhaps the most striking and well-known difference between the tissues of a young animal and those of an old one is that those of the former are tender (e.g. lamb) and those of the latter tough (e.g. mutton). The basic change, that accounts for the alteration in the physical characteristics of the older tissue, is that, as the animal ages, there is a progressive diminution in the amount of amorphous intercellular substance (which is jelly-like, see p. 94) and a proportionate increase in the formed fibrous variety. The same is true in Man.

As a person grows older, the connective tissue cells attempt to replace the intercellular substances, but the complete removal and substitution of old intercellular substance by new is beyond the capacity of the body's cells. This is particularly true of formed intercellular substance (see p. 94) which tends to persist and to deteriorate as it ages.

As a person ages, the collagen fibres in connective tissues increase in size and number, and the physical properties of elastic fibres are altered by the impregnation with mineral salts, which makes them harder and less elastic.

This is illustrated very clearly in the changes that occur with age in the skin, which becomes inelastic and sags in an old person. This is particularly noticeable in the skin of the neck, which does more to give away a person's age than almost any other physical attribute. Most others are easily falsified with cosmetics and dyes.

A consequence of loss of elasticity and deposition of mineral salts in elastic tissue, which is of greater clinical importance, is the rôle which this ageing process plays in hardening of the arteries. Added to this is the fact that arteries have difficulty in getting rid of colloids that accumulate over the years in the tissue spaces of their walls. This difficulty exists because colloids, that accidentally escape into tissue fluid, are usually disposed of by way of the lymphatics draining the tissue. However, as the wall of an artery is under constant tension because of the pressure of the blood within the vessel, it is difficult for lymphatics to function and colloids tend to accumulate in the arterial walls. This is possibly the basis of atheroma and, in conjunction with the loss of elasticity and hardening of elastic fibres, leads to **atherosclerosis.** No excuse is made for stressing these aspects of ageing, because about 60% of adults eventually die of degenerative or ageing diseases of the cardiovascular system.

The relative increase in formed intercellular substance which occurs in old age with its attendant loss of plasticity results in the impeding of cell movement. This accounts, at any rate in part, for the loss of the power of regeneration and repair in the tissues of old people.

It should however be realized that, in addition to changes in the intercellular substance with ageing, there are, as was stated above, also changes in the cells of the body, evidenced by histological changes in the organelles and in the nucleus of cells.

MENOPAUSAL CHANGES

The **menopause**, or 'change of life', usually refers to the fairly dramatic changes that occur in a woman's physiology at the end of her reproductive period of life. It should be pointed out that men often suffer from comparable changes, but they are much more variable and usually occur at a much later age. In a woman the 'change' is often heralded by irregularity of the menses (periods) before they finally stop, but it is interesting to note that the menopause is often preceded by a relatively short period of increased fertility before sterility sets in. It is not uncommon for a middle-aged woman, who has had a number of pregnancies earlier in life, to pass through a relatively infertile phase before conceiving again unexpectedly just before the menopause.

Attendant upon the cessation of menses, which is itself determined by the cessation of ovulation, there are usually psychological disturbances and disturbances of cardiovascular control (hot flushes and palpitations).

The inability of the ovaries to respond effectively to pituitary stimulation leads perhaps to an over secretion of pituitary trophic hormones (p. 518) and to hormonal imbalance. This may account for the development of cystic changes in the epithelial tissue of the breasts and to disorders of the connective tissue and smooth muscle of the uterus.

After a period of imbalance, a physiological equilibrium is usually re-established. This is associated with a reduction of the metabolic rate, atrophic changes in the genitalia, coarsening of the skin and hair, and a tendency to the deposition of fat and consequent gain in weight.

In an old man, the main manifestation of a 'menopausal' hormone imbalance is the change in the prostate which is usually referred to as senile enlargement of the prostate. There may be psychological changes too.

CHANGES IN GENERAL BODY STRUCTURES OCCURRING WITH AGEING

One of the earliest ageing changes to affect an individual is the diminution of water content in the nucleus pulposus of intervertebral discs (see p. 161). This diminution is considerable in old age and, with the increased curvatures of the spine, accounts for loss of stature when a person grows old (Fig. 237). Diminution of water content probably starts in the thirties and is thought to be related to the increased susceptibility of invertebral discs to injury, once an individual reaches the age of 30.

Loss of elasticity of the skin has already been described and there are changes in the appendages of the skin. Nails become more brittle and there is loss of hair. In males, this may lead to baldness, but the picture is complicated by the fact that heredity plays an important part, especially in premature baldness. It seems that it is also necessary for male hormones to be circulating in the body for baldness to occur, because women (except those with masculinizing diseases) never become really bald, nor do eunuchs.

The bones are affected in old age in that they become lighter, less dense and more brittle, and therefore break more easily.

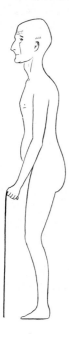

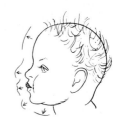

Fig. 237 (*left*). Silhouette of an old man showing some of the characteristic changes of old age. The cheeks fall in and the chin becomes more prominent because the teeth have fallen out. There is increased curvature of the vertebral column and the limbs are bent with resulting loss of stature. There is impairment of balance.

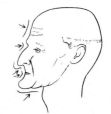

Fig. 238 (*right*). The profile of a young infant compared with that of an old man. Although both individuals lack teeth, the contours bulge out in the infant, because of abundant subcutaneous fat and well-developed 'suctorial' pads in the cheeks, whereas the corresponding contours fall in and the skin becomes wrinkled in the old man. This is because in old age there is a relative absence of subcutaneous fat, there is loss of water from the tissues and a loss of elasticity in all connective tissues, including that of the dermis of the skin.

Teeth tend to fall out, if they have not already been extracted, and the shape of the mandible is changed considerably. There is a flattening of the angle between the body and ramus, the body becomes attenuated and the coronoid process becomes slender and long. In addition there is resorption of the alveolar (toothbearing) margin of the body of the mandible so that it becomes more slender.

As a person ages, the hyaline cartilage of the body, especially in costal cartilages, becomes calcified and many fibrous and cartilaginous joints (e.g. the sutures of the skull and the sternal joints) become ossified.

INDEX